N TO

lar

Physiology

FOURTH EDITION

AN INTRODUCTION TO
Cardiovascular
Physiology

J. Rodney Levick DSc MA DPhil MRCP BM BCh (Oxon)

Professor of Physiology
St George's Hospital Medical School
University of London, UK

ARNOLD

A member of the Hodder Headline Group
LONDON

First edition published in Great Britain in 1991 by
Butterworth Heinemann; reprinted 1992
Second edition 1995; reprinted 1996, 1998
also by Butterworth Heinemann
German translation *Physiologie des Herz–Kreislauf-Systems* by
Fischer-Barnicol & Seller published in 1998 by Bath Verlag, Heidelberg
Third edition 2000
by Arnold, reprinted 2001
This fourth edition published in Great Britain in 2003 by
Arnold, a member of the Hodder Headline Group,
338 Euston Road, London NW1 3BH

http://www.arnoldpublishers.com

Distributed in the United States of America by
Oxford University Press Inc.,
198 Madison Avenue, New York, NY10016
Oxford is a registered trademark of Oxford University Press

Whilst the advice and information in this book are believed to be true and
accurate at the date of going to press, neither the author nor the publisher
can accept any legal responsibility or liability for any errors or omissions
that may be made. In particular (but without limiting the generality of the
preceding disclaimer) every effort has been made to check drug dosages;
however it is still possible that errors have been missed. Furthermore,
dosage schedules are constantly being revised and new side-effects
recognized. For these reasons the reader is strongly urged to consult the
drug companies' printed instructions before administering any of the drugs
recommended in this book.

British Library Cataloguing in Publication Data
A catalogue record for this book is available from the British Library

Library of Congress Cataloging-in-Publication Data
A catalog record for this book is available from the Library of Congress

ISBN 0 340 80921 3
2 3 4 5 6 7 8 9 10

Commissioning Editor: Joanna Koster
Production Editor: Anke Ueberberg
Production Controller: Deborah Smith
Cover Design: Stewart Larking

Typeset in 10.5/12 Bembo by Charon Tec Pvt. Ltd, Chennai, India
Printed and bound in Italy

To Charles Michel, following his retirement; in gratitude to my
college tutor of many years ago, and an inspirational colleague
and friend ever since

Contents

Preface to the fourth edition

A major stimulus for bringing out this edition has been the desire to upgrade the illustrations. Over 70 figures have been redrawn and 38 new ones added. Also, following the transfer of the book to a modern PC, I have taken the opportunity to revise the entire text, pruning detail in some areas, rebalancing and updating the chapters and shortening the text by around 6000 words despite some new material. New material includes the contribution of wave reflection to systolic hypertension, the role of vascular kinases in contraction, a fuller account of myocardial ischaemia and advances in understanding cardiac failure and arrhythmogenesis.

Detail should not be allowed to obscure concepts, so many chapters begin with an Overview, all end with a bulleted Summary, and new Concept Boxes outline key cardiovascular concepts. Along with revised Learning Objectives at the start of each chapter and statement subheading, these changes should help the hard-pressed student at examination time. Another new addition is a summary of the main cardiovascular parameters in Appendix 1.

Concepts are built on experimental observations. As the 1st edition stated, one of my aims is 'to show how our knowledge is derived from experimental observation. The latter not only puts flesh on the didactic bones, but ultimately keeps the student and the writer in contact with reality'. I make no apology therefore for presenting real data in place, warts and all, or for outlining evidence and techniques. Many new references have been added.

I wish to thank the referees to the 4th edition for helpful suggestions. I also want to thank the many medical students who have given me feedback on the book, including my own daughter Christina, whose uninhibited criticisms of Dad's book led to some of the above 'student friendly' improvements.

Revising a book may sound like a simple task, but this is far from the truth. Although the 4th edition is a little bigger, the text is actually shorter. The extra pages are due to new figures and Concept Boxes, which will hopefully help rather than hinder. My aim, successful or not, is to provide a readable, reasonably complete but not over-detailed account of the fascinating world of cardiovascular physiology.

Rodney Levick
Division of Physiology
St George's Hospital Medical School
May 2003

A note on active and problem-based learning

One may read a textbook and gain a primary level of understanding; but to master the subject thoroughly *it is essential to practice active, self-expression*. To this end, learning objectives and clinical problems are included.

Using the learning objectives

Traditional methods of promoting active learning include essay writing and question-and-answer tutorials. The *Learning Objectives* at the start of each chapter can be used as short-answer questions (e.g. 'Draw and explain a delayed afterdepolarization') or essay topics (e.g. 'Describe the roles of endothelium in inflammation'). The sections containing the answers are cited after each learning objective. Another excellent way to learn actively is to make brief notes on each learning objective.

The notes will prove handy when revising for examinations.

Problem-based learning

To encourage active, relevant learning, many medical schools and physiology departments include clinical problems in their teaching methods. Clinical cases are challenging because they bring together many different topics and cut across many different chapters of the book. For example, heart failure (Case 1) involves altered cardiac excitation–contraction coupling (Chapters 3 and 18), Starling's law of the heart (Chapter 6), haemodynamics (Chapter 8), micro-vascular fluid exchange (Chapter 11) and extrinsic control of the circulation (Chapter 14). Clinical cases are therefore presented at the end of the book, followed by questions, outline answers and links to the main text.

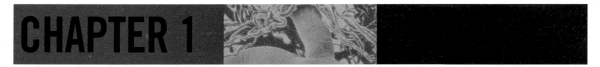

CHAPTER 1

Overview of the cardiovascular system

Learning objectives

After reading this chapter you should be able to:

- Outline the distance limitation of diffusional transport and the roles of diffusion and convection in circulatory transport (1.1).
- State the features that distinguish the pulmonary from the systemic circulation (1.3).
- Draw a graph to show how blood pressure, velocity and total cross-sectional area changes from the aorta to microcirculation to vena cava (Figure 1.9).
- Write down the basic law of flow (1.5) and apply it to the above graph to show where vascular resistance is chiefly located.
- Sketch the structure of the blood vessel wall (Figure 1.10) and state the roles of endothelium, elastin, collagen and vascular smooth muscle.
- Name five main functional categories of vessel and their roles (1.7).
- Define a 'portal circulation' and state its functional significance (1.8).

The heart and blood vessels evolved to transport oxygen, nutrients, waste products and heat around the body at high speed. Small, primitive organisms lack a circulatory system because their oxygen needs are satisfied by diffusion from the environment. Even in big animals such as man, diffusion is a vitally important transport mechanism, both inside the cells and between the cells and the bloodstream. Why, then, do we need a cardiovascular system? The answer lies in the limitations of diffusional transport.

1.1 Diffusion: its virtues and limitations

Diffusion is due to a molecular 'drunkard's walk'

Diffusion is a passive process. That is to say, it is driven by the random thermal motion of molecules, not by metabolic energy. When a concentration gradient is present, the randomly directed steps of individual solute molecules leads to a net movement of the solute down its concentration gradient, i.e. a net diffusional transport, as demonstrated in Figure 1.1.

Distance dramatically delays diffusion

The rate of diffusional transport is important because nutrient delivery must keep up with cellular demand. Unfortunately, the time t that it takes randomly jumping particles to move a distance x in a specific direction increases as the square of distance, as shown by Einstein:

$$t \propto x^2 \qquad (1.1)$$

As a result, diffusional transport is fast over short distances but horribly slow over large distances. Over a short distance such as the neuromuscular gap, 0.1 μm, diffusional transport takes only 5 millionths of a second. Across the 1 cm thick wall of the left ventricle diffusion would take more than half a day (Table 1.1).

Sadly, nature often gives us a practical reminder of Einstein's basic physics. Figure 1.2 shows a section through a human heart after a coronary artery thrombosis (clot) had obstructed blood flow to the left ventricle wall. The pale area is cardiac muscle that died from lack of O_2. The cells died even though the adjacent chamber was full of oxygenated blood. In other words, the patient died because a distance of a few millimetres reduced the rate of diffusional O_2 transport to a grossly inadequate level.

Convection provides fast transport over long distances

A faster transport system is clearly needed over distances greater than ~0.1 mm. This is provided by

Table 1.1 Time taken for a glucose molecule to diffuse a specified distance in one direction.

Distance (x)	Time (t)*	Comparable distance *in vivo*
0.1 μm	0.000005 s	Neuromuscular gap
1.0 μm	0.0005 s	Capillary wall
10.0 μm	0.05 s	Cell to capillary
1 mm	9.26 min	Skin, artery wall
1 cm	15.4 h	Ventricle wall

* Einstein's equation is $t = x^2/2D$. 'D' is the solute diffusion coefficient. For glucose at 37°C, D is 0.9×10^{-5} cm^2/s. For O_2 in water, 37°C, D is 3×10^{-5} cm^2/s.
(Einstein, A. (1905) *Theory of Brownian Movement* (trans. and ed. by R. Fürth and A. D. Cowper, 1956), Dover Publications, New York.)

Compartment A   Compartment B

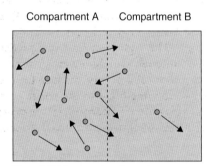

Time 1 (before random jumps):
concentration A = 8, concentration B = 2,
concentration difference ΔC = 6

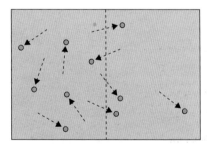

Time 2 (after random jumps):
concentration A = 6, concentration B = 4,
concentration difference ΔC = 2

Figure 1.1 Random molecular steps cause a net movement of solute molecules (pink dots) down a concentration gradient. As the density of solute molecules is greater in compartment A than B, the probability of a chance movement from A to B is greater than from B to A. Note that some molecules (one in this sketch) 'make it' into the opposite chamber; diffusion is multi-directional.

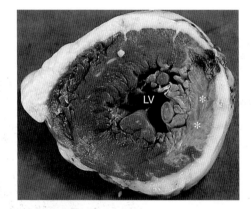

Figure 1.2 Section of human left ventricle after a coronary thrombosis, stained for a muscle enzyme. Pale area is an 'infarct' – an area of muscle badly damaged or killed by O_2 lack. The pallor is due to the loss of enzyme from dying muscle. The infarct was caused by coronary artery obstruction, which halted convective O_2 delivery. O_2 diffusion from blood in the main chamber (LV) is unaffected, yet only a thin rim of adjacent tissue (about 1 mm) survived. (Courtesy of the late Professor M. Davies, St George's Hospital Medical School, London.)

the cardiovascular system (Figure 1.3). The cardiovascular system still relies on **diffusion** to take up O_2 across the thin air-to-blood membrane inside the lungs; but the absorbed O_2 is then washed rapidly along in a stream of pumped fluid, covering large distances in seconds. This is called bulk flow or **convective transport**. The energy for convective transport is provided by the contraction of the heart. In humans it takes only 30 seconds for convective transport to carry O_2 a metre or more from the lungs to the smallest blood vessels of the limbs (capillaries). Diffusion would take more than 5 years! Over the final $10-20\,\mu m$ between the capillary and tissue parenchymal cell, diffusion is again the main transport process.

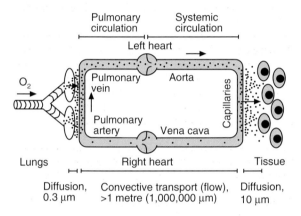

Figure 1.3 Overview of human circulation, showing roles of diffusion and convection in O_2 transport.

1.2 Functions of the cardiovascular system

- The primary function of the cardiovascular system (CVS) is the **rapid convective transport** of oxygen, glucose, amino acids, fatty acids, vitamins, drugs and water to the tissues; and the rapid washout of metabolic waste products such as carbon dioxide, urea and creatinine.
- The CVS is also a **control system**. It distributes hormones to the tissues and secretes a hormone itself, namely atrial natriuretic peptide.
- The CVS is crucial for **body temperature regulation**. It transports heat from deep organs to the skin surface for dissipation.
- In **reproduction** the CVS provides the hydraulic mechanism for genital erection.

1.3 The circulation of blood

The heart consists of two intermittent muscular pumps, the right and left ventricles (Figure 1.4). Each pump is filled from a contractile reservoir, the right or left atrium. The right ventricle pumps deoxygenated blood through the pulmonary artery to the lungs (Figure 1.5). Pulmonary veins return oxygenated blood from the lungs to the left side of the heart, completing the short **pulmonary circulation**. The left ventricle pumps out an equal volume of

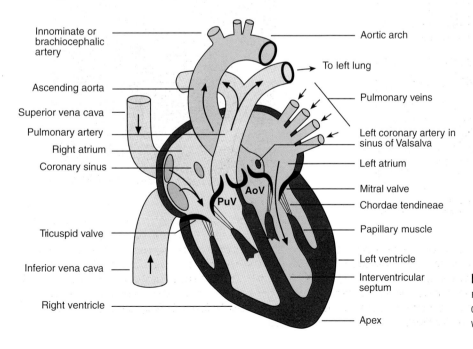

Figure 1.4 Structure of mammalian heart. Pink denotes oxygenated blood; AoV, aortic valve; PuV, pulmonary valve.

oxygenated blood to the rest of the body, and deoxygenated blood returns via two great veins, the superior vena cava and inferior vena cava, to the right atrium to complete the **systemic circulation**. The operation of one-way valves in the heart and veins ensures that blood follows this circular pathway, as was first proved by the London physician William Harvey. Harvey's ground-breaking introduction of experimentation into physiology and medicine is described in his book *De Motu Cordis* (Concerning the Motion of the Heart, 1628).

The right heart perfuses the pulmonary circulation

Venous blood enters the right atrium from the superior and inferior venae cavae, then flows through the tricuspid valve into the right ventricle. The ventricle is composed mainly of cardiac muscle and it receives the blood while the muscle is relaxed. Cardiac relaxation is called **diastole** (pronounced dia-stol-i). Contraction then follows, called **systole** (pronounced sis-tol-i). Systole expels some of the blood at a low pressure into the pulmonary artery, which divides and supplies the lungs. In the tiny air sacs of the lungs, or alveoli, gas exchange occurs by diffusion. Inhaled oxygen diffuses into the blood, raising its oxygen content from ~150 ml/l in mixed venous blood (at rest) to ~195 ml/l; and carbon dioxide diffuses from blood into the alveolar gas to be exhaled. The oxygenated blood returns through the four pulmonary veins and passes through the left atrium into the left ventricle.

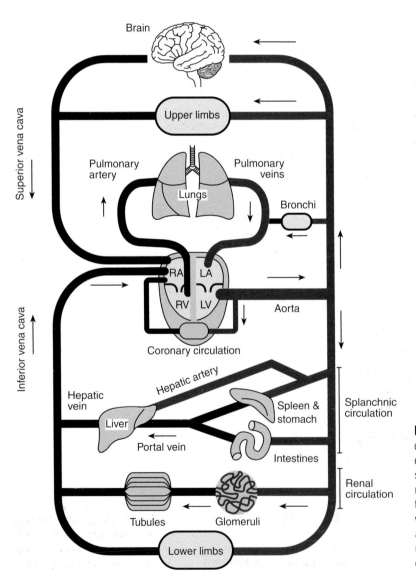

Figure 1.5 Stylized arrangement of the circulation. Systemic and pulmonary circulations are in series. Circulation to most systemic organs are in parallel (brain, myocardium, limbs, etc.), but liver and renal tubules have an in series supply. Bronchial venous blood drains anomalously into left atrium. RA and LA, right and left atrium, respectively; RV and LV, right and left ventricle, respectively.

The left heart perfuses the systemic circulation

The left ventricle contracts virtually simultaneously with the right ventricle and ejects the same volume of blood, but at a much higher pressure. The blood flows through the aorta, which gives off the major, named branches shown in Figure 1.6. Repeated arterial branching leads, ultimately, to the formation of millions of microscopic, thin-walled tubes called capillaries (Figure 1.7). Here the ultimate function of the cardiovascular system is fulfilled; dissolved gases and metabolites diffuse between the capillary blood and the cells of the body. The deoxygenated blood returns through a convergent system of veins that in general accompany the named arteries and drain into the superior and inferior venae cavae (Figure 1.5).

1.4 Cardiac output and its distribution

The cardiac output is the volume of blood ejected by one ventricle in one minute. Cardiac output is the product of **stroke volume** (the volume ejected per contraction) and **heart rate** (the number of contractions per minute). In a resting adult the stroke volume is typically $70-80\,ml$ and the heart rate $60-75\,beats/min$. Thus the resting cardiac output is $\sim 75\,ml \times 70$ per min, or 5 litres per min.

Cardiac output is not fixed; it adapts rapidly to changing internal or external circumstances. In strenuous exercise, for example, the human heart responds to the increased demand for O_2 with a $4-5$ fold increase in output. The cardiac response is driven by internal distension and extrinsic, autonomic nerves as described in later chapters.

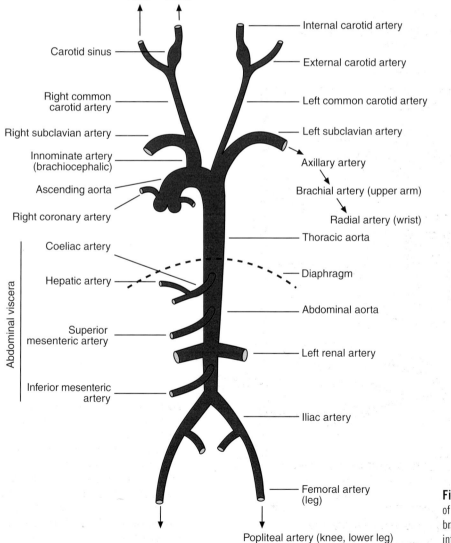

Figure 1.6 Simplified anatomy of human aorta and its largest branches. The paired thoracic intercostal arteries are not shown.

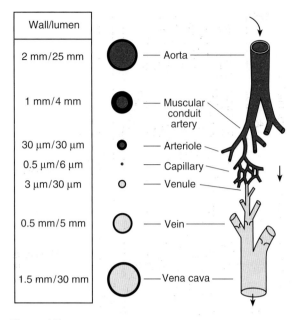

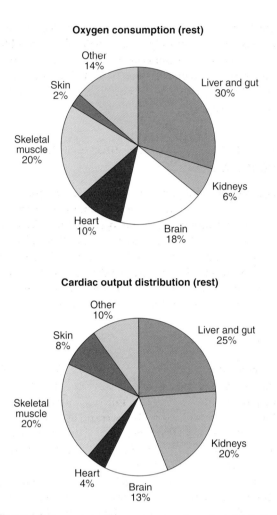

Figure 1.7 Thickness of the wall relative to the diameter of the lumen in different blood vessels. The ratio varies, however, with blood pressure and vascular tone. The large-vessel dimensions are for man. (Sources as for Table 1.3.)

Cardiac output is distributed according to metabolic and functional demand

As a rough rule the output of the left ventricle is distributed to the peripheral tissues in proportion to their metabolic rate. Skeletal muscle, for example, accounts for ~20% of human O_2 consumption at rest and receives ~20% of the cardiac output (Figure 1.8). This egalitarian principle is overridden, however, in the kidneys, because their excretory function demands a high blood flow. The kidneys account for only 6% of total O_2 consumption but receive 20% of the cardiac output for the purposes of water and urea excretion. Since renal flow is disproportionately large, some other tissues are less well supplied and, surprisingly, cardiac muscle is one of them. To compensate, the cardiac muscle extracts an unusually high proportion of the O_2 from the coronary blood, namely 65–75%.

The distribution of the cardiac output can be actively adjusted to match changing regional demands. For example, in exercise the proportion of the output going to skeletal muscle can increase to ~80%. The redistribution of the output is brought about by a widening of tiny arterial vessels called arterioles (Figure 1.7) inside the active muscle. This **vasodilatation** allows blood to flow more easily into the active muscle.

Figure 1.8 Comparison of O_2 usage and cardiac output distribution in humans at rest. (Data from Wade, O. L. and Bishop, J. M. (1962) *Cardiac Output and Regional Flow*, Blackwell, Oxford.)

1.5 Introducing 'hydraulics': flow, pressure and resistance

Gradients of pressure drive the flow

What drives blood along a blood vessel? The chief factor is the **gradient of blood pressure**. Ventricular ejection raises the aortic blood pressure to ~100 mmHg above atmospheric pressure, whereas the pressure in the great veins is close to atmospheric pressure. The pressure difference drives the blood from artery to vein. Units of 'mmHg above atmospheric pressure' are used because human blood pressure is usually measured with a mercury column, taking atmospheric pressure as the reference or zero level (see Appendix 2, 'Pressure').

Arterial pressure is **pulsatile**, because the heart ejects blood intermittently. Between successive ejections the systemic arterial pressure decays from a peak of ~120 mmHg to a trough of ~80 mmHg. At the same time pulmonary pressure decays from 25 mmHg to 10 mmHg (Figure 1.9). This is conventionally written as 120/80 mmHg and 25/10 mmHg respectively.

A simple law links flow, pressure and conductance

Although arterial pressure is pulsatile, many aspects of the circulation can be understood simply by considering the **average** pressure and **average** flow. To get at the basic rules, let us consider a steady flow of water or plasma along a long rigid tube, driven by a steady pressure head. Under these conditions the flow $\dot{Q}$ is proportional to the pressure difference between the inlet, pressure P_1, and the outlet, pressure P_2:

$$\dot{Q} \propto P_1 - P_2 \qquad (1.2)$$

Flow is often represented by a dotted Q because Q stands for quantity of fluid and the dot denotes rate of passage in Newton's original calculus notation. Note that **flow is, by definition, a rate**; flow is the volume transferred per unit time. The often-heard expression 'rate of flow' is both tautologous and dimensionally incorrect.

If we insert a proportionality factor, K, into the above relation, we obtain an equation that tells us how much flow a given pressure difference produces:

$$\dot{Q} = K(P_1 - P_2) \qquad (1.3)$$

The proportionality factor K is called the **hydraulic conductance**. The bigger the conductance, the bigger the flow generated by a given pressure gradient. Conductance depends on tube width, so a large artery has a much bigger conductance than an arteriole.

Resistance is opposition to flow

We often need to think about how much **difficulty** the blood experiences in passing through a vessel. For this purpose we use the concept of hydraulic resistance. Resistance, or opposition to flow, is simply the inverse of conductance, which is ease of flow. In other words, resistance R is $1/K$. Thus we can re-write the basic flow law as:

$$\dot{Q} = \frac{P_1 - P_2}{R} \qquad (1.4)$$

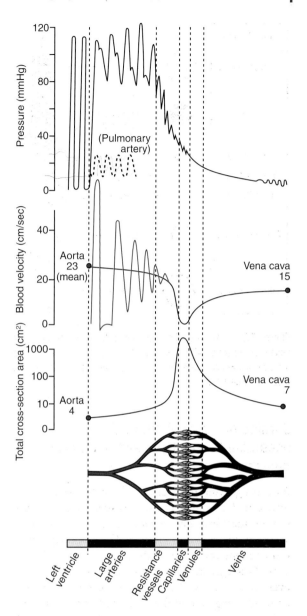

Figure 1.9 Profile of pressure and blood velocity in systemic circulation of a resting human. The same volume of blood passes each dashed line per minute, namely the cardiac output. The mean blood velocity (black line) is the flow divided by the cross-sectional area of the vascular bed. The red line shows the pulsation of velocity. The large fall in pressure across terminal arteries and arterioles (diameter 30–500 μm) proves that they are the main resistance vessels.

This is **Darcy's law of flow**. (It may be helpful to note its similarity to Ohm's law, namely flow of electrical current = voltage drop/resistance.) Darcy's law tells us that resistance is the difference in pressure needed to drive one unit of flow in the steady state, i.e. mmHg per ml/min. The bigger the resistance, the bigger the difference in pressure need to drive a given flow. Resistance is low in wide vessels such as the named arteries and veins, and high in narrow vessels such as arterioles.

The resistances of tubes in series summate

When two tubes are linked in series, their individual resistances simply add up. Consequently, although the resistance of the aorta is low, the resistance of the entire systemic circulation is high due to the addition of the resistances of the narrow arterioles and capillaries. (The complication introduced by multiple tubes linked in parallel is considered in Chapter 8.) The total resistance of the human systemic circulation is around 0.02 mmHg per ml/min. The resistance of the pulmonary circulation is much lower, ~0.003 mmHg per ml/min, so a low pulmonary artery pressure suffices to drive the cardiac output through the lungs.

Active changes in small-vessel calibre adjust resistance and local blood flow

The law of flow enables us to understand how the blood flow to an organ is regulated. There are only two ways to raise the flow: either the driving pressure must increase or the vascular resistance must decrease. In general the arterial blood pressure is maintained within narrow limits by nervous reflexes, so **local blood flow is regulated by changes in vascular resistance**. For example, when we salivate, the blood flow to the salivary gland increases 10-fold, and it does so because the vascular resistance in the gland is reduced to 1/10th of its former value through arteriolar vasodilatation. The arterial pressure driving the flow is unchanged. Changes in vascular resistance are brought about by the contraction and relaxation of the narrow, terminal branches of the arterial system, so we must next consider vessel structure.

1.6 Blood vessel structure

The aorta divides into a set of named conduit arteries (Figure 1.6). These branch progressively to form tiny arteries of diameter 0.1–0.5 mm, then even narrower vessels of very high resistance called arterioles (Figure 1.7). Arterioles branch into a vast number of fine, thin-walled capillaries. Capillaries converge to form venules, which converge into veins.

Vessel branching slows down the blood

The total cross-sectional area of the vascular system at a given level of branching (e.g. the capillaries) is the number of vessels n times the cross-sectional area of an individual vessel, πr^2. As blood spreads out along the arterial tree, the increase in n due to branching more than outweighs the reduction in vessel size, πr^2. As a result, **the total cross-sectional area of the circulation increases from the aorta to the capillary bed** (Table 1.2). It then falls again as venous vessels converge.

The broadening of the circulation with arterial branching is important because it slows down the blood. We can see an analogous effect when strolling beside a river: the current slows down wherever the river banks widen. The blood **velocity** (cm/s) at a particular level of branching is the total flow through the branches, i.e. the **cardiac output** (cm^3/s), divided by the **total cross-sectional area** of the branches (cm^2). As a result of area expansion, the blood velocity in capillaries is ~1/200th of that in major arteries (Figure 1.9). This is particularly important in the lungs, where the slow passage through the capillaries **allows time for the blood to equilibrate with the alveolar gas**.

Table 1.2 Average dimensions of blood vessels in dog mesentery*.

Vessel	Number	Length (mm)	Diameter (mm)	Total cross-sectional area† (mm²)	Volume (% of total)
Main artery	1	60	3	7	2.5
Arterioles and smallest arteries	1 380 000	1.5–2	0.024–0.031	739	8.1
Capillaries	47 300 000	0.4	0.008	2378	5.7
Venules	2 100 000	1.0	0.026	1151	6.9
Small veins	180 000	1–14	0.075–0.28	1019	21.3
Large veins	61	39–60	1.5–6	174	46.7

* The vessels are easily seen here for counting, unlike most circulations.
† Note that largest area and therefore slowest flow is in the capillaries. Largest volume is in the veins. (After Scleier, J. (1918) *Archiv Gesamte Physiologie*, **173**, 172.)

The vascular wall has three layers

The walls of all blood vessels except capillaries are made up of three layers (Figure 1.10): the tunica intima (innermost coat), tunica media (middle coat) and tunica adventitia (outer coat).

The **intima** is a sheet of flattened endothelial cells resting on a thin layer of connective tissue. The endothelial layer is the main barrier to the escape of plasma. It also actively secretes vasoactive agents such as the antithrombotic vasodilator agent nitric oxide.

The **media** supplies mechanical strength and contractile power. It consists of spindle-shaped smooth muscle cells arranged helically in a matrix of elastin and collagen fibres. Two sheets of elastin, called the internal and external elastic lamina, mark the boundaries of the media. In places the intimal endothelial cells project through the internal elastic lamina to make contact with smooth muscle cells and transmit signals between the intima and media.

The **adventitia** is a connective tissue sheath with no distinct outer border. Its role is to tether the vessel loosely to the surrounding tissue. The adventitia of large arteries contains small blood vessels called **vasa vasorum** (literally 'vessels of vessels') which nourish the thick media. The adventitia of the limb veins also contain **nociceptive nerve fibres** that mediate the pain of thrombophlebitis.

1.7 Functional classes of vessel

The circulation is constructed on the economical principle that each vessel must fulfil at least one extra role besides conducting blood. Based on the extra role the following classes of vessel are recognized:

- elastic arteries
- conduit (muscular) arteries
- resistance vessels
- exchange vessels
- capacitance vessels.

In each class of vessel the wall is specifically adapted to its role, as follows.

Elastic arteries receive the stroke volume and smooth the flow

The largest arteries such as the aorta and iliac arteries (diameter 1–2 cm in humans) have very distensible walls because the tunica media is rich in elastin (Table 1.3). **Elastin** is an extracellular protein that is six times more extensible than rubber. Elastin enables the elastic arteries to expand by ~10% during each heart beat and thereby accommodate the

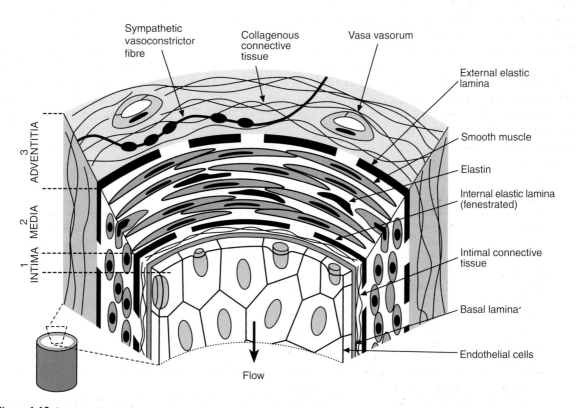

Figure 1.10 Structure of wall of a muscular artery.

ejected blood. The recoil of the elastic vessels during diastole converts the stop−go flow in the ascending aorta into a continuous flow through the more distal arteries (Figure 1.9). **Collagen** is an extracellular protein that forms a network of strong fibrils in the media. Collagen is 100 times stiffer than elastin and prevents over-distension of the vessel.

Conduit (muscular) arteries deliver blood to the organs

In medium to small arteries such as the radial, cerebral and coronary arteries (diameter 0.1−1.0 cm in humans), the tunica media contains more smooth muscle and is thicker, relative to the lumen, than in elastic arteries (Figure 1.7, Table 1.3). The thick wall prevents collapse at sharp bends such as the elbow and knee.

The muscular arteries can contract and relax, and have a rich autonomic innervation. Dilatation of the conduit artery supplying an active skeletal muscle facilitates the local increase in blood flow during exercise (Figure 13.7). Contraction of muscular arteries occurs physiologically in diving animals (Chapter 17). Contraction can be life-saving in accidents, as shown by a motor-cycle crash victim brought into Casualty with one leg severed at the knee. The popliteal artery was torn in half but was scarcely bleeding: an intense contraction had prevented the patient from bleeding to death. Less beneficial is the vasospasm of diseased coronary arteries, which accounts for some cases of angina (cardiac pain; Figure 15.6).

Pressure falls sharply across terminal arteries and arterioles

The **vascular pressure profile is fundamental to understanding the circulation** (Figure 1.9). Mean blood pressure falls very little along the elastic and conduit arteries because the large lumen offers little resistance to flow. The drop in mean pressure from the ascending aorta to radial artery is only 2 mmHg or so. (The curious 'peaking' of the pressure wave in peripheral arteries, evident in Figure 1.9, is explained in Chapter 8.) The **major drop in pressure occurs across the smallest, terminal arteries** (diameter 100−500 μm) **and arterioles** (diameter 10−100 μm). The law of flow, eqn 1.4, shows that there is only one possible explanation for a large drop in pressure; the vessels must offer a large resistance to flow. The terminal arteries and arterioles are therefore called the **resistance vessels**.

The proximal resistance vessels, i.e. the terminal arteries, are richly innervated by sympathetic vasoconstrictor nerve fibres and have a thick, muscular wall relative to the lumen (Figure 1.7). The terminal arterioles are poorly innervated and have 1−3 layers of smooth muscle cells in the media. Some workers define an arteriole as a vessel with just one layer of muscle, while others define it as any arterial vessel of diameter <100 μm. The terminal arteries and arterioles have a high resistance because the lumen is narrow and the number of vessels is relatively low (Table 1.2).

The resistance vessels act as taps that control local blood flow and capillary perfusion

Since resistance vessels dominate the resistance to flow, they serve as the taps of the circulation; they can turn local blood flow up or down to match local demand. When the resistance vessels dilate (**vasodilatation**), resistance falls and local blood flow increases. Conversely, **vasoconstriction** raises local resistance and reduces the local blood flow. The terminal arterioles also adjust the number of capillaries perfused with blood. This task used to be attributed to an imaginary 'precapillary sphincter', but it is now generally accepted that true sphincters rarely exist.

Exchange vessels transfer O_2 and metabolites to the tissue

Gas and metabolite exchange takes place chiefly in the **capillaries**. Capillaries are so numerous and tiny

Table 1.3 Composition of the blood vessel wall (%).

	Endothelium	Smooth muscle	Elastic tissue	Collagenous tissue
Elastic artery	5	25	40	27
Arteriole	10	60	10	20
Capillary	95	0	0	5 (basal lamina)
Venule	20	20	0	60

(After Caro, C. G., Pedley, T. J., Schroter, R. C. and Seed, W. A. (1978) *The Mechanics of the Circulation*, Oxford University Press, Oxford; and Burton, A. C. (1972) *Physiology and Biophysics of the Circulation*, Year Book Medical Publishers, Chicago.)

(diameter 4–7 μm) that most tissue cells are within 10–20 μm of a capillary. The wall of a capillary is merely a single layer of endothelial cells ~0.5 μm thick, which facilitates the rapid passage of gases and metabolites.

Some exchange also takes place in the next vessels downstream, the **postcapillary or pericytic venules** (diameter 15–50 μm). These are microscopic venules that lack a complete smooth muscle coat. Some O_2 also passes through the walls of arterioles. Strictly speaking, therefore, the term **exchange vessel** embraces microvessels on both sides of the capillary network.

Although capillaries are very narrow, the capillary bed as a whole has a surprisingly low resistance to flow and a relatively modest pressure drop (Figure 1.9). This is due to the very large numbers of capillaries in parallel array (Table 1.2), their shortness (~1 mm) and a special flow pattern called bolus flow (Chapter 8). The large cross-sectional area of the capillary bed slows the blood velocity to 0.5–1 mm/s (Figure 1.9). As a result each red cell takes ~0.5–2 s to traverse a systemic capillary. This **transit time** is sufficiently long for a red cell to unload O_2 and take up CO_2 from the tissue.

Arteriovenous anastomoses regulate heat exchange

A few tissues, notably the skin and nasal mucosa, possess wide shunt vessels of diameter 20–130 μm that connect the arterioles directly to the venules, bypassing the capillaries. The shunts are called arteriovenous anastomoses (singular, anastomosis). Their thick muscular walls are richly innervated by sympathetic nerves. In the skin they are involved in the control of body temperature. In the nasal mucosa they help to warm the inspired air. Arteriovenous anastomoses are not common in other tissues.

Capacitance vessels are venous vessels that act as blood reservoirs

Venules (diameter 50–200 μm) and veins differ chiefly in size and number. The thin wall comprises an intima, a thin media of smooth muscle and collagen, and an adventitia. The intima of limb veins possesses pairs of **semilunar valves**, discovered by Harvey's teacher, the gloriously named Hieronymous Fabricius ab Aquapendente, in 1603. The semilunar valves prevent the backflow of venous blood in limbs (Figure 8.23). The large central veins and the veins of the head and neck lack functional valves.

Venules and small veins are more numerous than the corresponding arterioles and arteries (Table 1.2),

so their net resistance is low. A pressure drop of 10–15 mmHg is sufficient to drive the cardiac output from the venules to the right atrium.

Because of their large number and size, veins contain about two-thirds of the circulating blood at any one instant (Figure 1.11). They are therefore called 'capacitance vessels'. Due to their thin walls they are easily distended or collapsed, so they act as a variable reservoir of blood. Moreover, many peripheral veins are innervated by vasoconstrictor nerve fibres, so the volume of blood in the venous reservoir can be actively controlled. At times of physiological stress the capacitance vessels constrict and displace blood into the heart and arteries.

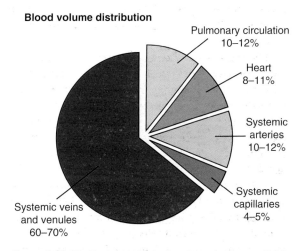

Blood volume distribution

Pulmonary circulation 10–12%

Heart 8–11%

Systemic arteries 10–12%

Systemic capillaries 4–5%

Systemic veins and venules 60–70%

Figure 1.11 Distribution of blood volume in a resting man (5.5 l). (From Folkow, B. and Neil, E. (1971) *Circulation*, Oxford University Press, London, by permission.)

Vascular resistance and conductance

■ Resistance to flow is the pressure difference needed to drive unit flow through a vessel or set of vessels. The basic law of flow (Darcy's law) tells us:

flow = pressure drop/resistance

■ Since the biggest pressure drop occurs across the terminal arteries and arterioles, these vessels must be the main sites of resistance to blood flow (resistance vessels).

■ The resistance vessels control local blood flow. When they dilate, resistance falls and blood flow to the downstream tissue increases.

■ Conductance is the inverse of resistance. If resistance falls, conductance and flow increase.

CONCEPT BOX 1

1.8 The plumbing

'In parallel' versus 'in series' circulations

The systemic circulation can be subdivided into specialized, individual circuits that supply the brain, heart wall, kidneys, intestines, etc. Usually the arterial supply to an organ arises more or less directly from the aorta, i.e. each organ is supplied directly with arterial blood. This form of plumbing is termed **in parallel** (Figure 1.5). A few organs, however, are connected **in series** with another organ; that is to say, they obtain their blood second-hand from the venous outflow of another organ. Such an arrangement is called a **portal system**.

Portal circulations provide a direct delivery service

The liver is the largest portal system in the body. Around 72% of the liver blood supply comes from the portal vein, which contains venous blood drained from the intestine and spleen (Figure 1.5). The portal vein enters the liver at the 'porta hepatis', or gateway of the liver, from which the term portal system originates. In addition the liver receives arterial blood directly from the hepatic artery, so its circuitry is partly in series and partly in parallel. Portal systems have the advantage of transporting a valuable commodity directly from one site to another. For example, the portal vein transports the products of digestion from the intestine directly to the liver for storage and processing.

Portal systems also exist in the kidney, where effluent blood from the glomerulus supplies the tubules: and in the brain, where a portal system carries regulatory hormones from the hypothalamus to the anterior pituitary gland.

A portal system has one serious drawback, namely the downstream tissue receives partially deoxygenated blood under a reduced pressure head. As a result the downstream tissue is vulnerable to damage during episodes of hypotension (low arterial pressure). For example, renal tubular damage is not an uncommon complication of severe hypotension.

1.9 Control systems

The contractile behaviour of the heart and blood vessels is continually adjusted to deal with changing external and internal demands, such as exercise, salivation, stress etc. This is achieved by nervous and endocrine reflexes, which are co-ordinated by the brain. One of the most important cardiovascular reflexes is the **arterial baroreceptor reflex**, which stabilizes arterial blood pressure and thereby safeguards the blood flow to the brain. The reflex is initiated by 'baroreceptors' in the walls of major arteries, which sense changes in blood pressure. Nerve impulses are sent to the brainstem. This elicits a reflex alteration in the activity of the autonomic nerves that control the heart and blood vessels. The resulting changes in cardiac output, peripheral resistance and venous capacitance restore the blood pressure to normal.

Where do we go from here? In a system as complex as the cardiovascular system there is a danger of not seeing the wood for the trees, but the above outline should help to avoid this. In Chapters 2–14 (cardiac electricity, haemodynamics, etc.) we bump into the trees and peep under the bark. In Chapters 15–18, we stand back to gain a broader perspective on how the system as a whole responds to physiological and medical challenges.

SUMMARY

■ The energy of the heart beat generates the rapid convective transport of O_2, nutrients, waste products, hormones and heat. The branching vascular tree delivers O_2 to within $10-20\,\mu$m of most cells. The final, short leg is covered by diffusion. Tissues die in the absence of convective transport (e.g. myocardial infarction, ischaemic foot) because diffusional transport time increases with the square of distance.

■ The right ventricle, filled via the right atrium, pumps deoxygenated blood at low pressure (mean $\sim 15\,$mmHg) through the pulmonary circulation for oxygenation. The left ventricle, filled via the left atrium, pumps oxygenated blood at high pressure (mean $\sim 90\,$mmHg) through the systemic circulation.

■ Resting human cardiac output is $\sim 5\,$l/min. Output equals heart rate (60–70 beats/min) times stroke volume (70–80 ml). The distribution to individual tissues is controlled by the local resistance vessels. In general blood flow is apportioned according to local metabolic activity, but the kidneys receive 20% of the cardiac output to satisfy their excretory role.

■ Blood flow $\dot{Q}$ is driven by the pressure drop from artery to vein, $P_A - P_V$. Darcy's law of flow states $\dot{Q} = (P_A - P_V)/R$, where R is resistance to flow. The main resistance is located in tiny terminal arteries and arterioles, as proved by the large pressure drop across them. These 'resistance vessels' actively constrict or dilate to match local blood flow to local demand.

■ The other functional categories of vessel are as follows. Elastic arteries (e.g. aorta) receive the intermittently ejected stroke volume and convert it into a continuous albeit pulsatile peripheral flow. Exchange vessels (capillaries, postcapillary venules) allow solute and water to exchange with the tissue. Capacitance vessels (venules, veins) contain about two-thirds of the circulating blood volume and act as controlled blood reservoirs.

■ Except in capillaries the vascular wall comprises three layers, the tunica intima (endothelium), tunica media (vascular smooth muscle, collagen and elastin) and tunica adventitia (connective tissue). The smooth muscle regulates the diameter of resistance and capacitance vessels, and thereby regulates local blood flow and blood volume distribution.

■ Vascular smooth muscle is controlled by autonomic nerves, circulating hormones and local factors. Autonomic nerves and circulating hormones also control the rate and force of the heart beat. The cardiovascular system is thus under the control of neural reflexes, such as the baroreflex. The baroreflex stabilizes the arterial blood pressure.

■ Most special circulations (coronary, cerebral, etc.) are plumbed in parallel to each other, so each one receives fully oxygenated blood. Portal circulations lie in series with an upstream tissue and receive venous blood. For example, the portal vein supplies the liver with venous blood from the intestine.

FURTHER READING

Fenger-Gron, J., Mulvany, M. J. and Christensen, K. L. (1995) Mesenteric blood pressure profile of conscious, freely moving rats. *Journal of Physiology*, **488**, 753–760.

Harvey, W. (1628) *On the Motion of the Heart and Blood in Animals* (trans. by R. Willis) (1993), Prometheus Books, Buffalo, New York.

Henderson, J. R. and Daniel, P. M. (1984) Capillary beds and portal circulations. In *Handbook of Physiology*, The Cardiovascular System, Vol. IV, Part 2 (eds Renkin, E. M. and Michel, C. C.), The American Physiological Society, Maryland, pp. 1035–1046.

Neil, E. (1983) Peripheral circulation: historical aspects. In *Handbook of Physiology*, Vol. III, Part 1 (eds Shepherd, J. T. and Abboud, F. M.), American Physiological Society, Maryland, p. 120.

Nichols, W. W. and O'Rourke, M. F. (1998) *McDonald's Blood Flow in Arteries. Theoretical, Experimental and Clinical Principles*, 4th Edition, Edward Arnold, London.

Rhodin, J. A. G. (1980) Architecture of the vessel wall. In *Handbook of Physiology, Cardiovascular System*, Vol. II (eds Bohr, D. F., Somlyo, A. P. and Sparks, H. V.), American Physiological Society, Bethesda, p. 132.

CHAPTER 2

The cardiac cycle

Learning objectives

After reading this chapter you should be able to:

- State the roles of the fibrotendinous ring, the four valves, papillary muscle, the ventricular wall thickness and the pacemaker (2.1).
- List the four phases of the ventricular cycle and the valve positions (2.2).
- Draw a graph to show the changes in atrial and ventricular pressures over one cardiac cycle (Figure 2.5).
- Draw a left ventricular pressure–volume loop for a resting adult, labelling each side and corner (Figure 2.6).
- Define 'ejection fraction' and state typical values (2.3).
- Give the relative timings of diastole and systole during rest and maximal exercise (2.4).
- State the origin of (i) the apex beat; (ii) the heart sounds; (iii) cardiac murmurs (2.5).
- State briefly the nature and use of electrocardiography, echocardiography, radionuclide angiography and cardiac catheterization (2.6).

An adult human heart weighs only 250–350 g, yet it pumps out ~200 million litres of blood over our allotted 'three score years and ten'. This chapter describes the mechanical events that generate this truly remarkable output.

2.1 Gross structure of the heart

The human heart is a roughly cone-shaped, four-chambered, hollow muscle, ~12 cm long by 9 cm wide. It lies obliquely across the midline of the chest with the tip of the cone (called the **apex** of the heart) behind the 5th left intercostal space (Figures 2.1, 2.2). The heart is rotated around its long axis so that the right atrium and right ventricle form the anterior surface. The four chambers are built around a ring of fibrous fatty tissue called the **annulus fibrosus**, which is situated at the atrioventricular junction. This region is called the **base** of the heart. Being tethered to the great vessels, the base moves relatively little. The apex moves substantially during contraction and produces the heartbeat (**apex beat**) that is felt through the chest wall.

The annulus fibrosus serves three roles. First, it acts as a mechanical base, the atria being anchored to its upper surface and the ventricles to its lower surface. Second, it is perforated by four apertures, each containing a valve. Third, it insulates the ventricles electrically from the atria.

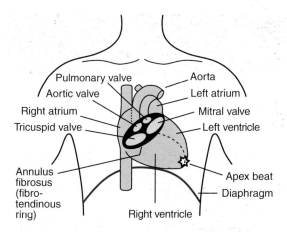

Figure 2.1 Orientation of heart and valves in human thorax. Heart lies obliquely, and is rotated so that right atrium and right ventricle form most of anterior surface. Fibrotendinous ring forms 'base' of heart. The tip of right ventricle forms 'apex'. Inferior surface and pericardium (not shown) rest on central tendon of diaphragm. The four valves are grouped closely in an oblique plane behind the sternum.

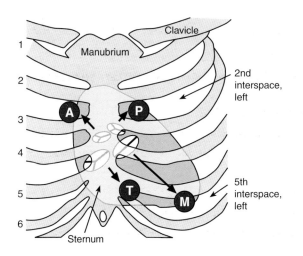

Figure 2.2 Location of cardiac valves and auscultation areas. A, aortic valve area; P, pulmonary valve area; T, tricuspid area; M, mitral area.

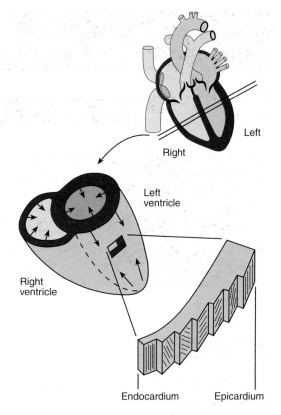

Figure 2.3 Schematic illustration of direction of ventricle wall motion during contraction (middle) and of orientation of muscle fibres in the wall (bottom).

The entire heart is enclosed in a fibrous sac or **pericardium** (peri, around). The sac is lined by a layer of mesothelium and is lubricated by pericardial fluid. The lower surface of the pericardium is fused to the diaphragm. Consequently, each time the diaphragm descends during inspiration, the heart is dragged into a more vertical orientation.

Right atrium and tricuspid valve

The right atrium is a thin-walled muscular chamber which receives the venous return from the venae cavae and the coronary sinus, the main vein draining the heart muscle (Figure 1.4). The **pacemaker**, which is the sparking plug that initiates each heart beat, is located in the right atrial wall close to the entrance of the superior vena cava.

The right atrium communicates with the right ventricle through a valve with three cusps, the tricuspid valve. Each cusp is a thin flap of connective tissue, ~0.1 mm thick, covered by endothelium. The free margins of the cusps are tethered by tendinous strings, the **chordae tendineae**, to inward projections of the ventricle wall called **papillary muscles** (Figure 1.4). The papillary muscles contract and tense the chordae tendineae during systole. This prevents the valve from inverting into the atrium as pressure builds up in the ventricle.

Right ventricle and pulmonary valve

The anterior wall of the human right ventricle is ~0.5 cm thick and resembles a pocket tacked around the septum (Figure 2.3). Expulsion of blood is produced chiefly by the free anterior wall approaching the septum, like an old-fashioned bellows. The outlet from the ventricle into the pulmonary artery is guarded by the pulmonary valve, which has three equal-sized, baggy cusps.

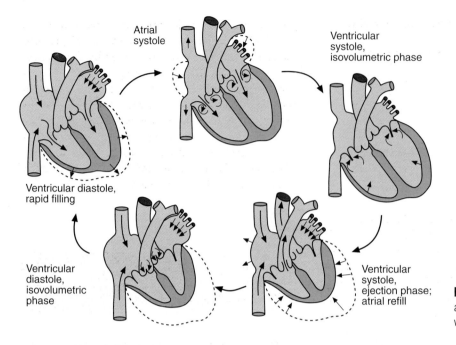

Atrial systole

Ventricular systole, isovolumetric phase

Ventricular diastole, rapid filling

Ventricular diastole, isovolumetric phase

Ventricular systole, ejection phase; atrial refill

Figure 2.4 Changes in valves, atrial volumes and ventricular volumes over the cardiac cycle.

Left atrium and mitral valve

The left atrium receives blood from the pulmonary veins and transmits it into the left ventricle through a bicuspid valve. The large anterior and small posterior cusps were thought to look like a bishop's mitre, hence the name mitral valve. The cusp margins are tethered by chordae tendineae to two papillary muscles in the left ventricle (Figure 1.4).

Left ventricle, apex beat and aortic valve

The chamber of the left ventricle is conical and blood is ejected by a reduction in both diameter and length. The wall is ~3 times thicker than in the right ventricle because the left side has to generate higher pressures. The muscle fibres are wrapped around the chamber somewhat like a turban, their orientation changing progressively with distance. The innermost (endocardial) muscle fibres are orientated longitudinally, running from the base of the heart (the fibrotendinous ring) to the apex, i.e. the tip of the left ventricle. The central fibres run circumferentially; the outermost or epicardial fibres again run longitudinally; and intermediate fibres run obliquely (Figure 2.3). When the chamber contracts, it twists forwards and the apex taps against the chest wall, producing a palpable **apex beat**. The apex beat is normally felt in the fifth, left intercostal space, about 10 cm from the midline (the mid-clavicular line). Cardiac enlargement can be detected by deviation of the apex beat from its normal location.

The root of the aorta contains a three-cusp valve. Occasionally it has only two cusps, and such valves are prone to narrowing (**stenosis**) in later life. Next to each cusp the root of the aorta bulges out into the **sinuses of Valsalva**. The two coronary arteries originate in the sinuses, just behind the valve leaflets (Figure 1.4).

2.2 The ventricular cycle

The cycle of atrial and ventricular contraction, the **cardiac cycle**, is illustrated in Figure 2.4. The ventricular cycle is divided into four phases, based on the positions of the inlet and outlet valves. We will begin, arbitrarily, with the moment when both the atria and ventricles are relaxed (**diastole**). The timings below refer to a human cycle lasting 0.9 s, equivalent to 67 beats/min. The data were acquired by echocardiography (Section 2.6), cardiac catheterization (Section 2.6), electrocardiography (Chapter 5) and cardiometry (Figure 6.8).

Ventricular filling

> Duration: 0.5 s (resting human)
> Inlet valves (tricuspid, mitral): open
> Outlet valves (pulmonary, aortic): closed

In a resting human, ventricular diastole lasts for nearly two-thirds of the cardiac cycle, giving ample time for refilling. The atria too are in diastole and blood flows passively from the great veins through the atria and open atrioventricular valves into the

Table 2.1 Mean pressures during the human cardiac cycle in mmHg*.

	Right	Left
Atrium	3	8
Ventricle –		
end of diastole	4	9
peak of systole	25	120

* Adult, resting supine.

ventricles. Filling is fast over the initial 0.15 s, as shown by the ventricular volume trace in Figure 2.5. The initial **rapid-filling phase** has a curious feature – the ventricular pressure actually falls at first even though ventricular volume is increasing. The reason is that the relaxing ventricle recoils elastically from its deformed end-systolic shape and thus sucks blood into its chamber. As the ventricle reaches its natural relaxed volume, the rate of filling slows down (**diastasis**). Further filling is due to venous pressure distending the ventricle, so ventricular pressure begins to rise.

In the final third of the filling phase **atrial contraction** pumps extra blood into the ventricle. In resting young adults atrial systole boosts the ventricular filling by only 10–20%. The atrial contribution increases with age, however, and reaches 46% by 80 years old. The atrial boost also becomes more important in exercise, because the high heart rate leaves less time for passive ventricular filling.

The volume of blood in a ventricle at the end of the filling phase is called the **end-diastolic volume** (EDV). The EDV is typically around 120 ml in an adult human (Figure 2.5). The corresponding **end-diastolic pressure** (EDP) is a few mmHg. As Table 2.1 shows, EDP is a little higher on the left side than on the right, because the left ventricle wall is thicker and needs a higher pressure to distend it. Since pressures are higher in the left atrium than right atrium, congenital defects in the atrial septum in neonates usually result in a left-to-right flow of blood. Such defects do not, therefore, deoxygenate the arterial blood or cause 'blue baby' syndrome.

Isovolumetric contraction

Duration:	0.05 s
Inlet valves:	closed
Outlet valves:	closed

The atrial boost is followed by ventricular systole. It lasts 0.35 s and is divided into a brief isovolumetric

phase and a longer ejection phase. As soon as the ventricular pressure rises just above atrial pressure, the atrioventricular valves are closed by the reversed pressure gradient. Backflow during closure is minimal because the cusps are already approximated in the late filling phase by vortices behind them (Figure 2.4, top). Since the ventricle is now a closed chamber, the tensing wall causes a steep rise in the pressure of the trapped blood. Indeed, the maximum rate of rise of pressure, dP/dt_{max}, is often used as an index of cardiac contractility (Figure 2.5).

Ejection

Duration:	0.3 s
Inlet valves:	closed
Outlet valves:	open

When ventricular pressure exceeds arterial pressure, the outflow valves are forced open and ejection begins. Three-quarters of the stroke volume is ejected in the first half of the ejection phase, the **phase of rapid ejection** (~0.15 s). Since the blood is ejected faster than it can drain away through the peripheral vessels, most of the stroke volume is accommodated temporarily by distension of the elastic arteries. The tension in the walls of the elastic arteries drives the pressure up to its maximum or 'systolic' level.

Vortices behind the cusps of the open aortic valve prevent them from blocking the adjacent entrances to the coronary arteries; the valve leaflets 'float' between midstream and the aortic wall. The vortices are caused by the outpouchings of the aortic wall, the **sinuses of Valsalva** (Figure 1.4).

As systole weakens, the rate of ejection slows down, as shown by the aortic velocity trace in Figure 2.5. The rate at which aortic blood flows away through the peripheral circulation now exceeds ejection by the ventricle, so pressure begins to fall. Although the ventricular pressure falls 2–3 mmHg below arterial pressure (Figure 2.5, top trace), the outward momentum of the blood prevents immediate closure of the aortic valve. The reversed pressure gradient progressively decelerates the outflow (Figure 2.5, velocity curve) until finally a brief backflow closes the outflow valve. Backflow is normally less than 5% of the stroke volume, though this figure increases greatly if the aortic valve is leaky (aortic incompetence). Valve closure creates a notch in the arterial pressure trace called the **incisura** or dicrotic notch. For the rest of the cycle, arterial pressure gradually declines as blood runs away into the periphery.

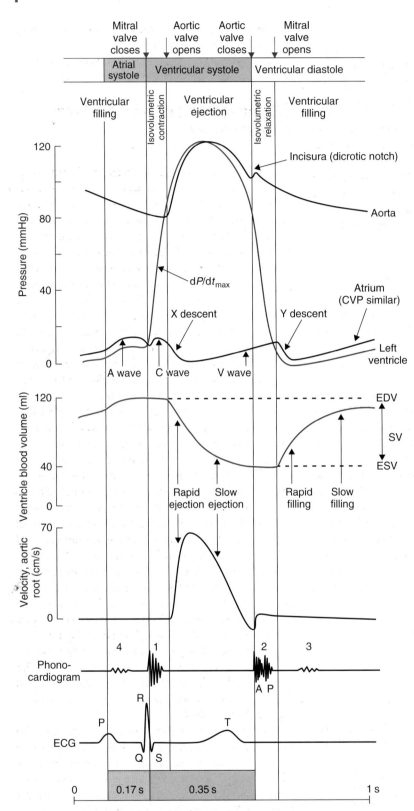

Figure 2.5 Changes in pressure, volume and flow in aorta, left ventricle and left atrium during human cardiac cycle. Right side (not shown) has similar patterns but lower pressures. **Jugular venous wave-form** in neck is like the left atrial waveform shown here. EDV, end-diastolic volume; ESV, end-systolic volume; SV, stroke volume. Second heart sound splits into aortic (A) and pulmonary (P) components. (After Noble, M. I. M. (1968) *Circulation Research*, **23**, 663–670.)

Only about two-thirds of the ventricular blood is ejected at rest. The ejected volume, or **stroke volume**, is 70–80 ml and the residual **end-systolic volume** is ~50 ml. The average **ejection fraction** at rest,

namely stroke volume/end–diastolic volume, is 0.67. The end-systolic volume serves as a reserve that can be used to increase the stroke volume in exercise. In other words, the ejection fraction increases in exercise.

Isovolumetric relaxation

Duration:	0.08 s
Inlet valves:	closed
Outlet valves:	closed

With closure of the aortic and pulmonary valves each ventricle is again a closed chamber. Ventricular pressure falls rapidly due to the elastic recoil of the deformed myocardium. When ventricular pressure has fallen just below atrial pressure, the atrio-ventricular valves open and blood floods in from the atria, which have been refilling during ventricular systole.

The ventricular pressure–volume loop

A plot of ventricular blood pressure versus volume forms a closed loop (Figure 2.6). This is a useful way of representing the ventricular cycle because it combines the volume and pressure traces of Figure 2.5 in one figure. Starting with the opening of the mitral valve at the bottom left corner of the loop, the bottom line represents ventricular filling. In the initial phase of rapid filling the pressure is falling due to the suction exerted by the elastic recoil of the ventricle. In the later, slow-filling phase (diastasis), the line coincides with the passive pressure–volume relation of the relaxed ventricle, the **compliance curve**.

With the onset of systole, the mitral valve closes (lower right corner) and isovolumetric contraction raises the ventricular pressure (vertical line). When ventricular pressure reaches diastolic blood pressure, the aortic valve opens (upper right corner). Volume then decreases as ejection occurs (top line). As the systole weakens, the aortic valve closes (upper left corner)

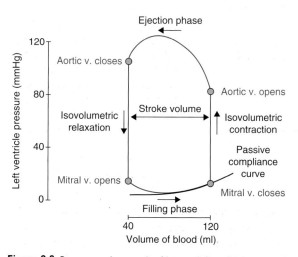

Figure 2.6 Pressure–volume cycle of human left ventricle.

and isovolumetric relaxation leads to mitral opening and refilling of the ventricle.

The atria refill with blood during ventricular systole, so we must consider next the atrial cycle.

2.3 The atrial cycle and central venous pressure waves

The atrial cycle produces a characteristic pattern of pressure changes in the jugular veins of the neck, because the neck veins are in open communication with the right atrium. The pattern is readily seen in a recumbent human and is inspected during routine clinical assessment. A direct recording of pressure in the atrium or jugular vein reveals two main pressure waves per cycle, the A and V waves, and a third smaller wave, the C wave (Figures 2.5, 8.20, 8.24). There are also two sharp falls in pressure called the X and Y descents.

The **A wave** is an increase in pressure caused by atrial systole; 'A' is for atrial. Atrial systole produces a slight reflux of blood through the valveless venous entrance, which briefly reverses the flow in the venae cavae and raises central venous pressure to its maximum point in the cycle, typically 3–5 mmHg. The backflow is slight, despite the absence of valves, because the returning venous blood has considerable inertia.

The next event, the **C wave**, occurs first in the atria and then in the neck. In the atria it is caused by the tricuspid and mitral valve cusps bulging back into the chamber as the valve closes. In the internal jugular vein, the C wave is caused partly by expansion of the carotid artery, which lies alongside the vein and presses on it during systole; 'C' stands for 'carotid'.

After the C wave comes a sharp fall in pressure, the **X descent**. The fall is caused by atrial relaxation and by a movement of the base of the ventricle as the ventricle ejects blood. Venous return into the atria reaches its peak velocity during this phase (Figure 8.24).

As the atria fill, atrial pressure rises, producing the **V wave**. 'V' refers to the concomittant ventricular systole. Finally, the atrioventricular valves open and the atria empty rapidly into the ventricles, producing the sharp **Y descent**.

The right atrial pressure cycle is mirrored in the internal and external jugular veins of the neck because there are no intervening valves. This enables the physician to assess the central venous pressure cycle simply by inspecting the neck of a recumbent subject (Figure 8.20). What the eye particularly notices are two sudden venous collapses, corresponding to the X and Y descents. Certain cardiac diseases produce characteristic abnormalities of the jugular venous pulse. **Tricuspid incompetence**, for example, produces exaggerated V waves in the neck, because ventricular systole forces blood back through the leaky valve into the right atrium and neck veins.

2.4 Altered phase durations as heart rate increases

The above timings refer to a resting human. When the heart is beating at 180 per min, close to the physiological maximum, all phases of the cycle have to be shortened because the entire cycle lasts only one-third of a second. The various phases do not, however, all shorten to an equal degree (Figure 2.7). Ventricular systole shortens moderately, to ~0.2 s. This leaves a mere 0.13 s for diastolic refilling. Passive filling remains important but atrial systole contributes relatively more than at rest. Even so, 0.13 s is close to the minimum interval that allows an adequate refilling of the human ventricle. Further increases in heart rate, such as the **pathological tachycardia** of Wolff–Parkinson–White syndrome (>250 beats/min), actually cause the cardiac output to decline because the diastolic interval is too short to refill the ventricle adequately. Diastolic interval is the chief factor limiting the maximum useful heart rate.

2.5 Heart sounds and valve abnormalities

The heart sounds are of great value to clinicians in assessing valve function.

The normal heart sounds

When a heart valve closes, the cusps balloon back as they check the momentum of refluxing blood. The sudden tensing of the cusps sets up a brief vibration, rather as a sail slaps audibly when suddenly filled by a gust of wind. The vibration is transmitted through the tissues to the chest wall and can be heard through a stethoscope. Provided that the valve is normal, only closure is audible. Opening is silent, as with a well-oiled door.

Two heart sounds are easily heard per beat, the first and second heart sounds. They are usually represented as lubb-dupp followed by a pause, roughly in waltz time; the first heart sound (lubb) is the one immediately after the pause. (Lubb-dupp should not be taken too seriously, for only English-speaking hearts go lubb-dupp. German ones go duhp-teup, and Turkish ones rrup-ta!) The heart sounds can be recorded by a microphone placed on the precordium, and a tracing of the sound is called a phonocardiogram (Figure 2.5). The **first heart sound** is a vibration of roughly

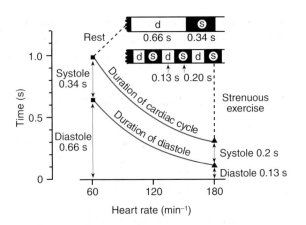

Figure 2.7 Effect of heart rate on the diastolic period available for filling. d, diastole; s, systole. Diastole is curtailed more than systole as heart rate increases. (Courtesy of Professor Horst Seller.)

100 cycles/s (100 Hz) caused by near-simultaneous closure of the tricuspid and mitral valves. The **second heart sound**, of similar frequency, is caused by closure of the aortic and pulmonary valves.

The second sound is sometimes audibly split into an initial aortic component and a fractionally delayed pulmonary component (**splitting of the second sound**). The first and split second sounds then sound like 'lubb-terrupp'. Splitting is best heard during inspiration due to two effects: (i) inspiration increases the filling of the right ventricle, which prolongs the right ventricular ejection time and delays pulmonary valve closure; (ii) inspiration also expands the lung's blood vessels and therefore transiently reduces the venous return to the left ventricle. This reduces the left ventricular stroke volume, shortens the left ventricle ejection time and hastens closure of the aortic valve. Splitting of the second sound is thus caused by equal and opposite movements of the aortic and pulmonary components.

Two additional sounds besides the first and second sounds can be detected by phonocardiography, but they are of low frequency and difficult for untrained ears to detect. The **third heart sound** is common in young people and is caused by the rush of blood into the relaxing ventricles during early diastole. The **fourth sound** occurs just before the first sound and is caused by atrial systole.

Each valve has a separate auscultation (listening) area

All four heart valves lie very close together under the sternum (Figure 2.2). Fortunately, each valve is best heard over a distinct, well separated auscultation area located over the chamber fed by the valve. The **mitral valve** is best heard in the mid-clavicular line of the fourth-fifth left intercostal space; the **tricuspid**

valve in the fifth interspace at the left sternal edge; the **aortic valve** in the second interspace at the right sternal edge; and the **pulmonary valve** in the second interspace at the left sternal edge.

Valve abnormalities cause murmurs

Valve abnormalities fall into two classes – incompetence and stenosis. **Incompetence** is a failure of the valve to seal properly, allowing blood to regurgitate through the valve. **Stenosis** is a narrowing of the open valve, as a result of which a high pressure-gradient is needed to drive blood through the valve (Figure 2.8).

In **aortic valve stenosis** the ventricular systolic pressure is increased. This raises the work of the ventricle. At the same time the aortic pressure, which feeds the coronary arteries, is reduced. The combination of increased ventricular work and reduced coronary O_2 supply can cause angina on exercise; angina is cardiac pain due to O_2 demand exceeding supply. Case 5 at the end of this book describes such a patient.

In both incompetence and stenosis the blood passes through the abnormal valve as a turbulent jet. This sets up a high-frequency vibration which is heard as a **murmur** through the stethoscope. Since there are four valves and two pathologies, there are eight basic valve murmurs. In **mitral incompetence**, for example, ventricular systole causes blood to regurgitate into the left atrium. This creates a murmur that extends throughout systole (pansystolic) and is loudest over the mitral area (Figure 2.8). The sound may be represented roughly as 'lu-shshshsh-tupp'. By contrast, **aortic valve stenosis** produces a systolic ejection murmur that rises and falls as ejection waxes and wanes (a crescendo–decrescendo murmur) and is loudest over the aortic area. **Aortic incompetence** produces an early diastolic murmur (Figure 2.8). Additional noises (clicks and snaps) can also develop.

Murmurs can have other causes than valve disease. Hypochondriac readers should note that a **benign systolic murmur** is common in the young. It is caused by turbulence in the ventricular outflow tract. Benign systolic murmurs are common during pregnancy, strenuous exercise and anaemia (Section 8.2). Ventricular septal defects too can cause murmurs.

2.6 Clinical assessment of the cardiac cycle

The cardiac cycle is assessed at the bedside by examining five of the physical signs described above, namely:

- the peripheral pulse (to assess heart rate and force)
- the systolic and diastolic arterial blood pressure

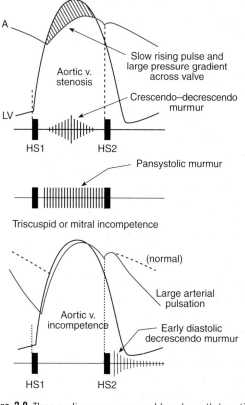

Figure 2.8 Three cardiac murmurs caused by valve pathology. (*Top*) Aortic valve stenosis creates a large pressure gradient between aorta (A) and left ventricle (LV) during ejection (hatched zone), causing a slow-rising arterial pulse and crescendo–decrescendo ejection murmur. (*Middle*) In tricuspid or mitral incompetence, regurgitation from ventricle to atrium in systole creates a pansystolic murmur. (*Bottom*) In aortic valve incompetence, diastolic leakage from aorta to ventricle causes a characteristic wide pulse pressure (systolic minus diastolic) and early diastolic, decrescendo murmur as the pressure head decays. Axes as in Figure 2.5. Duration of systole exaggerated for clarity.

- the jugular venous pulse
- the apex beat
- the heart sounds.

If pathology is suspected, more specialised investigations may be undertaken, as follows.

Electrocardiography

The electrocardiogram (ECG) is a recording of cardiac electrical events from the body surface. The ECG is covered in Chapter 5, so here we will simply note its relation to the key events of the cardiac cycle (Figure 2.5). The **P wave** is produced by electrical activation of the atria and marks the onset of atrial contraction. The **QRS complex** is produced by electrical activation of the ventricles, so it is followed almost immediately by the onset of ventricular contraction and the first heart sound. The **T wave** is produced by electrical recharging of the ventricles, and since this marks the onset of diastole it is closely followed by the second heart sound.

Echocardiography

Echocardiography is a non-invasive tool for observing the motion of the walls and valves of the human heart. A beam of ultra-high frequency sound is directed across the heart from a precordial emitter, namely a piezoelectric crystal emitting 1000 brief pulses per second. Reflections of the sound from the heart walls and valve cusps are collected during millisecond 'listening' intervals between each microsecond pulse. The reflected sound is processed to build up a picture of cardiac structure and motion.

In **M-mode** (motion mode) the changing position of anatomical structures in the sound beam is plotted against time. This gives a linear display of the motion of the heart walls and valve leaflets; see Figures 2.9 and 6.24.

In **2-D mode** (2-dimensional mode) an anatomical image of a slice through the heart is displayed at successive instants in time. This gives a moving image of the valve leaflets and heart wall and reveals valve lesions, abnormal wall motion due to infarction, and hypertrophic cardiomyopathy (pathological wall thickening). The systolic change in left ventricular dimension is used as a measure of the ejection fraction and hence cardiac contractility (Table 2.2).

During echocardiography, the frequency of the reflected ultrasound is altered by the moving blood cells. This **Doppler shift** is used to construct a colour-coded map of local blood flow in the chamber and around valves. In this way a non-invasive, semi-quantitative estimate can be made of regurgitation across a leaky valve.

Cardiac catheterization

This is a powerful but invasive investigation. Under local anaesthesia a fine catheter is threaded through the antecubital vein in the crook of the elbow and advanced under X-ray guidance through the right atrium into the right ventricle or pulmonary artery. The aorta, coronary arteries and left ventricle can be reached by a catheter introduced through the femoral artery. An intracardiac catheter can be used as follows.

Cine-angiography

A radio-opaque contrast medium is injected through the catheter and the progress of the medium through the cardiac chambers is followed by X-ray

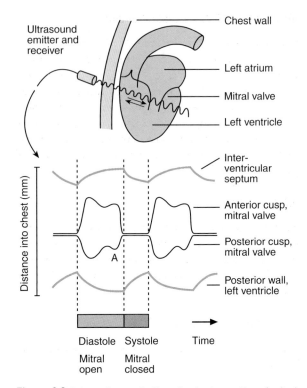

Figure 2.9 Echocardiogram in M-mode showing motion of mitral valve cusps and walls of the left ventricle. Note phases of fast filling in early ventricular diastole and fast shortening in early systole. Atrial systole (A) increases cusp separation in late ventricular diastole.

Table 2.2 Echocardiography results for a normal human left ventricle.

Wall or septum thickness	0.7–1.1 cm
End-diastolic internal diameter	3.5–5.6 cm
End-systolic internal diameter	1.9–4.0 cm
Ejection fraction (from cubed diameter change)	62–85%
Aortic valve orifice	1.6–2.6 cm

Data from Swanton, R. H. (1998) *Cardiology*, Blackwell Science, Oxford.

cinematography (cardiac angiography). This displays the movement of the heart wall and reveals any valvular regurgitation. It also reveals atheromatous obstructions in the coronary arteries.

Radionuclide angiography

The gamma-ray emitting isotope technetium is injected into a central vein. The gamma emission from the heart is then recorded by a scintillation camera over the precordium. Images of the heart in diastole and systole are computed, and the ejection fraction is calculated from the fall in counts per ejection.

Intracardiac pressure measurement

Chamber pressures can be recorded through an external pressure transducer or by mounting a miniature transducer in the catheter tip. The pressure drop across a closed valve is used to test valvular competence. Elevated pressure gradients across open valves, as in Figure 2.8 top, indicate stenosis. A pulmonary artery catheter can be wedged in the pulmonary arterioles and the wedge pressure taken as an estimate of pulmonary capillary pressure.

Intracardiac pacing

This is a therapeutic rather than diagnostic application. A wire catheter is wedged in the ventricle and used to stimulate each heart beat from an external electrical device, thereby replacing the heart's own pacemaker.

Measurement of cardiac output

This use of cardiac catheters is described in Section 7.2.

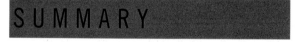

SUMMARY

◼ The four muscular chambers of the mammalian heart are built upon a fibrotendinous ring. The ring has four apertures, each occupied by a valve. The ring isolates the atria electrically from the ventricles.

◼ The ventricular cycle comprises four phases of unequal duration, with the right and left sides essentially in synchrony.

◼ In the **filling phase** the ventricle is in diastole. The arterial outlet valves (aortic and pulmonary) are closed. The atrio-ventricular inlet valves (tricuspid and mitral) are open. Initial rapid, passive filling is aided by elastic recoil. Filling then slows (diastasis). Late filling is boosted by **atrial systole**, especially in exercise and the elderly.

◼ In the **isovolumetric contraction phase** the onset of ventricular systole raises ventricular pressure, which closes the atrio-ventricular valves and creates the **first heart sound**. Pressure in the closed chamber then rises rapidly. The phase is quickly terminated by opening of the arterial outlet valves and onset of the **ejection phase**. Two-thirds of the ventricular blood (the **ejection fraction**) is expelled at rest.

◼ As the ejection rate wanes, pressures fall until the outlet valves are closed by a slight back-flow. The attendant **second heart sound** is split during inspiration. In the **isovolumetric relaxation phase** ventricular pressure falls rapidly until below atrial pressure. The atrio-ventricular valves then open and rapid filling begins.

◼ The ventricular **pressure–volume loop** depicts the cycle as, approximately, a rectangle. Each corner represents a valve action and each side a phase.

◼ The right atrial cycle is reflected in the jugular veins, which can be inspected in the neck. The **A wave** (atrial systole) and **C wave** (closure of tricuspid valve) are followed by the **X descent** (atrial diastole). Pressure rises again due to continuing venous return (**V wave**), then falls as the opening tricuspid valve dumps the atrial contents into the ventricle (**Y descent**).

◼ Ventricular diastole occupies two-thirds of the cycle at rest but only one-third at high heart rates. The restricted diastolic time for refill limits the maximum useful heart rate to 180–200 beats/min in man.

◼ Abnormalities of the human cardiac cycle can be detected by inspection of the jugular venous pulse, measurement of arterial blood pressure, palpation of the apex beat and auscultation of the heart sounds. **Murmurs** are caused by valve stenosis or incompetence. Special investigations include electrocardiography, echocardiography, radionuclide angiography and diagnostic cardiac catheterization.

FURTHER READING

Benavidez, O., Goldblatt, A. and Lilly, L. S. (1998) Heart sounds and murmurs. In *Pathophysiology of Heart Disease* (ed. Lilly, L. S.), Williams and Wilkins, Baltimore, pp. 25–38.

Horesh, S., Pendse, S. and Come, P. C. (1998) Diagnostic imaging and catheterisation techniques. In *Pathophysiology of Heart Disease* (ed. Lilly, L. S.), Williams and Wilkins, Baltimore, pp. 39–64.

Nishikawa, Y., Roberts, J. P., Tan, P., Klopfenstein, C. E. and Klopfenstein, H. S. (1994) Effect of dynamic exercise on left atrial function in conscious dogs. *Journal of Physiology*, **481**, 457–468.

Udelson, J. E., Bacharach, S. L., Cannon, R. O. and Bonow, R. O. (1990) Minimum left ventricular pressure during beta-adrenergic stimulation in human subjects: evidence of elastic recoil and diastolic 'suction' in the normal heart. *Circulation*, **82**, 1174–1182.

CHAPTER 3

The cardiac myocyte: excitation and contraction

Learning objectives

After reading this chapter you should be able to:

- State the key ultrastructural features and functions of the sarcomere, sarcoplasmic reticulum, transverse tubules and gap junctions (3.1).
- Explain how actin–myosin interaction produces shortening/tension and the role of Ca^{2+} in this process (3.2).
- Sketch a ventricular action potential, labelling the resting potential, depolarization, plateau and repolarization (3.3).
- Outline the ions and channels responsible for the above features (3.3, 3.5).
- State the link between the plateau and contractility (3.6).
- Describe the myocyte Ca^{2+} cycle and identify what governs the size of the SR store (3.7).
- State the effect of diastolic length on contractile force (3.8).
- Outline the effect of the following agents on contractile force: catecholamines; calcium channel blockers; phosphodiesterase inhibitors; digoxin (3.7, 3.8).
- Draw and explain a delayed afterdepolarization (3.9).

Overview. The heart beat is initiated by an electrical system within the heart wall called the pacemaker–conduction system, which is composed of modified muscle, not nervous tissue. An electrical discharge is initiated by the pacemaker and is conducted from cell to cell by currents flowing through local circuits. When the electrical discharge reaches the muscle fibres that form the bulk of the heart, each fibre is excited and fires an action potential. The action potential initiates a rise in intracellular calcium ion concentration, which activates the contractile machinery of the cell.

Cardiac muscle fibres thus fall into two categories. The majority do mechanical, contractile work and are simply called cardiac **myocytes**. Such myocytes will not contract until they are stimulated electrically by the pacemaker–conduction system. This chapter describes the properties of the 'workhorse' cells, the myocytes, and Chapter 4 describes the pacemaker–conduction system.

3.1 Ultrastructure

The human myocyte is $10-20\,\mu m$ in diameter by $50-100\,\mu m$ long. The cell is sometimes branched and possesses a single, central nucleus.

Junctions provide mechanical and electrical connectivity

Adjacent myocytes are attached end-to-end by a stepped junction, the intercalated disc. Within the intercalated disc there are two classes of junction, the gap junction and the desmosome (Figure 3.1).

The **gap junction** or nexus is oddly named in that the adjacent myocyte membranes actually approach each other very closely, to $2-4\,nm$. Gap junctions are crucially important because they transmit ionic currents and thus electrical excitation from one myocyte to the next. A gap junction is built up from the protein connexin. Six connexin subunits unite to form a hollow tube or 'connexon'. The connexon spans the narrow intercellular gap and opens into the cytoplasm on either side. Since ions can flow through the connexon from cell to cell, **the myocardium behaves as an electrically continuous sheet**. This is crucially important, because it ensures that myocytes throughout the ventricle wall are activated almost simultaneously. When coronary artery disease causes myocardial ischaemia, the rise in intracellular acidity and Ca^{2+} causes closure of some connexons, leading to poor electrical coupling.

Desmosomes serve to rivet the cells together, and consist of plaques of cadherin molecules. Cadherin is a transmembrane glycoprotein that spans the $25\,nm$ wide space between the adjacent myocyte membranes. Cytoskeletal filaments are anchored internally to the desmosomes and run the through the myocyte, giving it tensile strength.

The fundamental contractile unit is called a sarcomere

The myocyte is packed with long contractile bundles of diameter $\sim 1\,\mu m$ called myofibrils. Each myofibril

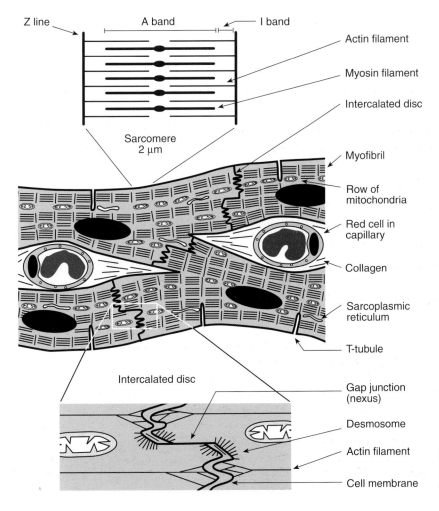

Z line

A band

I band

Actin filament

Myosin filament

Intercalated disc

Sarcomere
2 μm

Myofibril

Row of mitochondria

Red cell in capillary

Collagen

Sarcoplasmic reticulum

T-tubule

Gap junction (nexus)

Desmosome

Intercalated disc

Actin filament

Cell membrane

Figure 3.1 Schematic section of myocardium parallel to fibre axis, based on electron micrographs.

is composed of units called sarcomeres joined end to end. Sarcomeres are aligned in register across the cell, giving the myocyte its characteristic stripy appearance.

The sarcomere is the basic contractile unit. It is 1.8–2.0 μm long at rest and comprises a set of filamentous proteins between two Z lines. The **Z line** is a thin partition formed by the protein α-actinin. Between the Z lines there are two kinds of filament – thick filaments made of the protein myosin, and thin filaments composed primarily of the protein actin.

The **thick**, **myosin filaments**, of diameter 11 nm and length 1.6 μm, lie in parallel in the centre of the sarcomere. This region is called the A band due to its anisotropic appearance under polarized light.

Interposed between the thick filaments lie the **thin actin filaments**, of diameter 6 nm and length 1.05 μm. One end of the thin filament is free in the A band and the other is rooted in the Z line, forming the pale I band (isotropic band). The I band is only ~0.25 μm wide because most of the thin filament protrudes into the spaces between the myosin rods in the A band. In other words, the actin and myosin filaments interdigitate. The thin filament is made of F-actin (filamentous actin), which is a polymer of globular actin subunits (G-actin) arranged like beads on a string. The thin filament consists of two such strings arranged as a two-stranded helix (Figure 3.3). The groove of the double helix contains the regulatory proteins **troponin** and **tropomyosin**, which are involved in the initiation of contraction.

The cell also contains non-contractile cytoskeletal filaments of **titin** which contribute to the mechanical stiffness and elasticity of the heart wall.

A transverse tubular system carries excitation into the interior

The surface membrane, or sarcolemma, is invaginated opposite each Z line into a set of fine transverse tubules (T-tubules) that run into the cell interior (Figure 3.2). The T-tubules transmit the electrical stimulus rapidly into the interior of the cell and thus help to activate the numerous myofibrils almost simultaneously. T-tubules are well developed in ventricular myocytes but are scanty in atrial and Purkinje cells.

Sarcoplasmic reticulum holds a store of releasable Ca^{2+}

Within the myocyte cytoplasm, or sarcoplasm, there is a second system of tubular structures called the sarcoplasmic reticulum (SR), which is derived from endoplasmic reticulum. The SR is a closed set of anastomosing tubes that course over the myofibrils and in places pass very close to the T-tubules and the sarcolemmal surface. SR is of major importance because it contains a store of Ca^{2+} ions, which is partially released into the sarcoplasm upon electrical excitation of the cell, leading to contraction. The

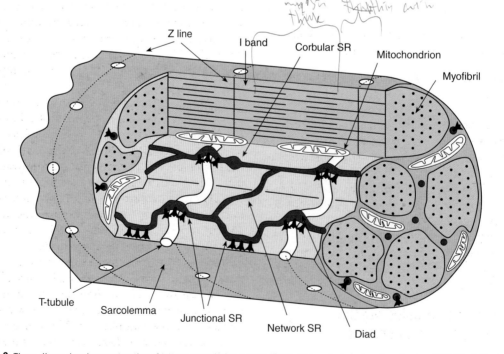

Figure 3.2 Three-dimensional reconstruction of transverse tubular system (T-tubules) and sarcoplasmic reticulum (SR). The latter is ~5% of the cell volume. The black 'feet' are Ca^{2+}-release channels or ryanodine receptors.

SR has three distinct regions (Figure 3.2) with different roles in Ca^{2+} handling, as follows.

Junctional SR approaches to within 15 nm of the sarcolemmal surface or a T-tubule, forming a 'diad' in the latter case. The lumen of the junctional SR contains a store of Ca^{2+} attached loosely to the storage protein calsequestrin. Tiny feet extend from the junctional SR towards the sarcolemma. Each foot is actually a gigantic protein called a **Ca^{2+} release channel**. The channels are also called **ryanodine receptors** because they bind the drug ryanodine, and **CICR channels** (calcium-induced calcium release channels) because they are activated by subsarcolemmal Ca^{2+}.

Corbular SR is a set of sac-like expansions of the SR in the I band, of diameter 50–100 nm. It too has a high content of Ca^{2+} and calsequestrin.

Network SR is responsible for the uptake of Ca^{2+} from the sarcoplasm. It comprises tubules of diameter 20–60 nm that run over the myofibrils. Unlike junctional SR, network SR has numerous **Ca^{2+}-ATPase pumps**. The pumps are regulated by the inhibitory protein **phospholamban**.

As indicated above, when the myocyte is excited electrically, Ca^{2+} is released from the SR store via the release channels and activates the contractile machinery. This brings us to the question of how the contractile machinery works.

3.2 Mechanism of contraction

The contraction of the heart is brought about by a shortening of each sarcomere, as follows.

Shortening is brought about by sliding filaments

The shortening of a sarcomere is brought about by the **sliding filament mechanism**; the thin filaments slide into the spaces between the thick filaments of the A band. This is evident from the observation that the I band shortens but the A band does not. The filaments are propelled past each other by the repeated making and breaking of biochemical bonds or **crossbridges** between the thin and thick filaments. The crossbridges are actually the heads of myosin molecules, which protrude from the side of the thick filament (Figure 3.3).

Ca^{2+} initiates shortening via the troponin–tropomyosin complex

Each actin subunit has a binding site for a myosin head, but the binding sites are blocked at rest by a

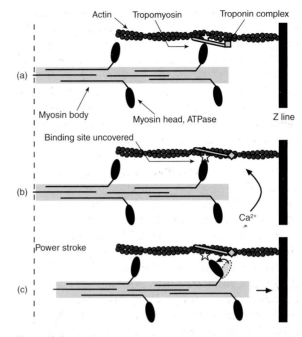

Figure 3.3 Three stages of crossbridge cycle. (a) Rest. Actin binding sites (one is shown as white star) are blocked by tropomyosin. (b) Displacement of troponin–tropomyosin by Ca^{2+} exposes actin binding sites. Myosin head forms a crossbridge. (c) Flexion of myosin head rows the thick filament towards the Z-line. Head then disengages and reattaches further along actin filament. Only one of numerous actin binding sites and four of the 400 myosin heads are shown.

ribbon-like protein, tropomyosin. Tropomyosin is a 42 nm long protein that lies in the groove of the F-actin double helix and overlies seven G-actin subunits. Each tropomyosin has a troponin complex attached to one end, composed of three units. Troponin C is a Ca^{2+}-binding protein; troponin I is inhibitory; and troponin T binds the complex to tropomyosin.

Exposure of the binding sites on actin is brought about by a sudden rise in the concentration of free Ca^{2+} in the sarcoplasm, due to Ca^{2+} release of the sarcoplasmic reticulum. Some of this Ca^{2+} binds to the troponin C of the troponin–tropomyosin complex. This causes a change in molecular configuration that shifts the tropomyosin–troponin complex deeper into the F-actin groove and exposes the myosin-binding sites on the actin. The myosin head can now bind to the actin, forming a crossbridge.

Force and movement are generated by a change in the angle of the attached myosin head, which advances the filament by 5–10 nm. After this the head disengages and the process repeats itself at a new actin site further along the thin filament. This process occurs with numerous myosin heads at numerous sites along the filament. Thus the thick filament rows itself into the space between the thin filaments.

The number of crossbridges determines contractile force

In skeletal muscle the sarcoplasmic Ca^{2+} concentration during excitation is so high that the troponin C is saturated and crossbridge formation is maximal. Each twitch of a single skeletal fibre therefore occurs at full power. In cardiac muscle this is not usually the case. The Ca^{2+} concentration is only sufficient to activate a fraction of the potential crossbridge sites, producing a **submaximal contraction**, typically ~40% maximal. As a result, anything that increases the amount of intracellular Ca^{2+}, such as adrenaline, will activate more crossbridges and cause the heart to beat more forcefully. In cardiac muscle **the force of the contraction is proportional to the number of crossbridges formed, and therefore to the sarcoplasmic Ca^{2+} concentration**.

ATP energizes the myosin head

The energy for contraction is provided by adenosine triphosphate (ATP). ATP binds to an ATPase site on the myosin head at the end of stage (c) of Figure 3.3. Energy is released immediately by hydrolysis to adenosine diphosphate (ADP) and inorganic phosphate. The energy immediately activates or energizes the myosin head by cocking it back into the high energy 'firing' angle shown in stage (a) of Figure 3.3. 'Firing', i.e. the power stroke in the sequence (b)–(c), is powered by the energy inherent in the cocked head.

Contractile performance is tightly linked to O_2 supply

Every cycle of crossbridge formation/detachment breaks down one ATP molecule, so a constant supply of ATP is necessary. To this end the myocyte has an exceptionally high mitochondrial density. The mitochondria lie in rows between the myofibrils and form 30–35% of the cell volume. ATP is manufactured in the mitochondria by oxidative phosphorylation, for which O_2 is obligatory. Cardiac performance is therefore heavily dependent on the supply of O_2 by the coronary arteries. The partial pressure of oxygen in the myocyte (P_{O_2}) is 5–20 mmHg. This establishes a large oxygen gradient from blood (P_{O_2} 100 mmHg) to cell to drive the diffusional process.

The sarcoplasm contains about 3.4 g/l **myoglobin**, an O_2-binding protein. The myoglobin provides a small reserve of O_2, being ~50% saturated at a P_{O_2} of 5 mmHg. It also facilitates the rapid diffusional transport of O_2 through the sarcoplasm.

The release of the SR Ca^{2+} store to activate the contractile machinery is triggered by an action potential, so we must consider next the electrical potentials in a myocyte.

3.3 Resting membrane potential

The potential difference between the interior and exterior of a myocyte can be measured by driving a fine microelectrode into the sarcoplasm. A **microelectrode** is a glass tube that has been heated, drawn out to a very fine point, filled with a conducting solution, and connected to an amplifier and voltmeter. The other lead of the voltmeter is connected to an extracellular electrode.

The **intracellular potential** at rest is −80 mV to −90 mV, that is to say, 80–90 mV below the potential of the extracellular fluid. In atrial and ventricular cells the resting potential remains stable until an external excitation reaches the cell (Figure 3.4a). In the pacemaker and many conduction fibres (Purkinje fibres) the potential is unstable and drifts towards zero with time (Figure 3.4b) – a complication that we will defer to Chapter 4.

The resting potential is generated by differences in ion concentration across the cell membrane, coupled with the presence of ion-selective trans-membrane channels. Ion channels have been identified using the **patch clamp method**. A tiny patch of cell membrane is glued to the end of a micropipette so that the electrical current through just a few channels can be recorded (Figure 4.3). The effects of different ions and blocking agents on the patch current allows specific ion channels to be identified. There are three main classes of cation-conducting channel, namely K^+, Na^+ and Ca^{2+} conducting channels, and many subtypes (Table 4.2). Channel selectivity is not absolute. The 'K^+ channel', for example, has a K^+/Na^+ permeability ratio of ~100/1.

Potassium ions generate the resting membrane potential

The resting potential is generated by a high intracellular concentration of potassium ions (140 mM) and the high permeability of the cell membrane to K^+ due to numerous open K^+ channels. The type of K^+ channel that exists in the open state at resting potential is called the inward rectifier channel, and its current is represented by i_{K1}. The Na^+ and Ca^{2+} channels, by contrast, are mostly closed at negative potentials. Since the intracellular concentration of K^+ is ~35 times higher than its extracellular concentration (Table 3.1), K^+ tends to diffuse out of the cell through the open K^+ channels. The negative intracellular ions,

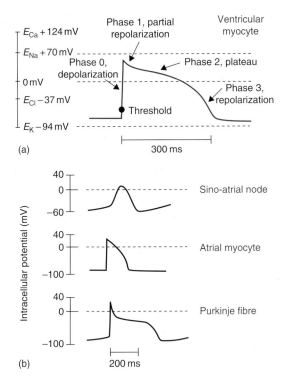

(a)

(b)

Figure 3.4 (a) Intracellular potential in a ventricular endo-cardial myocyte during action potential. Resting potential is −80 mV. Equilibrium potentials of main ions are shown for comparison. (b) Different forms of cardiac action potential. SA node and some Purkinje fibres have unstable resting potentials. The atrial potential is triangular in many species (shown) but spike-and-plateau in *humans*.

Table 3.1 Concentration of ions in myocardial cells.

	Intracellular (mM)	Extracellular (mM)	Nernst equilibrium potential (mV)
K^+	140	4	−94
Na^+	10	140	+70
Ca^{2+}	0.0001*	1.2†	+124
Cl^-	30	120	−37**
pH	7.0–7.1	7.4	–

* Value at rest.

** At −80 mV resting potential, Cl^- channels carry Cl^- efflux. During action potential, e.g. +20 mV, Cl^- channels carry Cl^- influx.

† The total Ca^{2+} concentration in plasma is about double this, but only 1.2 mM is in the ionic form.

mainly organic phosphates and charged proteins, cannot accompany the K^+ because the cell membrane is impermeable to them (Figure 3.5). The outward diffusion of a small number of K^+ ions quickly creates a tiny separation of charge, which leaves the cell interior negative with respect to the exterior. The electrical charge on a single ion is very large (see Faraday's constant, Appendix 2), and just one excess negative intracellular ion per 10^{15} ion pairs is enough to generate the resting potential. This minute imbalance is far too tiny to be detected by chemical analysis.

Nernst's equation predicts the K^+ equilibrium potential

If the intracellular potential were exactly the right magnitude, namely −94 mV, the negative potential attracting K^+ ions into the cell would exactly counterbalance the tendency of intracellular K^+ to diffuse out of the cell down its concentration gradient. There would then be no net movement of K^+ out of the cell. The **electrical potential** at which this would happen is called the potassium equilibrium potential, E_K. This potential is, by definition, equal in magnitude to the outward-driving effect of the concentration gradient, or **chemical potential**. The chemical potential depends on the ion concentration outside (C_o) and inside the cell (C_i). The relation between the equilibrium potential of **any** ionic species X (E_x) and the ionic concentration ratio is given by the **Nernst equation**:

$$E_x = (RT/zF) \log_e(C_o/C_i) \qquad (3.1a)$$

where z is the ionic valency, R is the gas constant (see Appendix 2), T is absolute temperature and F is Faraday's constant. For a monovalent ion at body temperature, namely 310°K, this works out in millivolts, after switching to 'ordinary' logarithms, as:

$$E_x = 61.5 \log_{10}(C_o/C_i) \qquad (3.1b)$$

Since the ratio C_o/C_i for potassium is 1:35, the K^+ equilibrium potential is −94 mV. Microelectrode measurements show that the resting membrane potential is close to E_K but never quite equal to it (Figure 3.6). If the extracellular K^+ concentration increases, as may happen in local ischaemia or renal failure, the resting potential declines, i.e. grows less negative, leading to cardiac arrhythmias. The membrane potential falls in proportion to the logarithm of the extracellular K^+ concentration (Figure 3.6), in agreement with the Nernst equation.

A Na^+ background current creates a non-equilibrium

Figure 3.6 shows that the resting membrane potential is not as big as the K^+ equilibrium potential. This is due to a small inward current of positive ions, mainly

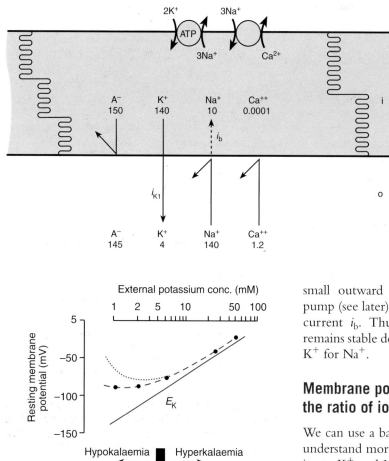

Figure 3.5 Chemical gradients and currents across the resting membrane (i, inside; o, outside). A⁻ inside cell refers to impermeant intracellular anions. Straight arrows show concentration gradients for ions permeating the sarcolemma. Reflected arrows indicate ions unable to penetrate the resting membrane. i_b is the inward background current and i_{K1} the outward background current. Cell membrane pumps are shown at the top.

Figure 3.6 Effect of extracellular K⁺ on resting membrane potential of myocyte (points) or Purkinje fibre (dotted line). Solid line is Nernst equilibrium potential E_K. Deviation from E_K is due to background inward current i_b. Increasing deviation in hypokalaemia is due to a fall in g_K and reduced outward current carried by 3Na⁺–2K⁺ pump. (Adapted from Noble, D. (1979) *The Initiation of the Heart Beat*, Clarendon Press, Oxford.)

Na⁺, referred to as **inward background current**, i_b. Although the permeability of the resting membrane to Na⁺ is only 1/10th to 1/100th of its permeability to K⁺, both the electrical and the chemical gradient for Na⁺ are directed into the cell (Table 3.1). The sum of the two gradients, the **electrochemical gradient**, drives a small inward current of Na⁺ into the cell (Figure 3.5). As a result, the resting potential is typically 10–20 mV more positive than the potassium equilibrium potential.

Since the resting potential is not quite negative enough to counteract fully the outward diffusion of K⁺ ions, there is a continuous trickle of K⁺ out of the cell, creating an **outward background current** i_{K1}. The outward current i_{K1}, along with another

small outward current generated by a Na⁺–K⁺ pump (see later), is equal and opposite to the inward current i_b. Thus the resting membrane potential remains stable despite a continuous slow exchange of K⁺ for Na⁺.

Membrane potential depends on the ratio of ionic permeabilities

We can use a basic law of electricity, Ohm's law, to understand more quantitatively how the permeability to K⁺ and Na⁺ affects the membrane potential. **Ohm's law** states that current i is proportional to potential difference ΔV and electrical conductance g (1/resistance). In other words, $i = g \cdot \Delta V$. The conductance of the cell membrane to a particular ion is proportional to its permeability to that ion (Appendix 2). For K⁺ the potential difference ΔV that drives the outward background current i_{K1} is the difference between the resting membrane potential V_m and the potassium equilibrium potential E_K. Therefore Ohm's law tells us that the potassium current i_{K1} is as follows:

$$i_{K1} = g_K(V_m - E_K) \qquad (3.2)$$

where g_K is the potassium conductance. By similar reasoning the inward background current of sodium ions i_b is given by:

$$i_b = g_{Na}(V_m - E_{Na}) \qquad (3.3)$$

where E_{Na} is the sodium equilibrium potential, about +70 mV. If the resting potential is stable, the inward and outward currents must be equal and opposite, so expressions (3.2) and (3.3) are equal, ignoring other minor currents. Combining the two, we get an expression for the resting potential called **the conductance equation**:

$$V_m = \frac{E_K + E_{Na} \cdot g_{Na}/g_K}{(1 + g_{Na}/g_K)} \qquad (3.4)$$

The conductance equation is a simple form of a more complex expression, the Goldman constant field equation, which deals with chloride currents too (Appendix 2). The conductance equation is ideal for the present purpose because it highlights the importance of **the ratio of sodium to potassium conductances, g_{Na}/g_K**, in determining the membrane potential. The conductance equation tells us that the resting potential is a potassium equilibrium potential ($-94\,mV$) that has been reduced by a fraction of the sodium equilibrium potential ($+70\,mV$). The fraction in question is 1/10th if the ratio of g_{Na} to g_K is 1:10. The conductance equation therefore predicts that the resting potential should be $(-94 + 7)/1.1$, or $-79\,mV$, which is close to the actual value. The conductance equation also tells us that if g_{Na} becomes bigger than g_K, as happens during an action potential, the membrane potential will become positive.

The current–voltage relations of ion channels are often non-linear

One problem in applying Ohm's law to ion channels is that the conductance g of an ion channel, unlike that of a strip of wire, often changes with the potential. Consequently, the current–voltage relation is non-linear. An Ohmic expression such as (3.2) or (3.3) tells us the current at a given conductance and potential but does not tell us the shape of the current–voltage relation. The K^+ channels chiefly responsible for the resting potential, **the inward rectifier K^+ channels**, provide an important example. Their conductance falls when the membrane is depolarized (loses charge), i.e. during the action potential (Figure 3.7). As a result, it is more difficult for K^+ to leak out of the myocyte during the action potential and current i_{K1} is reduced. This is called inward rectification and is important in **conserving the intracellular K^+ during the long cardiac action potential**.

3.4 Role of pumps and exchangers

A Na$^+$–K$^+$ pump preserves the intracellular ion levels

The myocyte is a chemical battery, and the chemical that powers the battery, K^+, slowly but continuously

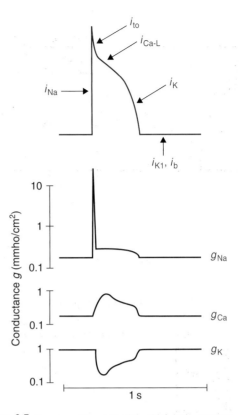

Figure 3.7 Myocyte action potential, chief ionic currents, and membrane conductance to Na^+, Ca^{2+} and K^+ (dissection of total membrane conductance of Figure 3.8). (Based on Noble, D. (1984) The surprising heart. *Journal of Physiology*, **353**, 1–50.)

leaks out of the cell. Unchecked, the concentrations of both K^+ and Na^+ would eventually equilibrate across the cell membrane, leaving the battery flat. This is prevented by active pumps in the sarcolemmal membrane, whose function is to preserve the chemical composition of the interior.

A sodium–potassium pump simultaneously transports Na^+ ions out of the cell and K^+ ions into the cell (Figure 3.5). The pumping rate is increased by a rise in intracellular Na^+ or extracellular K^+ concentration. Pumping is an active process and consumes metabolic energy in the form of ATP. The pump itself is an ATPase.

Three Na^+ ions are pumped out of the cell for every two K^+ ions pumped in. The pump therefore generates a net flow of positive charge out of the cell and is said to be electrogenic. The contribution to the resting potential is trivial, however, as shown by blocking the pump with ouabain. Ouabain reduces the membrane potential by only $2–4\,mV$.

A **Na$^+$–H$^+$ exchanger** regulates intracellular pH by transporting protons out of the cell, in exchange for a flow of Na^+ into the cell down the gradient set up by the Na^+/K^+ pump. The Na^+–H$^+$ exchanger is of major significance in ischaemia (Section 3.9 and Figure 6.22).

Calcium transporters regulate diastolic Ca²⁺ and stored Ca²⁺

The myocyte expels intracellular Ca^{2+} ions that enter the cell during the course of an action potential (see below). The predominant Ca^{2+} transporter in the surface membrane, or sarcolemma, is the **sodium–calcium exchanger**. This transmembrane protein allows three extracellular Na^+ ions to enter the cell in exchange for the expulsion of one intracellular Ca^{2+} ion (Figure 3.5). The entry of the excess Na^+ ion creates a small inward current. The $3Na^+$–Ca^{2+} exchanger is not powered by ATP but is driven by the downhill Na^+ concentration gradient, rather as a water-wheel is turned by a water gradient. Calcium expulsion thus depends indirectly on the active Na^+–K^+ pump, which maintains the Na^+ gradient. This point is important for understanding the action of the cardiac drug digoxin (Section 3.7). Sodium–calcium exchangers account for around three-quarters of Ca^{2+} expulsion from myocytes and are particularly abundant in the sarcolemma adjacent to the junctional SR.

The sarcolemma also has a relatively small number of ATP-powered **calcium pumps**, which account for about a quarter of the Ca^{2+} expulsion. Calcium pumps are very abundant, however, in the network SR, where they are of major importance in building up the internal store of Ca^{2+}. Together the active and passive Ca^{2+} transporters reduce the cytosolic Ca^{2+} concentration to an extremely low level in the resting myocyte, namely 10^{-7} M (0.1 μM).

3.5 Cardiac action potentials

The cardiac action potential has five phases

An action potential is an abrupt reversal of the membrane potential to a positive value (Figure 3.8). It is initiated by an action potential in the pacemaker–conduction system or an adjacent myocyte. The triggering action potential draws charge from the resting membrane by a process described later (Section 4.3), reducing the negative resting potential. When the potential reaches a **threshold** of −60 mV to −65 mV, the sarcolemmal conductance to Na^+ suddenly increases (Figure 3.8, middle trace). A sudden inward pulse of Na^+ ions (Figure 3.8, bottom trace)

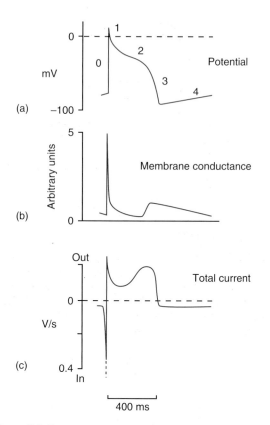

Figure 3.8 Changes in net electrical conductance of the myocyte cell membrane (b) during an action potential (a). This is a Purkinje cell with an unstable resting potential. (c) Net electrical current, with inward current directed downwards. (Wiedmann's seminal observation of 1956, redrawn from Noble, D. (1979) *The Initiation of the Heartbeat*, Clarendon Press, Oxford, by permission.)

causes the cell to **depolarize** extremely quickly and flip to a positive potential of +20 mV to +30 mV. This is called the **overshoot** (top trace; phase 0).

In human ventricular epicardial myocytes, atrial myocytes and Purkinje fibres, the membrane immediately begins to repolarize (phase 1), as a result of which the action potential has a spike-and-plateau shape. The early repolarization is only partial, however. When the membrane potential reaches 0 to −20 mV, it becomes relatively stable for a long period, 200–400 ms. This is called the **plateau** (phase 2). Due to the plateau the cardiac action potential lasts around a hundred times longer than in a nerve or skeletal muscle (1–4 ms). Endocardial myocytes lack a marked phase 1, so their action potential is more rectangular (Figure 3.4a). Finally the membrane **repolarizes** (phase 3), though at only 1/1000th of the rate of depolarization. Phase 4 is the resting potential.

The **shape** of the cardiac action potential differs according to site and species (Figures 3.4, 3.7–3.10). Atrial potentials last only 150 ms and are triangular

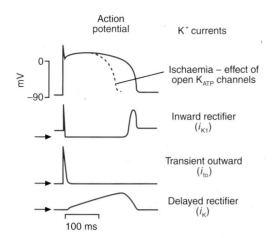

Figure 3.9 K^+ currents responsible for repolarization. Arrows indicate zero. In acutely ischaemic myocytes (dashed line) the increased open probability of K_{ATP} channels shortens the action potential. Glibenclamide, a blocker of K_{ATP} channels, abolishes the hypoxic shortening. (Adapted from Sanguinetti and Keating (1997); see Further Reading, by permission.)

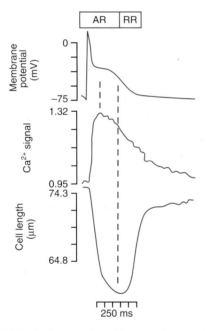

Figure 3.10 Relation between electrical, chemical and mechanical events in a single myocyte (rat). The myocyte was loaded with a fluorescent dye to measure free sarcoplasmic Ca^{2+}. Note the time sequence of the peaks – electrical, chemical and mechanical. AR, absolute refractory period (extends to -50 mV repolarization); RR, relative refractory period (-50 mV to full repolarization). Rat myocytes have an unusually low plateau potential. (Records from Spurgeon et al. (1990) *American Journal of Physiology*, **258**, H574–586.)

in many non-human species. Ventricular potentials are longer (400 ms) and more rectangular due to a distinct plateau at $+30$ mV to 0 mV. The phase 1 repolarization spike is well developed in epicardium

but not endocardium. The Purkinje cells of the conduction system have the longest action potentials (up to 450 ms), a pronounced phase 1 spike and a low plateau potential at around -20 mV.

The action potential is generated by a sequence of changes in sarcolemmal permeability to Na^+, Ca^{2+} and K^+ which allow ionic currents to flow down electrochemical gradients, as described next.

Fast Na^+ channels cause rapid depolarization (phase 0)

Depolarization is caused by an extremely rapid increase in sarcolemmal permeability to Na^+, due to the opening of **fast sodium channels** at a threshold of -60 to -65 mV. The fast Na^+ channel is said to be **voltage-dependent** because it opens at a critical or threshold potential, and **time-dependent** because its open state lasts only a very short time. Several drugs used to treat human arrhythmias, such as lignocaine, procaine and quinidine, inhibit the Na^+ channels.

Activation of the fast Na^+ channels raises the membrane conductance ~100-fold (Figure 3.7) and allows a rapid influx of Na^+ down its large electrochemical gradient. This generates the **first inward current**, i_{Na}. Current i_{Na} drives the potential towards the Nernst equilibrium potential for sodium, E_{Na}, which is $+70$ mV (Table 3.1). The potential never actually reaches E_{Na} because a small outward current of K^+ is still flowing. The situation at the **overshoot** is thus a mirror image of the resting situation. Equation 3.4 predicts an overshoot potential of $+55$ mV for a Na:K conductance ratio of 10:1.

The overshoot is brief because the Na^+ channels automatically **inactivate** after a very short time. The activation and inactivation mechanisms are illustrated in Figure 3.11. The Na^+ channel is formed by a single, very long polypeptide chain (i.e. a protein) that loops repeatedly across the cell membrane. There are four identical sets (domains I–IV) of six transmembrane loops (S_{1-6}). The 24 loops create a hollow channel, rather as do the staves of a barrel. The internal opening of the channel is guarded by two gates. The **m** or **activation gate** closes the inner mouth of the channel at resting potentials, and is probably formed by the S_6 loops. The activation gate opens quickly at threshold potential, causing a sudden rise in sodium permeability. Opening of the gate is driven by an outward shift of the positively charged, voltage-sensitive S_4 loops. The **h** or **inactivation gate** is open at resting potential, and begins to close at the same time as the activation gate opens, but it moves less quickly. The inactivation gate closes the channel automatically

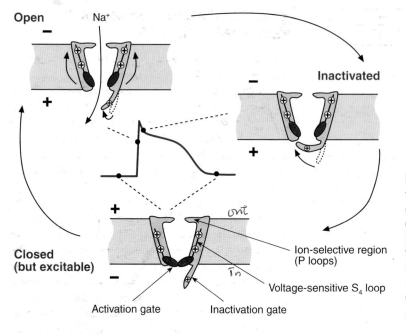

Open

Inactivated

Closed (but excitable)

Ion-selective region (P loops)

Voltage-sensitive S₄ loop

Activation gate   Inactivation gate

Figure 3.11 Activation–inactivation cycle for the voltage-sensitive Na⁺ channel. A depolarization-induced outward displacement of the charged S₄ loops causes the activation gate (S₆ loops) to open. The slower inactivation gate is a hinged lid; it is the intracellular loop that links domains III and IV of the molecule. The myocyte is refractory (incapable of re-excitation) as long as the inactivation gates are closed.

after a few milliseconds. The inactivation gate appears to be a hinged lid over the channel entrance, formed by a positively charged intracellular polypeptide loop linking domains III and IV.

Transiently open K⁺ channels cause early repolarization (phase 1)

In myocytes with a marked phase 1, such as epicardial myocytes and Purkinje fibres, the membrane next undergoes a rapid but incomplete repolarization (Figures 3.7–3.10). This is brought about by a transient outward current of K⁺ ions, i_{to}. Current i_{to} is carried by a class of K⁺ channel that opens transiently in response to depolarization, then quickly inactivates (Figure 3.9). The channel structure is broadly similar to that of a Na⁺ channel but with a different entrance selectivity and a ball-and-chain inactivation device rather than a hinged lid.

An influx of chloride ions through chloride channels also contributes to i_{to}. The partial repolarization in phase 1 serves to enhance the electrochemical force driving Ca²⁺ entry in the next phase.

L-type Ca²⁺ channels cause the plateau (phase 2)

The myocyte next displays its unique feature, the plateau, which lasts 200–400 ms. The plateau is generated by a small but long-lasting inward current of Ca²⁺ ions, i_{Ca}. The Ca²⁺ current is the second

inward current of the action potential (i_{Na} being the first) and it prevents the myocyte from repolarizing rapidly like a nerve. The existence of two distinct inward currents, i_{Na} and i_{Ca}, can be demonstrated using tetrodotoxin, a highly poisonous toxin from the Japanese puffer fish. Tetrodotoxin blocks the Na⁺ channels and selectively abolishes the initial spike of the action potential (Figure 3.12). Figure 3.12 also shows that the plateau current i_{Ca} is increased by the cardiac stimulant, adrenaline.

The Ca²⁺ ions flow into the cell down their electrochemical gradient through voltage-gated channels of a type called **long-opening** or **L-type Ca²⁺ channels**. Channel activation is rapid (though not as rapid as i_{Na}) and the current i_{Ca} has already climbed to 40% of its peak during phase 1. The current peaks at 2–7 ms but continues to flow at a declining rate for a long period afterwards, due to the slowness of Ca²⁺ channel inactivation. The prolonged elevation of Ca²⁺ conductance is shown in Figure 3.7. The structure of the Ca²⁺ channel is broadly similar to the Na⁺ channel, but an additional feature is that the inactivation process is enhanced by intracellular Ca²⁺. The rise in intracellular Ca²⁺ during the action potential thus helps to terminate Ca²⁺ channel opening.

The total conductance of the Ca²⁺ channels is low, so i_{Ca} is a small current. The small i_{Ca} counterbalances the repolarizing effect of a small outward K⁺ current, and thus holds the potential in the region of 0 mV for a long time.

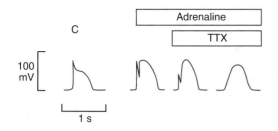

Figure 3.12 Effect of adrenaline and tetrodotoxin (TTX) on the action potential of calf Purkinje fibre. The control recording (C) shows a normal Purkinje action potential. Adrenaline enhances the plateau calcium current. Tetrodotoxin abolishes the initial spike depolarization because it blocks the fast sodium channels. The remaining action potential is quite like that in the SA node (see Figure 3.4). (After Carmeliet, E. and Vereeke, J. (1969) *Pfluger's Archiv*, **313**, 303–315.)

The **outward K$^+$ current i_{K1} is reduced** during most of the plateau due to the sudden fall in K$^+$ conductance when the cell depolarized (Figures 3.7, 3.9) – the phenomenon of inward rectification described earlier. This is a useful economy measure, because it minimizes the number of K$^+$ and Ca^{2+} ions that are exchanged and thus reduces the eventual energy cost of the action potential.

The Na$^+$–Ca^{2+} exchanger contributes to the late plateau

The inward current that maintains the late plateau is carried partly by Na$^+$ ions. For example, if Na$^+$ is removed from the fluid bathing an isolated myocyte, the plateau becomes shorter. The plateau Na$^+$ current is generated by the Na$^+$–Ca^{2+} exchanger (Figure 3.5), not the fast Na$^+$ channels. The exchanger creates a net inward current because it lets three Na$^+$ ions into the cell for every one Ca^{2+} expelled. The exchanger turns over at an increased rate during the plateau because the cytosolic Ca^{2+} concentration has increased, which reduces the uphill concentration gradient for Ca^{2+} expulsion. Since the exchanger transfers net positive charge into the cell, it is also influenced by membrane potential; it is speeded up by negative intracellular potentials and slowed down (or even reversed) by positive potentials. As a result, the exchanger contributes more to sustaining the late plateau in myocytes with a plateau at a negative potential, as in Purkinje fibres (Figure 3.4b), than in myocytes with a relatively positive plateau, such as ventricular myocytes (Figure 3.4a).

Due to its responsiveness to membrane potential, the exchanger may briefly go into reverse during the positive overshoot of the action potential, i.e. it helps to move Ca^{2+} into rather than out of the cell for a brief period (Appendix 2).

Potassium channel opening causes repolarization (phase 3)

The depressed net potassium conductance begins to increase as the plateau progresses (Figure 3.7). The increase is caused by the gradual opening of a class of slowly activating, voltage-operated K$^+$ channel called the **delayed rectifier** (Figure 3.9). As the Ca^{2+} channels inactivate, the delayed rectifier K$^+$ current dominates and initiates repolarization, aided in the final stages by the restored inward rectifier conductance.

The size of the K$^+$ current determines the duration of the plateau. When the heart rate is increased by sympathetic nerve stimulation, an increase in the repolarizing K$^+$ current induces early repolarization (Section 4.6). This shortens the action potential – an essential adaptation if there are to be more action potentials per minute. Action potential duration can also change in pathological conditions; it shortens during hypoxia (Figure 3.9 top) and lengthens in chronic heart disease (Section 3.6).

Absolute and relative refractory periods

The myocyte is electrically inexcitable, or refractory, throughout its long period of depolarization – the **absolute refractory period**. Since contraction lasts only 200–250 ms, contraction is weakening by the time the cell becomes repolarized and re-excitable (Figure 3.10). Consequently, the mechanical response of the myocardium is limited to a single twitch. A fused series of twitches, such as generate a sustained contraction in skeletal muscle, is not possible in myocardium. This seems an excellent arrangement, since a sustained myocardial contraction would quickly be fatal!

By the time repolarization reaches −50 mV, many but not all of the fast Na$^+$ channels have reset from the inactivated state to the closed but activatable state (Figure 3.11). That is to say, the inactivation gate reopens and the activation gate is closed. As a result, the cell partially regains electrical excitability at this point; but needs a larger-than-normal excitatory stimulus because only a fraction of the channels have reset. The period between −50 mV and full repolarization is therefore called the **relative refractory period** (Figure 3.10).

A relatively small quantity of ions is exchanged per action potential

The ionic currents are small and **the change in intracellular ion concentration resulting from a single action potential is tiny**. Students often assume,

Table 3.2 Chief ionic current in a myocardial work cell (for subdivision of currents, see Table 4.2).

Current	Ion	Direction*	Function	Blocker
$i_{K, total}$	K^+	Outward	1. Resting membrane potential 2. Repolarization	Ba^{2+} Tetraethyl ammonium 4-aminopyridine
i_b	Na^+ (mostly)	Inward	Inward background current keeping resting membrane potential less than E_K	–
i_{Na}	Na^+	Inward	Rapid depolarization	Tetrodotoxin
i_{Ca}	Ca^{2+}	Inward	1. Excitation–contraction coupling 2. Plateau maintenance	Mn^{2+} Verapamil, Nifedipine
i_{Na-Ca}	$3Na^+$ in $1Ca^{2+}$ out	Net inward current (Na–Ca exchanger)	Sustains late plateau and removes intracellular Ca^{2+} Responsible for arrhythmogenic 'afterdepolarizations' in ischaemic Ca^{2+} overload	–

* 'Inward' means from the extracellular to the intracellular compartment.

Cardiac potentials are due to ionic gradients and sequential activation of ion channels

▪ The resting potential, −80 mV, is created by the tendency of K^+ to diffuse out of the myocyte through K^+ channels, leaving behind a slight excess of negative charge.

▪ The resting potential approaches a Nernst equilibrium potential for K^+, modified by a small background Na^+ current.

▪ Voltage-gated Na^+ channels admit a brief influx of positive ions into the cell at the start of an action potential, depolarizing the cell.

▪ The overshoot of the action potential (+30 mV) approaches a Nernst equilibrium potential for Na^+, modified by a small background K^+ current.

▪ The activation of long-opening Ca^{2+} channels then allows an influx of Ca^{2+} (i_{Ca}) that approximately balances an outward K^+ current. This generates a long plateau on the action potential.

▪ The plateau is terminated by an increasing efflux of K^+ ions through delayed rectifier K^+ channels. K^+ efflux repolarizes the cell. Large K^+ currents shorten the plateau and small K^+ currents lengthen it.

a myocyte contains about 200 000 million Na^+ ions, the rise in concentration is a mere 0.02%. For intracellular K^+ the change is even smaller, 0.001% (Appendix 2, 'Quantity of ions'). The Na^+–K^+ and Na^+–Ca^{2+} transporters are therefore able to restore the chemical composition of the sarcoplasm without excessive expenditure of metabolic energy.

The main ionic currents are summarized in Table 3.2. Channel subtypes are summarized in Table 4.2.

3.6 Physiological and pathological changes in action potentials

Catecholamines enhance plateau current i_{Ca} and force

The plateau not only establishes a long refractory period but also **influences the strength of contraction**. Numerous studies have shown that the force of contraction is proportional to the plateau current i_{Ca}. The plateau current i_{Ca} is increased physiologically by the catecholamines, i.e. circulating **adrenaline** and local **noradrenaline** released by cardiac sympathetic nerves. The increase in i_{Ca} creates a more dome-shaped plateau (Figure 3.12). An increase in i_{Ca} causes a bigger free Ca^{2+} transient, which in turn increases the force of contraction. This is called the **inotropic** (strengthening) action of catecholamines. The biochemical steps that lead to the rise in i_{Ca} are described in Section 4.5, and the way in which i_{Ca} influences the size of the cytosol Ca^{2+} transient is described in Section 3.7.

wrongly, that the 'rush' of Na^+ into the cell must raise the intracellular Na^+ concentration substantially – but this is to mistake speed for quantity. Around 40 million Na^+ ions enter a myocyte during depolarization. Since

L-type calcium channel blockers such as verapamil and nifedipine have the opposite effect to catecholamines. The calcium channel blockers attenuate i_{Ca} and thus weaken the heartbeat.

Acute ischaemia shortens the action potential via K_{ATP} channels

The duration of the plateau is shortened by local, acute hypoxia, for example during a coronary artery thrombosis (Figure 3.10, top). Another class of K$^+$ channel (is there no end to them?) called the K_{ATP} channel is responsible. At normal ATP levels, ~5 mM, the open probability for K_{ATP} channels is low; but the open probability increases as ATP falls and as ADP, adenosine and H$^+$ concentrations rise, as happens in hypoxic cells. The resulting increase in K$^+$ conductance induces early repolarization and thus shortens the plateau phase. This in turn reduces the calcium entry per action potential. This might be helpful in that it reduces the workload for the Ca^{2+}-expelling pumps during hypoxia.

Chronic heart disease lengthens the action potential

In contrast to the shortening during acute hypoxia, the action potential is prolonged in chronic conditions such as severe cardiac failure, hypertrophy and chronic infarction. Prolongation is caused by the reduced expression of K$^+$ channel genes. A reduced K$^+$ current leads to delayed repolarization, a longer plateau and a high frequency of arrhythmias in these hearts.

The importance of the timing of repolarization is vividly demonstrated by a genetic abnormality of the delayed rectifier K$^+$ channel (**long Q–T syndrome**). This causes a prolonged action potential and long Q–T interval on ECG recordings. The long plateau can lead to Ca^{2+} overload and afterdepolarizations (Section 3.9), which may trigger arrhythmia and sudden death in young, apparently healthy individuals.

3.7 Excitation–contraction coupling and the Ca^{2+} cycle

Both extracellular and intracellular Ca^{2+} ions are essential for cardiac contraction. The need for extracellular Ca^{2+} was discovered by a London physiologist, **Sidney Ringer**, in 1883, and as with many seminal discoveries chance played a part. It was the job of Ringer's assistant to prepare solutions of (apparently) sodium and potassium chloride, which maintained the beating of an isolated frog heart for many hours. When the 'same' solution was made up in distilled water in later experiments, however, the heart quickly weakened and failed. Ringer discovered that in the earlier experiments his assistant had been using the local London tap water – which has a high Ca^{2+} content!

Thus it has been known for over a century that extracellular Ca^{2+} is essential for cardiac contraction. Indeed, rapid washout of extracellular Ca^{2+} from around an isolated myocyte causes the very next beat to fail. The reason is that the entry of extracellular Ca^{2+} into the subsarcolemmal space during the early part of i_{Ca} is needed to trigger the release of the SR Ca^{2+} store, which in turn initiates crossbridge formation.

A sarcoplasmic Ca^{2+} transient initiates contraction

The arrival of an action potential triggers a sharp rise in the sarcoplasmic concentration of free Ca^{2+}, from 0.1 μM in diastole to ~0.5–2 μM in systole, and some of the Ca^{2+} binds to troponin C to activate contraction (Figure 3.3). The correlation between contraction and the rise in free Ca^{2+} has been elegantly demonstrated by introducing Ca^{2+}-sensitive fluorescent dyes into the myocyte. The fluorescent signal begins to rise immediately after depolarization, and is quickly followed by contraction (Figure 3.10).

To prove the causal relation between sarcoplasmic Ca^{2+} and contractile force, Fabiato and Fabiato performed a classic experiment in 1975. The sarcolemma was stripped from the myocyte so that intracellular Ca^{2+} could be equilibrated with a known Ca^{2+} concentration in the bathing fluid. The 'skinned' cell was found to relax at 0.1 μM Ca^{2+}, contract moderately at 1 μM Ca^{2+}, and contract maximally at >10 μM Ca^{2+}. Intact myocytes have proved to be more sensitive to Ca^{2+} than the skinned fibres, and the free Ca^{2+} during a normal, sub-maximal twitch is probably ~0.55–0.75 μM.

How does the action potential induce an order-of-magnitude increase in the free Ca^{2+} concentration? As Figure 3.13 shows, the Ca^{2+} come from two sources: the sarcoplasmic reticulum store (the major source, ~75%) and the plateau current i_{Ca} (~25%).

Calcium-induced calcium release from SR is the main source of the Ca^{2+} transient

Junctional SR contains a concentrated store of Ca^{2+} (~1 mM) and is studded with Ca^{2+}-release channels. Each release channel is a giant protein of molecular mass 2.3 million daltons. The protein forms a 'foot' with a T-shaped tube through its centre, through which Ca^{2+} is presumably released. The foot terminates only nanometres from the sarcolemma of the T-tubules or cell surface, and is thus extremely close to L-type Ca^{2+} channels (Figure 3.13). The Ca^{2+}-release channels are activated by a rise in free Ca^{2+} concentration in their local, subsarcolemmal environment due to the opening of an adjacent L-type Ca^{2+} channel. This is called **calcium-induced calcium release** (CICR). The ratio of L-type Ca^{2+} channels to Ca^{2+}-release channels in the junctional region is roughly 1 to 10.

In diastole the free intracellular Ca^{2+} concentration is so low that the release channels are closed, except for occasional random discharges or 'sparks' (see below). With the arrival of an action potential the local current i_{Ca} through a sarcolemmal Ca^{2+} channel, called the **trigger calcium**, quickly raises the Ca^{2+} concentration in the adjacent sub-sarcolemmal space (Figure 3.13). The trigger calcium from a single L-type channel probably activates a cluster of 6–20 release channels. The sarcolemmal L-type Ca^{2+} channel and adjacent cluster of Ca^{2+}-release channels behave as a

functional unit. The sporadic activation of a cluster in diastole can be seen as a tiny, local **calcium spark** when a myocyte is loaded with a Ca^{2+}-sensitive fluorescent dye. Most sparks occur close to the T-tubules, while others arise from junctional SR coupled to the surface sarcolemma. The arrival of an action potential evokes thousands of such unitary sparks. The sparks summate in space and time to release a substantial fraction of the total SR store, typically ~50%. This raises the sarcoplasmic Ca^{2+} concentration to its peak level in ~50 ms. The released Ca^{2+} diffuses rapidly into the sarcomere and the cell begins to develop tension (Figure 3.10).

Gradation of response

An early conceptual problem with CICR was its inherent positive feedback nature, which could in principle cause an all-or-none discharge of the entire store. This clearly does not happen; experiments show that a small i_{Ca} causes a small free Ca^{2+} transient and weak contraction, while a big i_{Ca} causes a large free Ca^{2+} transient and strong contraction. This graded

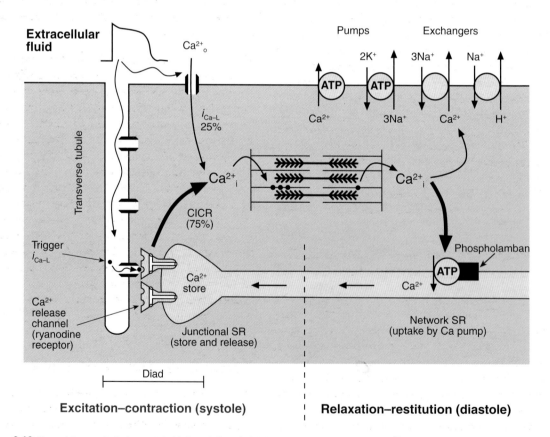

Figure 3.13 The calcium cycle during systole (*left*) and diastole (*right*). The sarcolemmal L-type Ca^{2+} channel forms a functional unit with the adjacent Ca^{2+}-release channels of junctional SR. The ratio is of the order 1 sarcolemmal Ca^{2+} channel to 10 Ca^{2+}-release channels. SR, sarcoplasmic reticulum; CICR, calcium-induced calcium release.

response is possible because the release channels are activated by **local subsarcolemmal Ca^{2+}**, not by the general cytosolic Ca^{2+}; nor does one cluster generally trigger its neighbours. Activation within a given cluster may be all-or-none due to positive feedback (the cluster bomb model) but **the number of clusters activated is proportional to the size of i_{Ca}**. The greater the number and duration of L-type Ca^{2+} channel opening events, the greater is the recruitment of subsarcolemmal release clusters and the greater the fraction of the store released.

After a rapid activation the release channel slowly inactivates over $\sim$100 ms. Inactivation is followed by a slow recovery of the initial sensitivity to Ca^{2+}.

Pumps in the network SR restock the store

Stimulated by the rise in free Ca^{2+}, the network SR then actively pumps most of the free Ca^{2+} back into the SR interior. The remainder, about 25%, is expelled by the sarcolemmal Na^{+}–Ca^{2+} exchanger (Figure 3.13). The amount expelled normally equals the amount that entered as i_{Ca}, so the cell Ca^{2+} content remains stable. As the free Ca^{2+} concentration falls, Ca^{2+} dissociates from the troponin–tropomyosin complex, leading to mechanical relaxation.

The Ca^{2+}-ATPase pumps of the network SR are regulated by an inhibitory protein **phospholamban**. The inhibitory effect of phospholamban is reduced by adrenaline and noradrenaline. Thus the catecholamines increase not only the Ca^{2+} store and contractility of myocytes (**inotropic action**) but also their rate of relaxation (**lusitropic action**).

Calcium uptake by the network SR is followed by restocking of the calsequestrin stores in the corbular and junctional SR (**restitution**). The restocking of the store is normally completed well before the next excitation.

Plateau current size (i_{Ca}) influences Ca^{2+} transient size and contractile force

After providing the trigger Ca^{2+} for store release, the continuing influx of extracellular Ca^{2+} as plateau current i_{Ca} itself contributes to the rise in free sarcoplasmic Ca^{2+}. The contribution is estimated to be 7–28%, depending on species. As noted above, the force of contraction correlates well with the amplitude and duration of i_{Ca}. When i_{Ca} is increased by **adrenaline** and **noradrenaline**, the free Ca^{2+} transient and contractile force increase proportionately. The reasons are twofold.

First, as explained earlier, an increase in trigger i_{Ca} in the subsarcolemmal space recruits more clusters of release channels. This releases a **greater fraction** of the total store. Second, over the duration of the plateau an enhanced i_{Ca} increases the amount of Ca^{2+} available for subsequent uptake into the SR store. This has a cumulative effect, and the **size of the Ca^{2+} store** increases over several beats. Together the increased store size and increased fractional release cause a bigger systolic free Ca^{2+} transient and stronger contraction. This focuses our attention on the question, 'What governs the size of the calcium store?'

Factors affecting the SR calcium store

The size of the store depends on the balance between the influx of extracellular Ca^{2+} during the plateau and its expulsion during diastole. The Ca^{2+} store therefore depends on:

1 the extracellular Ca^{2+} concentration;

2 the size of the plateau current, which is increased by adrenaline and noradrenaline; and

3 heart rate, which affects the duration of systole (Na^{+} and Ca^{2+} influx) relative to diastole (Na^{+} and Ca^{2+} expulsion). The increase in force with heart rate, or Bowditch effect, is described in Section 6.11.

The SR store can be manipulated using several pharmacological agents. The therapeutic drug **digoxin** is described below. **Caffeine** at high concentrations promotes Ca^{2+}-release channel activation. This can lead to contracture, i.e. a sustained contraction, *in vitro*. At therapeutic levels, however, its chief action is to inhibit phosphodiesterase enzymes. The drug **milrinone**, used in the treatment of cardiac failure, is likewise a phosphodiesterase inhibitor. The **phosphodiesterases** are a group of enzymes that degrade cyclic adenosine monophosphate (cAMP), the intracellular messenger that mediates the effect of adrenaline and noradrenaline (Figure 4.8). Caffeine and milrinone elevate cAMP and thus mimic the actions of adrenaline and noradrenaline.

Ischaemic heart disease can cause overloading of the SR store, which can trigger arrhythmia (Section 3.9).

Digoxin causes bigger Ca^{2+} transients

Digoxin is a cardiac glycoside produced by foxgloves. It has been used for over two centuries to treat heart failure because it enhances myocardial contractile force. Digoxin increases contractility by increasing the size of the systolic Ca^{2+} transient (Figure 3.14). Its direct pharmacological action, however, is not on

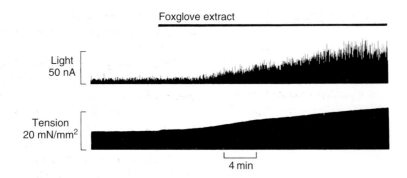

Figure 3.14 In 1785 William Withering reported that a folklore remedy based on an infusion of foxglove leaves (*Digitalis*) was beneficial in the treatment of 'dropsy' (cardiac failure). This experiment, to mark the bicentennial, shows how the extract increases both twitch force and the concentration of free intracellular calcium ions during contraction in ferret papillary muscle. The light emission from aequorin-injected muscle (*top trace*) is a function of calcium concentration. Aequorin is a protein from luminescent jellyfish and emits blue light in the presence of free Ca^{2+}. (From Allen, D. G., Eisner, D. A., Smith, G. L. and Wray, S. (1985) *Journal of Physiology*, **365**, 55P, by permission.)

CONCEPT BOX 3

Contractile force is proportional to crossbridge activation

■ A crossbridge is a myosin head linking the thick (myosin) and thin (actin) filaments. Flexion of the myosin head generates contraction.

■ Contractile force is increased by increasing the number of crossbridges.

■ Crossbridge formation is induced by a rise in sarcoplasmic free Ca^{2+} concentration.

■ The free Ca^{2+} transient is due chiefly to the partial discharge of the sarcoplasmic reticulum (SR) Ca^{2+} store. Store discharge is triggered by extracellular Ca^{2+} entry (current i_{Ca}) at the start of an action potential (calcium-induced calcium release).

■ During a quiet heart beat the free Ca^{2+} transient is only big enough to activate a fraction of the potential crossbridges.

■ Sympathetic stimulation increases i_{Ca} and store size, leading to a bigger free Ca^{2+} transient, more crossbridge formation and increased contractile force.

■ Stretching the cell increases crossbridge formation and force by increasing the sensitivity to Ca^{2+}.

Ca^{2+} but on the sarcolemmal Na^+–K^+ pump, which it inhibits. As a result, the subsarcolemmal Na^+ concentration rises. This reduces the Na^+ gradient across the sarcolemma. Since the Na^+ gradient drives the Na^+–Ca^{2+} exchanger, the expulsion of Ca^{2+} slows down. As a result, the Ca^{2+} store builds up and the contractility of the failing heart improves.

Toxic doses of digoxin can raise $[Na^+]_i$ so much that the Na^+–Ca^{2+} exchanger switches into reverse when the cell is depolarized during the action potential (Appendix 2). This drives yet more Ca^{2+} into the cell and causes store overload, a potent trigger for afterdepolarization and arrhythmia (Section 3.9).

3.8 Regulation of contractile force

The extent to which the contractile machinery is 'switched on' during systole is continually adjusted by physiological mechanisms in day-to-day life (Chapter 6). During a quiet heart beat only a fraction of the potential actin–myosin crossbridges are activated (~40%), so the heart beat is gentle. Contractile force can be increased during exercise or stress by increasing the number of crossbridges. There are two fundamentally different ways to achieve this:

1 The **systolic Ca^{2+} transient** can be increased, as described above. In normal life this is brought about by the release of noradrenaline from sympathetic nerve terminals in the myocardium, and by the secretion of adrenaline from the adrenal gland.

2 **Stretching the myocyte** in diastole provides a second, different way of increasing the contractile force. In normal life the myocardium can be stretched by increasing the diastolic filling of the heart, e.g. by lying down. Stretch acts by increasing the **sensitivity to Ca^{2+}** rather than the Ca^{2+} concentration. This is the basis of the fundamental **Starling law of the heart** or **length–tension relation** described in Chapter 6. An account of the underlying mechanism is deferred to that chapter.

3.9 Afterdepolarization, a trigger for arrhythmia

Cardiac ischaemia is usually due to coronary artery disease. It often initiates an arrhythmia such as ventricular fibrillation (Chapter 5). The trigger for ischaemic arrhythmia is **overloading of the SR calcium store**. Ischaemia raises the Ca^{2+} content by multiple mechanisms:

1 Intracellular Na^+ concentration increases due to reduced Na^+/K^+ pumping and acidotic stimulation of the Na^+-H^+ exchanger. This reduces the Na^+ gradient driving the Na^+-Ca^{2+} exchanger, so Ca^{2+} accumulates in the cell (Figure 6.22).

2 Increased sympathetic nerve activity, which is a reflex response to cardiac ischaemia, raises the plateau current i_{Ca} and hence Ca^{2+} entry. High sympathetic nerve activity in ischaemic hearts can thus lead to afterdepolarization (see below) and arrhythmia. Conversely, it is difficult to induce ventricular fibrillation by regional ischaemia in chronically denervated hearts.

An overloaded SR store is prone to discharge partially during early diastole, raising the sarcoplasmic Ca^{2+}. This stimulates the expulsion of Ca^{2+} by the sarcolemmal $3Na^+-1Ca^{2+}$ exchanger. Since Ca^{2+} expulsion entails a net inward flow of positive charge, it causes an afterdepolarization (Figure 3.15). If the afterdepolarization reaches threshold, a premature action potential ensues and may trigger an arrhythmia. The afterdepolarization may occur when the cell is fully repolarized (**delayed afterdepolarization, DAD**) or during the repolarization phase (**early afterdepolarization, EAD**). Delayed afterdepolarizations probably trigger most of the arrhythmias associated with digoxin, ischaemia and chronic cardiac failure.

Since increased i_{Ca} contributes to store overload and afterdepolarization, the risk of sudden death from arrhythmia after myocardial infarction can be reduced by blockers of L-type Ca^{2+} channels, for example verapamil and diltiazem, and by β-adrenoceptor blockers such as propranolol. It is necessary, however, that heart failure be absent, since these drugs also reduce contractile force.

SUMMARY

■ The myocyte resting potential, $-80\,mV$, approximates to a K^+ equilibrium potential, modified by a small inward background current of Na^+. The $3Na^+-2K^+$ pump preserves the intracellular ionic composition but contributes only $2-4\,mV$ to the potential.

■ Contraction is initiated by an action potential. Voltage-dependent Na^+ channel activation allows a rapid inward current of Na^+, i_{Na}, which depolarizes the myocyte (spike of action potential, phase 0). Following the rapid inactivation of Na^+ channels there is an early partial repolarization through K^+ efflux (i_{to}, phase 1). Next a second inward current, carried chiefly by extracellular Ca^{2+}, causes a long depolarized plateau lasting $200-400\,ms$ (i_{Ca}, phase 2). An inward Na^+ current through the $3Na^+-1Ca^{2+}$ exchanger helps to maintain the late plateau. Contraction begins during the plateau, and the cell is absolutely refractory to re-excitation.

■ Repolarization by an outward K^+ current terminates the plateau (i_K and i_{K1}, phase 3), and also determines its duration. Increased i_K shortens the plateau during tachycardia and hypoxia; reduced i_K lengthens it in chronic heart disease.

■ Immediately following depolarization, extracellular trigger Ca^{2+} passes through sarcolemmal L-type Ca^{2+} channels (early i_{Ca}) into the subsarcolemmal space. This local Ca^{2+} activates clusters of Ca^{2+}-release channels in the junctional sarcoplasmic reticulum (calcium-induced calcium release). The release of a fraction (about half) of the SR Ca^{2+} store quickly raises sarcoplasmic free Ca^{2+} to $\sim 1\,\mu M$.

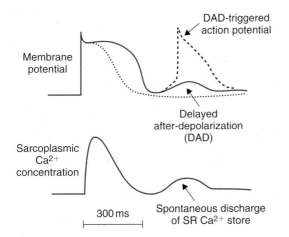

Figure 3.15 Delayed afterdepolarization (DAD, *upper trace*) initiated by partial discharge of over-loaded internal Ca^{2+} store (*lower trace*). This stimulates the electrogenic $3Na^+-1Ca^{2+}$ exchanger, causing a net inflow of positive charge (Na^+). The *dotted line* shows effect of replacing external Na^+ by Li^+, which impairs the exchanger. The plateau is shortened (showing that exchanger current normally contributes to late plateau) and the DAD is abolished. (Based on Benardeau, A., *et al.* (1996); see Further Reading.)

■ Some Ca^{2+} binds to the troponin–tropomyosin complex on actin filaments, leading to the exposure of myosin-binding sites. As a result, myosin heads form crossbridges between the thick and thin filaments. The myosin heads swivel and row the thick myosin filaments into the spaces between the thin actin filaments, producing tension and shortening. Recocking of the myosin head consumes ATP and O_2, so mitochondrial density is high.

■ Contractile force, typically ~40% maximal, depends on the fraction of the potential crossbridges that is activated. Crossbridge activation is regulated by two factors:

(i) Stretch of the sarcomere in diastole increases the **sensitivity** of the contractile machinery to Ca^{2+}. This leads to greater crossbridge activation and contractile force (the length–tension relation).

(ii) The **size** of the systolic Ca^{2+} transient also determines crossbridge activation. The Ca^{2+} transient is increased by adrenaline and noradrenaline. These agents increase i_{Ca}, which increases the store size over several beats, and also supplies more trigger Ca^{2+} so that a greater fraction of the store is released.

■ Overloading of the SR Ca^{2+} store occurs in ischaemia, especially when catecholamine stimulation is high. Spontaneous partial discharge of the overloaded store in diastole evokes afterdepolarization due to $3Na^{+}$–$1Ca^{2+}$ exchange. A large afterdepolarization can trigger a premature action potential leading to arrhythmia.

FURTHER READING

Reviews and chapters

Bers, D. M. (2001) *Excitation–Contraction Coupling and Cardiac Contractile Force*, Dordrecht, Kluwer.

Blaustein, M. P. and Lederer, W. J. (1999) Sodium/calcium exchange: its physiological implications. *Physiological Reviews*, **79**, 764–854.

Brady, A. J. (1991) Mechanical properties of isolated cardiac myocytes. *Physiological Reviews*, **71**, 413–442.

Cannell, M. D., Cheng, H. and Lederer, W. J. (1995) The control of calcium release in heart muscle. *Science*, **268**, 1045–1049.

Coraboeuf, E. and Escande, E. (1990) Ionic currents in the human myocardium. *News in Physiological Sciences*, **5**, 28–31.

Eisner, D. A., Trafford, A. W., Diaz, M. E. and Overend, C. L. (1998) The control of Ca release from the sarcoplasmic reticulum: regulation versus autoregulation. *Cardiovascular Research*, **38**, 589–604.

Fabiato, A. (1989) Appraisal of the physiological relevance of two hypotheses for the mechanism of calcium release from the mammalian cardiac sarcoplasmic reticulum: calcium-induced release versus charge-coupled release. *Molecular and Cellular Biochemistry*, **89**, 135–140.

Hiraoka, M. and Furukawa, T. (1998) Functional modulation of cardiac ATP-sensitive K^+ channels. *News in Physiological Sciences*, **13**, 131–137.

January, C. T. and Fozzard, H. A. (1988) Delayed afterdepolarizations in heart muscle: mechanisms and relevance. *Pharmacological Reviews*, **40**, 219–227.

Jongsma, H. J. and Gros, D. (1991) The cardiac connection (gap junction). *News in Physiological Sciences*, **6**, 34–40.

Nichols, C. G., Makhina, E. N., Pearson, W. L., Sha, Q. and Lopatin, A. N. (1996) Inward rectification and implications for cardiac excitability. *Circulation Research*, **78**, 1–7.

Niggli, E. (1999) Ca^{2+} sparks in cardiac muscle: is there life without them? *News in Physiological Sciences*, **14**, 129–134.

Sanguinetti, M. C. and Keating, M. T. (1997) Role of delayed rectifier potassium channels in cardiac repolarization and arrhythmias. *News in Physiological Sciences*, **12**, 152–157.

Solaro, R. J. and Rarick, H. M. (1998) Troponin and tropomyosin; proteins that switch on and tune in the activity of the cardiac myofilaments. *Circulation Research*, **83**, 471–480.

Sommer, I. R. and Johnson, E. A. (1979) Ultrastructure of cardiac muscle. In *Handbook of Physiology, Cardiovascular System*, Vol. 1, The Heart (ed. Berne, R. M.), American Physiological Society, Bethesda, pp. 113–186.

Wiers, W. G. and Balke, C. W. (1999) Ca^{2+} release mechanisms, Ca^{2+} sparks, and local control of excitation–contraction coupling in normal heart muscle. *Circulation Research*, **85**, 770–776.

Zipes, D. P. and Jalife, J. (1995) *Cardiac Electrophysiology from Cell to Bedside*, W. B. Saunders, Philadelphia. [Encyclopaedic!]

Research papers

Bernardeau, A., Hatem, S. N., Rucker-Martin, C., LeGrand, B., Mace, L., Dervanian, P., Mercadier, J-J. and Coraboeuf, E. (1996) Contribution of Na^{+}–Ca^{2+} exchange to action potential of human atrial myocyte. *American Journal of Physiology*, **271**, H1151–H1161.

Joergensen, A. O., Broderick, R., Somlyo, A. P. and Somlyo, A. V. (1988) Two structurally distinct calcium storage sites in rat sarcoplasmic reticulum: an electron microprobe analysis study. *Circulation Research*, **63**, 1060–1069.

Lawrence, J. H., Yue, D. T., Rose, W. C. and Marban, E. (1991) Sodium channel inactivation from resting states in guinea-pig ventricular myocytes. *Journal of Physiology*, **443**, 629–650.

O'Neill, S. C. and Eisner, D. A. (1990) A mechanism for the effects of caffeine on Ca^{2+} release during diastole and systole in isolated rat ventricular myocytes. *Journal of Physiology*, **430**, 519–536.

Sah, R., Ramirez, R. J., Kaprielian, R. and Backx, P. H. (2001). Alteration in action potential profile enhances excitation–contraction coupling in rat cardiac myocytes. *Journal of Physiology*, **533**, 201–214.

Shacklock, P. S., Wier, W. G. and Balke, C. W. (1995) Local Ca^{2+} transients (Ca^{2+} sparks) originate at transverse tubules in rat heart cells. *Journal of Physiology*, **487**, 601–608.

Sun, L., Fan, J-S., Clark, J. W. and Palade, P. T. (2000) A model of the L-type Ca^{2+} channel in rat ventricular myocytes: ion selectivity and inactivation mechanisms. *Journal of Physiology*, **529**, 139–158.

Wan, X., Bryant, S. M. and Hart, G. (2000) The effects of $[K_o]$ on regional differences in electrical characteristics of ventricular myocytes in guinea pig. *Experimental Physiology*, **85**, 769–774.

Initiation and nervous control of heartbeat

Learning objectives

After reading this chapter you should be able to:

- Sketch the anatomy of the excitation–conduction system of the heart, label it and state the role of each component (4.1).
- Explain what is meant by 'dominance' (4.1) and what happens to pacing in heart block.
- Draw a sino-atrial node potential over one cardiac cycle and state the ionic basis of each phase (4.2).
- Explain how depolarization propagates through the myocardium (4.3).
- State the chronotropic actions of (i) the sympathetic and (ii) the parasympathetic nerves, and outline their ionic mechanisms (4.5–4.6).
- Explain the inotropic and lusitropic effects of sympathetic stimulation (4.5).
- Describe the deleterious effect of hyperkalaemia (4.7).
- State the actions of (i) β-blockers and (ii) Ca^{2+}-channel blockers on the heart, and name an example of each (4.8).

Overview. If the heart is excised from a cold-blooded animal and placed in a beaker containing an appropriate solution of electrolytes, the heart continues to beat for a long period. This simple experiment proves that the heartbeat is initiated from within the heart itself. Unlike skeletal muscle, extrinsic nerves are not necessary to initiate contraction. The heartbeat is initiated by an intrinsic electrical system composed of modified myocytes, not nerves. These specialized myocytes are organized into (i) a group of cells in the sino-atrial node, the 'pacemaker', which discharge spontaneously at regular intervals to initiate the heartbeat; and (ii) elongated cells called conduction fibres that conduct the electrical impulse quickly to the ventricle wall. The conduction fibres trigger action potentials in the ventricular myocytes, and contraction follows. Although the firing of the pacemaker does not require any nervous input, its frequency is regulated by autonomic nerves. Autonomic nerves also regulate the force of contraction and hence stroke volume. Both components of the cardiac output, namely heart rate and stroke volume, are thus under nervous control.

4.1 Organization of pacemaker–conduction system

The sino-atrial node initiates the heartbeat

The sino-atrial node (SA node, pacemaker) is a strip of myocytes, roughly 20 mm long and 4 mm wide in man, located on the posterior wall of the right atrium close to the superior vena cava (Figure 4.1). The mammalian sino-atrial node is so called because it evolved from the sinus venosus, an antechamber to the right atrium in lower vertebrates. The node is made up of small myocytes that have scanty myofibrils and an unstable membrane potential. Human nodal cells fire an action potential spontaneously, approximately once every second at rest. This excites the adjacent atrial myocytes. The transmission of the action potential from myocyte to myocyte causes a wave of depolarization to sweep across both atria. The wave travels at ~1 m/s and initiates atrial systole.

The atrioventricular node delays ventricular excitation

The electrical impulse quickly reaches the atrioventricular node (AV node), which is a small mass of cells and connective tissue in the lower, posterior region of the atrial septum. The AV node is the starting point of the only electrical connection across the annulus fibrosus, which otherwise completely insulates the atria from the ventricles (Section 2.1). The impulse is delayed in the node for ~0.1 s at resting heart rates. The delay is caused by the complex local circuitry and the small diameter of the cells, 2–3 μm, which reduces the conduction velocity to ~0.05 m/s. The delaying role of the AV node is important because it allows time for atrial contraction to occur before ventricular contraction begins.

The bundle of His and its branches excite the ventricles

The function of the ventricular conduction system is to excite the whole ventricular wall as near simultaneously as possible. A bundle of fast-conducting muscle fibres, the **bundle of His**, conveys the electrical impulse from the AV node through the annulus fibrosus into the fibrous upper part of the interventricular septum. Here the bundle turns forwards and runs along the crest of the main, muscular part of the septum (Figure 4.1). The main bundle gives off a **left bundle branch**, which comprises two sets of fibres, one anterior and one posterior. These course down the left side of the muscular septum and supply the left ventricle. The remaining bundle, the **right bundle branch**, runs down the right side of the interventricular septum and supplies the right ventricle.

The bundle fibres are wide, fast-conducting myocytes arranged in a regular, end-to-end fashion. They terminate in an extensive network of large fibres in the subendocardium, described by the Hungarian histologist Purkinje in 1845. The **Purkinje fibres** are the widest cells in the heart, and their large diameters (40–80 μm) confer a high conduction velocity (3–5 m/s). Their role is to distribute the electrical impulse rapidly to the endocardial myocytes. From the endocardium the impulse passes from myocyte to myocyte at ~0.5–1 m/s in a generally outward, epicardial direction until the whole wall has been excited. This takes ~90 ms.

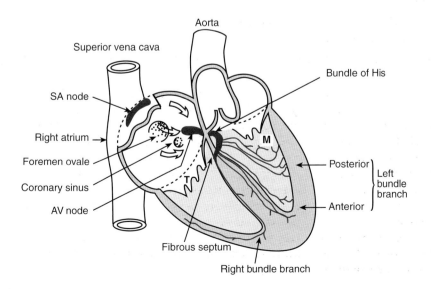

Figure 4.1 Diagram of the cardiac conduction system. The posterior fibres of the left bundle branch are seen *en face*, running just within the septal wall, then curling round within the left ventricular wall. The broad arrows show conduction through atrial muscle. Note the proximity of the valves (T, tricuspid; M, mitral) to the bundle of His; valvular lesions can affect the main bundle. The foramen ovale is the remnant of the fetal connection between right and left sides. The coronary sinus is the outlet of the main coronary vein.

The fastest pacemaker dominates a hierarchy of slower, latent pacemakers

There are other potential pacemaker sites besides the SA node but they have slower intrinsic frequencies of firing. The SA node normally sets the heart rate because its cells have the fastest intrinsic frequency, and thus excite the heart before other pacemakers have yet reached their firing threshold. If the SA node is destroyed, myocytes in the AV node or atrium take over as the new pacemaker, because they have the next highest rate of firing. The bundle of His too is capable of spontaneous firing, but only at ~40 beats/min. Purkinje cells have an even slower spontaneous frequency, ~15 beats/min, which is too slow to maintain an adequate cardiac output. There is thus a **gradient of intrinsic pacemaker frequencies along the cardiac electrical system**. The lower centres are normally excited from the SA node before they have time to fire spontaneously. This is called **dominance**.

The existence of an alternative slower pacemaker is revealed in a pathological condition called **heart block**. In heart block a failure of electrical transmission through the annulus fibrosus prevents the sino-atrial pacemaker from dominating the bundle of His. Cells in the bundle then take over as the pacemaker for the ventricles, driving them at ~40 beats/min (Figure 5.4e). This is too slow for many daily activities and such patients usually benefit from insertion of an artificial pacemaker.

4.2 Electrical activity of pacemaker

The decay of the pacemaker potential determines heart rate

The membrane potential of the SA node cells is small and unstable. The initial potential is only −50 to −70 mV because nodal cells possess few inward rectifier K^+ channels, which are responsible for the big, stable resting potentials of atrial and ventricular myocytes. The pacemaker cell possesses delayed rectifier K^+ channels, however (Tables 4.1, 4.2), and the efflux of K^+ ions through these channels generates the initial potential of about −60 mV.

The membrane potential then decays spontaneously with time (Figure 4.2). The slowly declining potential is called the **pacemaker potential**. When the pacemaker potential reaches a threshold of −40 to −55 mV, it triggers an action potential, which sparks off the next heartbeat.

The slope of the pacemaker potential is vitally important, because its **rate of decay determines the time taken to reach threshold, and thus determines the interval between heartbeats**. The steeper the slope, the sooner the threshold is reached and the shorter the interval between beats. Thus a steeply decaying pacemaker potential causes a high heart rate.

Multiple ionic currents cause the decay

The decay of the pacemaker potential is brought about by several different inward currents and by a decay of the outward current, as follows:

1 A small current of Na^+ ions flows into the cell, slowly depolarizing it. The current may be partly the inward background current i_b, described in Chapter 3. In addition many SA node cells possess a specialized pacemaker current called the **funny current**, i_f. Current i_f is only active at potentials negative to about −50 mV, and is funny-peculiar in that the channel is activated by hyperpolarization rather than depolarization.

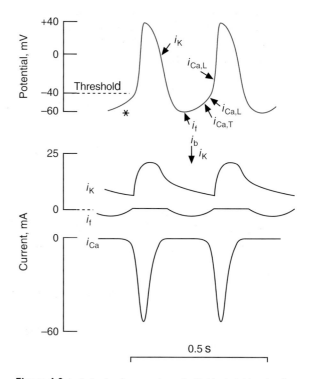

Figure 4.2 Ionic basis of pacemaker potential (asterisk) and action potential in sino-atrial cell. Slope of pacemaker potential determines time to reach threshold, and hence heart rate. Inward currents down, outward currents up. i_K, potassium current; i_f, 'funny' Na^+ current; i_b, background Na^+ current; $i_{Ca,T}$, *Transient* Ca^{2+} channel current; $i_{Ca,L}$, *Long-lasting* Ca^{2+} channel current. (Based on Petit-Jacques J., *et al.* (1994) and Noble, D. (1995); see Further Reading.)

The channel is actually non-selective between Na$^+$ and K$^+$, but i_f is chiefly an inward Na$^+$ current because at -50 mV or more the electrochemical gradient favours a Na$^+$ influx. Caesium ions block i_f and slow the rate of pacemaker depolarization. Caesium does not stop the pacemaker decay completely, however, which indicates that additional pacemaking currents exist.

2 The delayed rectifier K$^+$ channels deactivate slowly with time. As a result the **depolarizing outward current i_K decays with time**, allowing the inward currents to become increasingly dominant (Figure 4.2). The decaying K$^+$ conductance accounts for the declining net electrical conductance of the membrane during phase 4 in Figure 3.8.

3 As the potential decays past -55 mV or so, an **inward current of Ca^{2+} ions begins** to contribute to the depolarization. Voltage-sensitive Ca^{2+} channels of the transient or **T-type** in the SA node have an increased probability of being in the open state at these membrane potentials (Figure 4.3). Also, sparks of calcium-induced calcium release from the sarcoplasmic reticulum activate the **3Na$^+$–1Ca^{2+} exchanger**, which contributes

additional net inward, depolarizing current. As the potential declines further, voltage-sensitive **L-type Ca^{2+} channels** also begin to open. L-type channels activate at more depolarized (**L**ower) potentials than the T-type. Thus Ca^{2+} influx accelerates the depolarization rate in the late stages and triggers the action potential.

Node action potentials are small, sluggish and Ca^{2+}-based

The nodal action potential is slow-rising and small in amplitude, resembling that of the tetrodotoxin-blocked myocyte in Figure 3.12. This is because the nodal cell has few fast Na$^+$ channels, and the few present are mostly inactivated at -60 mV. The nodal action potential is generated solely by an inward Ca^{2+} current (Table 4.1). The same is true for AV node cells. Calcium-channel blockers, such as verapamil, reduce both the size of the nodal action potential and the rate of pacemaker decay.

Repolarization is brought about by an outward current of K$^+$ through delayed rectifier K$^+$ channels. These voltage-gated channels are activated rather slowly by depolarization (time constant $300-400$ ms) so they open gradually during the action potential. Conversely they inactivate slowly upon repolarization, thus contributing to the next pacemaker cycle.

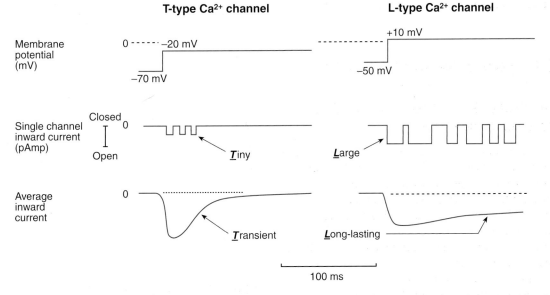

Figure 4.3 Currents through single Ca^{2+} channels in patch of myocyte membrane recorded by patch clamp method. Depolarization beyond -55 mV (*left, top*) caused a single T-type channel to flicker open sporadically (*left, middle*), admitting *T*iny pulses of current. After a short time, this stops. The average current passed by hundreds of such channels (*left, bottom*) is thus *T*ransient. When the membrane is depolarized to a greater extent (*right, top*), a single, higher threshold L-type Ca^{2+} channel opens sporadically, admitting *L*arger pulses of current (*right, middle*), and keeps on doing so. The average current passed by hundreds of such channels is thus *L*ong-lasting (*bottom, right*), although it does gradually inactivate. (Redrawn from Nilius, B., *et al.* (1985) *Nature*, **316**, 443–446.)

Table 4.1 Main ionic currents in nodal pacemaker cells.

Current	Ion	Direction	Function	Blocker
(i_{Na})	–	–	Fast Na^+ channels are largely absent	–
i_{Ca}	Ca^{2+}	Inward	1. Slow action potential 2. Last one-third of pacemaker potential	Mn^{2+}, verapamil, nifedipine
i_K	K^+	Outward	Delayed rectifier channels 1. Decays during pacemaker potential 2. Repolarization	Ba^{2+} –
i_f^* and i_b	Na^+	Inward	Supply inward depolarizing current during pacemarker potential	Cs^+ (i_f)

* i_f is a 'funny' current; i_b is 'background' current.

4.3 Transmission of excitation

Propagating currents spread the excitation

The spread of excitation through the atria, conduction system and ventricles is brought about by local electrical currents that act ahead of the action potential (Figure 4.4). In the active depolarized region, the interior of the membrane is positively charged, while the resting zone ahead is negative. The two regions are connected by a conducting pathway, the sarcoplasm and the **gap junctions** between cells. Positive charge therefore flows into the resting membrane, depolarizing it. Externally the converse applies; positive charge flows in the opposite direction through the extracellular fluid, reducing the charge on the outside of the resting membrane. The process is in fact the **passive discharge of a capacitor**, the lipid membrane. When the resting membrane potential reaches threshold, an action potential is triggered, setting up fresh local currents to excite the next region. Since the membrane to the rear is in its **refractory period**, excitation normally proceeds unidirectionally.

Conduction rate depends on fibre diameter and local current magnitude

The transmission of excitation is fastest in the widest cells, namely the Purkinje fibres, because a wide diameter confers a low axial electrical resistance. This allows the local circuits in Figure 4.4 to reach out further ahead of the active region.

Conduction rate also depends on the size and rate of rise of the action potential. Conduction is fast in myocytes with large, rapidly-rising action potentials such as ventricular myocytes, because such potentials generate big propagating currents, and big currents

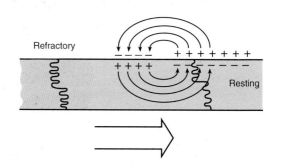

Figure 4.4 The spread of excitation through myocardium by local currents acting ahead of the action potential. The external current flows through the extracellular fluid and the internal current through the sarcoplasm and intercalated junctions. This discharges the cell membrane.

can extend well ahead of the active region. The **rate of depolarization**, i.e. the steepness of the initial Na^+-mediated spike of the action potential (500 volts/second, phase 0), is particularly important for the generation of big propagating currents, and hence for the secure propagation of excitation. Nodal cells have small, slow-rising action potentials, so they generate small propagating currents and have a poor **safety margin for conduction**. Conduction is slow and easily blocked in nodal tissue. The same is true for ventricular cells during ischaemia and hyperkalaemia (Section 4.7).

4.4 Regulation of heart rate

The human heart beats 50–100 times per minute at rest. Between species, heart rate is proportional to $1/mass^{0.25}$: the shrew's heart beats at 600/min and the elephant's at 25/min! The heart rate is controlled by sympathetic and parasympathetic autonomic nerves, which innervate the pacemaker.

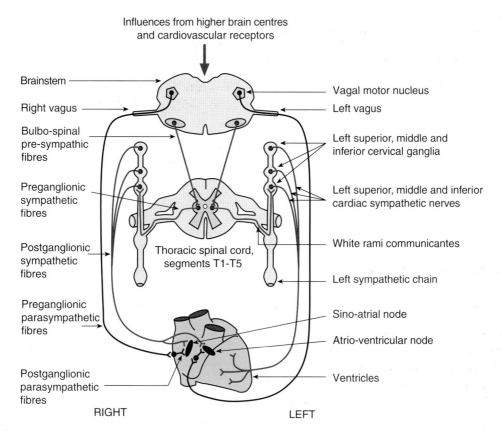

Influences from higher brain centres
and cardiovascular receptors

Brainstem

Right vagus

Bulbo-spinal
pre-sympathic
fibres

Preganglionic
sympathetic
fibres

Postganglionic
sympathetic
fibres

Preganglionic
parasympathetic
fibres

Postganglionic
parasympathetic
fibres

Vagal motor nucleus

Left vagus

Left superior, middle and
inferior cervical ganglia

Left superior, middle and inferior
cardiac sympathetic nerves

White rami communicantes

Left sympathetic chain

Sino-atrial node

Atrio-ventricular node

Ventricles

Thoracic spinal cord,
segments T1-T5

RIGHT

LEFT

Figure 4.5 Innervation of heart by sympathetic fibres (red) and vagal parasympathetic fibres (black). The sympathetic outflow arises from the intermedio-lateral horns of the thoracic spinal cord, segments T1–T5.

Sympathetic fibres innervate the whole heart

Preganglionic cardiac sympathetic fibres originate in the spinal cord at segments T1 to T5 (Figure 4.5). The short preganglionic fibres synapse in the paravertebral sympathetic ganglia. The long post-ganglionic fibres run along the surface of the great vessels to reach the heart. Unlike the parasympathetic system, the sympathetic fibres richly innervate the ventricular muscle as well as the atria and pacemaker–conduction system. The pacemaker and heart rate are controlled chiefly by fibres from the right paravertebral ganglia, while the contractile force of the ventricles is controlled chiefly by fibres from the left paravertebral ganglia.

Parasympathetic fibres have a more restricted distribution

The cardiac parasympathetic fibres originate in the vagal motor nuclei of the brainstem (Figures 4.5, 16.13, 16.14, 16.15). The preganglionic fibres travel

in the right and left vagus nerves. In general the right vagus supplies the pacemaker and the left vagus the AV node, although there is considerable anatomical variation. Unlike the sympathetic system, long preganglionic fibres synapse with the postganglionic parasympathetic neurons within the myocardium itself, mostly in the vicinity of the SA and AV nodes (Figure 4.5). Short postganglionic fibres innervate the nodes. There is only a sparse parasympathetic innervation of the ventricles.

Autonomic nerves continuously modify the intrinsic pacemaker rate

The nerve fibres are tonically (continuously) active, so the pacemaker firing rate is continuously modified by autonomic nerve activity, even at rest. Increased sympathetic activity speeds up the heart rate (**tachycardia**) (Figure 4.6). Increased parasympathetic activity slows it down (**bradycardia**) (Figure 4.7).

Both sets of autonomic nerve are tonically active, but **parasympathetic inhibition predominates at rest**. This is proved by the finding that the human

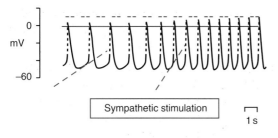

Sympathetic stimulation

1 s

Figure 4.6 Effect of continuous sympathetic stimulation (boxed interval) on pacemaker potential, leading to a relatively sluggish onset of tachycardia. The dashed gradients highlight the increased slope of the pacemaker potential. The upper double-dashed line draws attention to the increased size of the action potentials, which is due to the enhancement of the inward calcium current by catecholamines. (From Hutter, O. F. and Trautwein, W. (1956) *Journal of General Physiology*, **39**, 715–733, by permission.)

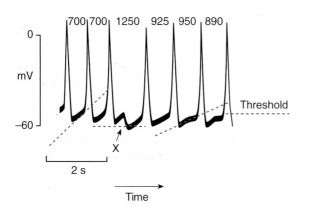

Threshold

X

2 s

Time

Figure 4.7 Effect of brief stimulation of vagus at X on pacemaker potential, leading to bradycardia. Note the brisk but poorly maintained hyperpolarization of the resting membrane and the more sustained, reduced slope of the pacemaker potential (dashed lines). Numbers at top are beat interval in ms. (After Jalife, J. and Moe, G. K. (1979) *Circulation Research*, **45**, 595–608.)

heart rate increases to ~105 beats/min if both divisions of the autonomic system are blocked, using **atropine** to block parasympathetic effects and **propranolol** to block sympathetic effects. The intrinsic pacemaker frequency is thus $\sim105\,min^{-1}$ in young humans.

Physiological changes in heart rate are usually brought about by **reciprocal changes in activity** of the sympathetic and parasympathetic fibres. The tachycardia of exercise, for example, is induced by increased sympathetic activity and reduced parasympathetic activity.

Parasympathetic regulation acts faster than sympathetic regulation

The tachycardia elicited by sympathetic stimulation is relatively sluggish in onset (Figure 4.6) and decays

The rate of decay of the pacemaker potential determines heart rate

☐ The negative potential of a pacemaker cell decays with time (becomes less negative) due to inward currents of Na^+ and Ca^{2+} and a falling K^+ conductance.

☐ The rate of decay (the slope) determines how long the pacemaker takes to reach the threshold for an action potential, which triggers the next heart beat. Decay rate thus determines the interval between heart beats.

☐ Sympathetic stimulation increases the decay rate, so threshold is reached sooner and the number of beats per minute (heart rate) increases.

☐ Parasympathetic stimulation reduces the decay rate, so it takes longer to reach threshold and the heart rate falls.

☐ Parasympathetic stimulation also rapidly hyperpolarizes the pacemaker cells, by activating acetylcholine-sensitive K^+ channels. This increases the time needed to decay to threshold, reducing the heart rate.

CONCEPT BOX 4

relatively slowly when stimulation ceases. By contrast the bradycardia elicited by parasympathetic stimulation has a very short latency (Figure 4.7), and resolves more quickly when fibre activity ceases. Thus changes in parasympathetic activity account for rapid changes in heart rate, such as the slowing of the heart with each expiration (sinus arrhythmia). The fast 'on' effect is due to a hyperpolarizing pathway activated by acetylcholine (see later). The fast 'off' effect is due to the rapid removal of acetylcholine by an enzyme, cholinesterase.

Temperature too affects heart rate

The pacemaker rate is influenced by **temperature**. A fever causes the heart rate to increase by ~10 beats/min per degree Centigrade. Conversely, cooling can be used to slow the heart during open heart surgery.

4.5 Effects of sympathetic stimulation

Sympathetic stimulation increases frequency, force and relaxation rate

The sympathetic fibres release the neurotransmitter noradrenaline ('norepinephrine' in the American literature). Noradrenaline binds to β_1-adrenoceptors on the cardiac cell membrane. The heart also possesses α- and β_2-adrenoceptors, but the β_1-receptors predominate. Activation of the β_1-receptors is followed over several beats by:

- an increase in heart rate (the **chronotropic effect**, Figure 4.6)

- increased AV node conduction velocity (the **dromotropic effect**)

- shortening of the myocyte action potential duration

- increased contractile force (the **inotropic effect**, Figure 6.18)

- increased rate of relaxation (the **lusitropic effect**, Figure 6.18).

The hormone **adrenaline** (epinephrine) acts similarly. Adrenaline is secreted into the bloodstream by the medulla of the adrenal gland in response to preganglionic sympathetic fibre activity. Adrenaline and noradrenaline are known collectively as the **catecholamines**.

The action of noradrenaline is terminated partly by diffusion into the bloodstream, which washes it away; and partly by reuptake into the sympathetic nerves. Since these processes are relatively slow, the recovery from sympathetic stimulation is slow.

The intracellular pathways that lead to the above dramatic changes in cardiac activity are as follows.

β_1–adrenoceptors activate the cAMP–PKA pathway

The activation of β_1-receptors triggers an intracellular biochemical cascade, the cAMP–protein kinase A pathway, that leads to changes ion channel and pump activity (Figure 4.8). The β_1-receptor is linked to an intramembrane G protein, G_s ('s' for stimulatory), which activates a membrane-bound enzyme, **adenylate cyclase**. This catalyses the conversion of ATP into the intracellular messenger **cyclic adenosine monophosphate (cAMP)**. cAMP has the following effects:

- cAMP interacts directly with **pacemaker i_f channels** to increase their open-state probability. The rise in i_f accelerates the pacemaker decay and contributes to the chronotropic effect.

- cAMP activates the intracellular enzyme **protein kinase A** (PKA). The PKA catalyses the **phosphorylation of L-type Ca^{2+} channels**, which increases the probability and duration of

the open state. In atrial and ventricular myocytes this contributes to the inotropic effect, and in the SA node to the chronotropic effect.

- PKA **phosphorylates the delayed rectifier K^+ channels**. The increased repolarizing outward current i_K shortens the ventricular action potential, thus permitting more excitations per minute.

- PKA **phosphorylates phospholamban**, reducing its inhibitory effect on the Ca^{2+}-ATPase pump of the network SR. The increased affinity of the pump for Ca^{2+} speeds up the uptake of free Ca^{2+} from the sarcoplasm into SR and accounts for most of the lusitropic effect.

The long, relatively slow transduction pathway accounts for the slow time-course of the 'on' response to sympathetic stimulation, which can be seen in Figure 4.6.

The above intracellular events combine to alter the performance of the whole heart as follows.

The chronotropic and dromotropic effects

1 **The rate of decay of the pacemaker potential is increased**, so the threshold is reached sooner and the heart rate increases (Figure 4.6). The increased decay rate is caused by the increase in depolarizing currents i_f, i_{Ca-L} and i_{Na-Ca}, and an increased rate of deactivation of the delayed rectifier K^+ channel. For the heart to function effectively at a higher pacing rate, it is also necessary for the entire cardiac cycle to be shortened. Sympathetic stimulation achieves this as follows.

2 **Conduction through the AV node is speeded up** by activated β_1-receptors in the AV node. This reduces the time lag between SA node firing and ventricular contraction.

3 **The action potential of atrial and ventricular myocytes is shortened**. Early repolarization is brought about by the increased repolarizing K^+ current i_K (Figure 4.8). The long plateau would otherwise severely limit the maximum heart rate.

The inotropic effect is due to an increased Ca^{2+} transient

The increase in the plateau Ca^{2+} current i_{Ca-L} is evident in Figures 3.12 and 4.6. The increased influx of extracellular Ca^{2+}, in conjunction with the increased affinity of the SR pumps for Ca^{2+}, increases the size of the SR store over several beats.

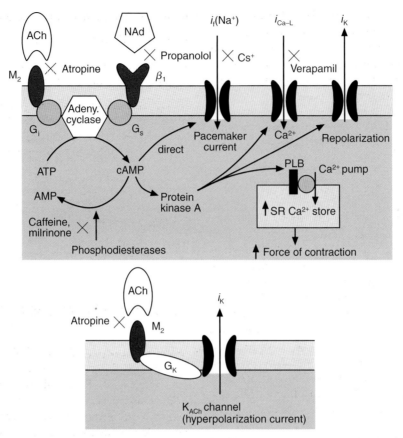

Figure 4.8 Intracellular signalling pathways for sympathetic noradrenaline (NAd) and parasympathetic acetylcholine (ACh) in myocardial and pacemaker cells (composite diagram). G_s, stimulatory guanosine triphosphate-binding protein; G_i, inhibitory guanosine triphosphate-binding protein; PLB, phospholamban; Adeny. cyclase, adenylate (or adenylyl) cyclase.

The **enlarged Ca^{2+} store** and **increased trigger Ca^{2+}** (increased i_{Ca-L}) cause a bigger systolic free Ca^{2+} transient (Sections 3.7, 3.8). This activates more cross-bridges and increases the force of atrial and ventricular systole.

The lusitropic effect is due to faster SR Ca^{2+} reuptake

The **duration of contraction is shortened** and **relaxation rate increased** at the end of systole. The shortening of systolic ejection and isovolumetric relaxation helps to **preserve the diastolic interval**. This is essential for the refilling of the heart (Section 2.4). These changes are chiefly due to the faster removal of sarcoplasmic Ca^{2+} by the stimulated Ca^{2+}-ATPase pumps in the network SR. In addition, phosphorylation of thin filament troponin I speeds up the crossbridge cycling, allowing a faster relaxation. However, studies using genetically engineered, phospholamban knock-out mice show that 85% of the lusitropy is attributable to pump stimulation by phosphorylated phospholamban.

Drugs that raise cAMP mimic sympathetic stimulation

The level of cAMP in the myocytes depends not only on its rate of production by adenylate cyclase but also on its rate of degradation by a group of enzymes, the **phosphodiesterases**. Agents that inhibit phosphodiesterase, such as **caffeine, theophylline** and **milrinone**, cause a rise in cAMP. They therefore mimic the effects of β_1-agonists, i.e. they increase the heart rate and contractility.

4.6 Effects of parasympathetic stimulation

The parasympathetic neurotransmitter is acetylcholine

Firing of the parasympathetic postganglionic fibres releases the neurotransmitter **acetylcholine** from the nerve terminal. Acetylcholine, discovered by Otto Loewi in 1921, was the first neurotransmitter to be identified. Loewi sampled fluid from a frog heart during vagal stimulation, and found that the fluid caused bradycardia when applied to an isolated frog heart. Acetylcholine acts by binding to **muscarinic M$_2$-receptors** on the myocyte membrane. The receptor initiates the intracellular cascade described below. Acetylcholine is quickly removed from the junctional region by the enzyme **cholinesterase**. Consequently, the heart rate picks up briskly when vagal activity is reduced.

Acetylcholine slows the pacemaker potential decay

Vagal stimulation produces bradycardia through two electrophysiological actions (Figure 4.7). The chief effect is to slow the rate of decay of the pacemaker potential. In addition the membrane is quickly hyperpolarized, i.e. made more negative. As a result of these two effects the potential takes longer to reach the threshold and the heart rate decreases. Of the two effects the reduction in slope is the more important over long periods, because it can be elicited by a lower concentration of acetylcholine and is better sustained. The chronic bradycardia of a trained athlete is an example of this effect.

M$_2$ receptors inhibit adenylate cyclase and activate K$_{ACh}$ channels

Acetylcholine reduces the pacemaker slope by reducing both the Na$^+$ current i_f and the L-type Ca^{2+} current i_{Ca-L}. The mechanism is in effect the reverse of that triggered by the β_1-adrenoceptors. The M$_2$ receptor is linked to an inhibitory G protein, G$_i$, which reduces the activity of adenylate cyclase (Figure 4.8). The ensuing fall in cAMP and protein kinase A activity reduces the activation of the i_f and L-type Ca^{2+} channels.

The hyperpolarizing effect of acetylcholine is mediated by M$_2$-receptors linked through a G protein, G$_K$, to a class of K$^+$ channel called the **K$_{ACh}$ channel**. Activation of K$_{ACh}$ channels by acetylcholine increases the outward K$^+$ current and shifts the membrane potential closer to the Nernst equilibrium potential for K$^+$, -94 mV (eqn 3.1). The directness of the receptor $-G_K-K_{ACh}$ linkage accounts for the rapidity with which vagal stimulation slows the heart.

Physiological roles

Examples of vagal bradycardia in man include:

- slowing of the heart during each expiration (sinus arrhythmia, Figure 5.4a)

- the low heart rate of a trained athlete

- slowing of the heart during a dive (Chapter 17)

- transient arrest of the heart at the onset of fainting (vasovagal attack, Chapter 18).

An extreme example of vagal bradycardia has given rise to the everyday expression, 'playing possum'. To fool a predator, the possum feigns death by collapsing and developing a profound bradycardia:

> Quoth Fox to Brer Possum
> 'You're due in my antrum'.
> Old possum smiled; he had a hunch
> His flaccid apnoe-a
> And bradycardee-a
> Would leave Fox in no mood for lunch.

4.7 Dangers of altered ionic environment

Severe disturbances of extracellular electrolyte concentration will in general be 'A Bad Thing' for cardiac function. As Ringer showed, **hypocalcaemia** reduces myocardial contractility. Extreme **hypercalcaemia** arrests the heart in systole. **Hypokalaemia**, a low extracellular K$^+$ concentration resulting from diarrhoea and vomiting or K$^+$-losing diuretics, hyperpolarizes the myocytes, leading to arrhythmia and even cardiac arrest. **Hyperkalaemia**, a raised concentration of extracellular K$^+$ ions, can develop in a number of clinical conditions and is potentially fatal, as described next.

Hyperkalaemia can cause arrhythmia

The K$^+$ concentration in extracellular fluid is normally $3.5-5.5$ mM. An increase to <7.5 mM can arrest the heart in diastole. In cardiac transplant surgery, for example, a solution of 20 mM K$^+$, called **cardioplegic solution**, is perfused through the donor heart to arrest it. An arrested heart uses less O$_2$, so is better able to survive the delay between donor and recipient.

Intermediate, **clinical hyperkalaemia** weakens the heartbeat and can lead to arrhythmia. Clinical hyperkalaemia can develop gradually during renal failure, acidosis or potassium overload, or acutely during haemolysis. Hyperkalaemia reduces the resting membrane potential, because it reduces the K$^+$ equilibrium potential (Figure 3.6). Secondary changes occur in the action potential, because the gradual reduction of the resting potential allows time for the inactivation gates of fast Na$^+$ channels to close.

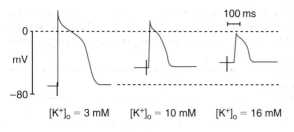

Figure 4.9 Effect of hyperkalaemia on the membrane potential of a Purkinje fibre (see text). The spike to the left of each action potential marks stimulation by an external impulse some distance away. Note the increasing conduction time, reduced resting potential, reduced action potential and slow rate of rise. (After Myerburg, R. J. and Lazzara, R. (1973) In *Complex Electrocardiography* (ed. Fisch, E.), Davis Co., Philadelphia.)

At a resting potential of $-70\,mV$ about half the inactivation gates are closed, while at $-50\,mV$ most are closed. As a result the action potential becomes increasingly dependent on i_{Ca-L}, and shows a sluggish rise and small amplitude (Figure 4.9). Small, slow-rising action potentials produce small propagating currents, so electrical transmission becomes impaired. This can lead to arrhythmia and heart block. Some of these changes also occur in **ischaemic myocardium**, because ischaemia causes a local increase in myocardial interstitial K^+ concentration (Figure 6.22).

Remarkably, despite the above catalogue of horrors, the plasma K^+ concentration of normal individuals can double to $8\,mM$ in severe exercise without evident harm. The K^+ is released by the exercising skeletal muscle. It appears that adrenaline and noradrenaline, the circulating levels of which can increase 20-fold in severe exercise, protect the myocardium against the hyperkalaemia. They probably do so by enhancing the Ca^{2+} current i_{Ca-L}.

H^+ and ischaemia weaken the heartbeat

Intracellular H^+ ions compete with Ca^{2+} for the troponin C binding site, so intracellular acidosis weakens the contraction. Intracellular pH is normally held at 7.1–7.2 by membrane transporters such as the Na^+–H^+ exchanger and Na^+–HCO_3^- importer. These can be overwhelmed, however, in ischaemia, leading to weak contractions (Section 6.12).

4.8 Pharmacological manipulation of the ion channels

β-blockers. The non-selective β-blockers propranolol and oxprenolol, and the specific β_1 blockers atenolol and metoprolol, block the tonic sympathetic influence on the heart. They therefore reduce the heart rate and contractile force. Since cardiac work is reduced, β-blockers are often used to treat hypertension and angina. Angina is ischaemic heart pain, usually provoked by exercise, caused by cardiac work exceeding the O_2 supply through diseased coronary arteries.

Ca^{2+}-channel blockers. Verapamil and nifedipine act on L-type Ca^{2+} channels to reduce the plateau current i_{Ca-L}. This shortens the action potential and has a negative inotropic (weakening) effect. Verapamil has a greater effect on the heart than nifedipine and is used to reduce cardiac O_2 demand in angina patients. Verapamil also slows AV node conduction, so it can suppress arrhythmias that depend on a 'circus' or re-entry mechanism (Section 5.8).

K^+-channel openers. The metabolically sensitive K_{ATP} channel, which we met in Section 3.6, is activated by the drugs cromakalim, pinacidil and nicorandil, leading to hyperpolarization of the cell. The main therapeutic effect of K_{ATP} activators, however, is the relaxation of blood vessels, which helps to relieve angina.

Adenosine is sometimes administered intravenously to terminate **supraventricular tachycardias**, pathologically high heart rates driven from the atria. Adenosine acts on purinergic A_1 receptors to activate nodal K^+ channels, leading to hyperpolarization. This reduces the heart rate and slows AV node conduction.

Na^+-channel blockers. Procainamide, lignocaine and quinidine are used as anti-arrhythmic drugs.

4.9 Stretch and mechano-electrical feedback

Mechanical stimuli can affect the electrical activity of the heart. For example, a thump on the chest will occasionally correct a pathological tachycardia (abnormally high heart rates). Likewise, a blow to the chest will sometimes restart an arrested heart. Stretch-activated ion channels (SACs) are responsible for these mechano-electric effects. SACs transmit an inward current and thus depolarize the cell. There are several classes of SAC, as summarized in Table 4.2. The following effects are attributed to SACs in the pacemaker and ventricles.

1 **The Bainbridge 'reflex'.** Bainbridge discovered in 1915 that the rapid infusion of a

Table 4.2 Types of ion channel in cardiac work and/or nodal cells. To paraphrase Professor Noble in 'The surprising heart', the description of ionic currents in the preceding text 'may already have exhausted the reader, but it certainly does not exhaust the mechanisms that have been found'. This table attempts to categorize the most important of these for the benefit of the more advanced student: ***first-year students should skip this table and finish reading this chapter!***

Channel and current	Properties and activator	Blocker	Role
Potassium			
Inward rectifier (i_{K1})	Allows little K^+ efflux at positive potentials; opens at negative potentials	Ba^{2+}	Supplies outward current for resting myocyte potential and repolarization from -20 to -80 mV. Few in SA node, hence small potential
Delayed rectifier (i_K) (or voltage-activated, i_{Kv})	Activated slowly on depolarization beyond -40 mV. Subtypes i_{Kr} (rapid) and i_{Ks} (slow) influence action potential duration	Ba^{2+}	Terminates action potential, supplying initial repolarization current to -20 mV. Slow inactivation causes falling g_K during pacemaker potential
Transient outward (i_{to})	Activated by depolarization	4-aminopyridine	Causes phase 1 repolarization spike in epicardium. Affects duration of action potential
Muscarinic (i_{K-ACh})	Activated by ACh. Some spontaneous opening. Inwardly rectifying like i_{K1}	Ba^{2+} (partially) (Pertussis toxin blocks the linked G-protein)	Hyperpolarizing effect of ACh and adenosine. Contributes to background K^+ current in SA node
ATP-K (i_{K-ATP})	Opened by low ATP (<0.1 mM), raised ADP, adenosine, H^+, nicorandil, cromakalim and pinacidil	Glibenclamide	Abundant. In ischaemia, opening of a small % terminates action potential early, reducing contractile force
Sodium			
Fast-inactivating (i_{Na})	Voltage- and time-dependent opening	Tetrodotoxin, local anaesthetics	Spike of myocyte action potential. Scarce in SA node so no spike
Hyperpolarization-activated (i_f)	Opens slowly at potentials negative to -60 to -45 mV	Cs^+ slows pacemaker depolarization by 10–40%	Depolarizing current of pacemaker. Increased by catecholamines via cAMP. Reduced by acetylcholine
Background (i_b)	Passive background current		Attenuates resting membrane potential
(Na–Ca exchanger, i_{NaCa})	Not a channel but allows $3Na^+$ into cell for $1Ca^{2+}$ expelled. Activated by rise in Ca_i^{2+}	Li^+, Cd^{2+}, La^{3+}	Supplies a net inward current in late plateau and in DADs. May reverse briefly after Na^+ spike, contributing to early Ca^{2+} influx
(Na–K pump i_{NaK})	Not a channel but $3Na^+$ pumped out of cell for $2K^+$ in	Digoxin, ouabain	Minor (2–4 mv) contributor to resting potential
Calcium			
L-type (i_{Ca-L})	Voltage-operated channel activated by depolarization '*L*'ong-lasting. i.e. >20 ms before inactivates	Cd^{2+}, verapamil, Ni^{2+}	Carries most of early plateau current and supplies trigger calcium for CICR. Also SA and AV node action potentials
T-type (i_{Ca-T})	Activated at more negative potentials than L-type, e.g. -55 mV. '*T*'ransient opening, i.e. fast inactivation	Ni^{2+}	Contributes to pacemaker depolarizing current. Insensitive to verapamil or β agonists
Chloride			
cAMP-dependent ($i_{Cl(AMP)}$)	Activated by cAMP and therefore by β_1 agonists		Contributes to phase 1 repolarization after β_1 activation, from +ve potentials down to E_{Cl}, -40 mV (Table 3.1)

(Continued)

Table 4.2 (*Continued*).

Channel and current	Properties and activator	Blocker	Role
Ca^{2+} dependent ($i_{Cl(Ca)}$)	Activated by cytosol Ca^{2+}	DiDS	Contributes to phase 1 repolarization and to pacemaker potential and to DADs (E_{Cl} is -40 mV)
Swelling activated	A stretch-activated channel		Opened by osmotic swelling of cell. Role in cell volume regulation
Stretch-activated channels (SAC)		Gd^{3+}	
Non-specific cation SAC	Activated by stretch		Mechanoelectric feedback
K$^+$-selective SAC	Activated by stretch		Mechanoelectric feedback
Cl$^-$-selected SAC	See under Chloride		See under Chloride

large volume of saline into the venous system causes a transient tachycardia (Section 16.3). The Bainbridge effect, which is of little physiological importance, may be due in part to the activation of pacemaker SACs.

2 **Stretch-induced depolarization.** Acute stretch of the atrium or ventricle, for example during cardiac catheterization, can trigger extra systoles and other arrhythmias. Gadolinium ions, Gd^{3+}, block some SACs and prevent stretch-induced arrhythmias.

SUMMARY

■ The sino-atrial node initiates atrial contraction. The atrioventricular node delays the transmission of excitation to the ventricle long enough to allow atrial contraction to precede ventricular contraction. The bundle of His and Purkinje system distribute the electrical impulse rapidly throughout the ventricular muscle mass.

■ The membrane potential of pacemaker cells decays with time (the pacemaker potential). Decay is due to multiple inward currents (Na$^+$ currents i_f, i_b, Ca^{2+} currents i_{Ca-T}, i_{Ca-L}, exchanger current i_{Na-Ca}) and a decaying delayed rectifier K$^+$ permeability. The potential decay rate determines the time taken to reach threshold and fire an action potential, which initiates the next heartbeat. Heart rate is thus controlled by the slope of the pacemaker potential. The nodal action potential is small, sluggish, and generated solely by L-type Ca^{2+} channels.

■ Sympathetic nerve fibres release noradrenaline, which activates cardiac β_1-adrenoreceptors.

β_1-activation in the SA node accelerates the decay of the pacemaker potential and thus increases heart rate (the chronotropic effect). Accelerated decay of the pacemaker potential is due to increases in the depolarizing pacemaker currents i_f and i_{Ca-L}, and a faster decay in K$^+$ permeability.

■ Activation of β_1-receptors on atrial and ventricular myocytes increases the open probability of L-type Ca^{2+} channels, leading to a bigger Ca^{2+} store and more forceful contraction (the inotropic effect). Reuptake of free Ca^{2+} by the SR pumps is enhanced, so systole is shortened and relaxation speeded up (the lusitropic effect). The effects of β_1-activation are mediated through the adenylate cyclase–cAMP–protein kinase A pathway.

■ Parasympathetic fibres from the vagi release acetylcholine, which activates muscarinic M$_2$-receptors. This slows the rate of decay of the pacemaker potential by reducing the inward pacemaker currents i_f and i_{Ca-L} (mediated by inhibition of the adenylate cyclase–cAMP–PKA chain). Muscarinic receptors also hyperpolarize pacemaker cells by activating K$_{ACh}$ channels. This produces a brisk fall in heart rate, e.g. on expiration, fainting.

■ Electrical activity can be altered by ionic environment and drugs. Hyperkalaemia depolarizes the myocytes, leading to conduction impairment and arrhythmias. β-blockers such as propanolol, and Ca^{2+}-channel blockers such as verapamil, reduce the plateau current i_{Ca}, which reduces contractile force and heart rate. Since this reduces myocardial O$_2$ demand, such drugs are used in ischaemic heart disease.

■ Cardiac ion channels are summarized in Table 4.2.

FURTHER READING

Reviews and chapters

Brown, A. M. (1991) Ion channels as G protein effectors. *News in Physiological Sciences*, **6**, 158–161.

Brown, H. and Kozlowski, R. (1997) *Physiology and Pharmacology of the Heart*, Blackwell Science, Oxford.

Caulfield, M. P. (1993) Muscarinic receptors – characterization, coupling and function. *Pharmacology Therapeutics*, **58**, 319–379.

DiFrancesco, D. (1993) Pacemaker mechanisms in cardiac tissue. *Annual Review of Physiology*, **55**, 451–467.

Hirst, G. D. S., Edwards, F. R., Bramich, N. J. and Klem, M. F. (1991) Neural control of cardiac pacemaker potentials. *News in Physiological Sciences*, **6**, 185–190.

Noble, D. (1995) Ionic mechanisms in cardiac electrical activity. In *Zipes and Jalife's Cardiac Electrophysiology* (see below), pp. 305–313.

Petit-Jacques, J., Bescond, J., Bois, P. and Lenfant, J. (1994) Particular sensitivity of the mammalian heart sinus node cells. *News in Physiological Sciences*, **9**, 77–79.

Sanguinetti, M. C. and Keating, M. T. (1997) Role of delayed rectifier potassium channels in cardiac repolarization and arrhythmias. *News in Physiological Sciences*, **12**, 152–157.

Simmerman, H. K. B. and Jones, L. R. (1998) Phospholamban: protein structure, mechanisms of action and role in cardiac function. *Physiology Reviews*, **78**, 921–947.

White, E. (1996) Length-dependent mechanisms in single cardiac cells (Mechano-electric aspects). *Experimental Physiology*, **81**, 885–897.

Zipes, D. P. and Jalife, J. (1995) *Cardiac Electrophysiology from Cell to Bedside*, W. B. Saunders, Philadelphia.

Research papers

Bassani, J. W. M., Yuan, W. and Bers, D. M. (1995) Fractional SR Ca release is regulated by trigger Ca and SR Ca content in cardiac myocytes. *American Journal of Physiology*, **268**, C1313–C1319.

Choate, J. K., Edwards, F. R., Hirst, G. D. S. and O'Shea, J. E. (1993) Effects of sympathetic nerve stimulation on the sinoatrial node of the guinea-pig. *Journal of Physiology*, **471**, 707–727.

DiFrancesco, D. and Mangoni, M. (1994) Modulation of single hyperpolarization-activated channels (i_f) by cAMP in the rabbit sino-atrial node. *Journal of Physiology*, **474**, 473–482.

Hussain, M. and Orchard, C. H. (1997) Sarcoplasmic reticulum Ca^{2+} content, L-type Ca^{2+} current and the Ca^{2+} transient in rat myocytes during β-adrenergic stimulation. *Journal of Physiology*, **505**, 385–402.

Kentish, J. C., McCloskey, D. T., Layland, J., Palmer, S., Leiden, J. M., Martin, A. F. and Solaro, R. J. (2001) Phosphorylation of troponin I by protein kinase A accelerates relaxation and crossbridge cycle kinetics in mouse ventricular muscle. *Circulation Research*, **88**, 1059–1065.

Lei, M., Brown, H. F. and Terrar, D. A. (2000) Modulation of delayed rectifier potassium current, i_K, by isoprenaline in rabbit isolated pacemaker cells. *Experimental Physiology*, **85**, 27–35.

Vinogradova, T. M., Bogdanov, K. Y. and Lakatta, E. G. (2002) β-Adrenergic stimulation modulates ryanodine receptor Ca^{2+} release during diastolic depolarization to accelerate pacemaker activity in rabbit sinoatrial nodal cells. *Circulation Research*, **90**, 73–79.

Wan, X., Bryant, S. M. and Hart, G. (2000) The effects of $[K^+]_o$ on regional differences in electrical characteristics of ventricular myocytes in guinea pigs. *Experimental Physiology*, **85**, 769–774.

Yano, M., Kohno, M., Tomoko, O., *et al.* (2000) Effect of milrinone on left ventricular relaxation and Ca^{2+} uptake function of cardiac sarcoplasmic reticulum. *American Journal of Physiology*, **279**, H1898–H1905.

Zaza, A., Robinson, R. B. and DiFrancesco, D. (1996) Basal responses of the L-type Ca^{2+} and hyperpolarization-activated (i_f) currents to autonomic agonists in the rabbit sino-atrial node. *Journal of Physiology*, **491**, 347–355.

CHAPTER 5

Electrocardiography and arrhythmias

Learning objectives

After reading this chapter you should be able to:

- Draw, label and scale a typical ECG trace and name the chosen lead (5.1).
- State the origin of the P, QRS and T waves, and the PR and ST intervals (5.2).
- Explain what a cardiac dipole is (5.4).
- Sketch out how the cardiac dipole changes with time in the frontal plane during ventricular depolarization (5.5).
- Explain why Leads I–III record different QRS patterns during the same systole (5.6).
- Give the meaning, mechanism and significance of:
  - sinus arrhythmia
  - ectopic beat
  - heart block
  - pathological tachycardia
  - atrial fibrillation
  - ventricular fibrillation.
- State the roles of afterdepolarization, vulnerable period, and re-entry circuits in arrhythmogenesis (5.8, 3.9).

5.1 Principle of electrocardiography

An electrocardiogram (ECG) is a record of potential changes at the skin surface that result from the depolarization and repolarization of heart muscle. The method was developed at the start of the 20th century by Willem Einthoven in Leiden, who invented the string galvanometer, and Augustus Waller in London, who applied the method to man, and whose demonstration to the Royal Society in 1909 provoked protests in Parliament (Figure 5.1). As noted in Section 4.3, the wave of excitation is spread through the myocardium by means of propagating currents in the extracellular fluid. The currents generate slight potential differences across the body surface, of the

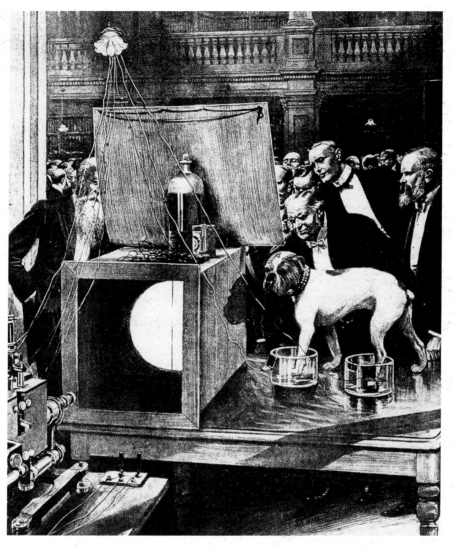

Figure 5.1 The electrocardiogram was demonstrated to the Royal Society by Waller's pet bulldog, Jimmie, in 1909. Jimmie has front and hind paws in pots of normal saline connected to a galvanometer. (From the *Illustrated London News*, May 22nd 1909.)

The Times newspaper of July 9, 1909 reported that Mr Ellis Griffith (MP for Anglesey) questioned the Secretary of State in Parliament over Waller's 'public experiment' on a dog with 'a leather strap with sharp nails secured around the neck, his feet being immersed in glass jars containing salts … connected by wires with galvanometers'. Had the Cruelty to Animals Act (1876) been contravened?
Mr Gladstone: 'I understand the dog stood for some time in water to which sodium chloride had been added or in other words a little common salt. If my honourable friend has ever paddled in the sea he will understand the sensation. (Laughter) The dog – a finely developed bulldog – was neither tied nor muzzled. He wore a leather collar ornamented with brass studs. Had the experiment been painful the pain would no doubt have been immediately felt by those nearest the dog. (Laughter).'
Mr MacNeill (Donegal South): 'Will the right honourable gentleman inform the person who furnished him with his jokes that there are members in this House who regard these experiments on dogs with abhorrence?' (Hear)
Mr Galdstone: 'I certainly shall not. The jokes, poor as they are, are mine own.' (Laughter and cheers) (From Waller, A.D. (1910) *Physiology the Servant of Medicine*, Hodder and Stoughton, London.)

order 1 mV. The potential difference can be recorded using metal electrodes in contact with the skin, connected to a sensitive voltmeter. The potential differences are recorded on a strip of moving paper or computer screen to produce the familiar ECG trace. Recording speed has become standardized at 25 mm/s or 0.2 s per large division.

The size of the skin potential depends on the size of the cardiac extracellular current, which in turn depends on the **mass of myocardium** that is activated. Consequently, the surface ECG detects the activity of atrial and ventricular muscle but not the tiny pacemaker–conduction system. The latter can only be recorded through a cardiac catheter.

5.2 Relation of ECG waves to cardiac action potentials

Figure 5.2 shows some typical human ECG recordings. There are three main deflections per cardiac cycle: the P wave, corresponding to atrial depolarization; the QRS complex, corresponding to ventricular depolarization; and the T wave, corresponding to ventricular repolarization. The trace returns to the baseline or **isoelectric state** during the PR interval and ST segment. The ECG waves are compared with the underlying cardiac action potentials in Figure 5.3 and with the events of the cardiac cycle in Figure 2.5.

The lettering of the waves has no particular meaning; letters were simply allotted alphabetically by Einthoven.

The P wave marks atrial excitation

The first electrical event to register is depolarization of the atrial myocytes, which produces a P wave lasting ~0.08 s. The P wave coincides with the upstrokes of the atrial action potentials. Atrial contraction occurs during the PR interval.

PR interval marks AV node delay

The interval between the start of the P wave and the start of the QRS complex is called the PR interval, even when it is strictly speaking a P–Q interval. The PR interval represents the time taken for excitation to spread through the atria, AV-node and His–Purkinje system into the ventricle. Much of the PR interval is caused by the delay at the AV node, which allows time for atrial systole to precede ventricular excitation. The PR interval should not exceed 0.2 s. Longer intervals indicate a defect in the conduction pathway called **heart block**, as in Figure 5.4c.

The ECG is isoelectric for much of the PR interval, even though there is a potential difference between the depolarized atria and the polarized ventricles. The recording is isoelectric because the insulating annulus fibrosus breaks the electrical circuitry shown in Figure 4.4, so no current flows.

Atrial repolarization does not register on the ECG, because it is sluggish (Figure 5.3) and asynchronous, and therefore does not generate sufficient extracellular current. It is often stated that the QRS complex obscures an atrial repolarization wave. However, recordings from patients with third degree heart block, where P waves are not followed by an 'obscuring' QRS wave (Figure 5.4e), prove that this explanation is a 'factoid' – something that is widely taught, eminently plausible, tenaciously believed, but demonstrably false!

QRS complex marks ventricular excitation

The rapid depolarization of a large mass of ventricular muscle produces a big deflection, the QRS complex

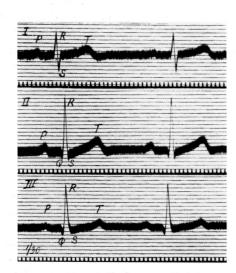

Figure 5.2 Human ECG, leads I–III. Lead II (60°) has the largest P, R and T waves. Lead I (0°) has the smallest R wave. This subject's electrical axis was between 60° and 90°. Ordinate divisions, 0.1 mV; time marks, 1/30th second. (From Sir Thomas Lewis's classic monograph *The Mechanism and Graphic Registration of the Human Heart*, 1920, Shaw and Sons, London. Thick baseline is an interference artefact of early string galvanometers, cf. Figure 5.4a.)

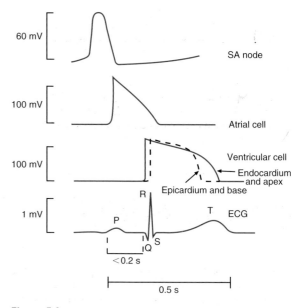

Figure 5.3 Timing of the ECG waves compared with intracellular recordings at different sites, including two sites in the ventricle (epicardium and endocardium). Note that the epicardium (dashed line) repolarizes before the endocardium. This is why the T wave is upright (Section 5.5).

(Figure 5.3). The Q wave is an initial downward spike, the R wave is an upward spike, and the S wave is a second downward spike. All three components are not necessarily present in every record – the complex may have just an RS configuration as in Lead I of Figure 5.2, or just a QR configuration. The complex normally lasts 0.1 s or less. Longer QRS complexes indicate bundle branch block or a ventricular ectopic beat (Figure 5.4b). The first heart sound follows just after the QRS complex (Figure 2.5).

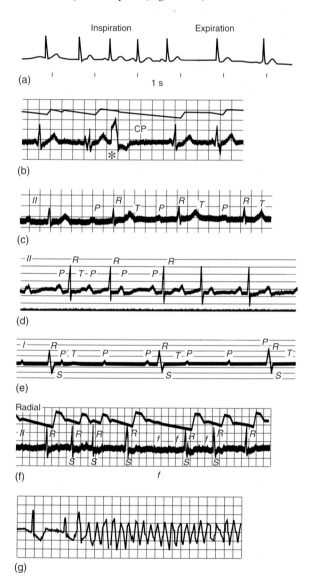

Figure 5.4 A cornucopia of arrhythmias. (a) Sinus arrhythmia in a healthy 19-year-old medical student. (b) The first example of an extrasystole (ventricular ectopic, asterisk) recorded by Einthoven (CP, compensatory pause). The upper trace is a radial pulse. (c–e) Progressive stages of heart block. (c) First-degree block. (d) Second-degree block. (e) Third-degree block. (f) Atrial fibrillation. (g) Ventricular fibrillation. (Records c–f are from Lewis' classic book, *The Mechanism and Graphic Registration of the Heart Beat*, Shaw, London, 1920.)

ST segment is shifted in ischaemic heart disease

The ST segment, from the end of the QRS wave to the start of the T wave, coincides with the plateau of the ventricular action potential and the rapid ejection phase. Since the ventricle is uniformly depolarized, no extracellular current is flowing and the ST segment is isoelectric. If a region of ventricular myocardium is damaged by ischaemia, however, the ST segment is no longer isoelectric. Immediately after **acute myocardial infarction** (a heart attack) the ST segment is elevated, while in **chronic myocardial ischaemia** the ST segment is depressed, as in the first beat in Figure 5.4g. The shifting of the ST segment is caused by **injury currents**. The myocytes in an ischaemic zone have a smaller resting potential and a smaller action potential than the surrounding healthy myocytes. The local differences in potential cause an injury current to flow, which shifts the level of the ST segment and/or the ECG baseline.

T wave marks repolarization

Ventricular repolarization is slower and less synchronous than depolarization, so it generates a broad, asymmetrical wave, the T wave (Figure 5.3). The second heart sound follows closely after the T wave.

Both the T wave and R wave are upright in most recording leads – which seems odd, given that repolarization is the electrical opposite of depolarization. The explanation (Section 5.5) is deferred until the concept of a 'cardiac dipole' has been introduced. Myocardial ischaemia not only shifts the ST segment but can also cause **T wave inversion** (e.g. first beat in Figure 5.4g).

5.3 Standard ECG leads

To understand the QRS complex we have to consider three things: (i) the position of the standard recording electrodes relative to the heart; (ii) the concept of the depolarizing ventricle as an electrical dipole; and (iii) the changes in dipole orientation as excitation spreads through the ventricles. Let us deal with the standard electrode positions first. The most basic ECG is recorded using three **limb electrodes**, one on each arm and one on the left leg (Figure 5.5). Wrists and ankles are usually used, but positioning makes no difference to the recording; the limb simply serves as a tube of conducting electrolyte solution (the extracellular fluid) connected to the torso.

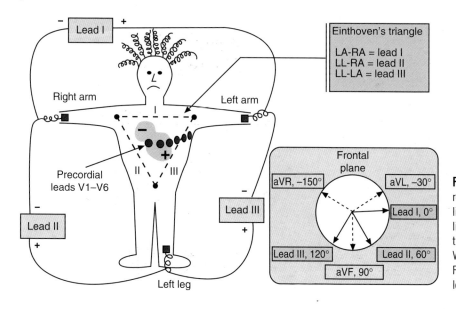

Figure 5.5 Electrode positions for recording a 12-lead ECG. The bipolar limb leads (I, II and III) and unipolar limb leads (aVL, aVR, aVF) record in the frontal plane. Precordial leads V1–V6 record in a transverse plane. For explanation of unipolar limb leads, see text.

There are three bipolar limb leads

Pairs of limb electrodes can be connected across a voltmeter in three different combinations, called the bipolar limb leads. If the left arm is connected to the positive terminal of the voltmeter and right arm to the negative terminal, this is a called a Lead I recording. If the potential on the left side of the body is more positive than on the right (due to the process of cardiac excitation), Lead I will record a positive potential. The three combinations are as follows.

Left arm (+) to Right arm (−) = LEAD I (0°)

Left leg (+) to Right arm (−) = LEAD II (60°)

Left leg (+) to Left arm (−) = LEAD III (120°).

The above wiring results in positive waves in all three leads.

Since each limb serves as an electrical conductor connected to the trunk, the three electrodes in effect record from the shoulders and the pelvis. They thus form a sensing triangle around the heart, called **Einthoven's triangle** (Figure 5.5). Each lead views the heart from a different angle in the frontal plane. Lead I, at the top of the triangle, is orientated horizontally across the chest. This angle is taken as zero. Lead II is angled at roughly 60° to Lead I, and Lead III at roughly 120°.

There are three unipolar limb leads

A cunning ruse allows the heart to be viewed from three more angles in the frontal plane using the same limb electrodes. The signal from several electrodes is fed simultaneously into one terminal of the voltmeter to produce an averaged signal coming, effectively, from the centre of Einthoven's triangle. When the signal from the left arm is connected to the other terminal, the angle of view is about −30°, i.e. from the left shoulder towards the centre of the chest (Figure 5.5). This is called unipolar limb Lead aVL; the 'a' stands for augmented. The three unipolar limb leads are:

Left arm to +ve terminal = aVL (−30°)

Right arm to +ve terminal = aVR (−150°)

Left foot to +ve terminal = aVF (90°).

Lead aVF is particularly useful for working out the electrical axis of the heart because it is at a right angle to Lead I (see later, Figure 5.6c).

There are six unipolar precordial leads

In clinical practice six skin electrodes are also placed at standardized points across the chest from the right side of the sternum to the left mid-axillary line. The six precordial leads view the heart in a plane perpendicular to the frontal plane. This is useful because the wave of excitation travels in 3 dimensions, not just the frontal plane 'seen' by the limb leads.

The ECG records an upward deflection when the positive pole of a potential difference is directed towards the left arm (Lead I) or left leg (Leads II and III), or towards any of the unipolar or precordial leads. We must therefore consider next the polarity of the heart during excitation.

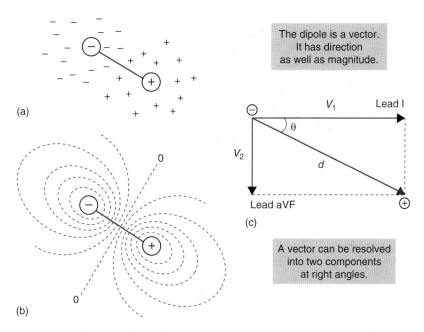

Figure 5.6 Properties of a dipole. (a) Representation of diffuse groups of opposite charge by a dipole (two points of electrical charge of opposite sign, such as the terminals of a battery). (b) Equipotential lines around a dipole. The zero potential runs across the middle of the dipole. (c) Resolution of dipole vector (red arrow) into two components at right angles. The length of the arrow is proportional to vector magnitude, d. The voltage difference V_1 detected by lead I depends on angle θ ($V_1 = d \cos \theta$). If V_1 and V_2 are drawn to match the sizes of the R waves in leads I and aVF, respectively, the *electrical axis* of the heart equals θ.

5.4 The cardiac dipole

Two clouds of charge can be represented by two poles

At any instant during the spread of excitation through the ventricle, there exists a resting zone with a diffuse cloud of positive extracellular charges and an excited region with a diffuse cloud of negative extracellular charges (Figure 5.6a). In the same way that a diffuse mass can be represented by a centre of gravity, so a diffuse charge can be represented as a single charge at its electrical centre or pole. Thus, during the spread of excitation the ventricles can be represented by one negative pole and one positive pole, i.e. by an electrical dipole.

The size of the ECG deflection produced by the dipole depends both on its **magnitude** and on its **orientation** relative to the recording lead, as explained next.

Detection of the dipole depends on the angle of recording leads

A dipole is surrounded by positive and negative potential fields, which grow weaker with increasing distance (Figure 5.6b). When the leads of a voltmeter are aligned with the two poles, the difference between the positive

The depolarizing ventricle is an electrical dipole

☐ For the 90 ms that it takes depolarization to spread through the ventricles, the excited region carries a cloud of negative extracellular charges (the negative pole) and the unexcited region a cloud of positive extracellular charges (the positive pole). A dipole thus forms across the heart.

☐ The dipole is biggest at mid-excitation, when roughly half the wall is negative and half positive.

☐ The direction in which the biggest dipole points is called the electrical axis of the heart. In the frontal plane it is typically 0–90° below the horizontal.

☐ An ECG lead detects the part of the dipole directed towards itself. Lead II, aligned at 60° to the horizontal, is roughly in line with the biggest dipole, so it usually has the biggest R wave.

☐ The dipole waxes and wanes, and swings anti-clockwise, as excitation sweeps through the ventricles. The changes in dipole size and orientation cause the Q, R and S waves.

and negative potential fields is recorded optimally. If, however, the leads are placed at right angles to the dipole, no potential difference is recorded, as is obvious from Figure 5.6b. Thus the potential difference

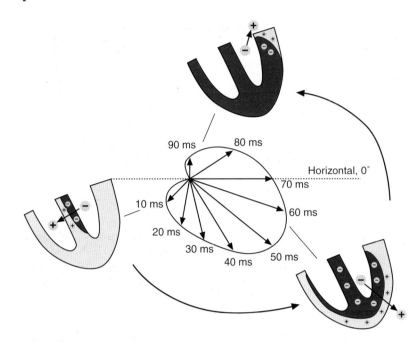

Figure 5.7 Changes in size and angle of cardiac dipole (straight arrows) with time during ventricular excitation. Grey areas are resting myocardium with positive *extracellular* charge; red areas are depolarized with negative extracellular charge. Cardiac vector rotates anticlockwise and waxes and wanes over ~90 ms. Electrical axis here is ~40°.

recorded by a voltmeter depends on the orientation of the recording electrodes relative to the dipole.

The dipole can be resolved into vectorial components

A dipole is a **vector quantity**; that is to say, it possesses direction as well as magnitude, just like a mechanical force. The symbol for a vector is an arrow whose length represents the size of the vector and whose direction represents the angle of the vector. Just as with a force vector, the electrical vector can be resolved into two components at right angles (Figure 5.6c). The voltmeter of the ECG registers **the magnitude of the component that is aligned with the recording leads**. This of course raises the question: in which direction does the cardiac dipole point?

5.5 The excitation sequence

Both the size and orientation of the cardiac dipole change continuously as excitation spreads through the ventricles. For simplicity, only the orientation in the frontal plane is described here, but it is worth repeating that the ventricles are three-dimensional bodies lying in an oblique, rotated position, so the dipole rarely lies purely in the frontal plane.

The dipole swings anticlockwise during depolarization

The first region to depolarize is the left side of the interventricular septum, which is activated by the left bundle branch (Figure 5.7). The resulting dipole is small because only a small mass is activated at this instant, and it is directed to the right, at about 120° to the horizontal. Next, the remaining septum and most of the endocardium depolarize; the epicardium is still polarized. The bulky left ventricle predominates and generates a large dipole pointing to the patient's left (your right) at about 60° to the horizontal. As excitation spreads, the last region to be reached by the advancing wave of depolarization is the base of the ventricles close to the annulus fibrosus, with the bulky posterior base of the left ventricle predominating. This results in a final dipole that is small and directed upwards. Thus the sequence of ventricular activation causes the cardiac vector to swing round in an anticlockwise direction, and to wax and wane in size. The entire sequence takes ~90 ms.

Repolarization occurs in reverse, creating an upright T wave

Why is the T wave upright? This seems odd, given that repolarization is a process of opposite sign to depolarization. The explanation is that the myocytes repolarize in roughly the reverse order to that in which they depolarized. In other words, the last myocytes to depolarize, namely the epicardium and the posterior base of the left ventricle (Figure 5.8, top), are the first to repolarize (Figure 5.8, bottom). This is because the myocytes in the epicardium and base have shorter action potentials than those in the endocardium and apex (Figure 5.3), due to differences in their K^+ channel populations. **Repolarization** begins in the

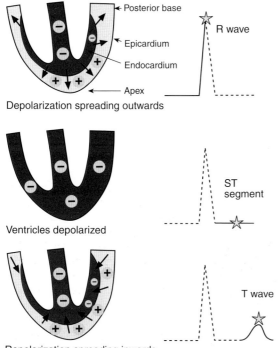

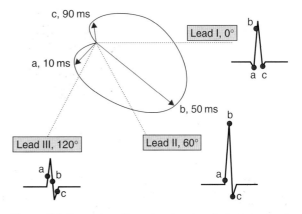

Figure 5.9 Illustration of how the changing dipole (red arrows) gives rise to different QRS complexes in different leads. The dipole is shown at three instants in time, a, b and c. The vectorial component recorded by leads I, II and III at each instant is marked by a red dot on the corresponding ECG trace.

Figure 5.8 Depolarization–repolarization pattern at three points in time – partial depolarization (red zone, R wave, *top*), full depolarization (ST segment, *middle*) and partial repolarization (grey zone, T wave, *bottom*). Signs refer to *extracellular* charge. Arrows show direction of advance of wavefront. As myocytes repolarize in reverse order to their depolarization sequence, the dipoles are in the same direction. Consequently, the T wave is upright.

epicardium and base, and spreads towards the endocardium, whereas **depolarization** does the reverse. As a result, the same polarity develops transiently across the heart during depolarization and repolarization (Figure 5.8). This is why the T wave is upright.

5.6 Why the QRS complex is complex

Knowing the lead and vector orientations, we can now work out why the QRS complex includes negative as well as positive waves, and why the same electrical event generates different shapes of QRS complex in different leads. Let us consider the dipole at three instants, the beginning, middle and end of ventricular excitation, as 'seen' by Leads I–III. In the example in Figure 5.9 the small initial dipole at ~120° (the little arrow) is directed obliquely away from Lead I. Resolving the vector, we find there is small component directed at 180°. Since its positive pole points away from Lead I (0°), Lead I records a small, negative deflection, i.e. a Q wave. At the same instant Lead III, which

detects the vectorial component directed at 120°, records a positive deflection, the start of an R wave.

After 50 ms the dipole has grown bigger and swung round to ~40°. The dipole now has a substantial vectorial component directed at Lead I, which records a substantial upward deflection, the R wave. Lead II registers an even larger R wave, because it 'looks' almost directly along the dipole axis at this instant. Thus **the biggest R wave is normally found in Lead II**. Lead III is almost at right angles to the dipole at this instant, and so Lead III records little potential difference.

By 90 ms the dipole has become smaller and swung round to about −100° in the case illustrated. Its vectorial components cause small negative deflections, i.e. S waves, in each lead.

Thus the same wave of ventricular excitation produced a QRS complex in Lead I, a small RS complex in Lead III, and a big RS complex in Lead II.

It is strongly emphasized that there are many variations on the illustrated QRS pattern, because the orientation of the heart and its dipole vary between individuals. For example, looking back at the subject in Figure 5.2, the R wave is biggest in Lead II but is bigger in Lead III than Lead I. This indicates a more vertically orientated electrical axis, and brings us to the issue of the electrical axis of the heart.

5.7 Electrical axis of the heart

The direction of the largest dipole in the frontal plane is called the electrical axis of the heart. In the case illustrated in Figure 5.9 the electrical axis is approximately 40° below the horizontal. The electrical axis can be calculated graphically from the size of the R waves in Leads I and aVF as shown in Figure 5.6c. More commonly the electrical axis is estimated roughly in the clinic as follows. (i) Compare the size of the R wave in Leads I–III. If the largest R wave is in Lead II, the electrical axis is closer to 60° than to 0° or 120°. (ii) Look for the lead with the smallest QRS complex and R and S waves of nearly equal height. This lead must be roughly at right angles to the electrical axis (e.g. Lead I in Figure 5.2).

The range of the normal electrical axis is wide, from −30° to +110°. The axis depends partly on the anatomical orientation of the heart, being more vertical in a tall person with a narrow thorax than in a short, broad-chested individual. The axis also becomes more vertical during each inspiration, because the descending diaphragm tugs on the pericardium and drags down the apex.

The electrical axis also depends on the relative thickness of the walls of the right and left ventricles. Hypertrophy of the left ventricle due to cardiomyopathy shifts the electrical axis to the left (**left axis deviation**). Hypertrophy of the right ventricle due to pulmonary disease produces **right axis deviation**.

5.8 Arrhythmia and arrhythmic mechanisms

The ECG is invaluable for the diagnosis of cardiac disorders such as myocardial ischaemia, ventricular hypertrophy and irregular rhythms (arrhythmia). Arrhythmias range from the benign and perfectly normal, through pathological but relatively harmless 'palpitations', to serious, life-threatening disorders. Many pathological arrhythmias, particularly in ischaemic heart disease, are triggered by **delayed afterdepolarization** following SR Ca^{2+} store overload (Section 3.9) and are sustained by a **re-entry (circus) mechanism** (see below).

Sinus arrhythmia

Sinus arrhythmia is normal. It is a regular physiological slowing of the heart during expiration and speeding up during inspiration. Sinus arrhythmia is especially marked in children and young adults. In the medical student of Figure 5.4a the heart rate slowed from 92 min^{-1} during each inspiration to 52 min^{-1} during each expiration. The inspiratory tachycardia helps to preserve cardiac output in the face of a fall in left ventricular stroke volume during inspiration. Stroke volume falls during inspiration because the

return of blood to the left heart is reduced by the inspiratory expansion of the pulmonary vascular bed.

Sinus arrhythmia is caused by a phasic rise in vagal activity during expiration, which slows the pacemaker. The phasic increase in vagal activity persists even when breathing is paralysed, because it is driven primarily by an input from the respiration centre to the vagal motor nuclei in the brainstem (Figure 16.15).

Ventricular ectopic beats

Aberrant myocytes may occasionally fire before the SA node, triggering a premature beat called an ectopic beat or extra systole. If the ectopic trigger is located in the ventricle (as opposed to the atria), the resulting QRS wave is broad and ill synchronized, because the excitation has not been distributed through the His–Purkinje system (Figure 5.4b). Moreover, the ensuing ill-co-ordinated contraction fails to eject blood, as shown by the blood pressure trace in Figure 5.4b. When the next normal impulse from the SA node arrives, the ventricular myocytes are still in their **refractory period**, so no contraction is elicited. This results in a long interval before the next normal beat, called the **compensatory pause**. The patient often notices this, commenting that 'My heart keeps missing a beat'. Occasional ectopic beats are not uncommon in normal individuals. Ventricular ectopics are increasingly common after a heart attack, probably due to **delayed afterdepolarizations** (DADs) in the ischaemic region (Section 3.9).

Heart block

The AV node, main bundle or one of the bundle branches may fail to transmit electrical excitation properly, due to ischaemic heart disease or fibrosis of the closely adjacent atrioventricular valves. Three degrees of main bundle block are readily diagnosed by ECG:

1 **First-degree heart block** is a lengthening of the PR interval, e.g. to 0.45 s in Figure 5.4c. This is caused by a slowing of conduction from the AV node to ventricular myocardium.

2 **Second-degree heart block** is an intermittent failure of excitation to pass from the atria to the ventricles. In Figure 5.4d there are four labelled P waves but only three corresponding QRS complexes. The PR interval lengthens with each beat, until a point is reached (at the 3rd P wave in this particular case) where transmission fails. The sequence then repeats.

3 In **third-degree heart block** electrical transmission from the atria to the ventricles fails

completely, so the atria and ventricles beat at entirely independent rates. In Figure 5.4e the atria (P waves) are beating at $72\,min^{-1}$, driven by the SA node, but the ventricles are beating at $30\,min^{-1}$, driven by a latent pacemaker in the bundle of His or Purkinje system, which is no longer dominated by the SA node. Such patients may experience sudden faints called **Stokes–Adams attacks** and will need an artificial pacemaker.

Re-entry (circus) mechanisms can cause/maintain pathological tachycardias

Sometimes an abnormal myocardial conduction pathway causes a wave of excitation to travel in a never-ending circle (**circus**, Figure 5.10) or spiral. Myocytes emerging from their refractory period find themselves at once re-excited by the return of the excitation wave, a process called **re-entry**. Re-entry mechanisms probably account for many tachycardias, and for maintaining fibrillation (see below) after it has been triggered by afterdepolarizations.

The unforgettably named **Wolff–Parkinson–White syndrome** is a well-documented example of a re-entrant arrhythmia. The syndrome is characterized by episodes of paroxysmal tachycardia or 'palpitations' at over 200 beats/min. The syndrome is caused by an extra electrical connection across the annulus fibrosus, besides the bundle of His, called the bundle of Kent. Under certain circumstances the wave of ventricular excitation re-enters the atria through the bundle of Kent and re-excites the AV node prematurely, producing a self-perpetuating tachycardia. Not only is the sensation of 'palpitations' alarming, but also the reduction in the diastolic filling interval leads to a fall in cardiac output, causing light-headedness and even collapse.

Treatment is aimed at disrupting the timing of re-entry by the use of inhibitors of fast Na^+ channels, (**procainamide, quinidine**), or of L-type Ca^{2+} channels (e.g. **verapamil**), or activators of hyperpolarizing K^+ channels (**adenosine**, Section 4.8).

A little applied physiology can sometimes halt a pathological tachycardia. **Massage of the carotid sinuses**, a reflexogenic area just below the angle of the jaw (Figure 16.2), elicits a reflex increase in vagal parasympathetic drive to the heart. This slows the pacemaker and reduces the conduction velocity through the AV node, terminating the tachycardia.

Atrial fibrillation

Fibrillation is an uncoordinated, repetitive excitation of myocytes that causes a writhing movement of

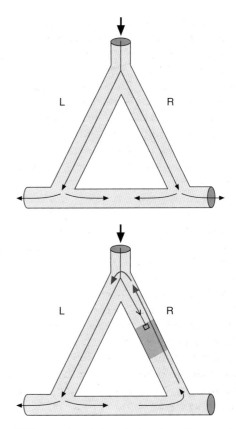

Figure 5.10 Circus (re-entry) mechanism of arrhythmogenesis. (*Top*) Normal spread of excitation. The divide might be around a blood vessel, for example. (*Bottom*) Pathology, for example ischaemia or chronic failure, causes a long refractory period and slow conduction velocity in the right-hand fibres (R). As excitation arrives at R, it finds the myocytes refractory from the previous impulse, so it propagates no further. By the time excitation has spread down L, across and up R retrogradely, R is no longer refractory. R conducts the impulse back up to the junction with L, which is re-excited (re-entry), setting up a self-perpetuating loop or 'circus'.

the wall with no effective ejection of blood. It is thought to result from multiple local re-entry circuits within the wall. Atrial fibrillation is a relatively mild condition in itself, quite common in the elderly and compatible with a sedentary life. Small, irregular oscillations called 'f' waves replace the normal P wave in the ECG (Figure 5.4f). Excitation is transmitted sporadically to the ventricles, resulting in a highly characteristic and easily diagnosed radial pulse, which is **irregularly irregular** in timing and variable in amplitude, as shown by the upper trace in Figure 5.4f. One of the chief dangers of atrial fibrillation is the formation of an organized blood clot or **thrombus** in a stagnant region of the atrium. Atrial thrombi can embolize, i.e. float away downstream, with serious consequences.

CONCEPT BOX 6

Afterdepolarization and re-entry underlie arrhythmia

☐ In ischaemic heart disease the overloaded SR calcium store may discharge in early diastole. This increases Ca^{2+} expulsion by the $3Na^+-1Ca^{2+}$ exchanger. The net positive charge transferred into the cell by the exchanger causes an afterdepolarization.

☐ A delayed afterdepolarization (DAD) can reach threshold, triggering an action potential and ventricular ectopic beat (extra systole).

☐ In the latter half of the T wave ('vulnerable period') an ectopic readily triggers ventricular fibrillation.

☐ Multiple local circus pathways develop readily in the vulnerable period, because some myocytes have repolarized while others have not. Ectopic excitation can travel through the repolarized myocytes and excite myocytes emerging from their refractory period, which re-excite the first group (re-entry), and so on. Re-entry underlies fibrillation.

Ventricular fibrillation

Fibrillation of the ventricle wall is a common, fatal sequel to myocardial ischaemia, anaesthetic overdose or electrocution. In Figure 5.4g, the existence of myocardial ischaemic disease is evident from two characteristic ECG abnormalities in the first two cardiac cycles on the record, namely ST segment depression and T wave inversion. After the second sinus beat a ventricular ectopic arises during the latter half of the T wave, which is called the **vulnerable period**. Ventricular ectopics in ischaemic hearts are commonly triggered by **delayed afterdepolarizations** (**DADs**, Section 3.9). The ventricle is particularly vulnerable to fibrillation if an ectopic site fires during the latter half of the T wave, because some of the myocytes have repolarized while others are still in their refractory period; consequently, multiple local circus pathways are readily triggered. These create numerous rapid, uncoordinated electrical waves and an ineffective rippling motion of the ventricle wall. With no cardiac output, death follows within minutes. 'Cardioversion' by a DC electric shock to the chest wall sometimes succeeds in restoring sinus rhythm.

frontal plane (three bipolar limb leads, three unipolar limb leads) and transverse plane (six precordial leads) of the chest.

■ The P wave is caused by atrial depolarization, the QRS complex by ventricular depolarization, and the T wave by ventricular repolarization.

■ The PR interval is due chiefly to slow transmission through the atrioventricular node and should not exceed 0.2 s in humans. The delay allows atrial systole to precede ventricular systole.

■ The isoelectric ST segment corresponds to the plateau of the ventricular action potential. It is displaced in ischaemic heart disease by injury currents.

■ The T wave is upright because repolarization occurs in reverse sequence to depolarization, due to the short action potentials of epicardial and basal myocytes.

■ When the ventricle is in the process of activation, its negative and positive charges represent an electrical dipole.

■ The QRS complex differs in each lead because each lead detects the dipole from a different angle. Lead I (left arm−right arm) is horizontal (0°), Lead II (left leg−right arm) is at 60° and Lead III (left leg−left arm) at 120° in the frontal plane. These three bipolar limb leads form Einthoven's triangle.

■ The three components Q (down), R (up) and S (2nd down wave) are caused by changes in the size and direction of the cardiac dipole as excitation spreads first across the interventricular septum, then out through the endocardium, and finally into the epicardium and base of the ventricle. The dipole is dominated by the left ventricle and, viewed in the frontal plane, rotates anti-clockwise, waxing and waning as it does so.

■ The angle of the largest dipole, usually 0−90°, is called the electrical axis of the heart.

■ The ECG is used to diagnose ischaemia, hypertrophy and cardiac arrhythmia. The principal mechanisms of arrhythmogenesis are conduction impairment (heart block), afterdepolarizations due to ischaemic overload of the SR calcium store circus (ectopic beats and trigger for fibrillation) and re-entrant circuits (tachycardias and fibrillation). Afterdepolarizations during the vulnerable period (late T wave) may trigger multiple re-entry circuits that cause fatal ventricular fibrillation.

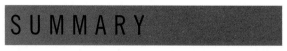

SUMMARY

■ The 12-lead electrocardiogram is a recording of small potential differences (~1 mV) across the

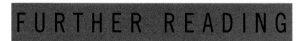

FURTHER READING

Billman, G. E. (1992) Cellular mechanisms for ventricular fibrillation. *News in Physiological Science*, **7**, 254−259.

Carmeliet, E. (1999) Cardiac ionic currents and acute ischemia: from channels to arrhythmias. *Physiological Reviews*, **79**, 917–1017.

Jalife, J. (2000) Ventricular fibrillation: mechanisms of initiation and maintenance. *Annual Review of Physiology*, **62**, 25–50.

Lilly, L. S. (ed.) (1997) *Pathophysiology of Heart Disease*, 2nd Edition, Williams and Wilkins, Baltimore.

Rowlands, D. J. (1996) The electrocardiogram. In *Oxford Textbook of Medicine*, 3rd Edition (eds Weatherall, D. J., Leddingham, J. G. G. and Warrell, D. A.), Oxford University Press, Oxford, pp. 2182–2191.

Scher, A. M. and Spach, M. S. (1979) Cardiac depolarization, repolarization and the electrocardiogram. In *Handbook of Physiology, Cardiovascular System*, Vol. 1, *The Heart* (ed. Berne, R. M.), American Physiological Society, Bethesda, pp. 357–392.

Volk, T., Nguyen, T. H-D., Schultz, J-H., Faulhaber, J. and Ehmke, H. (2001) Regional alterations of repolarizing K^+ currents among the left ventricular free wall of rats with ascending aortic stenosis. (Epicardial versus endocardial potentials and T wave.) *Journal of Physiology*, **530**, 443–455.

Waldo, A. L. and Wit, A. L. (1993) Mechanisms of cardiac arrhythmias. *Lancet*, **341**, 1189–1193.

Zipes, D. P. and Jalife, J. (eds) (1995) *Cardiac Electrophysiology: From Cell to Bedside*, 2nd Edition, W. B. Saunders, Philadelphia.

CHAPTER 6

Control of stroke volume and cardiac output

Learning objectives

After reading this chapter you should be able to:

- Outline the mechanisms behind the length–tension relation (6.2–6.3).
- State the Starling law of the heart and its effect on stroke volume (6.4).
- Draw a ventricular function (Starling) curve and define stroke work (6.4–6.5).
- List the chief factors influencing central venous pressure (6.6).
- State the roles of the Frank–Starling mechanism in man (6.7).
- Use Laplace's law to explain why cardiac distension is harmful in heart failure (6.8).
- State the direct and secondary effects of arterial pressure on stroke volume (6.9).
- Define contractility and draw a graph to show how altered contractility affects the Starling curve (6.10).
- List the effects of sympathetic stimulation on cardiac performance (6.10).
- Draw a ventricular pressure–volume loop and sketch the effect of (i) increased filling pressure; (ii) increased contractility; (iii) increased arterial pressure (afterload); and (iv) exercise (6.5, 6.10).
- Name two important inotropic hormones and two classes of inotropic drug (6.11).
- Outline the negative inotropic and arrhythmogenic effects of acute myocardial ischaemia (6.12).
- Outline the co-ordinated cardiac and peripheral vascular responses to exercise (6.13).
- Explain the tight link between myocardial performance and coronary blood flow (6.14).

6.1 Overview

The cardiac output of a resting human adult is 4−7 l/min, depending on body size. The **cardiac index**, which takes size into account, is 3 l/min per square metre of body surface area. The latter is ~1.8 m^2 for a 70 kg adult.

The cardiac output is continually adjusted in response to external and internal events. For example, sleep reduces cardiac output by ~10% and standing reduces it by ~20%. A heavy meal, excitement or stress can increase the output by 20−30% and pregnancy raises it by up to 40%. Heavy exercise can raise the output 4−6 fold, though the increase is much less in ischaemic hearts (Table 6.1).

Changes in output usually involve changes in both heart rate and stroke volume. The control of **heart rate** by autonomic nerves was described in Chapter 4. In this chapter we concentrate on the control of stroke volume and on the co-ordination of changes in stroke volume, heart rate and peripheral blood vascular tone to raise cardiac ouput.

Table 6.1 Output of human heart (l/min ± standard deviation).

	Rest	Exercise
Normal adult	6.0 (±1.3)	17.5 (±6.0)
Coronary artery disease	5.7 (±1.5) *	11.3 (±4.3)

* The output of the diseased heart was within the normal range at rest but became inadequate during exercise to 85% of maximum heart rate or to onset of angina. (After Rerych, S. K., Scholz, P. M., Newman, G. E., *et al.* (1978) *Annals of Surgery*, **187**, 449–458.)

Stroke volume is influenced by two opposing factors, namely the energy of contraction and the arterial pressure that must be overcome to expel the blood (Figure 6.1). A highly energetic contraction produces a large stroke volume. A high arterial pressure, on the other hand, opposes ejection and reduces the stroke volume in the absence of compensatory changes.

The **energy of contraction** can be raised by two mechanisms. (i) Stretching the myocardium in diastole, through a rise in end-diastolic pressure, enhances the contractile energy. This is called **Starling's law of the heart**. (ii) The strength of contraction at a given stretch can be increased by sympathetic stimulation and circulating adrenaline. This is called an increase in **contractility**.

Arterial pressure depresses stroke volume because ejection cannot begin until ventricular pressure exceeds aortic pressure. If arterial pressure is high, much of the contractile energy is consumed in raising ventricular blood pressure during the isovolumetric phase, leaving less energy for the ejection phase.

Stroke volume thus depends on the interplay of three factors:

- diastolic stretch, which depends on venous filling pressure;

- contractility, which is regulated by sympathetic fibres and hormones, and reduced by cardiac disease;

- arterial pressure, which opposes ejection.

This chapter considers first the effect of stretch (Sections 6.2−6.8), then arterial pressure (Section 6.9), then contractility (Sections 6.10−6.12).

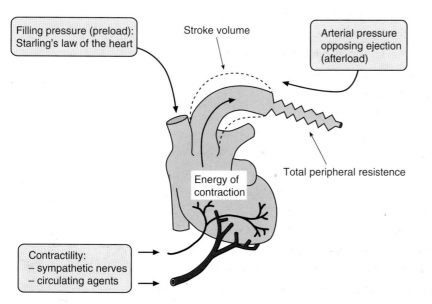

Figure 6.1 Schematic representation of factors regulating stroke volume. Peripheral resistance is represented by the narrow tube in series with the aorta.

6.2 Contractile properties of isolated myocardium

The response of an isolated strip of myocardium to stretch is fundamental to understanding the behaviour of the more geometrically complicated intact heart. Papillary muscle is often used *in vitro* because its fibres are fairly straight. These studies led to the introduction of the terms 'preload' and 'afterload'.

Preload increases active force; the isometric length–tension relation

A relaxed muscle can be stretched to a known length by hanging a weight from it, called the **preload** (Figure 6.2). If the ends of the muscle are anchored at the preloaded length to rigid points, electrical excitation causes active tension (force) to develop without shortening. This is called an **isometric contraction** (iso-, same; -metric, length). Remarkably, the active tension increases with stretch (Figures 6.2a, 6.3). This effect is called the **length–tension relation**.

In the intact ventricle the **diastolic filling pressure** governs fibre stretch and preload. **Isovolumetric contraction** is roughly equivalent to isometric contraction. The increase in contractile energy with the distension in an intact heart is called **Starling's law of the heart** (Section 6.4).

Afterload reduces shortening; the isotonic afterload–shortening relation

To study shortening *in vitro*, one end of the muscle is left free. As the muscle begins to shorten, it lifts a weight called the **afterload**. This ensures that the

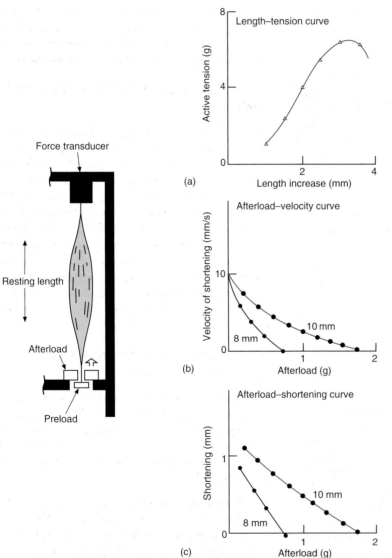

Figure 6.2 Contractile behaviour of isolated cat papillary muscle. Preload weight sets resting length. If preload is clamped, contraction is isometric (no shortening, (a)). If the muscle is allowed to shorten and lift a second weight (the afterload), contraction is isotonic. Isotonic contractions are shown for 8 and 10 mm initial stretches. (After Sonnenblick, E. H. (1962) *American Journal of Physiology*, **202**, 931–939.)

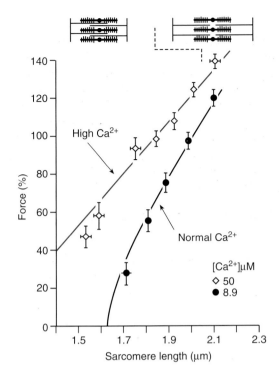

Figure 6.3 Effect of resting sarcomere length on contractile force of 'skinned' myocardium. The sarcolemma has been permeabilized by a detergent and exposed to a physiological Ca^{2+} concentration (8.9 μM) or a saturating one that produces maximal contracture at each length (50 μM). The lower but steeper curve resembles that of intact, unskinned cardiac muscle. Sketches at top show change in resting actin–actin overlap with stretch. (From Kentish, J. C., ter Keurs, H. E. D. J., Ricciardi, L., Bucx, J. J. J. and Noble, M. I. M. (1986) *Circulation Research*, **58**, 755–768, by permission.)

muscle contracts at a constant, known tension (**isotonic contraction**; iso-, same; -tonic, force). An increase in the afterload reduces both the rate and degree of shortening (Figure 6.2). This is called the **afterload–shortening relation**. If the starting length is increased by a higher preload, the isotonic contraction achieves a greater velocity and degree of shortening (Figure 6.2, red curves), because stretch increases contractile energy.

In an intact heart the moment when the ventricle pushes open the outlet valve is equivalent to the moment when isolated muscle begins to move the afterload. The **arterial pressure** is one of the determinants of afterload. The **ejection phase** is roughly equivalent to isotonic shortening; and the **pump-function curve** (Section 6.9) is roughly equivalent to the afterload–shortening relation. The qualifier 'roughly' is used because the afterload is not actually constant in an intact heart; it waxes and wanes as arterial pressure peaks and falls. This is called an **auxotonic contraction**. The afterload–shortening

relation underlies the use of arterial pressure-reducing drugs to improve the stroke volume of failing hearts.

6.3 Mechanisms of length–tension relation

Sarcomere stretch leads to increased contractile energy

Measurements of sarcomere length in living myocytes by laser diffraction show that each sarcomere is lengthened by preload. There is a steep relation between diastolic sarcomere length and contractile force, reaching maximum force at sarcomere lengths of 2.2–2.3 μm (Figure 6.3). Beyond 2.3 μm the contractile force decays. It is difficult to stretch sarcomeres beyond 2.3 μm due to increasing stiffness, so sarcomere length probably never exceeds 2.3 μm *in vivo*. In intact hearts at normal end-diastolic pressures, the sarcomere length is less than 2.2 μm. Therefore **myocytes normally operate on the ascending part of the length–tension curve**.

Stretch can raise contractile force without raising Ca^{2+}

Figure 6.4 shows the effect of diastolic stretch on twitch contractions and on the simultaneous cytosolic Ca^{2+} transients. Stretch causes an immediate increase in contractile force without any increase in the free cytosolic Ca^{2+} transient – in complete contrast to the effect of catecholamines (Sections 3.8, 4.5). If the stretch is maintained, there is a further, slow increase in force over ~5 minutes which *is* associated with increased Ca^{2+} transients. The immediate rise in force accounts for 60% of the eventual response and is the basis of the length–tension relation. The later, Ca^{2+}-mediated **slow force response** underlies the **Anrep effect** in intact hearts (see later).

Stretch reduces filament overlap and raises Ca^{2+} sensitivity

How does stretch increase contractile force without an increase in the Ca^{2+} transient? Two mechanisms contribute, namely changes in filament overlap and increased sensitivity to Ca^{2+}. The latter mechanism is the more important one in cardiac muscle, unlike skeletal muscle.

1 **Filament interference.** Since each actin filament is 1 μm long, the opposed filaments overlap in sarcomeres shorter than 2.0 μm. This interferes with actin–myosin crossbridge formation. At even

shorter lengths, <1.6 μm, the myosin filament hits the Z lines. Stretch between 1.6 μm and ~2 μm reduces these interference problems (Figure 6.3, top) and thus enhances contractile force. This is an incomplete explanation, however, because the same interference effects occur in skeletal muscle yet the **cardiac muscle is much more sensitive to stretch than skeletal muscle**. The length–tension curve is much steeper for cardiac than skeletal muscle (Figure 6.5). An additional, more important mechanism must therefore exist in cardiac muscle.

2 **Increased sensitivity to Ca^{2+}.** The upper curve of Figure 6.3 shows the length–tension relation for cardiac muscle when all the crossbridges available at a given sarcomere length are activated by a supra-normal Ca^{2+} level. The less steep increase in active tension with length resembles that in skeletal muscle and is due to the filament interference effect. At a physiological Ca^{2+} level (lower curve), the active tension is smaller because only a fraction of the potential crossbridges is activated; but the force increases much more steeply with stretch, approaching closer and

closer to the full activation line. This shows that **stretch increases the fraction of crossbridges activated by a given Ca^{2+} level**. In other words, stretch increases the sensitivity of the contractile machinery to Ca^{2+}.

The effect of stretch on Ca^{2+} sensitivity is confirmed by a plot of force versus Ca^{2+} concentration at two different stretches (Figure 6.6). Stretch shifts the curve to the left; in the stretched myocyte, less Ca^{2+} is needed to produce 50% of maximal tension.

The cause of length-dependent Ca^{2+} sensitivity is controversial

Some evidence favours a **lattice spacing hypothesis** to explain the length-dependence of Ca^{2+} sensitivity. Since cell volume is fixed, any increase in length reduces the cell diameter. This reduces the side-to-side separation of the actin and myosin filaments, which may allow crossbridges to form more readily. In support of this hypothesis, hyperosmotic solutions that reduce the myocyte diameter also increase their contractile force. Other evidence indicates, however, that the magnitude of this effect may be too small to explain the physiological Ca^{2+} sensitization. We have to conclude that the mechanisms underlying the stretch effect are still unclear.

Having defined the properties of isolated muscle, we can now turn to the intact heart and the role of stretch in regulating stroke volume.

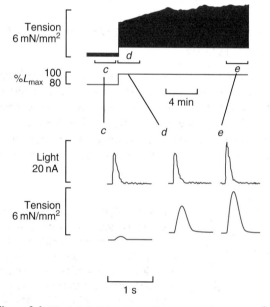

Figure 6.4 Effect of stretch on isometric contractile force and Ca^{2+} transients in isolated papillary muscle. The muscle was stretched from 80% of optimum length (L_{max}) to 100%. Note immediate, large increase in force at d, then a smaller, slow force response. Averaged light signals from the Ca^{2+}-sensitive protein aequorin show that the big initial response, d, does not involve a change in the Ca^{2+} transient, whereas the slow force response at e does (Anrep effect). (After Allen, D. G., Nichols, C. G. and Smith, G. L. (1988) *Journal of Physiology*, **406**, 359–370.)

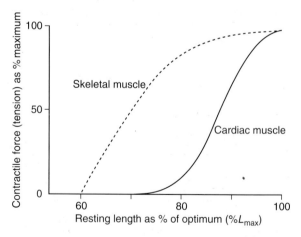

Figure 6.5 Relation between resting length and active tension for cardiac muscle and skeletal muscle. The relation is much steeper for cardiac than skeletal muscle at physiological lengths (80–100%, L_{max}), even though filament overlap is the same. The Ca^{2+} sensitivity of cardiac fibres increases with stretch. (Adapted from Fuchs, F. and Smith, S. S. (2001); see Further Reading.)

6.4 The Frank–Starling law of the heart

The isovolumetric contracting heart

The isometric length–tension relation (Figure 6.5) operates in intact hearts too, as the German physiologist Otto Frank demonstrated in a seminal experiment in 1895. The aorta of a frog heart was ligated so that the contraction was purely isovolumetric, similar to an isometric contraction. When the ventricle wall was stretched by increasing the diastolic fluid volume (raised preload), systolic pressure generation increased (Figure 6.7a). Therefore, **the energy of contraction of the intact heart increases as a function of diastolic distension** (Figure 6.7b, red curve). The isovolumetric contraction curve of Figure 6.7b

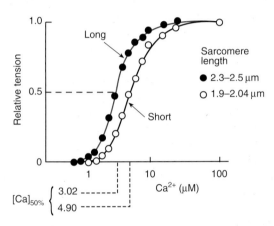

Figure 6.6 Effect of stretch on contractile response to calcium. Ca^{2+} was varied in the solution bathing chemically skinned rat ventricular muscle at submaximal (right) and maximal sarcomere lengths (left). Stretch reduced the Ca^{2+} concentration need for 50% maximum contraction, $[Ca]_{50\%}$. (From Hibberd, M. G. and Jewell, B. R. (1982) *Journal of Physiology*, **329**, 527–540.)

will be shown later to form the maximum upper limit of a pressure–volume loop (Section 6.5).

The ejecting heart

A more physiological state, namely ventricular ejection, was studied by Ernest Starling and his co-workers in London at the start of the 20th century. In their classic experiment the isolated heart and lungs of a dog were perfused with warm oxygenated blood from a venous reservoir (Figure 6.8). The height of the reservoir controlled the central venous pressure (CVP), which is the pressure at the entrance to the right atrium. This determines the right ventricular end-diastolic pressure (RVEDP) and resting distension. **Changes in CVP thus represent changes in right ventricular muscle preload**. Similarly, pulmonary vein pressure governs left ventricle end-diastolic pressure and preload. A useful general term for these pressures is **filling pressure**. Since aortic pressure influences afterload, it was held constant by a variable resistance called a Starling resistor. The combined stroke volume of the two ventricles was recorded by a bell cardiometer. Being isolated and denervated, the heart–lung preparation was free from any extrinsic nervous or hormonal influences. The chief findings were as follows.

Raising central venous pressure increases stroke volume

When CVP is raised, the RVEDP and volume increase, which stretches the right ventricle fibres. The ventricle develops a greater contractile energy and ejects a greater stroke volume. The left ventricle quickly follows suit, because the increased right ventricular output raises the pressure in the pulmonary

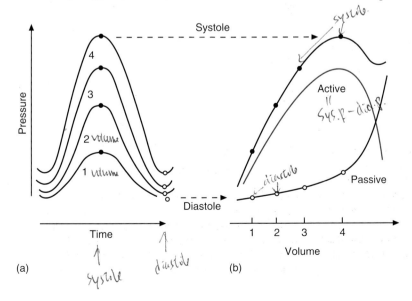

Figure 6.7 Effect of diastolic volume on energy of contraction, as measured by systolic pressure in an isovolumetric frog ventricle (aorta ligated). (a) Active pressure generated between diastole (open circles) and systole (closed circles) increases as ventricular volume is raised from 1 to 4 (arbitrary units). (b) Effect of volume plotted out. Bottom curve shows passive pressure–volume relation: note the increasing stiffness (upswing) as the ventricle is distended. Top curve shows systolic pressure as a function of diastolic volume. Red curve shows pressure generated actively, i.e. systolic pressure minus diastolic pressure. (After Otto Frank's seminal experiment of 1895.)

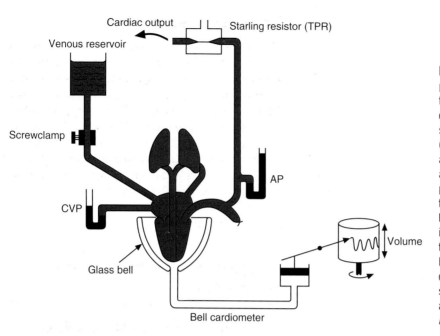

Figure 6.8 Isolated dog heart–lung preparation of Starling. The height of the venous reservoir and the screw-clamp regulated central venous pressure (CVP). CVP and arterial pressure (AP) were measured by manometers and AP was held constant by a variable resistance equivalent to the total peripheral resistance (TPR). Ventricular volume was measured by Henderson's bell cardiometer (an inverted glass bell), which is attached to the atrioventricular groove by a rubber diaphragm. Beat-by-beat volume changes were recorded on a rotating smoked drum. (After Knowlton, F. P. and Starling, E. H. (1912) *Journal of Physiology*, **44**, 206–219.)

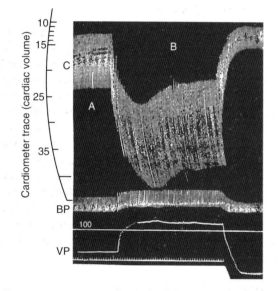

Figure 6.9 Volume of the ventricles recorded beat-by-beat in the isolated heart–lung preparation; note the inverted volume scale (ml): diastolic volume is at the bottom of the volume excursion, systolic volume is at the top. Stroke volume is the distance from top to bottom of the trace. There was a 64% rise in stroke volume upon raising central venous pressure (VP) from 9 cmH$_2$0 (period A) to 15 cmH$_2$0 (period B). There is a modest reduction in ventricular distention later on without any fall in stroke volume. This indicates a small rise in contractility (the *Anrep effect*). (From the original smoked-drum recordings of Patterson, S. W., Piper, H. and Starling, E. H. (1914) *Journal of Physiology*, **48**, 465–511, by permission.)

The ventricular function curve reaches a plateau in humans

A plot of stroke volume versus filling pressure is called a ventricular function curve or Starling curve (Figure 6.10). The stroke volume increases as a curvilinear function of filling pressure from zero to 10 mmHg – the **ascending limb** of the curve. In the human heart *in vivo* the curve reaches a **plateau** above 10 mmHg filling pressure (Figure 6.10b). A human subject in a standing or sitting position has a left ventricular end-diastolic pressure (LVEDP) of 4–5 mmHg, so the human heart is generally on the ascending limb. A supine human has a higher LVEDP, 8–9 mmHg, due to a redistribution of blood from the lower body, and the heart is then operating close to the plateau.

In the isolated dog hearts studied by Starling the stroke volume declined at CVPs above 25 mmHg, producing a **descending limb** on the ventricular function curve (Figure 6.10a). It is unlikely, however, that human hearts ever reach the descending limb. Stroke volume declines in the over-distended isolated heart because the atrioventricular valves begin to leak and because the reduced curvature of the wall impairs the conversion of wall tension into blood pressure (Laplace's law, see later).

A bewildering variety of plots are called 'ventricular function curves'. Any graph whose ordinate (y-axis) is a measure of contractile energy (e.g. stroke volume) and whose abscissa (x-axis) is an index of resting fibre length is a ventricular function curve. CVP is often plotted on the abscissa because it is easily measured by catheterization. Other indices include RVEDP,

circulation. This increases the filling pressure and stretch of the left ventricle, raising its contractile energy. Thus a rise in CVP causes an increase in the output of both ventricles (Figure 6.9).

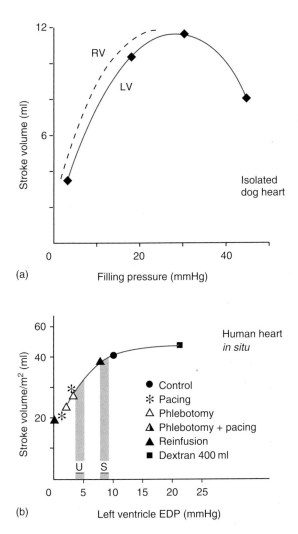

Figure 6.10 The ventricular function curve. (a) Effect of filling pressure on the stroke volume of an isolated dog heart pumping against a constant arterial pressure. The solid line shows Starling's data for left ventricular (LV) stroke volume and left atrial pressure. Dashed line is right ventricle (RV). (b) Human ventricular function curve. LV end-diastolic pressure (LVEDP) was varied *in vivo* by phlebotomy (venous bleeding) and other manoeuvres, and the effect on stroke volume per unit body surface area observed (stroke index). Normal range of human LVEDP in supine position (S) and upright position (U) are shown. Human ventricle *in situ* reaches a virtual plateau above 10 mmHg. (From Parker, J. D. and Case, R. B. (1979) *Circulation*, **60**, 4–12, by permission.)

LVEDP, and echocardiographic ventricle diameter. For the ordinate, stroke volume is a reasonable measure of contractile energy if the mean arterial pressure is held constant, as in Starling's heart–lung preparation. However, it takes more energy to raise a given stroke volume to a high pressure than to a low pressure. Therefore, stroke volume × mean arterial pressure, or *stroke work*, is a better measure of contractile energy *in vivo* (Section 6.5).

The 'law of the heart'

The results in Figure 6.10 establish that **the greater the stretch of the ventricle in diastole, the greater the stroke work achieved in systole**. As Patterson, Piper and Starling concluded in 1914, 'The energy of contraction of a cardiac muscle fibre, like that of a skeletal muscle fibre, is proportional to the initial fibre length at rest'. This statement is now honoured as **Starling's law of the heart**. Its physiological and pathophysiological roles in humans are described in Section 6.7. Before this, however, we need to consider the concept of stroke work and its relation to Starling's law.

6.5 Stroke work and the pressure–volume loop

Stroke work depends on stroke volume and arterial pressure

The energy expended by the myocardium in systole is converted partly into heat and partly into useful mechanical work in the form of an increase in blood pressure and volume in the arterial system. We can discover how much work is involved by starting from the definition of work, namely force F times the distance moved L. One joule of work is 1 newton of force displaced over 1 metre. The active force exerted on the blood by the ventricle in systole is the rise in pressure ΔP times the wall area A, since pressure is force per unit area. If the wall then moves a distance L, the volume ΔV displaced into the aorta is $L \times A$. This is illustrated by the top manikin in Figure 6.11. Thus the work per stroke W is given by:

$$W = F \times L = (\Delta P \times A) \times L$$
$$= \Delta P \times (A \times L)$$
$$= \Delta P \times \Delta V$$

In other words, the stroke work is the average increase in ventricular pressure times stroke volume.

Stroke work is the area inside a pressure–volume loop

The pressure–volume loop introduced in Section 2.2 is a convenient way of representing stroke work and will be used later to describe changes in cardiac performance. Since stroke work is the displaced volume × gain in pressure, **stroke work is the area inside the ventricular pressure–volume**

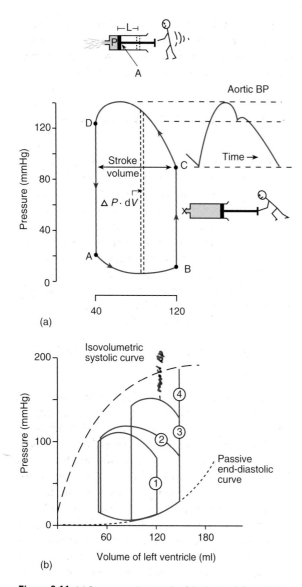

Figure 6.11 (a) Pressure–volume cycle of the human left ventricle. A, opening of mitral valve; AB, filling phase; B, closure of mitral valve at onset of systole; BC, isovolumetric contraction; C, opening of aortic valve; CD, ejection phase; D, closure of aortic valve; DA, isovolumetric relaxation. Since systolic pressure reaches 140 mmHg here, this subject is probably middle-aged. The *mechanical work* performed equals the sum of all the $\Delta P \cdot dV$ strips within the loop, i.e. *total loop area*. The sketches indicate how the isovolumetric phase produces no external work despite large energy expenditure by the myocardial manikin. (b) Factors influencing the pressure–volume cycle. The lower border is set by the passive pressure–volume curve of the relaxed ventricle. The upper boundary is set by the systolic pressure that would be produced in a purely isovolumetric contraction from a given end-diastolic volume; this line represents the Frank–Starling mechanism. Loop 1 represents a control state. Loop 2 shows the effect of increasing the end-diastolic volume; stroke volume increases, provided arterial pressure is held steady. If arterial pressure is then raised (loop 3), stroke volume decreases, provided end-diastolic volume is held steady. Line 4 depicts a purely isovolumetric contraction.

loop (Figure 6.11). During the isovolumetric contraction phase B–C the heart is 'working' in the everyday sense (it is consuming O_2 and generating force) but no blood is entering the aorta, so no external work is being accomplished. This phase is like a man trying to push over a house; he accomplishes no external work but consumes a lot of O_2! At point C the aortic valve opens because diastolic arterial pressure has been reached. The ejection phase C–D is loosely equivalent to an isotonic contraction, or more strictly an auxotonic contraction.

The pressure–volume loop is confined by active and passive boundary curves

The ventricular pressure–volume loop is constrained by two boundaries (Figure 6.11b). The lower boundary is the **passive compliance curve** of the ventricle, which relates end-diastolic volume to end-diastolic pressure. Every contraction starts from this line. The passive pressure–volume relation is not linear but curves upwards, because the ventricle is more stretchy (compliant) at low pressures than at high pressures (like a car tyre). Changes in CVP in the physiological range, 0–10 mmHg, evoke bigger changes in stretch and stroke volume than do changes above ~10 mmHg.

The upper boundary is the **isovolumetric pressure relation**, i.e. the systolic pressure that would be generated by a non-ejecting ventricle, as in Frank's experiment (Figure 6.7). This curve has an ascending limb and plateau due to the Frank–Starling mechanism; the greater the end-diastolic volume, the greater the contractile energy and pressure generation. In an ejecting heart the systolic pressure never reaches the isovolumetric boundary because some of the contractile energy is used to eject the blood.

Figure 6.11b illustrates how preload and afterload alter the loop width within the upper and lower boundaries. Loop 1 represents a normal left ventricular cycle with a stroke volume of 70 ml at normal pressure. In loop 2, the end-diastolic volume and pressure have been raised, for example by lying down, so corner B is shifted up the passive compliance curve. The increased preload raises the stretch, and hence the contractile energy through the Frank–Starling mechanism. Consequently the stroke volume and loop area (stroke work) increase. Note that the operation of the Frank–Starling mechanism involves the ventricle getting bigger both at end-diastole (side BC) and, to a lesser degree, at end-systole (side DA).

Loop 3 illustrates the deleterious effect of **afterload**, starting from the same end-diastolic stretch as loop 2. Afterload can be raised by raising the arterial pressure, using a vasoconstrictor drug. More energy is consumed in raising the ventricular pressure to a higher level, so less energy remains for ejection. As a result, the stroke volume falls. If ejection were totally prevented, as in line 4, maximum systolic pressure would be generated, but zero stroke volume and stroke work.

6.6 Central venous pressure and cardiac filling

Any circumstance that alters the central venous pressure (CVP), such as a blood transfusion or a haemorrhage, will alter the stroke volume through the Frank–Starling mechanism. The CVP depends on the total volume of blood in the circulation, and on how the volume is distributed between the peripheral and central veins. Venous volume distribution is affected by gravity, peripheral venous tone, the skeletal muscle pump and breathing. The distribution of blood between the central veins and central arteries is also influenced by the pumping action of the heart.

Low blood volume reduces filling pressure

About two-thirds of the entire blood volume is located in the venous system (Figure 1.11). Consequently, a fall in blood volume (hypovolaemia) due to **haemorrhage** or **dehydration** will tend to reduce the CVP. The resulting fall in stroke volume accounts for the hypotension associated with severe hypovolaemia. Conversely, a blood transfusion raises the CVP and improves the stroke volume after a haemorrhage.

The upright posture reduces CVP

In a standing human, gravity redistributes ~500 ml of blood from the thorax into the veins of the lower limbs. This is called **venous pooling**. Venous pooling reduces the CVP. As a result, human stroke volume is reduced in the upright position. Conversely, lying down redistributes venous blood from the lower part of the body into the thorax, which raises the CVP and stroke volume substantially (Figure 6.10b).

Sympathetic nerves regulate peripheral venous tone

The veins of the skin, kidneys and splanchnic system are innervated by sympathetic venoconstrictor fibres. Blood displaced from the peripheral veins by sympathetic venoconstriction is shifted into the central veins, which gives the nervous system a degree of control over the cardiac filling pressure (Figures 14.5, 14.4). Venoconstriction occurs during exercise, stress, deep respiration, haemorrhage, shock and cardiac failure. Conversely, venodilatation occurs in the skin in hot environments for reasons of temperature regulation, with an attendant, incidental fall in CVP and stroke volume.

The venous muscle pump boosts CVP in exercise

Rhythmic exercise repeatedly compresses the deep veins of the limbs, displacing their blood centrally due to the venous valves (Figure 8.23). This raises the CVP and stroke volume slightly during dynamic exercise. Conversely, soldiers standing at attention for long periods in hot weather have an inactive muscle pump, leading to an embarrassing propensity to faint. The combination of gravitational venous pooling, heat-induced venodilatation and lack of muscle pump activity reduces the CVP and stroke volume, leading to cerebral hypoperfusion and fainting.

Increased cardiac output reduces filling pressure

The heart pumps blood out of the venous system and into the arterial system. It is easy to forget that pumping not only increases the volume and pressure of blood in the arterial system but also **reduces the volume and pressure of blood in the central veins** (Figure 6.12). Stimulation of the cardiac output, for example by the sympathetic system, speeds up the transfer of blood out of the central veins and into the arteries, so it tends to reduce the filling pressure (reduced preload). Along with the rise in arterial pressure (increased afterload) this becomes a brake that limits the stroke volume, unless compensatory changes are brought into play (Section 6.13). Conversely, **if cardiac output is suddenly reduced by acute cardiac failure, for example following a heart attack, the filling pressure rises**.

Respiration causes oscillation of cardiac extramural pressure, filling and output

Ventricular filling is affected not only by the internal filling pressure but also by the external pressure around the heart. The true filling pressure is the difference between the internal and external pressures, or **transmural pressure** (trans-, across; -mural, wall). The external pressure is normally the intrathoracic pressure, which oscillates between $-5\,cmH_2O$ at end-expiration and $-10\,cmH_2O$ at end-inspiration.

Inspiration makes the intrathoracic pressure more negative and the intra-abdominal pressure more positive due to the descent of the diaphragm. This

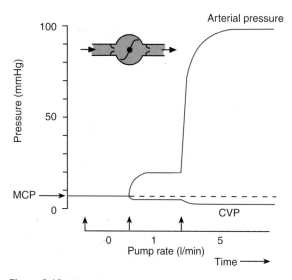

Figure 6.12 Effect of a pump on input and output pressure. Volume transfer lowers the input pressure, as well as raising output pressure. At zero pumping rate, the central venous pressure (CVP) and arterial pressure would be equal (mean circulatory pressure, MCP). CVP changes less than arterial pressure because venous compliance (volume accommodated per unit pressure change) is greater than arterial compliance. (Based on Levy, M. N. (1979) *Circulation Research*, **44**, 739 and Berne, R. M. and Levy, M. N. (1997) *Cardiovascular Physiology*, Mosby, St Louis, by permission.)

promotes the filling of the thoracic venae cavae (Figure 8.24, top) and **enhances right ventricular filling and stroke volume**. At the same time, however, the lung expansion increases the pulmonary blood pool, which temporarily reduces the return of blood to the left ventricle. Consequently, **left ventricle stroke volume falls transiently during each inspiration**. The effect of this on output is partially countered by sinus arrhythmia, i.e. by the tachycardia of inspiration (Section 5.8). Expiration reverses all these effects. As a result, respiration causes synchronous oscillations in arterial pressure called **Traube–Hering waves**.

Increased extramural pressure impairs filling

Forced expiration, such as a bout of coughing or the Valsalva manoeuvre (Section 17.2), raises intrathoracic pressure to positive values. This reduces the ventricular transmural pressure. The attendant fall in ventricular filling and cardiac output can cause dizziness.

The extramural pressure can become dominated by the pericardium in certain diseases. The pressure around the heart can be raised by a **pericardial effusion** or by **constrictive pericarditis**. The impaired ventricular filling severely reduces the cardiac output.

6.7 Operation of Starling's law in humans

The single most important role of the Frank–Starling mechanism is to **balance the outputs of the right and left ventricles** (see below). It also contributes to an **increase in stroke volume in exercise** (Chapter 17). It mediates **postural hypotension**, which is a fall in cardiac output and blood pressure on standing, leading to dizziness. It also mediates **hypovolaemic hypotension** after a haemorrhage (Chapter 18) and the **fall in stroke volume during forced expiration** (see above).

The Frank–Starling mechanism equalizes right and left outputs

It is essential that the right ventricular output should equal the left ventricular output over any interval greater than a few beats. Imagine a right ventricular output that is merely 1% greater than left ventricular output. The pulmonary blood volume, normally 0.6 litres, would increase with every heart beat and reach 2 litres within half-an-hour, causing a catastrophic pulmonary congestion and oedema. In heavy exercise, with outputs around 25 l/min, catastrophic congestion would build up within minutes. Conversely, a sustained excess of left ventricular output would quickly drain the pulmonary vessels dry.

The Frank–Starling mechanism prevents such catastrophes by equalizing the two outputs. If right ventricular output starts to exceed left ventricular output, the increase in pulmonary blood volume raises the pressure in the pulmonary veins, which increases the filling of the left ventricle. By Starling's law this raises the left ventricular output until balance is restored. The opposite happens if left ventricular output transiently exceeds right output. The two outputs are thus automatically equalized in the long term.

Imbalances do occur, but only transiently. On standing up the right output is less than left output for a few beats, due to venous pooling. Also, as noted above, the effect of respiration on right and left outputs causes a regular, alternating imbalance synchronous with the respiratory cycle.

CVP is a truer determinant of stroke volume than 'venous return'

'Venous return' is the flow of blood into the right atrium. In an intact circulation, venous return equals cardiac output in the steady state, because the circulation is a closed system of tubes: any inequality can only be transient. Under steady state conditions the venous return is simply the cardiac output observed in veins rather than arteries. The popular notion that venous return 'controls' the cardiac output seems an unhelpful and literally circular viewpoint, because venous return **depends** on cardiac output. Imagine a plot of cardiac output as a 'function' of venous return; it would be a straight line of slope 1.0! CVP by contrast is an **independent** variable; it can be adjusted independently of cardiac output, for example by changes in venoconstrictor tone or blood volume. CVP is thus an independent determinant of the stroke volume.

The Guyton cross-plot highlights the role of CVP

The pivotal role of CVP is illustrated by an ingenious cross-plot devised by the American physiologist Guyton (Figure 6.13). The '**cardiac output curve**' on the plot represents the positive effect of CVP on stroke volume through Starling's law. The other line, the '**venous return curve**', shows a negative effect of CVP on venous return. This stems from the basic law of hydraulics; any rise in CVP will reduce the pressure gradient from the capillaries to central veins, which in itself tends to reduce venous flow. The venous return curve reaches zero at ~7 mmHg because 7 mmHg is the **mean circulatory pressure** – the pressure of blood when flow is stopped and all pressures have equilibrated throughout the circulation. In the steady state *in vivo*, **the cardiac output and venous return must be equal**, and this happens at only one point on the plot, namely where the two curves cross. The stable intersection occurs at the CVP that provides an identical cardiac output and venous return.

The Starling curve is depressed in heart failure

Guyton's cross-plot provides insights into many pathophysiological states, including cardiac failure (Figure 6.13). In cardiac failure the output curve (Starling curve) is depressed by a reduction in contractility. However, there is a concomitant rise in mean circulatory pressure due to venoconstriction and fluid retention. This displaces the venous return curve upwards. The new steady state for the failing heart is at the new intersection. The failing output is, surprisingly, only slightly below normal, because the CVP is greatly increased. These are indeed the characteristic features of moderate ventricular failure (Chapter 18).

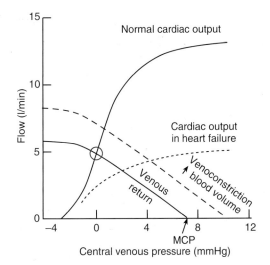

Figure 6.13 Guyton's analysis of the circulation. The cardiac output–CVP relation follows Starling's law of the heart, at constant heart rate. The venous return curve shows blood flow from the peripheral vasculature into the central veins (see text). MCP is mean circulatory pressure at zero flow. The normal operating point is where the two lines cross, i.e. output equals return (open circle). The output curve is shifted downwards in heart failure by a fall in contractility (short dashes). The venous return curve is shifted upwards if MCP is increased by venoconstriction or increased plasma volume (long dashes); or downwards if MCP is reduced by hypovolaemia (not shown). (After Guyton, A. C., Jones, C. E. and Coleman, T. G. (1973) *Circulatory Physiology: Cardiac Output and its Regulation*, W. B. Saunders, Philadelphia.)

6.8 Laplace's law and swollen hearts

Chamber radius is the link between wall tension and pressure

The radius of the ventricle affects the conversion of active muscle tension into blood pressure. This is important in failing hearts, which become very swollen. The radius or curvature of any hollow chamber links the wall tension to the internal pressure, as pointed out by the French mathematician, the Marquis de Laplace, in 1806 – in a treatise on celestial mechanics! Laplace's law for a hollow sphere states that the internal pressure P is proportional to the wall tension T and is inversely proportional to the internal radius, r:

$$P = \frac{2T}{r} \qquad (6.1)$$

Tension is a force. The tension equals the wall stress S times wall thickness w. Stress is by definition

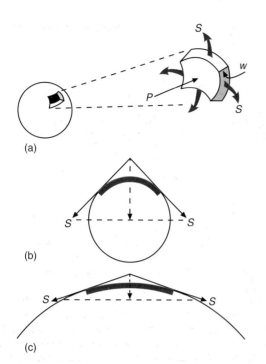

Figure 6.14 Laplace's law: the relation between wall stress (S), pressure (P) and curvature of a hollow sphere; stress is force per unit cross-sectional area of wall. In the ejecting heart, S is the 'afterload' on the myocytes; w, wall thickness. (a) Depicts a hollow sphere, such as a tennis ball, with an 'exploded' segment showing the two circumferential wall stresses. (b) Shows, in two dimensions, how the wall stresses (tangential arrows) give rise to an inward stress equal and opposite to pressure. Arrow length is proportional to stress magnitude. The thick line represents a muscle segment exerting tension. (c) Shows how an increase in radius reduces the inward component of the wall stress.

force per unit cross-sectional area of wall. Laplace's law can therefore be written as:

$$P = \frac{2Sw}{r} \qquad (6.2)$$

The involvement of radius is readily understood by considering the wall's curvature (Figure 6.14). As the radius increases, curvature decreases; consequently a smaller component of the wall tension is angled towards the cavity, generating less pressure. In other words, the curvature of the ventricle wall determines how effectively the active wall tension is converted into intraventricular pressure.

Laplace's law affects cardiac performance in several ways, as follows.

The Laplace relation facilitates late ejection

The afterload on the myocytes (Section 6.2) is the stress S during ejection. Laplace's law tells us that the ventricular afterload S equals the ejection pressure × radius/2w. Thus **afterload depends on chamber radius** as well as on arterial pressure. Since the radius of the chamber falls as ejection proceeds, afterload falls too, facilitating ejection. In other words, ejection gets easier as it proceeds.

Ventricular distension has advantages and disadvantages

The Laplace effect and Frank–Starling mechanism act in opposition. Distension of the ventricle raises its contractile force through the Frank–Starling mechanism but reduces the pressure generated by a given force through Laplace's law, reducing mechanical efficiency. Fortunately, in a healthy heart the gain in contractile energy on the ascending limb of the Starling curve greatly outweighs the Laplace effect. This is not the case, however, in the failing heart, as described next.

The dilated, failing heart operates at low mechanical efficiency

The failing heart is often grossly dilated (Figure 18.11) and the Laplace problem becomes dominant. Increases in radius in this state cause little to no increase in contractile force, because the heart is on the plateau of the Starling curve; instead, an increase in radius reduces systolic pressure generation and ejection through the operation of Laplace's law. Therefore, **an important therapeutic goal in heart failure is to reduce the cardiac distension**, thereby improving the conversion of contractile force into pressure. This is usually achieved by diuretics, which lower the cardiac filling pressure.

Summary of Starling and Laplace laws in man

Few summaries of the operation of Starling's law in man could be more memorable than Professor Alan Burton's rhyme, 'What goes in, must come out':

> The great Dr. Starling, in his Law of the Heart
> Said the output was greater if, right at the start,
> The cardiac fibres were stretched a bit more,
> So their force of contraction would be more
>   than before.
> Thus the larger the volume in diastole
> The greater the output was likely to be.
>
> If the right heart keeps pumping more blood
>   than the left,
> The lung circuit's congested; the systemic bereft.
> Since no-one is healthy with pulmo-congestion,
> The Law of Doc Starling's a splendid suggestion.
> The balance of outputs is made automatic

And blood–volume partition becomes
   steady–static.

When Guardsmen stand still and blood pools
   in their feet
Frank–Starling mechanics no longer seem neat.
The shift in blood volume impairs C–V–P,
Which shortens the fibres in diastole.
Contractions grow weaker and stroke volume
   drops,
Depressing blood pressure; so down the Guard
   flops.

But when the heart reaches a much larger size,
This leads to heart failure, and often demise.
The relevant law is not Starling's, alas,
But the classical law of Lecompte de Laplace.
Your patient is dying in decompensation,
So reduce his blood volume or call his relation.

(From Physiology and Biophysics of the Circulation (1972), Year Book Medical Publishers, Chicago, by courtesy of the publishers. With apologies to Alan Burton's spirit for the addition of verse 3.)

6.9 Effect of arterial pressure on the heart

Arterial blood pressure affects the output of the heart through several opposing mechanisms. Overall, a high arterial pressure has an adverse effect, depressing the output in the short term and leading to ventricular hypertrophy and failure in the long term.

Stroke volume falls with increasing afterload; the pump function curve

It will be recalled that the greater the afterload on a muscle strip *in vitro*, the less the shortening (Figure 6.2c). In the intact heart the equivalent of an increase in afterload is an increase in arterial pressure; and the equivalent of reduced shortening is a fall in stroke volume. Thus **a rise in arterial pressure impairs stroke volume**, as in loop 3 of Figure 6.11b.

A plot of stroke volume as a function of arterial pressure is called a **pump function curve** (Figure 6.15). The pump function curve for any pump operating at a fixed power, be it the heart or a laboratory roller pump, shows maximal stroke volume at zero pressure; a decline in stroke volume as the pressure opposing outflow is raised (point W to point 1, Figure 6.15); and maximal pressure generation at zero stroke volume. The pressure intercept is the maximum, isovolumetric systolic pressure, as in loop 4 of Figure 6.11b. If the energy of the

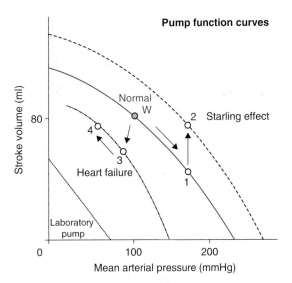

Figure 6.15 Pump function curves for a normal heart, failing heart and laboratory roller pump. W, normal working pressure. Raising the outflow pressure depresses stroke volume (point 1) if end-diastolic volume is held constant. Otherwise ventricular distension restores stroke volume by shifting the pump function curve to a higher energy level (point 2) (Frank–Starling mechanism, see Figure 6.16). Impaired contractility (heart failure) shifts curve to a lower energy level (point 3), but the stroke volume can be improved by pressure-reducing drugs (point 4). (Adapted from work of Elzinga, G. and Westerhof, N. (1979) *Circulation Research*, **32**, 178–186, and Nichols, W. W. and O'Rourke, M. F. (1998); see Further Reading, Chapter 8.)

pump is increased, for example by the Frank–Starling mechanism, the curve is shifted upwards (point 1 to 2, Figure 6.15). If energy is reduced by heart failure, the curve is shifted downwards (point W to point 3).

Arterial pressure depends partly on the resistance of the peripheral circulation, so stroke volume is influenced by peripheral resistance. This is put to practical use in the treatment of heart failure. **The stroke volume of a failing heart can be improved by lowering the peripheral resistance**, using vasodilator drugs. The fall in peripheral resistance reduces arterial pressure, which reduces ventricular afterload and allows the stroke volume to increase (point 4, Figure 6.15).

Increased arterial pressure evokes conflicting secondary effects

1 **Compensation through the Frank–Starling mechanism**. Following an acute rise in arterial pressure, the reduced ejection leads to the accumulation of an increased ventricular end-diastolic blood volume over a few beats (Figure 6.16). This distends the ventricle and increases the contractile energy through the

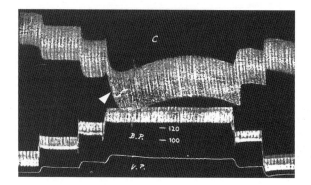

Figure 6.16 Three effects of raising arterial pressure (middle trace, *B. P.*) on stroke volume (excursion of upper trace) and ventricular end-diastolic volume (EDV) (lower border of upper trace) in a Starling heart–lung preparation. Volume record is inverted as in Figure 6.9; time scale is the same. (i) White arrowhead marks immediate reduction in stroke volume on raising arterial pressure (the **pump function relation**). (ii) As blood accumulates, venous pressure (*V. P.*) and EDV increase (volume scale is inverted), restoring stroke volume (**length–tension relation**). (iii) At *C*, a slow reduction in EDV without a fall in stroke volume indicates a slow increase in contractility (**Anrep effect**). (From Patterson, S. W., Piper, H. and Starling, E. H. (1914) *Journal of Physiology*, **48**, 465–511, by permission.)

Frank–Starling mechanism. The pump function curve is shifted to a higher level and the stroke volume improves (point 2, Figure 6.15).

2 **Compensation through the Anrep response**. Figure 6.16 shows a further adaptation over the next 5–10 min. The contractility of the ventricle increases, so that the stroke volume is maintained at a lower end-diastolic volume. This is called the Anrep response and is the equivalent of the **slow force response** of isolated myocardium (Figure 6.4). The Anrep response appears to be due to the local release within the myocardium of inotropic (strengthening) agents, namely myocardial angiotensin II and endothelin 1, which act in an autocrine/paracrine fashion.

3 **Depression of output by baroreflex**. In the intact animal an acute rise in arterial pressure triggers the baroreceptor reflex (Chapter 16). The baroreflex reduces cardiac sympathetic nerve activity, which reduces ventricular contractility, stroke volume and heart rate (Figure 6.17).

The effect of an acute rise in arterial pressure on stroke volume thus depends on the interplay of two negative effects (increased afterload and the baroreflex) and two compensatory effects (the Starling and Anrep responses) as shown in Figure 6.17. The net outcome is in general a reduction of the stroke volume.

'Preload' and 'afterload' in the ventricle

☐ *Preload* is defined as the force per unit cross-sectional area (stress *S*) applied to resting muscle. *In vitro* it can be set by a weight dangling from a muscle strip.

☐ In the intact ventricle the diastolic wall stress (preload) depends on the diastolic pressure *P*, chamber radius *r* and wall thickness *w* (Laplace's law; $S = Pr/2w$). The *end-diastolic pressure* itself is often referred to, inaccurately, as the preload.

☐ *Afterload* is the force per unit cross-sectional area (stress) that opposes the shortening of an isotonically contracting muscle strip. *In vitro* it can be set by a weight that the muscle picks up as it begins to shorten.

☐ In the intact ventricle, the systolic wall stress (afterload) depends on arterial pressure, chamber radius and wall thickness (Laplace's law.) *Arterial pressure* itself is often referred to, inaccurately, as the afterload.

Chronic hypertension causes concentric ventricular hypertrophy

Chronic elevation of the arterial pressure, as in clinical hypertension, has further, long-term effects. The left ventricle undergoes concentric hypertrophy, in which the wall grows thicker without any increase in chamber size (in contrast to the effect of endurance training, where chamber size increases). Myocyte hypertrophy is induced by local growth factors, including angiotensin II and endothelin, which trigger kinase pathways (the MAP kinase cascade) leading to the activation of nuclear transcription factors. Hypertrophy increases the contractile force for a while, helping the ventricle to cope with the hypertension. In the longer term, however, the overloaded ventricle often goes into failure (Figure 6.17). This is one of several reasons why hypertension, although symptomless, should be treated.

6.10 Sympathetic regulation of contractility

The meaning of contractility or inotropic state

Up to this point we have been concerned with changes in contractile energy caused by changes in

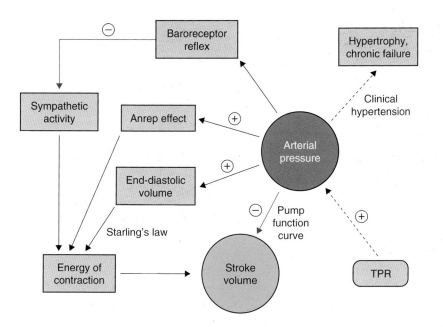

Figure 6.17 Schematic representation of multiple pathways by which arterial pressure influences stroke volume. TPR, total peripheral resistance.

resting fibre length. This is sometimes called 'intrinsic regulation'. Contractile energy is also regulated, however, by external chemical factors, or 'extrinsic regulation'. **A change in contractile energy that is not due to changes in fibre length is called a change in contractility.** This definition of contractility specifically excludes the Frank–Starling mechanism. The term 'inotropic state' is synonymous with contractility.

The most important inotrope normally is the sympathetic neurotransmitter noradrenaline. Others include circulating adrenaline, angiotensin II and extracellular Ca^{2+} ions.

Sympathetic stimulation produces a shorter, stronger beat

Sympathetic activity is increased during exercise, orthostasis (standing up), stress and haemorrhage. The left sympathetic fibres innervate the atrial and ventricular myocardium, and the right fibres innervate the pacemaker–conduction system (Figure 4.5). The release of noradrenaline from the sympathetic terminals activates myocyte β_1-adrenoceptors. These trigger the G_s–adenylate cyclase–cAMP–protein kinase A–phosphorylation cascade (Figure 4.8). The ensuing increase in Ca^{2+} current i_{Ca} raises the sarcoplasmic reticulum (SR) Ca^{2+} store and the trigger Ca^{2+} at the start of each contraction. As a result the magnitude of the **cytosolic free Ca^{2+} transient is increased**, causing more crossbridge formation and force development. At the same time stimulation of the SR Ca^{2+} uptake pumps by phosphorylated phospholamban

Contractility (inotropism)

☐ Contractility is the force of contraction achieved *from a given initial fibre length*.

☐ Contractile force can be increased *either* by increased contractility *and/or* by increasing the resting fibre length (end-diastolic stretch, the Frank–Starling mechanism).

☐ Positive inotropes (factors that increase contractility) include the sympathetic neurotransmitter noradrenaline, adrenaline, β_1 agonist drugs, phosphodiesterase inhibitors, digoxin and beat interval.

☐ Negative inotropes include acute myocardial ischaemia (acting through intracellular acidosis), chronic cardiac failure, anaesthetics, parasympathetic fibre activity (a minor effect), β_1 receptor antagonists and Ca^{2+} channel blockers.

shortens the Ca^{2+} transient and contraction period. Sympathetic stimulation thus causes a shorter, more forceful contraction of the myocyte, with the following effects on gross cardiac performance:

- **Ventricular pressure** rises more rapidly and reaches a higher systolic pressure (Figure 6.18a). Systolic pressure increases because the elastic arteries are expanded by an increased stroke volume over a shorter time. The maximum rate of pressure increase, dP/dt_{max}, has been used as an index of myocardial contractility, although it

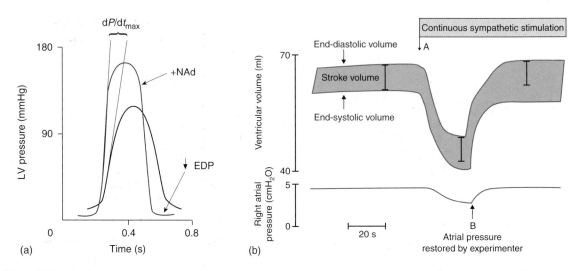

Figure 6.18 Effect of sympathetic stimulation or noradrenaline on cardiac performance. (a) Left ventricular pressure wave shows increased rate of climb (dP/dt_{max}), increased peak pressure, reduced EDP and reduced duration. (b) Combined stroke volume recorded by a cardiometer with heart rate held constant. The left cardiac sympathetic nerves were stimulated continuously from point A onwards. An increase in ejection fraction caused right atrial pressure and cardiac volume to fall, and the Frank–Starling mechanism then largely prevented any rise in stroke volume. Enhanced contractility is evident from a slightly increased stroke volume despite a smaller end-diastolic volume. At B the filling pressure was artificially restored to its previous level, allowing the effect of contractility on stroke volume to be fully expressed. Vertical bar represents size of original stroke volume. (Adapted from Linden, R. J. (1968) *Anaesthesia*, **23**, 566–584, by permission.)

is also increased by the Frank–Starling mechanism (Figures 6.2b, 6.7).

- **Ejection fraction** is increased. This is a favourite clinical index of contractility.

- **Diastolic volume** falls, because systolic ejection is more complete. Thus increased contractility makes the ventricle **smaller in diastole and systole** (Figure 6.18b). With the Frank–Starling mechanism, by contrast, diastolic and systolic volumes increase.

- **Stroke volume** increases, but the size of the increase is attenuated by the reduced end-diastolic volume (hence reduced Frank–Starling effect) and increased arterial pressure (increased afterload). The full increase in stroke volume is only expressed when these adverse changes are prevented (Figure 6.18b). During exercise, peripheral vascular adjustments minimize such checks and allow fuller expression of the stimulated stroke volume.

- The **duration of systole** shortens (Figure 6.18a), preserving diastolic filling time. The increased contraction velocity enables the stroke volume to be ejected during the shorter period.

The net effect of sympathetic nerve stimulation, therefore, is to increase arterial pressure, stroke volume

and ejection fraction, and to reduce ejection time, end-diastolic pressure and ventricle size.

Graded sympathetic activity generates a family of ventricular function curves

Because sympathetic stimulation enhances the contractile energy at a given end-diastolic length, the entire ventricular function curve is shifted upwards (Figure 6.19). Sarnoff showed in the 1960s that the shift is graded according to the level of sympathetic activity. Thus the heart operates not on one ventricular function curve but on an entire family of ventricular function curves. Stroke volume can be altered by moving along a curve (change in contractile energy, the Frank–Starling mechanism), and/or by moving from one curve to a higher one (change in contractility). A combination of both events is common *in vivo*. For example, upright exercise raises the filling pressure (movement along a curve) and increased contractility (movement to a higher curve).

The pressure–volume loop is widened and shifted left

Sympathetic stimulation steepens the upper confine of the pressure–volume loop, i.e. the isovolumetric systolic pressure line, because isovolumetric contractions are strengthened by the raised contractility

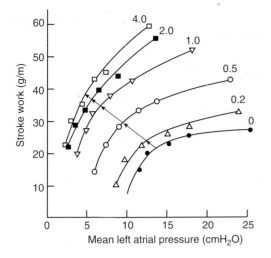

Figure 6.19 Family of ventricular function curves generated by graded sympathetic stimulation of dog heart. Sympathetic activity in range 0–4 s^{-1} increased contractility in a graded fashion. Arrows show how enhanced contractility reduces filling pressure as well as raising stroke volume. (From Sarnoff, S. J. and Mitchell, J. H. (1962) *Handbook of Physiology Cardiovascular System*, Vol. 1, American Physiological Society, Baltimore, pp. 489–532, by permission.)

(Figure 6.20). Peak pressure, stroke volume, ejection fraction and stroke work (loop area) are all increased within the expanded boundary. The loop is shifted to the left, however, by the reduced end-diastolic volume, causing the Frank–Starling mechanism to limit the gain in stroke volume (Figure 6.20a, loop 2). *In vivo*, the end-diastolic volume can be prevented from falling, or even raised, by peripheral venoconstriction and the muscle pump, e.g. in upright exercise. This widens the loop in both directions, resulting in a larger increase in stroke volume and stroke work (Figure 6.20b, loop 3).

6.11 Other positive inotropic influences

Adrenaline and other β-agonists

The human adrenal medulla secretes adrenaline and noradrenaline in the ratio of approximately 4:1. Adrenaline activates cardiac β$_1$-adrenoceptors, with the same effect as noradrenaline. The plasma concentrations of both substances increase ~20 times in maximal exercise. Even so, the cardiac response to exercise is normally dominated by the powerful cardiac sympathetic nerves rather than circulating catecholamines.

Other β-agonists such as isoprenaline, dopamine (a precursor of adrenaline) and the synthetic analogue dobutamine have similar inotropic and chronotropic effects. They can be used to support an acutely failing heart for a short period.

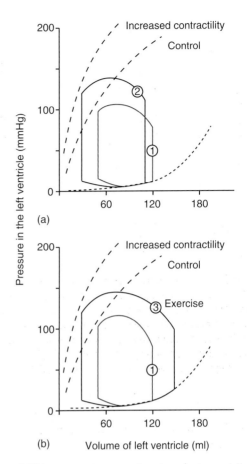

Figure 6.20 Schematic pressure–volume loops for human left ventricle when myocardial contractility is increased. The upper dashed confine is the relation between systolic pressure and end-diastolic volume for a purely isovolumetric contraction (Frank–Starling mechanism). (a) Loop 1 represents a basal state. Loop 2 represents a state of increased contractility. Ejection fraction is increased, so end-diastolic volume falls unless actively regulated. Loop area (stroke work) is increased. (b) During exercise (loop 3), contractility is raised by sympathetic activity and end-diastolic volume is raised by peripheral circulatory adjustments (venoconstriction, muscle pump). The increase in stroke volume is now much greater.

The phosphodiesterase inhibitors **caffeine**, **theophylline** and **milrinone** raise intracellular cAMP and thus mimic the effects of β-agonists (Figure 4.8).

Angiotensin II

Angiotensin II is a circulating hormone, described in Section 14.8. The greater part of its positive inotropic effect is achieved through neuromodulation; that is to say, angiotensin binds to sympathetic nerve terminals and facilitates the release of noradrenaline (Figure 14.2). It also acts directly on the myocyte to enhance i_{Ca}. Angiotensin II levels increase in exercise and heart failure.

Other circulating inotropes

The hormones thyroxine, insulin, glucagon and corticosteroids all have a long-term, positive inotropic effect. The inotropic drug **digoxin** inhibits the sarcolemmal Na^+–K^+ pump, leading to a rise in intracellular Ca^{2+} (Section 3.7).

The interval–tension relation

The American physiologist Bowditch observed in 1871 that shortening the interval between the heart beats causes a gradual increase in contractile force. If the frequency of electrical stimulation is increased, there is one weakened beat, then the beats grow progressively stronger in a 'staircase' pattern until a new steady state is reached. Conversely, if beat

interval is increased, there is one stronger beat, then the contractions weaken (Figure 6.21a).

The increased contractility with rate is due to increased free Ca^{2+} transients (Figure 6.21a), caused by an increased SR Ca^{2+} store. The store is increased by (i) the reduced diastolic interval for Ca^{2+} expulsion and (ii) an increase in intracellular Na^+ due to increased action potential frequency, which slows the expulsion of Ca^{2+} by the Na^+–Ca^{2+} exchanger. Although the Bowditch rate effect is interesting, it contributes only a little to the increased contractility of exercise, which is due chiefly to sympathetic stimulation.

The first beat after an interval reduction, unlike the rest, is weaker rather than stronger. Similarly, a **premature (ectopic) beat** in humans produces a weak beat, even if it follows the normal conduction pathway. The beat after the ensuing compensatory pause is stronger than normal (**post-extrasystolic potentiation**, Figure 6.21b). The patient may notice the post-extrasystolic potentiation and complain 'My heart gives a jump, Doctor'. Increased filling time and hence increased end-diastolic volume contribute to the post-extrasystolic potentiation in patients. This does not, however, explain the same phenomenon in isolated myocardium. The weak premature beat is due to the slow recovery of SR Ca^{2+} release channels from their inactivated state. A premature beat finds them partially refractory. By the next beat the SR Ca^{2+} store has increased.

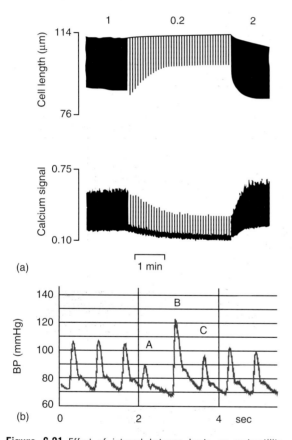

(a)

(b)

Figure 6.21 Effect of interval between beats on contractility. (a) Twitches of isolated rat ventricular myocyte stimulated at 1, 0.2 and 2 beats/s. Calcium signal is from intracellular fluorescent dye Fura-2. (b) In a patient with heart failure a premature systole (beat A) is feeble but the beat after the compensatory pause, beat B, is stronger than usual (**post-extrasystolic potentiation**). ((a) From Frampton, J. E., Orchard, C. H. and Boyett, M. R. (1991) *Journal of Physiology*, **437**, 351–375, by permission; (b) From Voss, A., Baier, V., Schumann, A., *et al.* (2002) *Journal of Physiology*, **538**, 271–278, by permission.)

6.12 Negative inotropism, ischaemia and arrhythmia

Negative inotropic influences are factors that reduce myocardial contractility. Aside from parasympathetic activity they are generally non-physiological. They include:

- parasympathetic (vagal) activity and cholinergic agonists;
- β-blockers such as propranolol, oxprenolol and atenolol (Section 4.8);
- calcium-channel blockers such as verapamil (Section 4.8);
- hyperkalaemia (Section 4.7);
- barbiturates and many anaesthetics;
- acidosis and hypoxia (ischaemic heart disease, see below);
- chronic cardiac failure (Section 18.5).

Parasympathetic fibres have only a weak effect on ventricular contractility

The vagi innervate the pacemaker–conduction system and the atrial muscle and have a powerful effect on heart rate, but their effect on ventricular contraction is weak. The human ventricles have parasympathetic fibres and muscarinic M_2 receptors, but maximal vagal stimulation weakens ventricular contraction by only 15–38%. Interestingly, there is a concomitant fall in noradrenaline in the coronary venous blood, because some parasympathetic fibres terminate close to sympathetic fibres and inhibit them. Conversely, sympathetic fibres release the neuropeptides neuropeptide Y and galanin, which inhibit the release of acetylcholine by vagal fibres. In the SA node this facilitates the increase in heart rate.

Ischaemia impairs contractility and causes arrhythmia

Ischaemia is a deficiency in O_2 supply to a tissue caused by vascular insufficiency. In the heart an atheromatous narrowing of one or more coronary arteries is usually responsible. The reduced blood supply leads to local hypoxia and intracellular acidosis. These in turn lead to the impairment of cardiac output, especially on exercise (Table 6.1), reduced exercise capacity, often angina, and sometimes fatal arrhythmias. The ECG may show ST segment depression at rest due to injury currents (Section 5.2). In mild cases ST segment displacement may only develop during an exercise stress test, which increases myocardial O_2 demand and thus aggravates the ischaemia. The multiple effects of ischaemia, some of which were described in earlier chapters, are brought together in Figure 6.22.

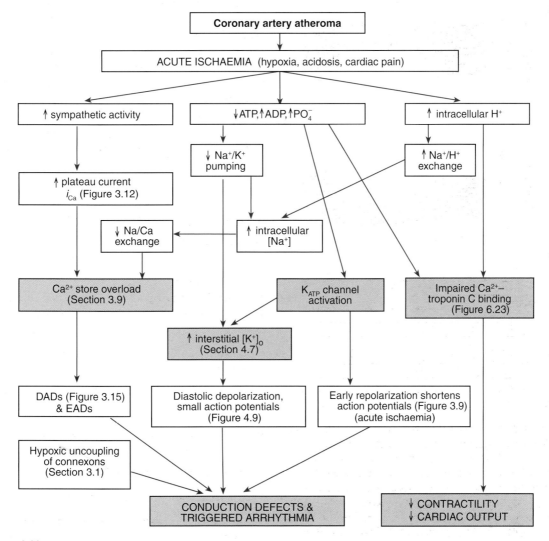

Figure 6.22 Summary of mechanisms by which acute ischaemia (usually due to coronary artery disease) impairs contractility and causes arrhythmia. For effects of chronic heart failure see Section 18.5.

Impaired contractility. The reduced mitochondrial oxidative metabolism leads to a fall in the creatine phosphate energy reserve, a rise in inorganic phosphate and ADP and eventually a fall in ATP. Pyruvate oxidation is diverted into lactic acid formation, causing intracellular acidosis.

Acidosis has a strongly negative inotropic effect (Figure 6.23), probably because H^+ ions compete with Ca^{2+} for the troponin C binding sites. The rise in inorganic phosphate also impairs contractility, though less strongly. A reduction in the open state probability of SR Ca^{2+}-release channels further impairs contractility.

Arrhythmia. The ischaemic heart is prone to conduction defects and arrhythmia due to multiple mechanisms (Figure 6.22). Acute ischaemia has the following arrhythmogenic effects:

- Resting membrane potential falls, due to an increase in interstitial $[K^+]$ following Na^+–K^+ ATPase rundown.

- Action potential size (phase 0) and duration (phase 2) are reduced, due respectively to the closure of some inactivation gates of Na^+ channels (effect of reduced membrane potential) and K_{ATP} activation (Figure 3.9).

- The conductivity of connexons is reduced.

- Intracellular $[Na^+]$ increases, due to increased Na^+–H^+ exchange (effect of the intracellular acidosis) and reduced Na^+–K^+ ATPase activity.

- Ca^{2+} influx i_{Ca} increases, due to a reflex increase in sympathetic activity.

- The SR Ca^{2+} store becomes overloaded, partly due to the increased i_{Ca}, and especially due to the reduced Ca^{2+} expulsion by the Na^+–Ca^{2+} exchanger, consequent upon the rise in intracellular Na^+.

The spontaneous discharge of an overloaded Ca^{2+} store transiently stimulates the $3Na^+$–$1Ca^{2+}$ exchanger, leading to an afterdepolarization that may trigger an ectopic beat (Figure 3.15). The impairment of action potential phase 0 and of connexons impairs the propagation of excitation, and since the abnormalities are not uniformly distributed, re-entry circuits can develop (Figure 5.10). Thus, an **afterdepolarization-triggered ectopic** during the **vulnerable period** (late T wave, some myocytes repolarized, others not) can trigger a **re-entrant arrhythmia** such as fibrillation (Figure 5.4g).

The paradox of myocardial ischaemia–reperfusion injury

An adequate O_2 supply is vital for myocardial survival. Yet, paradoxically, the reperfusion of ischaemic myocardium with oxygenated blood increases the cellular damage (**necrosis**). Re-oxygenation enables the Na^+–K^+ ATPase to restore the Na^+ gradient that drives the sarcolemmal Na^+–H^+ exchanger, which in turn leads to the rapid correction of intracellular acidosis and restoration of contractility. If the intracellular Ca^{2+} overload has not yet been corrected, the restored contractility causes a severe, sustained **contracture**. Contracture can damage the cytoskeleton, disrupt cell membranes and cause tissue necrosis (cell death).

Reperfusion injury can be substantially reduced in experimental animals by pharmacological inhibition of the Na^+–H^+ exchanger using amiloride. The resulting prolongation of the intracellular acidosis causes the 'natural' inhibition of contraction to continue longer. This purchases time for the myocyte to restore its normal, extremely low free Ca^{2+} concentration, and thus avoid contracture.

Reperfusion injury is exacerbated by the formation of toxic, **oxygen-derived free radicals**, as described later (Section 13.9). The oxygen-derived free radicals damage the sarcolemma, with arrhythmic consequences.

Even if reperfusion does not lead to tissue necrosis, it can lead to **myocardial stunning**. 'Stunning' refers to hours to days of decreased contractile function despite normal Ca^{2+} transients and energetic status. Stunning is caused by troponin I degradation, which reduces the thin filament responsiveness to Ca^{2+}.

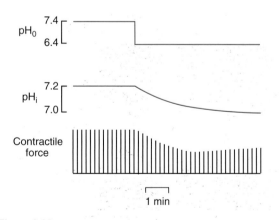

Figure 6.23 Strongly negative inotropic effect of intracellular acidosis (pH_i); pH_i was altered in this experiment by extracellular acid (pH_0). A pH_i reduction of only 0.2 units approximately halves the contractility. (Based on Hongo, K., White, E. and Orchard, C.H. (1995) *Experimental Physiology*, **80**, 701–712; and Bountra, C. and Vaughan-Jones, R. D. (1989) *Journal of Physiology*, **418**, 163–187.)

6.13 Co-ordinated control of cardiac output

An uncoordinated stimulus is relatively ineffective

In the intact animal the effective regulation of cardiac output is achieved through a co-ordinated set of changes in multiple factors. It is illuminating to see how ineffective a single uncoordinated stimulus can be. For example, if the pacing frequency is turned up in a patient with an artificially paced heart, the cardiac output increases remarkably little at rates above $100\ min^{-1}$, and actually declines at high pacing rates due to a fall in stroke volume. The stroke volume falls at high pacing rates because the reduction in diastolic interval curtails re-filling. Thus, changes in a single cardiac parameter are relatively ineffective. The co-ordinated, co-operative changes needed to increase the cardiac output effectively are well illustrated by the response to exercise.

Exercise involves co-ordinated cardiac and vascular changes

Human cardiac output increases by ~6 l/min for every extra litre of O_2 consumed per min. The increased output is achieved by various combinations of tachycardia and increased stroke volume, as shown by echocardiography and aortic Doppler flowmetry. The relative contributions of heart rate and stroke volume to the increase varies with exercise intensity, posture and age, but tachycardia is generally the

major factor. Human heart rate increases in proportion to O_2 consumption to a maximum of 180–200 beats/min. In upright exercise, stroke volume too can increase, by 50–100% (Table 6.2 and Figure 6.24). In the supine position stroke volume is already high at rest, so the increase during exercise is less pronounced.

The co-ordinated cardiac and peripheral vascular changes that underlie the large increases in output can be summarized as follows:

1 Sympathetic stimulation and reduced vagal activity **raise the heart rate** and **shorten systole**. A **reduction in diastolic filling interval** is countered by the sympathetically mediated increase in **atrial contractility**, which enhances the atrial contribution to ventricular filling.

Table 6.2 Typical cardiac response to upright exercise in a non-athlete.

	Rest	Hard exercise
Oxygen consumption (l/min)	0.25	3.0
Cardiac output (l/min)	4.8	21.6
Heart rate (beats/min)	60.0	180.0
Stroke volume (ml)	80.0	120.0
End-diastolic volume (ml)	120.0	140.0
Residual volume (end-systolic)	40.0	20.0
Ejection fraction	0.67	0.86
Cycle time (s)	1.0	0.33
Duration of systole (s)	0.35	0.2
Duration of diastole (s)	0.65	0.13

(After Rerych, S. K., Scholz, P. M., Newman, G. E., *et al.* (1978) *Annals of Surgery,* **187**, 449–458.)

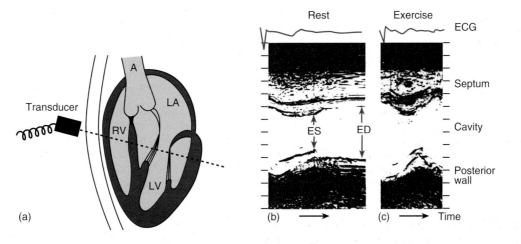

Figure 6.24 (a) Ultrasound beam directed across ventricle, in sagital section. M-mode echocardiograms of human left ventricle during rest (b) and upright exercise (c). Resting end-diastolic dimension (ED) *increased* on average by 2 mm and end-systolic dimension (ES) *fell* by 5 mm. The change in dimension upon contraction serves as an index of stroke volume and increased by 24% during exercise. (From Amon, K. W. and Crawford, M. H. (1979) *Journal of Clinical Ultrasound,* **7**, 373–376, by permission.)

2 Sympathetic stimulation, and to a lesser degree adrenaline, increase ventricular contractility, leading to rises in **stroke volume** and ejection fraction and a **fall in end-systolic volume** (Figure 6.24).

3 Sympathetic vasomotor nerves induce **venoconstriction** in the splanchnic circulation. Also, the **skeletal muscle pump** compresses veins in the limbs. The resulting transfer of blood into the central veins prevents the **CVP** from falling, as it otherwise would with increased cardiac pumping. The CVP can increase by a mmHg or so during exercise in the upright position, **raising end-diastolic volume** (Figure 6.24). This enables the **Frank–Starling mechanism** to contribute to the increase in stroke volume, particularly during sudden, intense, upright exercise and in the elderly.

4 **Vasodilatation** in the exercising skeletal muscle reduces the peripheral vascular resistance, which prevents arterial pressure from rising excessively. Stroke volume is therefore not limited by a big increase in afterload.

The increased cardiac output of exercise thus involves a co-ordinated interaction between changes within the heart (rate and contractility) and outside it (regulating CVP and systemic vascular resistance).

Transplanted and artificially paced hearts respond to exercise

Cardiac transplantation necessarily entails denervation. The impairment of exercise performance is surprisingly moderate, however, due to a **redundancy of control mechanisms**. Astonishingly, racing greyhounds with denervated hearts experience only a 5% reduction in track speed. Although the denervated heart lacks the usual immediate tachycardia at the start of exercise, its stroke volume increases rapidly due to a rise in CVP as the leg muscle pump becomes active, and a fall in arterial pressure (reduced afterload) as muscle resistance vessels dilate. Moreover, the heart rate and contractility increase over the next 1–2 min, due to increases in circulation adrenaline and angiotensin II. The track performance of the denervated greyhound only deteriorates substantially if the adrenergic back-up system is blocked by a β-antagonist (Figure 17.7).

Like the greyhound, patients with transplanted hearts or an artificial pacemaker benefit from the redundancy of cardiac control systems. Even at a fixed pacing rate, exercise increases the stroke volume, due to the skeletal muscle pump, peripheral vasodilatation and adrenaline-enhanced contractility. This may not make for Olympic records, but it enables thousands of people to walk in the park, do the shopping and generally lead a full life.

6.14 Cardiac energetics and metabolism

Pressure work exceeds kinetic work

Part of the energy expended in ventricular systole is 'useful', in the sense that it achieves mechanical work on an external system, the arteries; the rest of the energy appears as heat. The useful, mechanical work takes the form of an increase in the mass, pressure and velocity of blood in the arterial system.

Pressure work (stroke work). As explained in Section 6.5, the work done by the ventricle in pressurising and displacing the stroke volume into the arteries is called the stroke work. Stroke work equals stroke volume $\Delta V \times$ mean increase in pressure ΔP, i.e. the area of the pressure–volume loop (Figure 6.11). If the left ventricle raises the pressure by 100 mmHg ($1.33 \times 10^4 \mathrm{N/m^2}$) and ejects 75 cm^3 of blood ($0.75 \times 10^{-4} \mathrm{m^3}$), it performs nearly 1 N·m or 1 joule of work. The arterial system gains 1 joule of potential energy, i.e. pressure energy.

Kinetic work. The ventricle imparts velocity to the ejected blood as well as pressure, so it adds **kinetic energy** KE, the energy of motion. Kinetic energy is proportional to velocity squared (v^2) and mass m. Total ventricular work W is the pressure work plus the kinetic work, i.e.

$$W = \Delta V \Delta P + KE = \Delta V \Delta P + mv^2/2$$

Under resting conditions 0.08 kg of blood is ejected at a mean velocity of 0.5 m/s during systole, so the imparted kinetic energy is 0.01 kg m^{2}s^{-2} or 0.01 joules for either ventricle. The kinetic work is only 1% of the pressure work of the left ventricle, but ~5% on the right side, where pressure work is lower.

Exercise. During heavy exercise the right and left ejection velocities increase ~five-fold to 2.5 m/s, whereas the pressure work increases only moderately. Kinetic energy now accounts for 14% of left ventricular work and 50% of right ventricular work.

Power. Power is rate of working, so cardiac power equals stroke work $\times$ heart rate. Cardiac power ranges from ~1.2 watts (joules/s) at rest to around 8 watts in heavy exercise – about a fiftieth the power of a small electric lawn mower.

Emotional stress and high blood pressure increase cardiac work

A high blood pressure increases the stroke work and therefore myocardial O_2 consumption. An angry, emotional scene causes a large rise in blood pressure, so it greatly increases myocardial O_2 demand. This is clearly something to be avoided by patients with **coronary artery insufficiency**. As the celebrated eighteenth-century anatomist John Hunter observed in relation to his own ischaemic heart, 'My life is at the mercy of any rascal who chooses to annoy me'. The couch on which Hunter expired following a stormy committee meeting can still be seen in the library at St George's Hospital Medical School in London.

Cardiac efficiency improves during exercise

The gross mechanical efficiency of a machine is the ratio of external work to energy expended. Cardiac mechanical efficiency is low in a resting subject, namely 5–10%, because a quarter of the energy expenditure goes into ionic pumping and because the tension generation during isovolumetric contraction consumes a lot of energy. Myocardial O_2 consumption is in fact dominated by internal work rather than external work, and correlates well with active tension multiplied by the time for which it is maintained (the **tension–time index**). This may seem odd until one recalls that the O_2 consumption of a tug-of-war team depends mainly on the huge tension they exert, rather than on the external work involved in shifting the opposition across a metre or so of ground. In cardiological practice the tension–time index is estimated as heart rate × systolic pressure.

Efficiency improves to ~15% during dynamic exercise, because flow increases much more than arterial pressure. There is relatively little increase in the energy-expensive isovolumetric phase. This is helpful to patients with cardiac disease. Isometric exercise such as weight lifting is best avoided by such patients, because it greatly increases arterial pressure.

Efficiency is reduced by cardiac dilatation

The improvement of cardiac efficiency is an important aim when treating heart failure. Heart failure leads to cardiac dilatation (Figure 18.11). **Laplace's law** tells us that to maintain a normal systolic pressure P, a heart of enlarged radius r has to exert a greater

contractile tension T, because $P = 2T/r$ (Section 6.8). Thus pressure generation in the dilated state entails more O_2 consumption and a low efficiency – the very things a failing heart can ill afford. **Excessive cardiac dilatation impairs efficiency**, and must be reduced by diuretic therapy.

Myocardial O_2 consumption and metabolism

High energy phosphate. Myocardial metabolism is normally aerobic. The immediate energy source for the actin–myosin machinery, ATP, is synthesized by oxidative phosphorylation in the abundant mitochondria. There is a small back-up store of high-energy phosphate bonds in **creatine phosphate**, but the total high-energy phosphate content is only enough for about 15 beats. As a result, the heart relies heavily on matching the ATP supply closely to demand.

Oxygen. The supply of ATP is tightly linked to the supply of O_2. There is only a small store of O_2 bound to myoglobin, so coronary O_2 delivery must keep pace with mitochondrial demand – especially as the heart cannot take a long rest, unlike skeletal muscle. At basal cardiac outputs, myocardial O_2 uptake is ~10 ml/min per 100 g. This is a high proportion, 65–75%, of the O_2 delivered in the coronary arterial blood, leaving little in reserve. In exercise, the **increased myocardial O_2 demand can only be met by corresponding increases in coronary blood flow**. As a result, myocardial performance is heavily dependent on coronary blood flow.

Metabolic substrates. The substrates consumed by myocardium have been worked out by analysing coronary sinus and arterial blood. Broadly speaking, **free fatty acids** supply 50–65% of the energy requirement, or more during endurance exercise. The rest is supplied by **glucose** and **lactate**. In contrast to skeletal muscle, well-oxygenated myocardium can oxidize blood lactate when it is available. This is a useful asset during hard exercise, because lactate is released into the bloodstream by the active skeletal muscle. If myocardium becomes hypoxic, however, it switches to the anaerobic production of lactate, leading to intracellular acidosis and impaired contractility.

Cardiac enzymology. Lactate is oxidized through the enzyme **myocardial lactic dehydrogenase** (LDH), an isotype specific to heart. When myocytes undergo ischaemic damage following coronary thrombosis, LDH and other intracellular enzymes such as **creatine phosphokinase** and **aspartate aminotransferase**, escape into the circulation. Their detection in plasma provides a valuable laboratory test for myocardial infarction.

SUMMARY

■ The heart meets increased peripheral demand through increases in heart rate and stroke volume. Stroke volume can be raised by (i) diastolic stretch, which increases contractile force; (ii) catecholamine-mediated increases in contractility; or (iii) a reduction of the arterial pressure opposing ejection.

■ Ventricular diastolic stretch is determined by the filling pressure, namely central venous pressure (CVP) on the right and pulmonary venous pressure on the left. Stretch increases myocyte Ca^{2+} sensitivity, leading to a stronger contraction and increased stroke work (stroke volume × pressure increment). This is called the length–tension relation/Frank–Starling mechanism/Starling's law of the heart.

■ The Frank–Starling mechanism equalizes right and left stroke volumes; helps raise stroke volume in upright exercise; and reduces stroke volume in orthostasis and hypovolaemia.

■ CVP, and hence stroke volume, is affected by blood volume, gravity (orthostasis), sympathetic-mediated peripheral venous tone, the skeletal muscle pump and breathing.

■ Excessive CVP in heart failure over-distends the heart. The reduced wall curvature impairs mechanical effectiveness, i.e. the conversion of wall tension T into internal pressure P (Laplace's law, $T = 2P/radius$). In heart failure the Laplace effect outweighs the weakened Frank–Starling mechanism, so one aim of treatment is to reduce CVP.

■ An increase in contractile force that is not due to increased stretch is called increased contractility or positive inotropism. The normal inotropes are the sympathetic neurotransmitter noradrenaline and circulating adrenaline. These activate the myocyte β_1-adrenoceptor–adenylate cyclase–cAMP–protein kinase A cascade, leading to an increase in the action potential Ca^{2+} current. The increased SR Ca^{2+} store and trigger Ca^{2+} raise the systolic free Ca^{2+} transient. Stimulation of the SR Ca^{2+} pumps shortens the Ca^{2+} transient.

■ The result is a stronger, briefer contraction. Stroke volume and ejection fraction increase. End-systolic volume falls. Systolic pressure rises, and relaxation is faster.

■ Increased contractility shifts the Starling curve (stroke work vs. filling pressure) upwards. The shift is graded in proportion to sympathetic activity. The heart thus operates on a 'family of ventricular function curves'. The pressure–volume loop becomes wider, taller and shifted to the left.

■ Other positive inotropic influences include β-agonists such as isoprenaline and dobutamine; phosphodiesterase inhibitors such as caffeine and milrinone; the Na^+–K^+ pump inhibitor digoxin; and increased beat frequency (the Bowditch effect). Premature beats (extra systoles) are weaker than normal and the beat after the compensatory pause is stronger than normal.

■ Negative inotropic influences include the hypoxia and acidosis of acute myocardial ischaemia, and chronic heart failure. This impairs exercise ability. Intracellular acidosis strongly impairs contractility. Arrhythmia is common, due to reduced membrane potentials, increased intracellular [Na^+], and Ca^{2+} store overload, which triggers afterdepolarization.

■ Paradoxically, the re-oxygenation of ischaemic myocardium can increase the tissue damage (myocardial stunning and ischaemia–reperfusion injury).

■ Increased arterial pressure raises 'afterload' and impairs stroke volume. This effect is represented by the pump function curve or afterload–shortening relation. Pressure reduction by vasodilator drugs improves the stroke volume, especially in heart failure.

■ Secondary effects of raised arterial pressure are diastolic distension (raising contractile force through Starling's law); the Anrep effect (raising contractility); the baroreflex (reducing sympathetic drive); and in the long term concentric ventricular hypertrophy leading to failure.

■ In exercise a co-ordinated response of the heart (sympathetic mediated tachycardia; increased stroke volume) and peripheral circulation facilitates the increased cardiac output. Stroke volume can double, due to increased end-diastolic volume and decreased end-systolic volume. Peripheral venoconstriction and the skeletal muscle pump maintain or raise the CVP and preload. Vasodilatation in active muscle minimizes the rise in arterial pressure and afterload. Transplanted and artificially paced hearts respond to exercise due to the redundancy of control mechanisms, e.g. circulating catecholamines, skeletal muscle pump.

■ Cardiac efficiency is at best 15%. Much of the energy goes into raising pressure. Emotional stress raises pressure and should therefore be avoided by patients with ischaemic heart disease.

■ The energy source is ⅔ to ¾ free fatty acid; the rest is glucose and lactate. The high-energy phosphate reserve is low, so increased myocardial performance is tightly dependent on increased coronary O_2 delivery.

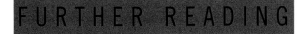

FURTHER READING

Reviews and chapters

Allen, D. G. and Kentish, J. C. (1985) The cellular basis of the length–tension relation in cardiac muscle. *Journal of Molecular and Cellular Cardiology*, **17**, 821–840.

Bonow, R. O. (1994) Left ventricular response to exercise. In *Cardiovascular Response to Exercise* (ed. Fletcher, G. F.), American Heart Association Monongraph, Futura Press, New York, pp. 31–47.

Brady, A. J. (1991) Mechanical properties of isolated cardiac myocytes. *Physiological Reviews*, **71**, 413–427.

Casadei, B. (2001) Vagal control of myocardial contractility in humans. *Experimental Physiology*, **86**, 817–823.

Cingolani, H. E., Perez, N. G. and Camilion de Hurtado, M. C. (2001) An autocrine/paracrine mechanism triggered by myocardial stretch induces changes in contractility. *News in Physiological Science*, **16**, 88–91 (The Anrep effect).

Fuchs, F. and Smith, S. S. (2001) Calcium, cross-bridges, and the Frank–Starling relationship. *News in Physiological Science*, **16**, 5–10.

Kleber, A. G. and Janse, M. J. (1995) Impulse propagation in myocardial ischemia. In *Cardiac Electrophysiology from Cell to Bedside* (eds Zipes, D. P. and Jalife, J. W. B.), W. B. Saunders, Philadelphia, pp. 156–161.

Lindpainter, K. and Ganten, D. (1991) The cardiac renin–angiotensin system: a synopsis of current experimental and clinical data. *News in Physiological Sciences*, **6**, 227–232.

Molkentin, J. D. and Dorn, G. W. (2001) Cytoplasmic signaling pathways that regulate cardiac hypertrophy. *Annual Review of Physiology*, **63**, 391–426.

Piper, H. M. (1997) Mechanism of myocardial injury during acute reperfusion. *News in Physiological Sciences*, **12**, 53–54.

Sagawa, K., Maughan, L., Suga, H. and Sunagawa, K. (1988) *Cardiac Contraction and the Pressure–Volume Relationship*, Oxford University Press, New York.

Starnes, J. W. (1994) Myocardial metabolism during exercise. In *Cardiovascular Response to Exercise* (ed. Fletcher, G. F.), American Heart Association Monongraph, Futura Press, New York, pp. 3–13.

te Keurs, H. E. D. J. and Noble, M. I. M. (1988) *Starling's Law of the Heart Revisited*, Kluwer Academic, Dordrecht.

Research papers

Balnave, C. D. and Vaughan-Jones, R. D. (2000) Effect of intracellular pH on spontaneous Ca^{2+} sparks in rat ventricular myocytes. *Journal of Physiology*, **528**, 25–37.

Banner, N. R., Guz, A., Heaton, R., Innes, J. A., Murphy, K. and Jacoub, M. (1988) Ventilatory and circulatory responses at the onset of exercise in man following heart or heart–lung transplantation. *Journal of Physiology*, **399**, 437–449.

Elliott, A. C., Smith, G. L. and Allen, D. G. (1994) The metabolic consequences of an increase in the frequency of stimulation in isolated ferret hearts. *Journal of Physiology*, **474**, 147–159 (The Bowditch effect).

Elstad, M., Toska, K., Chon, K. H., Raeder, E. A. and Cohen, R. J. (2001) Respiratory sinus arrhythmia: opposite effects on systolic and mean arterial pressure in supine humans. *Journal of Physiology*, **536**, 251–259.

Kentish, J. C. and Wrzosek, A. (1998) Changes in force and cytosolic Ca^{2+} concentration after length changes in isolated rat ventricular trabeculae. *Journal of Physiology*, **506**, 431–444.

Konhilas, J. P., Irving, T. C. and de Tombe, P. P. (2002) Myofilament calcium sensitivity in skinned rat cardiac trabeculae: role of interfilament lattice spacing. *Circulation Research*, **90**, 59–65.

Lewis, M. E., Al-Khalidi, A. H., Bonser, R. S., *et al.* (2001) Vagus nerve stimulation decreases left ventricular contractility in vivo in the human and pig heart. *Journal of Physiology*, **534**, 547–552.

Ruiz-Meana, M., Garcia-Doarado, D., Julia, M., *et al.* (2000) Protective effect of HOE642, a selective blocker of $Na^{+}-H^{+}$ exchange, against the development of rigor contracture in rat ventricular myocytes. *Experimental Physiology*, **85**, 17–25.

Sullivan, M. J., Cobb, F. R. and Higginbotham, M. B. (1991) Stroke volume increases by similar mechanisms during upright exercise in normal men and women. *American Journal of Cardiology*, **67**, 1405–1412.

CHAPTER 7

Assessment of cardiac output and peripheral pulse

Learning objectives

After reading this chapter you should be able to:

- Define the Fick principle (cf. Fick's law of diffusion!) (7.1).
- Apply the Fick principle to estimate pulmonary blood flow from O_2 uptake (7.1).
- Draw a typical concentration or temperature vs. time plot for the indicator or thermal dilution method, and explain how cardiac output is derived from it (7.2).
- Outline three common 'high-tech' methods for estimating human stroke volume (7.3, 7.5).
- Describe the relation between pulse pressure and stroke volume (7.4).
- Define arterial compliance and state three major factors that affect it (7.4).

Overview. The cardiac output is the volume of blood ejected by one ventricle in one minute, and equals stroke volume $\times$ beats per minute. Many ways of measuring the cardiac output have been devised over the years, partly for research purposes, such as investigating an athlete's response to training, and partly for medical purposes, such as quantifying the severity of cardiac disease with a view to treatment.

Human cardiac output can be measured as a whole using the **Fick's principle** or the **dilution method**. Alternatively, the stroke volume can be measured separately by the **Doppler ultrasound**, **radionuclide counts** or **echocardiography** methods, and then multiplied by the heart rate. The latter can be counted by palpation or recorded using a device such an ECG or pulse oximeter.

The above methods all involve complex technology and a laboratory setting. By contrast, much the commonest, albeit least direct, way of making a rough assessment of the stroke volume is to examine the **arterial pulse** at the patient's bedside.

We will begin with the gold-standard, but most invasive, method, which introduces an important general principle of transport called Fick's principle.

7.1 Fick's principle and pulmonary oxygen transport

Adolf Fick pointed out in 1870 that the rate at which the circulation absorbs O_2 from the lungs must equal the change in O_2 concentration in the pulmonary blood multiplied by the pulmonary blood flow. Since the pulmonary blood flow is the output of the right ventricle, O_2 uptake measurements provide a way of determining the cardiac output.

Fick's principle quantifies O_2 uptake from the lungs

Fick's principle is more than just a methodology – it is basic to understanding O_2 transport from the lungs to blood, one of the major functions of the cardiovascular system (Figure 7.1). The amount of O_2 carried into the lungs in venous blood per minute is the blood flow $\dot{Q}$ times venous oxygen concentration C_V:

$$\frac{O_2 \text{ in venous blood entering}}{\text{the lungs per minute}} = \dot{Q}C_V$$

Similarly, the amount of O_2 carried out of the lungs per minute in oxygenated blood equals the blood flow times the arterial oxygen concentration C_A:

$$\frac{O_2 \text{ in arterialized blood leaving}}{\text{the lungs per minute}} = \dot{Q}C_A$$

The amount of O_2 taken up by the blood as it passes through the lungs is the difference between the above two quantities, so:

$$\frac{O_2 \text{ uptake by pulmonary}}{\text{blood per minute}} = (\dot{Q}C_A) - (\dot{Q}C_V)$$

In a steady state, the oxygen uptake by blood must equal the oxygen removed from the alveolar gas in the lungs, $\dot{V}_{O_2}$ so:

$$\frac{\text{Removal of alveolar}}{O_2 \text{ per minute}} = \frac{\text{Uptake by pulmonary}}{\text{blood per minute}}$$

or in symbols:

$$\dot{V}_{O_2} = (\dot{Q}C_A) - (\dot{Q}C_V)$$

Re-arranging this in terms of the arteriovenous concentration difference $C_A - C_V$:

$$\dot{V}_{O_2} = \dot{Q}(C_A - C_V)$$

This is **Fick's equation**. It tells us that the rate of O_2 uptake from alveolar gas, in ml O_2/min, equals pulmonary blood flow (in l/min) times the arteriovenous difference in O_2 concentration (in ml O_2/l blood).

Since pulmonary blood flow $\dot{Q}$ is right ventricular output, we can rearrange the expression to give the cardiac output, thus:

$$\text{Cardiac output } \dot{Q} \text{ (l/min)} =$$

$$\frac{\text{Oxygen uptake rate } \dot{V}_{O_2} \text{ (ml/min)}}{\text{Arterial } O_2 \text{ conc. } C_A - \text{Venous } O_2 \text{ conc. } C_V \text{ (ml/l)}}$$

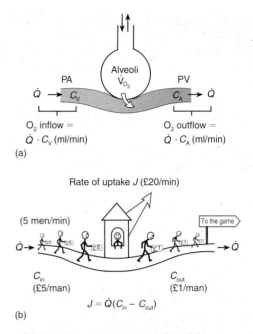

Figure 7.1 The Fick principle. (a) Application to measurement of pulmonary blood flow; PA, pulmonary artery containing venous blood; PV, pulmonary vein with arterialized blood. (b) Application to measure flow of supporters through a football turnstile. The supporters could equally well represent red cells giving up CO_2 in the lungs, or plasma giving up glucose to the brain.

For example, a resting human absorbs ~250 ml O_2 per minute from the alveolar gas ($\dot{V}_{O2}$). Arterial blood contains 195 ml O_2 per litre and the mixed venous blood entering the lungs contains 145 ml O_2 per litre. Each litre of blood therefore takes up 50 ml O_2, i.e. $(C_A - C_V) = 50$ ml/l. To take up 250 ml O_2, 5 l of blood are required (i.e. 250/50). Since this uptake occurs in 1 min, the pulmonary blood flow must be 5 l/min.

Fick's method involves cardiac catheterization

Fick's method was not practicable until the 1940s, when progress in cardiac catheterization allowed **mixed venous blood** to be sampled from the right ventricle. Mixed venous blood gives the average concentration of O_2 in blood entering the lungs. Peripheral venous blood is no good for this purpose because its O_2 concentration varies widely (e.g. 170 ml/l in renal venous blood, 70 ml/l in coronary venous blood). Venous blood only becomes fully mixed and uniform in the right ventricle and pulmonary artery. The problem of sampling mixed venous blood was solved by the German physician Werner Forssman, who in 1929 passed a ureteric catheter through his own arm vein and into the right heart, watching its progress on an X-ray screen. This brave act founded human cardiac catheterization, won Forssman the disapproval of his head of department and, later, the Nobel prize.

The Fick method is now as follows. The subject's resting O_2 consumption, $\dot{V}_{O2}$, is measured for 5–10 min by spirometry or by collecting expired air in a Douglas bag. During this period an arterial blood sample is taken from the brachial, radial or femoral artery, and a mixed venous sample is taken from the pulmonary artery or right ventricle outflow tract by a cardiac catheter, introduced through the antecubital (elbow) vein. The O_2 content of each blood sample is measured and the cardiac output calculated as above.

The Fick method has several limitations

Although Fick's method is the yardstick by which new methods are judged, it takes 5–10 min to perform, so beat-by-beat changes in stroke volume cannot be resolved. Also, the method is only valid in the steady state, so rapidly changing cardiac outputs cannot be resolved. The method is invasive and is not used during severe exercise because the cardiac catheter may provoke arrhythmia in a violently beating heart. The **indirect Fick method** avoids cardiac catheterization and estimates C_V by the analysis of re-breathed gas. This may be used in special circumstances, as was recently the case in an orbiting space laboratory!

The Fick principle is very general

The Fick principle is an important, general physiological principle that applies to the exchange of any material in any perfused organ – for example, glucose transport from microcirculation to muscle or brain (Section 10.10). In general terms, the flux J of a material between the fluid and the perfused organ equals the fluid flow Q multiplied by the concentration difference between the inlet, C_{in}, and outlet, C_{out};

$$J = Q(C_{out} - C_{in})$$

As Figure 7.1b shows, the Fick principle even applies to the influx of money at the turnstile of a football ground. In physiology Fick's principle is widely used to work out the rate at which an organ is consuming a nutrient such as glucose from measurements of blood flow and the arteriovenous concentration difference.

7.2 Indicator and thermal dilution methods

It is usual, nowadays, for cardiac departments to use the thermal dilution method rather than its parent, the indicator dilution method. We will consider the indicator method first, however, because it is easier to understand quantities of dye than quantities of 'cold'.

Indicator dilution method

A known mass of a foreign substance, the indicator, is injected rapidly into a central vein or the right heart. The indicator should be confined to the bloodstream and easy to assay – dyes such as Evans blue or indocyanine green that bind to plasma albumin, for example; or albumin labelled with radio-iodine. The indicator becomes diluted in the returning venous blood, passes through the heart and lungs and is ejected into the systemic arteries (Figure 7.2a). Arterial blood is sampled from the radial or femoral artery, and its indicator content is plotted against time.

For simplicity, let us first suppose that the indicator concentration in the ejected bolus is uniform, as in Figure 7.2b. The time-concentration plot tells us: (i) the time t taken by the bolus to pass a given point; and (ii) the average concentration of indicator in the bolus. Concentration C is by definition the injected mass m divided by the volume of plasma in which the indicator has become distributed, V_D: in other words, $C = m/V_D$. The distribution volume V_D is thus:

$$V_D = m/C$$

For example, if 1 mg of indicator produces a bolus plasma concentration of 1 mg/l, its volume of distribution is 1 l. If this volume takes t seconds to pass the sampling point, the left ventricle is pumping plasma along at rate V_D/t. In Figure 7.2b the rate is 1 l in 20 s or 3 l/min. Thus the cardiac output of plasma can be calculated as:

$$\text{Cardiac output of plasma} = \frac{V_D}{t} = \frac{\text{Mass of indicator } (m)}{\text{Mean concentration } C \times \text{Passage time } (t)}$$

The output of blood is calculated as output of plasma divided by 1 – haematocrit. Haematocrit is the fraction of blood made up of cells.

Note that the denominator $C \times t$ in the above expression is the area under the plot of concentration versus time. Thus the expression simplifies to:

$$\text{Cardiac output of plasma} = \frac{\text{Mass of indicator } (m)}{\text{Area under } C - t \text{ plot}}$$

In reality the $C-t$ plot is not a square wave but a curve that rises to a peak and then decays exponentially (Figure 7.2c). Dye concentration decays

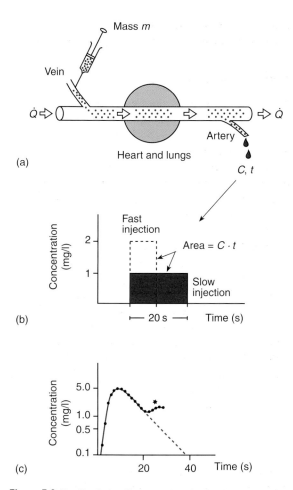

(a)

(b)

(c)

Figure 7.2 Hamilton's dye-dilution method. (a) Arterial concentration *C* depends on the mass of indicator injected (*m*) and the volume of blood in which it became diluted. (b) Idealized plot of arterial concentration against time. Although the shape of the plot depends on injection rate, the area $C \times t$ (20 mg·s·l^{-1}) does not; the increase in concentration produced by a fast injection is offset by the shorter duration of the bolus. If the injected mass of dye is 1 mg, the cardiac output of plasma is 1/20 = 0.05 l/s, or 3 l/min. For a haematocrit of 0.4, the cardiac output of blood is 5 l/min. (c) The grim reality. True shape of the concentration curve, with concentration plotted on a log-arithmic scale to linearize the decay and allow extrapolation past the recirculation hump (asterisk). Area under the extrapolated curve is used to calculate the cardiac output. (After Asmussen, E. and Nielsen, M. (1953) *Acta Physiologica Scandinavica*, **27**, 217.)

transit of the myocardial circulation, which is the shortest circulation in the body.

The above area-under-curve expression is still applicable to real indicator curves, but it is necessary to find the area under a $C-t$ curve uncomplicated by recirculation. To do this, the early part of the decay curve is extrapolated past the recirculation hump. A semi-logarithmic plot converts the exponential decay into a straight line, which can then be extrapolated to a negligible concentration (usually 1% of the peak) as in Figure 7.2c. The area under the corrected $C-t$ curve is used to calculate the cardiac output.

A modern, computerized version of the method uses an intravenous injection of **lithium ions**, which are detected in the arterial blood by an ion-sensitive electrode. It appears that lithium loss during passage through the lungs is negligible.

Pros and cons of dye dilution

Dye dilution results agree with Fick's direct method to within 5%. The dilution method has a better time resolution (30 s) that Fick's method (5–10 min) and can be used in exercise because ventricular catheter-ization is not required. The error involved in extrapolating the decay curve is, however, a draw-back. In diseased hearts, where the initial part of the decay curve may be short and distorted, this can be a serious limitation.

Thermal dilution method

This is a variant of the dilution method that is widely used in cardiac departments. Instead of a dye, temperature is used as the indicator. A known mass of cold saline is injected quickly into the right atrium, right ventricle or pulmonary artery. The dilution of the cold saline in the warm, flowing blood of the pulmonary artery is recorded through a Swan–Ganz catheter, the tip of which is advanced into the distal pulmonary artery and contains a ther-mistor. Cardiac output is calculated as the injected amount of heat (i.e. cold) divided by the area under the temperature–time plot.

Pros and cons of thermal dilution

A major advantage of thermal dilution is that the recirculation problem is circumvented, because the saline has warmed up to body temperature before it returns to the right side. Heat transfer across the walls of the right ventricle and pulmonary artery can cause over-estimation of the distribution volume and hence cardiac output, but a computed correc-tion can be made for this.

exponentially because the ventricle only ejects about two-thirds of its contents per systole. The residual indicator in the ventricle is diluted by indicator-free venous blood returning during the next diastole, and the diluted blood is in turn only partially ejected in systole – and so on. After about 15 seconds the decay curve is interrupted by a recirculation hump. The hump is caused by blood with a high indicator content returning to the heart after one complete

7.3 Aortic flow by pulsed Doppler method

To assess the stroke volume, repeated pulses of ultrasound are directed down the ascending aorta from a transmitter crystal at the suprasternal notch (Figure 7.3, top). Reflected ultrasound from the red cells is collected and analysed for a shift in frequency, which is caused by the high velocity of the cells during ejection. This is the Doppler shift effect, analogous to the change in pitch of a police car siren as it speeds past. The mean blood velocity across the aorta is computed for each successive millisecond of the cardiac cycle and plotted against time (Figure 7.3, bottom). The velocity curve is interpreted as follows.

Stroke distance is distance advanced along the aorta per ejection

The area under the velocity–time curve represents the distance advanced by the blood along the aorta during one systole (because distance is velocity × time). This is called the **stroke distance**. To convert this into stroke volume, the cross-sectional area of the aorta must be measured by echocardiography (see Section 2.6). The area, in cm^2, is then multiplied by the stroke distance in cm to give the stroke volume in cm^3

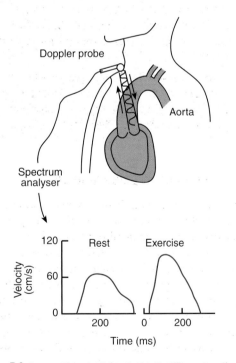

Figure 7.3 Transaortic pulsed Doppler method for measuring the mean velocity of blood across the aorta at each instant of systole. (From Innes, J. A., Simon, T. D., Murphy, K. and Guz, A. (1988) *Quarterly Journal of Experimental Physiology*, **73**, 323–341, by permission.)

(minus the volume that escaped through the coronary arteries).

Pros and cons of Doppler method

The Doppler method is difficult to calibrate and has 'noise' problems. On the other hand it has the enormous advantage of non-invasiveness and high temporal resolution. Unlike the Fick or dilution methods, it records every instant of every ejection.

7.4 Peripheral pulse and its relation to cardiac output

The oldest, cheapest, quickest and easiest way to assess the cardiac output is to feel the radial pulse at the wrist. **Heart rate** can be counted and the **strength of the pulse** estimated subjectively. A strong pulse is associated with a large stroke volume – for example during exercise; and a weak pulse is associated with a low stroke volume, for example after a haemorrhage. What the finger actually detects is the expansion of the artery as pressure rises during systole. The rise in pressure, or **pulse pressure**, is systolic pressure minus the diastolic pressure, and this is easily measured objectively by brachial artery sphygmomanometry (Section 8.5).

Arterial compliance links stroke volume and pulse pressure

The relation between stroke volume and arterial pressure is one of the key haemodynamic relations of the circulation. It is introduced here (Figure 7.4) and reviewed further in Chapter 8. During the ejection phase most of the stroke volume, about 70–80% in a resting subject, is accommodated in the elastic arteries, because the ventricle ejects blood faster than it can drain away. The distension of the artery wall raises the blood pressure, generating the systolic pressure. The rise in pressure, or pulse pressure, thus depends on the distensibility or **compliance** of the arterial system and on the **stroke volume**. Compliance is defined as change in volume per unit change in pressure:

$$\text{Arterial compliance} = \frac{\text{Increase in blood volume}}{\text{Increase in arterial pressure}}$$

In a young adult the arterial compliance is ~2 ml per mmHg at normal blood pressures.

The increase in arterial blood volume during systole equals the stroke volume minus the volume that runs off during the ejection period. Therefore, the pulse pressure is related to stroke volume as follows:

$$\text{Pulse pressure} = \frac{(\text{Stroke volume} - \text{Initial runoff})}{\text{Arterial compliance}}$$

On this basis, changes in pulse pressure have long been used as a guide to changes in stroke volume.

Arterial compliance is not a fixed quantity

There are certain problems inherent in the above approach, arising from the fact that arterial compliance is not a constant. The compliance changes both acutely and chronically, as follows.

1 Arterial compliance (distensibility) falls as pressures and volume increase. This causes the upward curvature of the arterial pressure–volume plot in Figure 7.4.

2 Compliance is reduced by high ejection velocities, because the artery wall is a viscoelastic material (see Appendix 2). During exercise the pulse pressure increases proportionately more than the stroke volume because there is less time for viscous relaxation of the wall during a fast ejection.

3 Compliance declines with advancing age due to a degenerative stiffening of elastic arteries called arteriosclerosis. As a result the pulse pressure increases with age, raising the work of the heart (Sections 8.4, 17.7). **Arteriosclerosis** is a diffuse stiffening of elastic arteries due to medial and intimal hypertrophy. It should not be confused with **atheroma** (Table 17.4).

Arterial compliance links pulse pressure and stroke volume

☐ Arterial compliance C is the increase in blood volume in the arterial system ΔV that produces unit increase in arterial pressure ΔP. Thus $C = \Delta V/\Delta P$. It is an objective measure of stretchiness.

☐ Pulse pressure is the increase in pressure between diastole and systole.

☐ From the above definitions, pulse pressure = stroke volume (minus run-off during ejection)/arterial compliance. Therefore pulse pressure can be increased by a rise in stroke volume (e.g. in exercise) or a fall in compliance.

☐ Arterial compliance falls as pressure increases, due to tensing of collagen in the walls. Consequently, a rise in *mean* arterial pressure causes a rise in *pulse* pressure.

☐ Arterial compliance falls with ageing due to arteriosclerosis, a diffuse stiffening of the media and intima of elastic vessels. As a result pulse pressure can double between youth and old age.

Pros and cons of pulse method

Because arterial compliance is not constant, and because the amount of run-off during ejection depends on the peripheral resistance, the pulse pressure is only an indirect measure of stroke volume, of limited value. Within its limitations, however, the changes in the peripheral pulse, recorded with nothing more sophisticated than a wrist watch and sphygmomanometer, gives a convenient bedside indication of changes in cardiac output in an individual patient from hour to hour – for example during recovery from an acute haemorrhage.

At a more sophisticated level, computer models have been developed that make reasonably accurate computations of acute changes in stroke volume

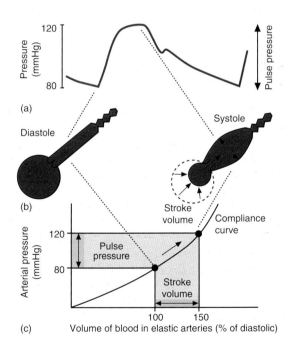

Figure 7.4 Relation between pulse pressure and stroke volume; lines join up coincident points. (a) Aortic pressure wave. (b) Ejection of left ventricle stroke volume into elastic arteries. (c) Pressure–volume relation (compliance curves) of young human aorta. Note increase in stiffness (steepening of slope) with pressure. (Based on Nichols, W. W. and O'Rourke, M. F. (1998); see Further reading.)

from recordings of peripheral arterial pressure. This has enabled **continuous computer monitoring** of stroke volume, heart rate and cardiac output in intensive care units.

Pulse oximetry monitors pulse rate

The pulse rate can be measured using a watch and palpation of the radial artery; or by a modern, miniaturised ECG that straps to the chest and transmits the heart rate to a wrist monitor; or by a **pulse oximeter**. An oximeter is a small device in which light is shone through a tissue, usually an ear lobe or finger. The transmitted light is detected by a photoelectric cell. Red cells absorb some of the light, and oxygenated haemoglobin absorbs a different wavelength of light to deoxygenated haemoglobin. As the arterial system expands with each pulse, the net light transmission changes. From this the pulse rate and oxygen saturation of the arterial blood are computed.

7.5 Radionuclide ventriculography, echocardiography and electromagnetic 'flow' meter

Radionuclide ventriculography

After an intravenous injection of radionuclide, the gamma count emanating from the ventricles is monitored by a precordial gamma camera. The radionuclide is commonly a compound of technetium that binds to red cells. The difference between the radioactive content of the ventricles in diastole and in systole is used to calculate the ejection fraction and stroke volume.

Echocardiography

The end-diastolic and end-systolic dimensions of the ventricle can be estimated by echocardiography (Figures 2.9, 6.24). These measurements can be converted into an estimate of stroke volume and ejection fraction if some assumptions are made about chamber shape. Typical human values are listed in Table 2.2.

Electromagnetic 'flow' meter

This technique is used in laboratory animals. A miniature, semicircular magnet is implanted at surgery, with the magnetic poles on either side of the blood vessel of interest, e.g. pulmonary artery. Blood is an electrical conductor, and as it cuts through the magnetic field it induces an electrical potential, which is measured. The potential is proportional to the blood velocity (cm/s), not flow. The internal diameter of the vessel is required to convert mean velocity to flow. Being small, an electromagnetic flowmeter can be left inside a conscious animal, transmitting a signal by telemetry (radio-waves). In this way much has been learned about the regulation of stroke volume in unfettered animals.

SUMMARY

■ The gold-standard method for humans is the **Fick principle**, namely, rate of uptake of solute = flow × concentration difference between incoming and outgoing blood. Applied to the lungs, the rate of uptake of O_2 is measured by spirometry or expired air collection. The O_2 content of mixed venous blood is measured in a sample obtained from the right ventricle by cardiac catheterization, and arterial blood is sampled from a systemic artery. Pulmonary blood flow, i.e. right ventricular output, is then calculated by the Fick principle.

■ The **indicator** and **thermal dilution methods** offer better time resolution. A known mass of dye or cold saline is injected quickly into the right ventricle or pulmonary artery, and the concentration or temperature is recorded at a point downstream. Concentration or temperature is plotted versus time. From the injected mass m and the average measured concentration C (or temperature) the volume of blood in which the indicator has distributed is calculated; $V_D = m/C$. The time taken for this volume of blood to pass the sampling point gives the cardiac output.

■ High-technology methods include the **pulsed Doppler ultrasound** measurement of aortic blood velocity. The area under the velocity−time plot gives the stroke distance. Stroke distance × aortic diameter (measured by ultrasound) gives the stroke volume.

■ In **radionuclide ventriculography** the stroke volume is calculated by comparing the radioactive counts present in the ventricle during end-diastole and end-systole.

■ In **echocardiography** changes in ventricular dimension are measured. With all methods that estimate stroke volume alone, the cardiac output is calculated as heart rate × stroke volume. The pulse rate can be monitored by **pulse oximetry**.

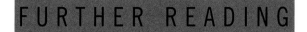 The simplest way to assess cardiac output at the bedside is to count the pulse and use sphygmomanometry to measure the **pulse pressure** (systolic minus diastolic pressure). Pulse pressure is proportional to stroke volume, although the relation is complicated by runoff, non-linear aortic compliance, dependence on ejection rate and age-related arterial stiffening (arteriosclerosis)

FURTHER READING

Band, D. M., Linton, R. A. F., O'Brien, T. K., Jonas, M. M. and Linton, N. W. F. (1997) The shape of indicator dilution curves used for cardiac output measurement in man. (Lithium dilution method.) *Journal of Physiology*, **498**, 225–229.

Crawford, M. H. and Flinn, R. S. (1994) Doppler echocardiographic assessment of left ventricular systolic and diastolic flow during exercise. In *Cardiovascular Response to Exercise* (ed. Fletcher, G. F.), Futura, New York, pp. 49–56.

Harms, M. P. M., Wesseling, K. H., Pott, F. and van Lieshout, J. J. (1999) Continuous stroke volume monitoring by modelling flows from non-invasive measurements of arterial pressure in humans under orthostatic stress. *Clinical Science*, **97**, 291–301.

Mehta, N., Iyawe, V. I., Cummin, A. R. C., Bayley, S., Saunders, K. B. and Bennett, E. D. (1985) Validation of a Doppler technique for beat-to-beat measurement of cardiac output. *Clinical Science*, **69**, 377–382.

Nichols, W. W. and O'Rourke, M. F. (1998) *McDonald's Blood Flow in Arteries. Theoretical, Experimental and Clinical Principles*, 4th Edition, Edward Arnold, London. [Pulse pressure and arterial compliance.]

Schelbert, H. R., Verba, I. W., Johnson, A. D., *et al.* (1978) Non-traumatic determination of left ventricular ejection fraction by radionuclide angiography. *Circulation*, **51**, 902–909.

CHAPTER 8

Haemodynamics: flow, pressure and resistance

Learning objectives

After studying this chapter you should be able to:

- Use Darcy's law to relate mean arterial pressure to cardiac output and peripheral resistance (8.1).
- Distinguish between laminar and turbulent flow and where they occur (8.2).
- State the relation between arterial pulse pressure, arterial stiffness and stroke volume (8.4, 7.4).
- Draw, label and scale the arterial pressure pulse and explain its main features (8.4).
- Explain why arterial stiffening raises cardiac work (8.4).
- List the main factors affecting mean arterial pressure (8.5).
- Describe how human blood pressure is measured using auscultation (8.5).
- Use Poiseuille's law to explain how arteriolar radius regulates flow and arterial pressure (8.7).
- Explain the relevance of Laplace's law to aneurysm formation (8.7).
- State the factors governing effective blood viscosity and their physiological/clinical significance (8.8).
- Draw a graph showing blood flow as a function of arterial pressure in (i) the absence and (ii) the presence of autoregulation (8.9).
- Sketch the manometric effect of gravity on arterial and venous pressures on standing (8.11).
- List the key factors affecting blood volume in peripheral veins (8.10).
- Explain how human central venous pressure is estimated by inspection of neck veins (8.10).
- Describe the skeletal muscle pump and three beneficial effects (8.12).

8.1 Hydraulic principles

The science of haemodynamics concerns the relation between blood flow, pressure and hydraulic resistance. The simplest guide to these issues is Darcy's law, which was introduced in Chapter 1.

Darcy's law relates flow to pressure difference

Darcy was a French engineer who studied the flow of water through the gravel beds of the fountains in Dijon. In 1856 Darcy reported that flow in the steady state, $\dot{Q}$, is linearly proportional to the pressure difference between two points, $P_1 - P_2$. That is to say:

$$\dot{Q} = K(P_1 - P_2) = \frac{(P_1 - P_2)}{R} \qquad (8.1a)$$

The proportionality coefficient K is called the hydraulic conductance – in effect the ease of flow. Its reciprocal is called the hydraulic resistance, R – the difficulty of flow. Darcy's law can be applied to channels of any geometry, including blood vessels. For example, blood flow through the kidney is equal to the pressure in the renal artery minus that in the renal vein divided by renal resistance.

Flow through the entire systemic circulation equals the cardiac output CO. The pressure difference is mean arterial pressure $\bar{P}_a$ minus central venous pressure CVP. The resistance is called total peripheral resistance, TPR. Putting these symbols into Darcy's law we find:

$$CO = \frac{(\bar{P}_a - CVP)}{TPR} \qquad (8.1b)$$

Since CVP is almost zero (i.e. close to atmospheric pressure), the expression simplifies to $CO \cong \bar{P}_a/TPR$. This can be re-arranged to answer the fundamental question, **What determines the mean blood pressure?** The answer is $\bar{P}_a = CO \times TPR$; in words, mean blood pressure is determined by the cardiac output and the peripheral resistance.

> Mean blood pressure =
> Cardiac output × Peripheral resistance

Bernoulli's theory incorporates other forms of fluid energy

Darcy's law deals with pressure, which is only one of three forms of mechanical energy that affect flow. The other two are gravitational potential energy and kinetic energy, as recognized by Bernoulli. Bernoulli was an 18th century Swiss physician who became a professor of mathematics at the age of 25. Bernoulli's theory states that the flow between points A and B in the steady state is proportional to the difference in the mechanical energy of the fluid between A and B; and that the mechanical energy is the sum of the pressure energy, potential energy and kinetic energy.

- **Pressure energy** is pressure $P \times$ volume V.

- **Potential (gravitational) energy** is the capacity of a mass to do work in a gravitational field by virtue of its height. The potential energy of blood relative to the heart equals its height above the heart $h \times$ gravitational force $g \times$ mass (which is volume $V \times$ density ρ).

- **Kinetic energy** is the energy that a moving mass, ρV, possesses due to its momentum. Kinetic energy increases in proportion to velocity squared (v^2) and equals $\rho V v^2/2$.

Adding the three energies together we have:

$$\text{Mechanical energy of unit volume blood} = \frac{P + \rho g h + \rho v^2}{2} \qquad (8.2)$$

It should be noted that both Darcy's and Bernoulli's law apply to flow that is not varying with time. If flow is pulsatile, as it is in arteries, the laws still apply to the mean flow; but they do not tell us how the flow is oscillating instant by instant.

Some applications of Bernoulli's theory to the circulation

Pressure falls inside a stenosed artery. Bernoulli's theory tells us what happens inside a stenosed, atheromatous artery (Figure 8.1). Any narrowing increases the fluid velocity v, so some of the fluid energy is converted into kinetic energy, reducing the pressure energy. Flow occurs from the narrowed segment into the wider outlet despite a contrary pressure gradient, proving that flow occurs down a gradient of total energy rather than pressure alone. The fall in pressure inside the stenosed, atheromatous segment exacerbates its collapse.

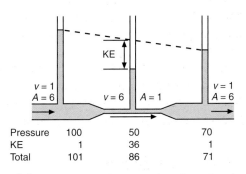

Pressure	100	50	70
KE	1	36	1
Total	101	86	71

Figure 8.1 Basic hydraulics; flow occurs down the total mechanical energy gradient. Where the cross-sectional area A narrows (e.g. arterial atheroma), velocity v increases, so pressure energy turns into kinetic energy KE. Where the tube widens, KE is reconverted to pressure. Flow from the narrow section to wide section is against the pressure gradient but down the total energy gradient.

A kinetic energy gradient aids cardiac filling. Kinetic energy is 1% of arterial fluid energy in a resting human (Section 6.14) but 12% of venous fluid energy, due to the low pressure energy in veins. On reaching the relaxed ventricle, the kinetic energy of venous blood falls virtually to zero. The kinetic energy gradient from vein to ventricle aids ventricular filling; or to put it another way, the momentum of the returning blood contributes to ventricular expansion.

Gravitational puzzles in humans. Although Darcy's law is generally adequate in vascular physiology, the more universal Bernoulli theory resolves some puzzles. For example, mean arterial pressure is typically 95 mmHg above atmospheric pressure in the aorta and 183 mmHg above atmospheric pressure in the dorsalis pedis artery of the foot during standing (Figure 8.2); yet blood flows from the aorta to the foot, apparently in defiance of Darcy's law. The explanation is, of course, that aortic blood has ~90 mmHg more gravitational potential energy than blood in the foot, so the energy of unit volume of aortic blood is 185 mmHg relative to the foot's 183 mmHg. The net energy difference of 2 mmHg drives the flow from the aorta to the dorsalis pedis artery.

8.2 Flow patterns

Three different patterns of flow are found in blood vessels: laminar flow, turbulent flow and single-file flow (Figures 8.3, 8.4). Laminar flow occurs in normal arteries, arterioles, venules and veins. Turbulent flow occurs in the ventricles and stenosed arteries. Single-file flow occurs in capillaries.

Laminar flow has smooth, parallel streamlines

During laminar flow through a cylindrical tube a liquid behaves like a set of infinitesimally thin concentric shells (laminae) that slide past each other. The lamina in contact with the vessel wall has zero velocity due to molecular cohesive forces – the **zero-slip condition**. The adjacent lamina slides slowly past the zero-slip lamina. The third lamina slides past the second lamina, and since the second lamina is itself moving, the third lamina has a higher velocity relative to the tube wall – and so on until maximum velocity is reached in the centre of the tube. Thus red cells have a higher velocity in the vessel centre than

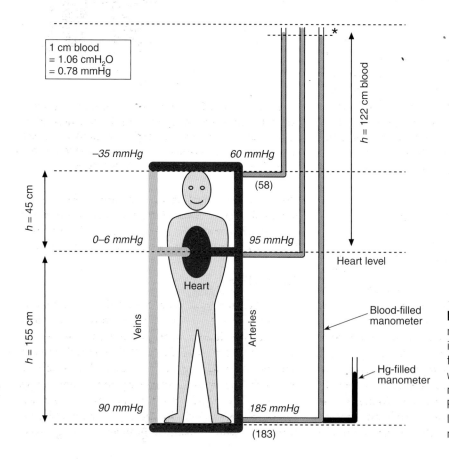

Figure 8.2 Effect of gravity on arterial and venous pressure in a standing human. Pink manometers are filled with blood, black (lower right) with mercury. Pressures in italics represent static effect of fluid column. Pressures in brackets are 2 mmHg lower (asterisk) due to slight arterial resistance to flow.

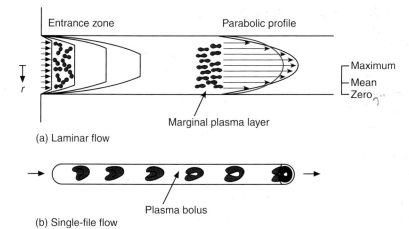

Entrance zone　　　　Parabolic profile

— Maximum
— Mean
— Zero

Marginal plasma layer

(a) Laminar flow

Plasma bolus

(b) Single-file flow

Figure 8.3 Blood flow patterns in a large vessel (a) and capillary (b). In (a), arrow length indicates the velocity (v) of each lamina. For a Newtonian fluid in fully developed laminar flow, velocity is a parabolic function of radial position (r): $v = v_{max}(1 - r^2/R^2)$, where R is tube radius. Mean velocity is $v_{max}/2$. The profile is blunter for a non-Newtonian fluid like blood (red line). The gradient of the velocity curve is called the '**shear rate**'. (b) In capillaries the red cells deform into parachute/slipper configurations (*left*) and folded shapes (*right*). (After Chien, S. (1992); see Further Reading.)

at the periphery. Similarly, the current is faster in the centre of a river than at its edges. In fully established laminar flow **the velocity profile across the tube is a parabola** for a simple fluid such as water. For a particulate suspension such as blood the profile is more blunted (Figure 8.3, red line). The profile is almost flat in the **entrance region**, as in the **ascending aorta**, and this simplifies the estimation of cardiac output by the Doppler method (Section 7.3).

The shearing of blood creates a marginal plasma layer

Shear is the sliding motion of one lamina past another. Shear causes the red cells to orientate preferentially in the direction of flow and move a little towards the central axis (**axial flow**). This leaves a thin, cell-deficient layer of plasma next to the vessel wall called the **marginal plasma layer**, of thickness $2-4\,\mu m$. The marginal plasma layer is functionally very important, because it greatly facilitates blood flow through the resistance vessels (the Fåhraeus–Lindqvist effect, Section 8.8).

Shear stress tugs on the endothelium

The friction between molecules in the sliding laminae causes each lamina to tug at its neighbour. The tugging force exerted by one layer on the next is called the **shear stress**. The size of the shear stress depends on the shear rate (rate of sliding) and fluid viscosity. At the vessel margin the shear stress tugs on the lining endothelium and stimulates the secretion of the regulatory vasoactive substance nitric oxide (Chapter 9).

In the proximal aorta the high shear stresses can tear the endothelium in susceptible individuals, namely those with hypertension, atheroma or Marfan's syndrome. This leads to a **dissecting aortic aneurysm**. Blood passes through the endothelial tear and tracks

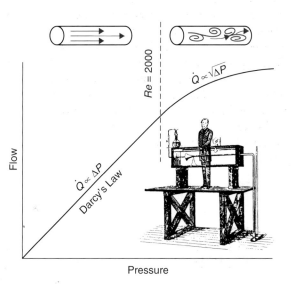

$Re = 2000$

$\dot{Q} \propto \sqrt{\Delta P}$

Flow

$\dot{Q} \propto \Delta P$
Darcy's Law

Pressure

Figure 8.4 Pressure–flow relation for a Newtonian fluid in a rigid tube. Darcy's law, represented by the straight line through the origin, breaks down when turbulence develops. Inset shows Sir Osborne Reynolds' apparatus for studying the onset of turbulence; the flow-pattern (top) was visualized by injecting dye into the fluid.

along the aortic wall in the subintimal plane, with potentially fatal results. An interim measure, prior to emergency surgery, is to reduce the wall shear stress by reducing the cardiac output pharmacologically.

Turbulence

As the pressure head driving fluid through a tube is increased, a point is eventually reached where the flow ceases to rise linearly with pressure and rises as the square-root of pressure (Figure 8.4). This is due to the transition from a laminar to a turbulent flow pattern in which chaotic cross-currents dissipate pressure energy as heat. The conditions that provoke turbulence were explored in 1883 by the engineer Sir Osborne Reynolds, who visualized turbulence using dyes.

Turbulence is encouraged by a high fluid velocity v, a large tube diameter D and a high fluid density (ρ, rho), because these three factors increase the fluid momentum and encourage the persistence of flow distortions. Turbulence is discouraged by a high viscosity (η, eta) because this damps out flow deviations. The ratio of the pro- to anti-turbulence factors is called the **Reynolds' number**, Re and is dimensionless:

$$Re = \frac{v\,D\,\rho}{\eta}$$

The critical Reynolds' number for the onset of turbulence during steady flow down a rigid, straight, uniform tube is ~2000. The critical value is less than 2000 in blood vessels because the flow is pulsatile and blood vessels are not rigid, straight or uniform. Even so, Re is well below the critical level in most blood vessels; in resistance vessels, for example, Re is ~0.5.

Turbulence is normal in the ventricles, where it helps to mix the blood and produce a uniform arterial gas content. Turbulence can also occur in the human aorta during peak flow, creating an **innocent systolic ejection murmur** (Section 2.5). Re reaches ~4600 during peak flow in the human aortic root, where the peak velocity v is 70 cm/s, diameter D is 2.5 cm, blood density ρ is 1.06 g/cm^3, and blood viscosity is 4 milliPascal-seconds or 0.04 g cm^{-1}s^{-1}.

Turbulence can also occur in leg arteries roughened by atheromatous plaques. The turbulence causes a **bruit** (local murmur audible through the stethoscope) and sometimes a palpable **thrill**. By contrast, normal laminar blood flow is silent.

Single-file (bolus) flow occurs in capillaries

The diameter of a capillary, 5–6 μm, is smaller than that of a red cell, 8 μm. As a result, red cells can only pass through capillaries in single file, and have to bend into a folded, parachute-like configuration to enter the capillary – a cartoon-like spectacle when seen through the microscope. Since the deformed red cell spans the full width of the capillary, parabolic flow is impossible; the plasma is trapped between the red cells and moves along as a bolus of uniform velocity (**bolus flow**). Bolus flow eliminates much of the internal friction that occurs during laminar flow, and thus offers a low resistance to flow.

As noted above, capillary flow is critically dependent on the **deformability of the red cells**. Deformability becomes impaired in **sickle cell anaemia**, because the red cells contain an abnormal haemoglobin that polymerizes in hypoxic situations. Polymerization causes the red cell to become rigid, sickle-shaped, and adhesive to the microvascular endothelium and other red cells. The rigidity and stickiness impair red cell passage through microvessels. The ensuing tissue ischaemia causes painful 'sickling crises'.

White cells (leukocytes) are rounder and stiffer than red cells. The leukocyte moves less freely along the microvessels and often creates a little traffic jam of red cells behind it. If leukocytes adhere to the vessel wall, as happens in small venules during inflammation, the local resistance to flow increases and impairs microvascular flow. This happens during inflammation, ischaemia, severe haemorrhagic hypotension, and in venous leg ulcers.

8.3 Measurement of blood flow

It is often necessary to measure blood flow quantitatively for research or clinical reasons – for example, to assess the flow impairment in an ischaemic leg following femoral artery atherosclerosis.

In anaesthetized animals the velocity of blood in large vessels can be measured using an **electromagnetic velocity meter** implanted surgically around the vessel (Section 7.5); or by **hot-wire anemometry**, in which the cooling of a heated wire in the bloodstream is proportional to the blood velocity. Blood flow in smaller regions can be assessed by giving a brief intra-arterial injection of **radiolabelled microspheres** of diameter ~15 μm. The microspheres are washed into the tissue in proportion to local blood flow and lodge in the terminal arterioles. The distribution of flow within the tissue can be assessed by excising it, dicing it into small pieces and counting the radioactivity of each piece.

In humans less direct methods are used as follows.

Doppler ultrasound measures large artery blood velocity

This non-invasive method, described in relation to the aorta in Section 7.3, is widely used to assess arterial flow in the feet of patients with ischaemic limb disease. It is also used to assess middle cerebral artery perfusion and placental perfusion in pregnancy.

A variant of the method, the **laser-Doppler fluxmeter**, employs a laser light beam rather than ultrasound to record the flux of red cells through the superficial dermis.

Fick's method measures organ blood flow

The Fick principle, introduced as a way of measuring pulmonary blood flow in Section 7.1, can also be applied to certain other organs. To measure **renal blood flow**, para-aminohippuric acid (PAH) is injected intravenously and its rate of appearance in urine is measured. PAH is almost completely cleared from renal blood, so renal venous concentration is taken as zero and the arterio-venous concentration difference is equated with the measured arterial concentration. Blood flow is calculated as excretion rate in urine (mg/min) divided by arterial concentration (mg/ml).

Venous occlusion plethysmography measures limb blood flow

Plethysmography is used in research laboratories to measure blood flow in a human limb, foot or digit (Figure 8.5). To measure forearm blood flow, an inflatable cuff is wrapped around the arm over the brachial vein and inflated quickly to 40 mmHg. This arrests the venous drainage from the arm but not the arterial inflow, so the arm begins to swell with blood. The initial swelling rate equals arterial blood flow. The swelling rate is measured using a mercury-in-rubber strain gauge, namely a mercury-filled elastic

tube wrapped around the limb. As the circumference of the limb increases, the mercury column is stretched and narrowed. The resulting increase in electrical resistance is measured and converted to change in forearm circumference by a calibration factor. (In former years, swelling was measured less conveniently by the displacement of air or water out of a rigid jacket around the limb, called a plethysmograph ('fullness record'). This is how the method's gargantuan name arose.)

Kety's tissue-clearance method measures microvascular flow

Radioisotope clearance provides a way of assessing microvascular blood flow in a small region of human tissue. A rapidly diffusing, radioactive solute is injected into the tissue as a local depot (Figure 8.6). It is gradually cleared from the depot by diffusion across the

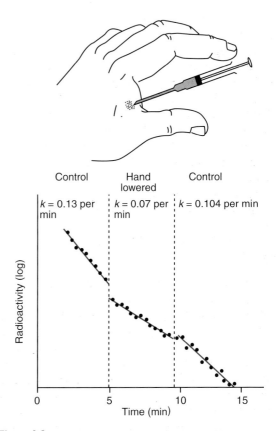

Figure 8.6 Tissue clearance method, using a cutaneous injection of xenon-133. With the hand at heart level the washout slope, k, was 13%/min (half-life 5.3 min; half-life is $0.693/k$). The calculated blood flow averaged 9 ml/min/100 ml. Lowering the hand 40 cm below heart level reduced blood flow to 7 ml/min/100 ml due to local arteriolar constriction (see Chapter 13). (After Lassen, N. A., Henriksen, U. and Sejrsen, P. (1983) In *Handbook of Physiology, Cardiovascular System*, Vol. 3, Part 1, *Peripheral Circulation* (eds Shepherd, J. T. and Abboud, F. M.), American Physiological Society, Bethesda, pp. 21–64.)

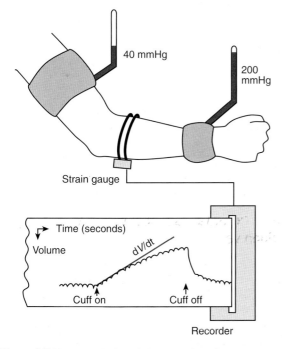

Figure 8.5 Venous occlusion plethysmography using a mercury-in-rubber strain gauge to record forearm circumference. The 'congesting cuff' (upper arm) occludes venous return and the wrist cuff eliminates hand blood flow from the measurement. The initial swelling rate (tangent to curve) measures forearm blood flow. Swelling rate tails off as venous back-pressure rises. After a few minutes (not shown here; see Figure 11.3) forearm blood volume stabilizes because venous pressure has exceeded cuff pressure, and venous outflow resumes.

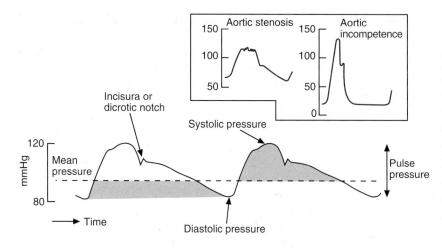

Figure 8.7 Pressure wave in human subclavian artery over two cycles recorded by an electronic transducer. The mean pressure, averaged over time, is the pressure at which the pink area above the mean ($\int P \cdot dt$) equals the pink area below the mean. Inset shows abnormal waveform in aortic valve stenosis (slow rise, prolonged plateau) and aortic incompetence (excessive pulse pressure, low diastolic pressure). (After Mills, C. J., Gale, I. T., Gault, J. H., *et al.* (1970) *Cardiovascular Research*, **4**, 405.)

walls of the capillaries into the bloodstream, which washes the solute away. If diffusion is fast enough, the rate of removal of solute is limited solely by the rate of capillary washout, i.e. clearance is proportional to blood flow (see 'Flow-limited exchange', Section 10.10). For this reason a fast-diffusing, lipid-soluble radioisotope such as xenon-133 or krypton-85 is employed. The removal rate is recorded by a gamma-counter over the depot. Kety pointed out in 1949 that, given flow-limited exchange, the isotope concentration declines exponentially with time, so a plot of the logarithm of concentration C against time t is linear (Figure 8.6). The slope of the logarithmic plot is called the removal rate constant k and is related to microvascular flow by the expression:

$$\log_e C = \log_e C_0 - kt$$

$$\text{where } k = \frac{\dot{Q}}{V\lambda} \qquad (8.3)$$

C_0 is concentration at time zero, V is the volume in which the solute is distributed, and λ (lambda) is the solute equilibrium partition coefficient between blood and tissue. The blood flow per unit volume, $\dot{Q}/V$, is calculated from the observed slope k.

8.4 The arterial pressure pulse

Basic shape of pulse in proximal arteries

The ventricle ejects blood into the proximal arterial system, namely the aorta and subclavian vessels, faster than it can flow away. This causes a steep increase in arterial pressure during systole (Figures 8.7, 8.8). Around 67–80% of the stroke volume is temporarily stored in the elastic arteries during systole, while 20–33% runs off through the peripheral resistance.

As ventricular ejection wanes, run-off begins to outpace ejection, so pressure begins to fall. When ejection ceases, a slight back-flow of aortic blood closes the aortic valve. Valve closure interrupts the descending limb of the pressure trace and produces an **incisura** or **dicrotic notch**. The notch is followed by a small, brief pressure oscillation due to vibration of the aortic valve cusps. As the run-off of arterial blood through the peripheral resistance continues, the blood pressure falls gradually towards its diastolic value. Diastolic pressure decay is slower than systolic pressure rise; the pulse is not symmetrical.

Pulse pressure increases with stroke volume and arterial stiffness

The size of the pressure oscillation between diastole and systole is called the **pulse pressure**. The factors governing pulse pressure were explained in Section 7.4. To summarize that section, the aortic pulse pressure depends primarily on:

- **stroke volume**, minus run-off during the ejection phase; and

- **arterial stiffness**, which is 1/compliance (Concept Box 9).

Thus the greater the stroke volume or arterial stiffness, the bigger the pulse pressure (Figure 8.8).

The arterial stiffness is influenced by the following three factors:

1 Mean blood pressure (because the arterial compliance curve gets steeper as pressure rises) (Figure 8.8).

2 Ageing (because arteriosclerosis accompanies ageing).

3 Rate of ventricular ejection (because the artery wall is visco-elastic).

An acute rise in mean pressure, ejection rate or ageing therefore leads to an increased pulse pressure. The effect of chronic hypertension on the pulse is considered later (Section 18.4).

The aortic pulse is transmitted rapidly to the peripheral arteries

If arteries had rigid walls, pressure would rise almost instantaneously throughout the arterial system; but arteries are not rigid, and as a result the pressure wave takes a finite time to spread along the arterial tree. The pulse travels at around 4–5 m/s in young people and 10–15 m/s in the elderly. This is an order of magnitude faster than the blood itself travels – the

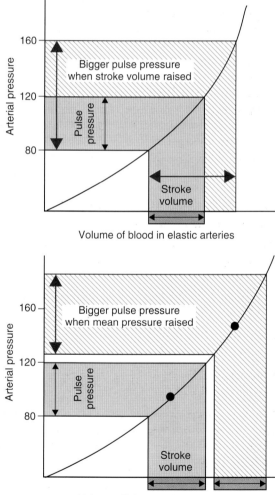

Figure 8.8 Non-linear pressure–volume relation of arteries and how it affects pulse pressure (schematic). (*Top*) A moderate increase in stroke volume doubles the pulse pressure, because the arteries get stiffer with stretch, steepening the curve. (*Bottom*) The same stroke volume ejected at a higher mean pressure (filled circles) causes a bigger pulse pressure.

mean blood velocity in the ascending aorta is only ~0.2 m/s.

One is reminded at this point of the White Queen's suggestion that Alice should practise believing at least six impossible things before breakfast. The difference between the pulse transmission velocity and blood velocity is, however, merely difficult to understand, not impossible (Figure 8.9). Since blood is essentially incompressible, the blood ejected into the proximal aorta has to create space for itself. It does this partly by distending the proximal aorta (which raises the pressure) and partly by pushing ahead the blood previously occupying the space. As the displaced blood moves forward, it too must make space for itself, partly by distending the wall downstream (which raises the pressure there) and partly by displacing the blood ahead. This shunting sequence repeats itself in rapid succession along the arterial tree. The process can be likened to a railway engine shunting trucks; the engine may only be moving at 3 mph, but a shock wave travels down the line of wagons much faster. The pulse is thus transmitted by a wave of wall distension at 4–15 m/s while the ejected blood itself advances only 20 cm (the **stroke distance**) in 1 second.

Since pulse propagation involves wall deformation, the transmission velocity is affected by wall stiffness. The **transmission velocity increases with wall stiffness**. As noted above, arterial stiffness increases with blood pressure and ageing. Consequently, pulse transmission is faster in hypertensive or elderly subjects. Human transmission velocity can be measured by timing the central and peripheral pulses, and from this the arterial distensibility can be calculated.

Pulse shape alters with ageing and pathophysiological state

The pressure wave in a proximal human artery may show two additional features besides those described earlier, depending on the age and pathophysiological condition of the individual. They are the **diastolic wave** and the **systolic inflection** (Figure 8.10).

Diastolic waves in the young

In children, young adults and animals such as dogs, the decay of pressure in diastole is interrupted by a small bump, i.e. a transient rise in pressure, called a diastolic wave. This is not seen in older people, in whom pressure falls off exponentially after the incisura. The diastolic wave is caused by **wave reflection**. The initial systolic pressure wave spreads so rapidly down the arterial tree that it reaches the major branches and resistance vessels in a fraction of a second. The branch points and resistance vessels partially reflect the wave, sending an attenuated pressure wave back up the arterial tree. The reflected wave arrives back in the proximal vessels during the diastole of the same heartbeat, creating the diastolic wave (Figure 8.10b). This is in some ways like wave reflection at a harbour wall; as the reflected wave travels back out to sea, it meets an incoming wave and the two waves summate briefly into a tall peak.

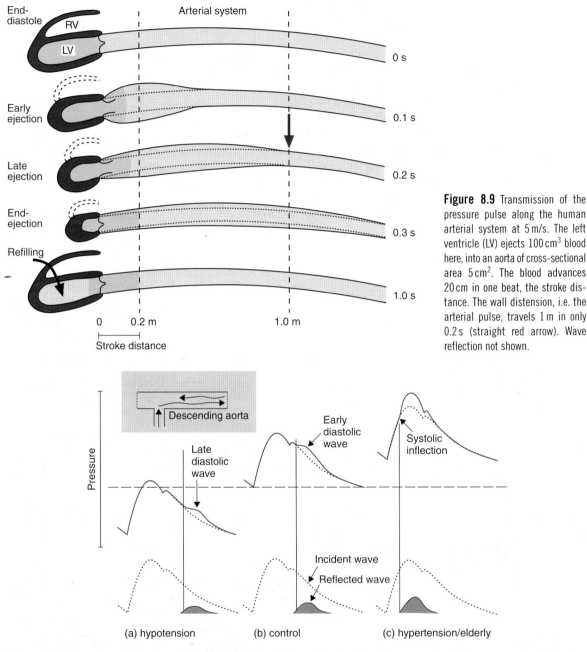

Figure 8.9 Transmission of the pressure pulse along the human arterial system at 5 m/s. The left ventricle (LV) ejects 100 cm^3 blood here, into an aorta of cross-sectional area 5 cm^2. The blood advances 20 cm in one beat, the stroke distance. The wall distension, i.e. the arterial pulse, travels 1 m in only 0.2 s (straight red arrow). Wave reflection not shown.

Figure 8.10 Effect of wave reflection on aortic pulse. *Red trace* is observed pulse. *Lower two curves* show its two components, the basic or 'incident' wave (dotted line) and the reflected wave (filled). Time from foot of incident wave to arrival of reflected wave is used to calculate transmission velocity. (a) Waveform in hypotension or after a vasodilator drug. Low pressure causes low arterial stiffness and slow propagation, so reflected diastolic wave is late. (b) Waveform at normal pressure in a young human or rabbit. Diastolic wave is earlier due to normal arterial stiffness and transmission velocity. Pattern (b) can be generated from (c) by vasodilator drugs, e.g. nitroglycerine. (c) Waveform in a hypertensive or elderly human, or a normal subject after a vasoconstrictor drug. High arterial stiffness and transmission velocity causes reflected wave to return quickly, creating a systolic inflection. *Inset*: model of arterial system as an asymmetric T-tube. Short limb on left represents all arteries of upper body; long limb on right represents lower body; ends represent the average of all the reflection sites in the upper and lower body, respectively. After Nichols and O'Rourke (1998); see Further Reading.

Systolic inflections in the elderly or hypertensive

The arteries of middle-aged and elderly humans are stiffer than those of young subjects, so the pressure wave and its reflection travel faster. As a result, the reflected wave arrives back in the aorta in late systole rather than diastole (Figure 8.10c). Elderly humans thus lack a diastolic wave. Instead, the reflected wave adds to the late part of the 'incident' (original) systolic wave, raising the peak systolic pressure and creating a kink or **inflection** in the systolic wave.

The process of wave reflection is illustrated in the inset to Figure 8.10. The human wave velocity is 4–15 m/s, the distance to major reflection sites such as the aortic bifurcation is ∼0.5 m, and each pulse lasts ∼1 s. Consequently there is time for a reflected wave to return and interact with the initiating or 'incident' wave. The measured time between the foot (start) of the incident wave and the inflection marking arrival of the reflected wave is typically 0.07 to 0.2 seconds in an adult, and can be used to estimate human arterial stiffness.

Changes in waveform with pathophysiological state

Whether the pulse shows a diastolic wave or a systolic inflection depends on (i) the magnitude of reflection by peripheral vessels, which is increased by vasoconstriction and reduced by vasodilatation; and (ii) the velocity of pulse transmission, which increases with ageing and mean blood pressure. Hypotension following a haemorrhage or vasodilator drug reduces the mean blood pressure and thus wall stiffness, which delays the reflected wave (Figure 8.10a). As a result, a diastolic wave can appear during hypovolaemia in middle-aged humans who normally have no such wave. Conversely, raising blood pressure by a vasoconstrictor drug causes the reflected wave to return faster, changing the pulse from one with a low systolic pressure and a diastolic wave (Figure 8.10a or b) into one with a high systolic pressure, a systolic inflection, and no diastolic wave (Figure 8.10c).

Wave reflection: does it matter?

Is the reflected wave of any functional importance? In young humans and animals such as dogs the augmentation of diastolic pressure by the slowly returning wave (the diastolic wave) enhances coronary artery perfusion without adding to ventricular work. By contrast, in patients with hypertension or elderly subjects the premature return of the reflected wave raises the pressure against which the ventricle has to eject blood in late systole. This adds to the ventricular afterload, cardiac work and O_2 demand.

Aortic stiffness increases cardiac O_2 demand

The high distensibility of the young aorta reduces systolic pressure, and hence cardiac work and O_2 demand. Conversely, ejection into a stiff arterial system elevates the systolic pressure, cardiac work and O_2 demand. The O_2 consumption of a dog heart ejecting through a rigid plastic tube is found to be much higher than when ejecting through the aorta. Since arterial stiffness increases with age, so does the O_2 cost of ejection. The return of the reflected wave during systole adds further to the energy cost of the late ejection phase.

Pulse shape alters in peripheral arteries

The shape of the pulse can change in a surprising way as it travels out to the periphery. The pulse of young humans and dogs, far from damping out as one might imagine, actually grows taller as it propagates along the named arteries (Figures 8.11, 1.9). As a result, systolic pressure in the brachial artery is higher than in the aorta. Four features of the wave alter.

- The incisura is damped out and disappears.

- The mean pressure falls slightly, by ∼2 mmHg from ascending aorta to radial artery.

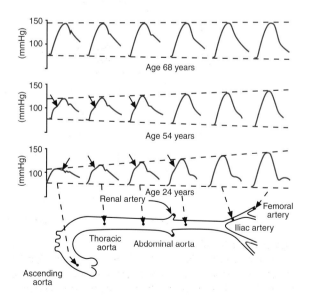

Figure 8.11 Pressure wave at different points along the arterial tree in three humans aged 24, 54 and 68 years. Pressure amplification with distance is ∼60% in the young and almost absent in the elderly. Arrows point to systolic inflection that marks arrival of reflected wave. After Nichols and O'Rourke (1998); see Further Reading.

- The systolic pressure wave grows taller, rather like a sea wave approaching the beach. This **pressure amplification** can be as much as 60% in the femoral artery of young humans. Pressure amplification is less marked in middle aged humans and is absent in the elderly.

- A new pressure wave appears in late diastole.

These complex changes are caused by a combination of increased arterial stiffness with distance, faster transmission of the higher pressure components, aortic taper (the abdominal aorta is roughly half as wide as the ascending aorta), and wave reflection.

The pulse pressure continues to increase as far as the third or fourth generation of arteries, such as the radial artery. Beyond this the pulse becomes progressively damped out by the viscous properties of the vessel wall and blood (Figure 1.9). The pressure oscillations dwindle and the flow becomes more continuous as the blood enters the resistance vessels.

Clinical abnormalities of pulse

In **aortic valve stenosis** the aortic valve is narrowed by fibrosis. As a result the arterial pressure rises sluggishly during ejection and has an abnormal plateau (Figure 8.7, inset; Figure 2.8).

In **aortic valve incompetence**, the pressure decays abnormally quickly during diastole, due to reflux into the ventricle. As a result the pulse pressure may be twice as big as normal, causing relaxed limbs to jerk in time with the throbbing pulse.

Pulsus paradoxus is a condition in which the pulse pressure falls by more than 10 mmHg during each inspiration. This is not really a 'paradox' but an exaggeration of normal events. Pulsus paradoxus is generally caused by cardiac tamponade (pressure around the heart) following constrictive pericarditis or an accumulation of a fluid in the pericardial cavity. Tamponade limits the combined volume of the two ventricles within the pericardial sac. During inspiration the fall in intrathoracic pressure increases the flow of venous blood into the right ventricle, raising the right ventricular volume. Since the pericardial space is limited by the tamponade, a rise in right ventricular volume reduces the left ventricular volume. Thus left ventricular stroke volume and systolic pressure decline excessively during inspiration.

In **pulsus alternans** the pulse is alternately strong and weak i.e. pulse pressure is reduced every other beat. This is generally a sign of severe left ventricular failure.

8.5 Mean arterial pressure and pressure measurement

What does 'mean' pressure mean?

Mean arterial pressure $\overline{P}_a$ is not simply the arithmetic average of the systolic and diastolic pressures, because the blood spends more time at diastolic levels than at systolic levels. The average pressure is nearer the diastolic value, and is the area under the pressure wave ($\int P \cdot dt$) divided by time (Figure 8.7). For clinical convenience the rule-of-thumb is to add a third of the pulse pressure to the diastolic pressure, as measured in the brachial artery:

$$\text{Mean blood pressure } \overline{P}_a = P_{\text{diast}} + \frac{(P_{\text{sys}} - P_{\text{diast}})}{3}$$

(8.4)

For example, if the brachial artery pressure is 110/80 mmHg, the pulse pressure is 30 mmHg and the mean pressure is ~90 mmHg.

What determines the mean pressure?

As explained in Section 8.1, Darcy's law tells us that two factors determine the mean arterial pressure:

$$\frac{\text{Mean blood}}{\text{pressure } \overline{P}_a} = \frac{\text{Cardiac output CO} \times}{\text{Total peripheral resistance TPR}}$$

(8.5)

This is called the **mean blood pressure equation** and states that mean pressure is governed by the size of the cardiac output and the total peripheral resistance. The mean pressure and the pulse pressure together determine how high the systolic pressure rises and how low the diastolic pressure falls.

Direct measurements of arterial pressure

Arterial pressure was first measured by Stephen Hales, the vicar of Teddington, near London, in 1773. Hales connected a vertical 3 metre glass tube to the carotid artery of a horse via a goose trachea, and noted the height to which the blood rose in the tube.

Principle of manometry

A century later the French medical physicist J. L. M. Poiseuille developed the smaller **mercury**

manometer, which is still in use today. The principle of manometry is that a vertical column of fluid in the manometer exerts a downward pressure which opposes the blood pressure, as in Figures 8.1 and 8.2. When the column reaches a stable height h, the pressure at the bottom of the column must be equal to the blood pressure. The pressure at the bottom of a column of fluid is ρgh (fluid density $\rho \times$ force of gravity $g \times h$). Since mercury is very dense, 13.6 g/ml, a column about 100 mm high balances the blood pressure at heart level. Using his new mercury manometer, Poiseuille proved that there is little change in mean pressure along the arterial system, and therefore little resistance to flow along arteries.

Electronic pressure transducers

The mercury manometer measures the mean blood pressure but not the pulse owing to the inertia of mercury. To record the pulse a fast-responding, electronic pressure transducer is needed. This was developed by the American scientists Lambert and Wood as a spin-off from aviation research during World War II. The transducer contains a metal diaphragm which deforms slightly under pressure, changing the electrical resistance. Since the latter can be measured electronically, the device is able to follow fast changes in pressure. The transducer has to be calibrated, however, by a column of liquid, so blood pressure is normally reported in mmHg or cmH$_2$O rather than Pascal. Conversion factors are given in Appendix 2 'Pressure'.

Measurement of human blood pressure by sphygmomanometry

The mercury manometer is employed throughout the world to measure human blood pressure, using an indirect method called sphygmomanometry (Figure 8.12). An inflatable rubber sac within a cotton sleeve, called a **Riva–Rocci cuff**, is wound around the upper arm. The inflatable sac must be located medially over the brachial artery and the artery must be at heart level. The cuff is inflated sufficiently to obliterate the radial pulse, which might require a pressure of >180 mmHg in an elderly subject. The cuff pressure is measured by a mercury manometer. The pressure is transmitted through the tissues of the upper arm and occludes the brachial artery. When a stethoscope is placed over the brachial artery in the antecubital fossa (inner aspect of elbow), no sound is heard because there is no blood flow. Cuff pressure is then gradually lowered, and the following sequence of sounds is heard.

1 When cuff pressure is just below systolic pressure, the artery opens briefly during each systole. The transient spurt of blood vibrates the artery wall downstream and creates a dull tapping noise called a **Korotkoff sound**. The pressure at which the Korotkoff sound first appears is conventionally accepted as systolic pressure, but is actually about 10 mmHg below the true value.

2 As cuff pressure is lowered further, the Korotkoff sounds grow louder, because the intermittent spurts of blood grow stronger.

3 When cuff pressure is close to diastolic pressure, the artery remains patent for most of the cardiac cycle and the vibration of the vessel wall diminishes. This causes a sudden diminution of the Korotkoff sounds. The cuff pressure at which this happens has been accepted as the diastolic pressure, although it is ~8 mmHg higher than true diastolic pressure. A faint Korotkoff sound may persist below this and complete silence may not be attained until 8–10 mmHg below the true diastolic pressure. The point of silence is currently recommended as the measure of diastolic pressure.

In some hypertensive patients there is a silent period within the systolic–diastolic pressure range, which could cause hypertension to be missed. It is important, therefore, when first inflating the cuff, to palpate

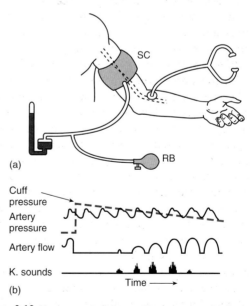

Figure 8.12 Measurement of human blood pressure. (a) Dashed line represents compressed brachial artery under the sphygmomanometer cuff (SC). Cuff pressure is controlled by the rubber bulb (RB) and measured by the mercury column. (b) Korotkoff sounds begin when cuff pressure is just below systolic pressure and diminish when cuff pressure is close to diastolic pressure.

the radial artery and note the pressure at which the pulse disappears. This is a good measure of systolic pressure and prevents missing a case of systolic hypertension.

How is brachial artery pressure related to aortic pressure? As noted earlier, the pulse pressure amplifies as it travels along the arterial tree (Figure 8.11), except in the elderly. The brachial artery systolic pressure overestimates the aortic systolic pressure by ~20 mmHg in resting young to middle-aged subjects, or more during exercise. Moreover, when blood pressure is changed by drugs, brachial artery measurements may underestimate the change in aortic pressure due to changes in wave reflection.

Automated indirect pressure measurement

Automated, oscillation-based systems such as the **Dinamap** report diastolic, systolic and mean pressure in the brachial artery. The arterial pulsation causes the pressure in a cuff around the arm to oscillate. With the cuff automatically inflated by an electrical pump to above systolic pressure, the oscillation in cuff pressure is slight. Cuff pressure is then automatically reduced. The oscillation begins to increase when cuff pressure equals systolic pressure, reaches a maximum at mean arterial pressure, and dies back to a minimum at diastolic pressure. These cues are used to record the pressures electronically.

The **Finapress** gives a continuous record of digital artery pressure, using a volume clamp method. The finger is enclosed in an inflatable cuff and the finger volume is monitored by infra-red light transmission. The volume normally oscillates slightly with each pulse of the artery. The volume signal is fed back to a pump, which increases its output to the finger cuff each time the artery pulses, just enough to 'clamp' the volume at a constant level. The cuff pressure is thus enslaved to the arterial pressure.

What is 'normal' blood pressure?

That mythological polymath 'every schoolboy' knows that 'normal' human blood pressure is 120/80 mmHg. For a young adult under certain conditions he would be right, but it is quite wrong to adopt 120/80 mmHg as the normal standard for a resting child, a pregnant woman in midterm or an elderly man. The lability of blood pressure is illustrated by the 24-h record shown in Figure 8.13, and some of the factors affecting blood pressure are as follows.

Age

Blood pressure increases progressively with age, averaging 100/65 mmHg at 6 years, 125/80 mmHg at 30 years, and 180/90 mmHg at 70 years (Figure 17.10). The increase in pulse pressure with age is due to arteriosclerosis (not to be confused with atheroma, Table 17.4). As a rule-of-thumb the systolic pressure equals 100 mmHg plus age in years.

CONCEPT BOX 10

What determines arterial pressure?

▪ *Mean* aortic pressure is determined by the cardiac output (*CO*) and the total peripheral resistance (*TPR*). From Darcy's law in Concept Box 1 mean pressure = $CO \times TPR$. Clinical hypertension is due to increased *TPR*. Hypotension is often due to a fall in *CO*.

▪ *Systolic* and *diastolic* pressures are determined by the size of the oscillation about the mean pressure.

▪ The size of the oscillation, or *pulse pressure*, is determined by the stroke volume *SV* and arterial compliance *C*. See Concept Box 9.

▪ In the long term the *kidneys* are crucial regulators of mean blood pressure, because they regulate the plasma volume and hence the cardiac filling pressure.

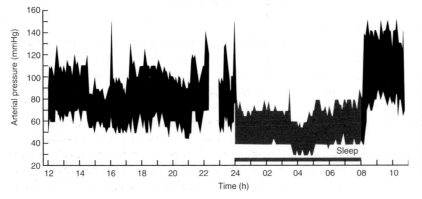

Figure 8.13 Arterial pressure in a normal subject recorded continuously for 24 h. Sleep (red period) lowered the pressure. A painful stimulus at 16.00 h and sexual intercourse at 24.00 h markedly raised pressure. (From Bevan, A. T., Honour, A. J. and Scott, F. H. (1969) *Clinical Science*, **36**, 329, by permission.)

Sleep and exercise

Blood pressure can fall to 80/50 mmHg or less during sleep (Figure 8.13). In heavy dynamic exercise the mean pressure increases by $10-40$ mmHg. In heavy resistive exercise such as weightlifting the pressure can increase by over 100 mmHg.

Standing and gravity – the giraffe's nightmare

Pressure increases to an equal degree in arteries and veins below heart level, due to the weight of the column of blood between the heart and the blood vessels (Figure 8.2). For a fluid column of height h the increase in pressure equals ρgh; see 'Principle of manometry', above. In a human foot 115 cm below heart level, arterial pressure will increase by 115×1.06 cmH$_2$O because blood is 1.06 times as dense as water. Since the density of mercury is 13.6 times that of water, the increase is equivalent to 90 mmHg. Therefore, if aortic pressure at heart level is 95 mmHg, arterial pressure in the foot will be nearly $90 + 95 = 185$ mmHg. It will actually be slightly less than this due to the slight arterial resistance to flow. Conversely, pressure is reduced in arteries above heart level. In the human brain it is 60 mmHg during standing. Our problem is small, though compared with that of the giraffe. Because the giraffe's head is so far above its heart, the heart has to generate an aortic pressure of $\sim$200 mmHg to ensure adequate cerebral perfusion.

Gravity: indirect effect

Upon moving from a lying position to standing, the arterial pressure at heart level changes due to changes in cardiac output and peripheral resistance. There is a transient fall in aortic pressure, which can produce a passing dizziness (postural hypotension), followed by a small but sustained reflex rise in pressure (Section 17.1).

Emotion and stress

Anger, apprehension, fear, stress and sexual excitement are all potent 'pressor' stimuli, i.e. they elevate blood pressure (see Figure 8.13). Attendance at a meeting may raise pressure by 20 mmHg. Since a visit to the doctor is stressful for many patients, a solitary high pressure measurement is not diagnostic of hypertension. The measurement needs to be repeated later with the patient relaxed. The pressor effect of stress is particularly harmful to patients with ischaemic heart disease, as the cautionary history of John Hunter in Section 6.14 illustrates.

Regular oscillations in mean pressure

Mean arterial pressure oscillates synchronously with respiration (**Traube–Hering waves**). The pressure falls by a few mmHg during each inspiration, because the left ventricular stroke volume declines as the lung vascular bed expands. Although there is a compensatory increase in heart rate during inspiration (sinus arrhythmia, Section 5.8), this only partially buffers the fall in stroke volume in humans. In dogs, by contrast, the pressure rises with each inspiration because the inspiratory tachycardia outweighs the fall in stroke volume.

In addition to oscillations in phase with respiration, blood pressure may show regular oscillations at a lower frequency, around 6/min, called **Mayer waves**. These are attributed to cyclic changes in sympathetic vasomotor tone, driven by a resonance in the baroreceptor reflex.

Other factors

The **Valsalva manoeuvre**, a forced expiration against a closed or narrowed glottis, causes a complex sequence of blood pressure changes (Section 17.2). In **pregnancy** the blood pressure falls and reaches a minimum at $\sim$6 months due to the expansion of the uterine and other vascular beds. Consequently, in obstetrical practice a pressure of 130/90 mmHg at 6 months gestation would cause grave concern, even though it is merely close to the upper limit of normal for a non-pregnant woman. Many **pathological processes** also alter arterial pressure, such as dehydration, haemorrhage, shock, syncope (fainting), chronic hypertension, acute heart failure and valvular lesions such as aortic incompetence.

It is clear from the above survey that **the yardstick used to assess a subject's blood pressure must be matched to their age, physiological and psychological condition**.

8.6 Pulsatile flow

Blood flow is stop–go in the aorta and major arteries (Figure 8.14); the flow almost ceases during diastole. Pressure rises first in the proximal aorta, creating a pressure gradient from the proximal aorta to the peripheral arteries, which accelerates the blood. The pulse then spreads distally, reaching the radial artery in $\sim$0.1 second. At this point in time the distal pressure is transiently higher than the proximal pressure, which is tailing off. As a result, the pressure gradient is now reversed, and this decelerates the flow. Thus,

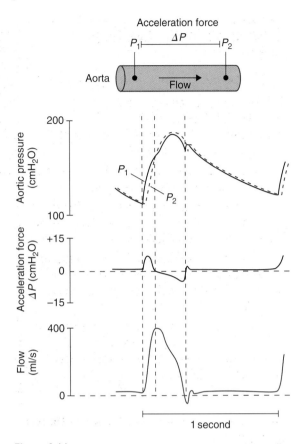

Figure 8.14 Flow and pressure gradients in the human ascending aorta. Pressure difference (ΔP) at first accelerates flow along the aorta, and then decelerates it. A brief back-flow closes the aortic valve. Proximal aortic flow is almost zero in diastole. (After Snell, R. E., Clements, J. M., Patel, D. J., Fry, D. L. and Luchsinger, P. C. (1965) *Journal of Applied Physiology*, **20**, 691.)

flow in the major arteries first accelerates and then decelerates over the initial third of the cardiac cycle. During the two-thirds of the cycle after aortic valve closure, flow is almost zero. The instantaneous flow is not governed by Darcy's law (which, as pointed out earlier, is a steady-state expression) but is governed by Newton's second law of motion, namely acceleration = force/mass.

The period of near zero flow gradually shortens as blood enters smaller arteries, and in the smallest arteries flow becomes continuous, albeit still pulsatile (Figure 1.9).

8.7 Peripheral resistance, Poiseuille's law and wall mechanics

The resistance of the circulation to flow arises chiefly in the tiny terminal arteries and arterioles

(Concept Box 1), and to a lesser degree the capillaries and venules. The total peripheral resistance as defined in eqn 8.1b is ~1 mmHg per ml per second in a resting adult, or 1 peripheral resistance unit.

Poiseuille's law describes the hydraulic resistance of a tube

Resistance to flow arises exclusively from the internal friction within a fluid; it has nothing to do with friction between the fluid and the tube wall, where there is no flow owing to the zero-slip condition (Figure 8.3). Resistance is nevertheless greatly affected by tube radius because, for a given flow, the shear rates are greater in a narrow tube than a wide tube. High shear rates require more force and thus a bigger pressure gradient; and resistance is by definition the pressure gradient required to produce unit flow.

The factors that govern tube resistance were elucidated by the Parisian physician Jean Leonard Marie Poiseuille around 1840 in a meticulous study of water flowing through glass capillary tubes. Poiseuille established that the resistance R to the steady laminar flow of a Newtonian fluid such as water (or plasma) along a straight cylindrical tube is directly proportional to the fluid viscosity η and the length of the tube L; and is **inversely proportional to tube radius raised to the fourth power, r^4**:

$$R = \frac{8\eta L}{\pi r^4} \qquad (8.6)$$

Combining this definition of resistance with Darcy's law (eqn 8.1a), and recalling that conductance K is 1/resistance, we get an expression for flow through a tube called 'Poiseuille's law':

$$\dot{Q} = (P_1 - P_2)K = (P_1 - P_2)\frac{\pi r^4}{8\eta L} \qquad (8.7)$$

Resistances in series vs. resistances in parallel

Poiseuille's law describes flow along a single tube. If several tubes are arranged in **series**, for example a terminal artery and an arteriole, their total resistance R_{total} is the sum of the individual resistances. This is written as ΣR ('Σ', Greek capital sigma, is shorthand for 'sum of all the individual values of −'). In a series array R_{total} equals ΣR.

If many tubes are arranged in **parallel**, as in a capillary bed, a given driving pressure will produce more flow than it would through a single tube, because the conducting capacities of the tubes summate. The net conductance is the sum of all the individual tube conductances, i.e. ΣK. Since resistance is the reciprocal of conductance, the net resistance of multiple tubes in parallel is $1/\Sigma K$. Thus, in parallel arrays $R_{total} = 1/\Sigma K$. The rule is 'For series arrays, add the resistances; for parallel arrays, add the conductances'. The summation of huge numbers of conductances in parallel partly explains why the capillary bed has a relatively low hydraulic resistance.

Armed with Poiseuille's law we can now consider the systemic resistance, which resides chiefly in the arterioles and tiniest arteries.

Arteriolar radius regulates local flow and central arterial pressure

Vascular resistance is exquisitely sensitive to radius due to the r^4 relation in Poiseuille's law. A fall in radius from 1 cm in the human aorta to 0.01 cm in an arteriole represents a one hundred million times increase in resistance. This is why the arterioles and terminal arteries are the main sites of resistance.

Arteriolar radius is actively controlled by the smooth muscle of the tunica media. Contraction narrows the lumen (vasoconstriction) and relaxation produces vasodilatation. If there is a widespread arteriolar constriction throughout the body, the total peripheral resistance rises. This provides a powerful way of regulating the **central arterial pressure** (eqn 8.5). If just the local arterioles in a small mass of tissue change calibre, **local blood flow** to the tissue is altered (eqn 8.1a) without much affecting the TPR or arterial pressure. The increase in blood flow to the salivary gland during eating is a good example of this; a mere 19% increase in the radius of the salivary gland resistance vessels doubles their flow conductance due to the r^4 effect.

The radius of a capillary is even smaller than that of an arteriole, so why does the capillary network not offer an even greater resistance than the arteriolar network? The resistance of a single capillary is indeed bigger than that of a single arteriole. Nevertheless, the pressure drop across the whole capillary bed, 20–30 mmHg, is smaller than that across the arteriolar bed, 40–50 mmHg. This is due to (i) the huge number of capillaries in parallel (as explained above R_{total} is $1/\Sigma K$); (ii) the shortness of capillaries (~500 μm); and (iii) bolus flow, which reduces the effective blood viscosity η inside capillaries, as explained later.

Poiseuille's law for flow through a tube

☐ Conductance is the flow per unit pressure drop.

☐ Poiseuille's law states that the conductance of a tube of radius r is proportional to r^4, and inversely proportional to fluid viscosity η and vessel length L. The conductance equals $\pi r^4/8\eta L$.

☐ The conductances of tubes in parallel add up. Thus the conductance of the capillary bed is high.

☐ The inverse of conductance is resistance. Resistance equals $8\eta L/\pi r^4$. The resistances of vessels in series add up, e.g. small arteries and arterioles.

☐ Due to the r^4 relation, active changes in arteriolar calibre have a powerful effect on local blood flow, and also on total peripheral resistance and mean arterial pressure.

☐ Blood viscosity η depends chiefly on the haematocrit. The effective viscosity falls in microvessels (the Fåhraeus–Lindqvist effect), thus reducing resistance and conserving cardiac energy.

Laplace's law relates radius, wall tension and pressure

The radius of an artery or arteriole is influenced by three mechanical factors (Figure 8.15):

1 the **internal pressure** distending it

2 the **external pressure** compressing it

3 the **circumferential tension** in the wall.

When the radius is stable (a state called mechanical equilibrium), the wall tension exactly counteracts the difference between the internal and external pressures, or **transmural pressure**.

Laplace's law tells us that the wall tension at mechanical equilibrium increases with the radius of the vessel. This is easily proved. Consider a tube whose walls are thin relative to the vessel radius. The circumferential tension T is the circumferential force per unit length of wall, F/L (Figure 8.15). This opposes the distending force generated by the internal pressure P_i. The distending force is $P_i \times$ area acted on in one direction (since pressure is force per unit area). For a tube of mean radius r and unit length, the area acted on in one direction is $2r$. Thus the internal distending force is $P_i \times 2r$. By similar reasoning the outer surface is compressed by the outside pressure P_o with a force $P_o \times 2r$. At mechanical equilibrium the sum of the wall tensions on each side of the tube,

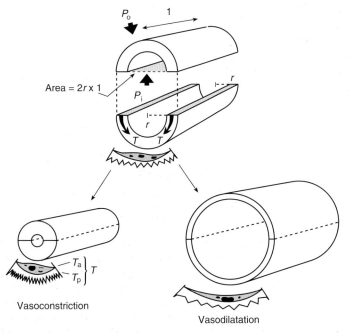

Figure 8.15 Wall mechanics. Internal pressure P_i acts on area $2r$ to push the two halves of the cylinder apart. This is opposed by external pressure P_o and wall tension T on each side of the cylinder. Tension T is the sum of active tension in smooth muscle, T_a, and passive tension in elastin/collagen fibres, T_p, shown as a spring. The spring on the left is in its relaxed state and that on the right is stretched and tense. T_a and T_p change in opposite directions during vasoconstriction to produce mechanical stability.

$2T$, must be equal and opposite to the transmural distending force $P_i 2r - P_o 2r$. The '2's cancel out to give Laplace's equation for a thin-walled tube:

$$T = (P_i - P_o)r \qquad (8.8)$$

Laplace's law shows that a capillary experiences a low wall tension; and that the wall tension is greater in the aorta than in smaller arteries even though their pressures are similar. This contributes to the development of an **aortic aneurysm**, a bulging of the weakened aortic wall that may rupture with catastrophic consequences.

A slightly more elaborate expression applies to vessels with thick walls, but leads to similar predictions. (See 'Love's equation', Appendix 2.)

Changes in wall tension bring about constriction and dilatation

The tension T in an arterial vessel has two components; there is the active tension of the smooth muscle cells and the passive tension of the elastin and collagen fibrils. When the smooth muscle contracts, its immediate effect is to raise the wall tension T. This produces a temporary mechanical disequilibrium and the radius begins to decrease. Laplace's law shows that, if the transmural pressure $P_i - P_o$ is constant and radius r falls, a new mechanical equilibrium can only be attained by reducing the **net** (total) wall tension T. A fall in net wall tension is achieved by unloading the passive fibrils, i.e. their tension falls as

the vessel radius is reduced by the contracting cells (Figure 8.15). There is in effect a transfer of tension from the passive fibres to the active muscle cells. Without this, vasoconstriction would be an extremely unstable process.

Conversely, vasodilatation is achieved by relaxation of the smooth muscle cells. This reduces the active tension, producing mechanical disequilibrium. The internal distending pressure then pushes the wall out to a bigger radius, until a point is reached where the increasing tension in the stretched collagen and elastin re-establishes a mechanical equilibrium (Figure 8.15).

8.8 Viscous properties of blood

Poiseuille's law shows that vascular resistance depends not only on radius but also on the viscosity of the perfusing liquid, namely blood. Blood viscosity is altered in many haematological diseases, with attendant effects on flow and pressure.

Viscosity represents the internal friction in a fluid

The word viscosity stems from 'viscum', Latin for mistletoe, because mistletoe berries contain a thick, glutinous fluid. Viscosity was defined by Isaac Newton as 'defectus lubricitatis', lack of slipperiness, because it represents the internal friction within a moving fluid, analogous to the friction between two moving solid surfaces. Viscosity is defined formally as the shear stress per unit shear rate (Appendix 2, Viscosity). **Shear stress** is the sliding force applied to a unit area of contact between two laminae of fluid, and is proportional to the pressure gradient along the vessel. **Shear rate** is the change in fluid velocity per unit distance across the tube, i.e. the slope of the velocity profile in Figure 8.3. The unit of viscosity is the Newton-s/m^2 or milliPascal-second, but it is often convenient to use **relative viscosity**, as below. The relative viscosity of blood or plasma is its viscosity divided by that of water.

Plasma viscosity is dominated by plasma proteins

The voluminous albumin and globulin molecules raise the viscosity of plasma to 1.7 times that of water. In **myeloma**, a cancer of globulin-secreting cells, the increased plasma globulin concentration raises the viscosity and may also cause the red cells to agglutinate (attach to each other) under cool conditions. In cold fingers the agglutination raises the blood viscosity and resistance to such a degree that perfusion is badly impaired, leading to necrosis of the fingertips (tissue death).

Blood viscosity is dominated by haematocrit

The addition of red cells to plasma greatly increases the internal friction within the liquid. Consequently, the viscosity of blood is proportional to its haematocrit (Figure 8.16). Haematocrit is the red cell volume expressed as a percentage of the blood volume. At a haematocrit of 47% the relative viscosity of human blood is ~4. The optimal haematocrit for O$_2$ delivery represents a compromise between raising the O$_2$-carrying capacity and raising the blood viscosity, which impairs flow. In humans the normal haematocrit is 40–45%. In camels the red cells are less flexible, so their viscous effect is greater and the camel's compromise haematocrit is only 27%.

Abnormalities of haematocrit have serious consequences, as follows.

Polycythaemia

Poly-(many)-cythaemia (blood cells) is a condition in which the haematocrit is abnormally high. Polycythaemia occurs as a physiological adaptation to chronic hypoxia in people at **high altitude**. It also occurs in the disease **polycythaemia rubra vera**, in which an overproduction of red cells can raise the haematocrit to 70%. At a haematocrit of 63% the red

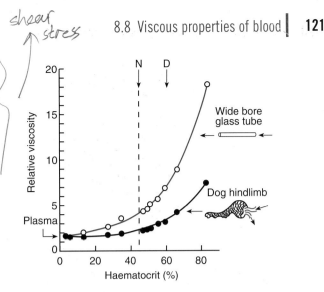

Figure 8.16 Effect of haematocrit on the viscosity of blood relative to water. Open circles: viscosity in a high-velocity glass viscometer. Closed circles: smaller effective viscosity in the vasculature of an isolated dog hindlimb, due to the Fåhraeus–Lindqvist effect – see text. N, normal haematocrit; D, haematocrit at which cells are packed so tightly that they deform even at rest. (After the classic experiment of Whittaker, S. R. F. and Winton, F. R. (1933) *Journal of Physiology*, **78**, 339–369.)

cells are so closely packed that viscosity and resistance are doubled. As a result, polycythaemia rubra vera causes hypertension and a sluggish blood flow, leading to cerebral or coronary thrombosis (strokes and heart attacks).

Anaemia

Anaemia by contrast reduces the blood viscosity and resistance. To maintain the blood pressure the cardiac output has to be increased (eqn 8.5). If the anaemia is prolonged this can lead to a form of cardiac failure called high-output failure. Homeostasis of blood viscosity is thus important for normal cardiovascular function.

Blood viscosity is non-Newtonian. I – Effects of tube radius

The viscosity of a simple fluid like water or plasma is unaffected by the radius of the conducting tube or by shear rate. Such a fluid is called a **Newtonian fluid**. Whole blood, by contrast, shows bizarre but physiologically helpful non-Newtonian behaviour.

Viscosity falls in microvessels (the Fåhraeus–Lindqvist effect)

In 1931 Fåhraeus and Lindqvist made the strange discovery that the viscosity of blood is lower in a narrow-bore viscometer than in a wide bore viscometers (Figure 8.17a). A viscometer is simply a fine glass tube through which the flow is timed. The same phenomenon evidently occurs in the circulation, because the effective viscosity of blood perfused through a dog hind limb is half that of blood in a wide-bore viscometer (Figure 8.16). Blood viscosity begins to fall at tube widths of <1 mm, e.g. small arteries. In tubes of width 30–40 μm, such as arterioles, the relative viscosity is only ~2.5. In tubes of width ~6 μm (capillaries) the viscosity reaches its minimum value, almost as low as that of plasma. This 'Fåhraeus–Lindqvist effect' accounts for the low effective viscosity of blood in the circulation (Figure 8.16). The Fåhraeus–Lindqvist effect is important because it greatly reduces the arterial pressure needed to perfuse the microcirculation. Without it the arterial pressure and cardiac work would need to be much higher.

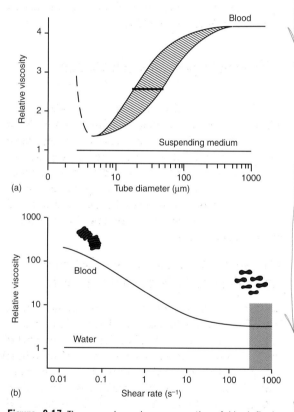

Figure 8.17 The anomalous viscous properties of blood flowing through glass tubing. (a) Fåhraeus–Lindqvist effect: viscosity decreases as tube diameter is reduced. The effective viscosity of blood in the intact circulation is approximately 2.5 (black bar), implying that the functional diameter of the resistance vessels is approximately 30 μm (arterioles). At diameters smaller than a blood capillary, viscosity rises again (dashed line). (b) Effect of shear rate on viscosity. Pink region shows typical shear rates *in vivo*. Sketches show red cell aggregation into rouleaux at low shear rates and disaggregation at high rates. ((a) After Gaetghens, P. (1981) In *The Rheology of Blood, Blood Vessels and Associated Tissues* (eds Gross, D. R. and Wang, N. H. C.), Sijthoff and Noordhoff, Amsterdam; (b) from Chien, S. (1992); see Further Reading.)

Several mechanisms underlie the Fåhraeus–Lindqvist effect. In capillaries, **bolus flow** reduces the viscosity. In arterioles, the viscosity is reduced by the **peripheral plasma stream** generated by axial flow (Figure 8.3). Since shear rates are highest close to the vessel wall, a reduction in friction close to the wall has a marked beneficial effect on viscosity. The effect is not noticeable in tubes of width >1 mm because the thickness of the marginal layer is then negligible relative to the tube width.

Haematocrit falls in microvessels (Fåhraeus effect)

Robin Fåhraeus described a further curious effect of tube radius. The concentration of red cells in blood passing through a narrow tube, called the **dynamic** or **tube haematocrit**, is lower than the central haematocrit in the feeding and draining vessels. In a tube of radius 15 μm fed from a reservoir with a central haematocrit of 40%, the dynamic haematocrit is only ~24%. This is a little hard to digest at first acquaintance! The explanation lies in the difference between axial and marginal stream velocities (Figure 8.3). Suppose, for example, that arterial blood of haematocrit 50% feeds an arteriole in which the cells have twice the velocity of the plasma due to their more axial location. If the haematocrit in the parent artery and vein is to remain at 50% (which it must, since the circulation is in a steady state) equal volumes of plasma and red cells must pass through the arteriole in a given time. Since the cell velocity is twice the plasma velocity in our example, equal volume flows are only possible if the concentration of red cells in the arteriole is half that in the parent blood. This is achieved by the red cells speeding away from the plasma at the tube entrance, thinning out like traffic entering a fast road from a congested slip road.

Blood viscosity is non-Newtonian. II – Shear thinning

The viscosity of blood also varies with flow, or more accurately shear rate (Figure 8.17b). Shear rate, it will be recalled, is the change in fluid velocity per unit distance normal to the direction of flow, and has the curious units of s^{-1}. Blood viscosity falls as flow and shear rate increase. This is called shear thinning. The same phenomenon occurs in non-drip paints. Shear rates are relatively high in the circulation (~1000 s^{-1}), so blood is normally in a shear-thinned state.

The shear thinning of blood is attributed to the deformation and lining-up of red cells along the flow lines, and to a tank-tread motion of the red cell membrane around its interior. At low flows in horizontal tubes, partial sedimentation of the cells within the tube contributes to the rise in viscosity.

Abnormally low flow allows the red cells to adhere to each other to form **rouleaux**, resembling stacks of coins. It is thought that such changes probably occur in veins *in vivo* if blood flow is sluggish. The tendency of red cells to aggregate in this way is related to the concentration of **fibrinogen** in the plasma.

8.9 Pressure–flow relations and autoregulation

Poiseuille's law is strictly valid for a steady flow (cf. pulsatile *in vivo*) of a Newtonian fluid (cf. non-Newtonian blood) in a long straight vessel (cf. irregular blood vessel anatomy) with rigid walls (cf. distensible blood vessels). Not surprisingly, therefore, blood flow shows some deviation from Poiseuille's law (Figure 8.18). For example, the pressure–flow relation is curved at low pressures in perfused lungs and in hindlimbs with little vascular muscle tone, although it is nearly linear in the physiological range (Figure 8.18, 'blood' curve). The direction of the curvature at low pressures indicates that resistance falls as pressure rises. This is caused by the shear thinning of blood and to a lesser degree distension of the resistance vessels as pressure rises. Shear thinning is

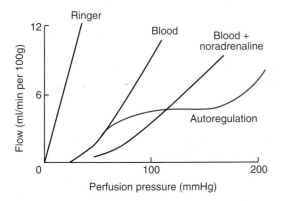

Figure 8.18 Pressure–flow curves for dog skeletal muscle. When the arterioles are in good physiological condition, *autoregulation* is present. When this is *abolished*, steeper curvilinear relations are seen: the curvature is caused by changes in resistance with pressure. *Noradrenaline* causes vasoconstriction and increases resistance. Perfusion with mammalian *Ringer's solution* (a physiological salt solution) produces a steeper line due to its low viscosity, and the line is almost straight because the anomalous viscous effect of blood is removed. (From Pappenheimer, J. R. and Maes, J. P. (1942) *American Journal of Physiology*, **137**, 187–199; and Stainsby, W. N. and Renkin, E. M. (1961) *American Journal of Physiology*, **201**, 117–122, by permission.)

probably the chief factor, because perfusion of a dog hindlimb with saline produces an almost linear pressure–flow relation (Figure 8.18).

Vascular beds with a high arteriolar tone show a very different, physiologically important pressure–flow relation that deviates wildly from Poiseuille behaviour. The relation is called an **autoregulation curve**. Blood flow increases with pressure up to a certain point, but a plateau then develops. Over the plateau the flow changes remarkably little with pressure, until the pressure exceeds ∼180 mmHg. A nearly constant flow in the face of a rising pressure, called autoregulation, indicates that resistance is rising in proportion to the pressure. Autoregulation is caused by an active constriction of the resistance vessels in response to pressure (Section 13.6). Autoregulation is an active response that stabilizes an organ's blood flow in the face of changes in arterial pressure, and occurs in most organs except the lung.

8.10 Venous pressure and volume

Peripheral veins and venules are thin-walled, voluminous vessels containing roughly two-thirds of the circulating blood. They serve as an adjustable reservoir of blood that can be used to top up the central veins, raising the CVP and hence stroke volume. The volume of blood in the peripheral veins depends both on the **venous blood pressure** and on the **tone of smooth muscle** in the tunica media (Figure 8.19).

The pressure–volume curve of veins is sigmoidal due to vein profile changes

Blood enters venules at ∼12–20 mmHg at heart level. The pressure falls to ∼8–10 mmHg in named veins such as the antecubital or femoral vein at heart level. Venous resistance is small, so 8–10 mmHg is enough to drive the cardiac output back to the right ventricle, where the diastolic pressure is 0–6 mmHg.

Venous pressure increases below heart level and decreases above heart level due to the effect of gravity (Figure 8.2). This has marked effects on local venous volume, because the cross-sectional profile of these thin-walled vessels changes with pressure. At transmural pressures below zero, for example in a hand raised above heart level, the vein collapses into a dumb-bell shaped profile and flow is confined to the narrow marginal channels. At a transmural pressure of 1 mmHg the vein assumes a narrow elliptical cross-section. As pressure rises towards 10 mmHg, the elliptical profile becomes progressively rounder.

The change in shape enables the vein to accommodate a large volume of blood for only a small change in pressure. The maximum distensibility (compliance) occurs at ~4 mmHg and is ~100 ml/mmHg for the human systemic venous system, or ~50 times greater than arterial compliance.

Above 10–15 mmHg the vein profile is fully circular and, since the stretched collagen in the wall is relatively inextensible, venous volume becomes less sensitive to pressure. Due to the collapse of veins at low pressure and their relative stiffness at high pressure, the venous pressure–volume curve is sigmoidal (S-shaped).

Venous smooth muscle tone regulates venous volume

The veins of the gastrointestinal tract, liver, kidneys and skin are innervated by sympathetic vasomotor nerves. Sympathetically excited venoconstriction greatly reduces the capacitance of these veins at a given pressure (Figure 8.19), displacing blood into the thoracic compartment. In this way the central nervous system is able to exert some control over the filling pressure of the heart.

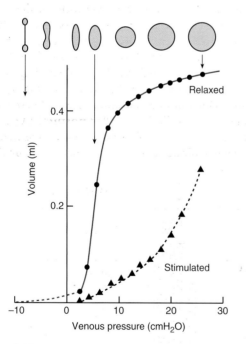

Figure 8.19 Venous pressure–volume curve, in relaxed state (filled circles) and at maximum venoconstriction (triangles). 'Capacitance' is volume V at a given pressure P; this is reduced by venoconstriction. 'Compliance' or distensibility is slope dV/dP. The change in cross-section of the vein with pressure is shown schematically above. (Canine saphenous vein, from Vanhoutte, P. M. and Leusen, I. (1969) *Pfluger's Archiv*, **306**, 341–353, by permission.)

Human CVP can be estimated by inspection of neck veins

In intensive care units the central venous pressure (CVP) is monitored through a catheter in the subclavian vein or superior vena cava. During routine clinical examination, the CVP is assessed indirectly by inspection of the neck veins (Figure 8.20). The external jugular vein runs over the sternomastoid muscle, and the internal jugular vein runs deep to the muscle. With the subject semi-supine, the lower part of the jugular vein is normally distended while the upper part is collapsed because its blood is at a sub-atmospheric pressure. The sub-atmospheric pressure is due to the effect of gravity on the column of venous blood 'hanging' from the head (Figure 8.2). From the sigmoidal pressure–volume curve we know that **transmural pressure is zero at the point of collapse of a vein**. Applying the principles of manometry described earlier, it follows that the CVP equals the pressure exerted by the vertical column of blood between the point of collapse and the right atrium.

A numerical example should make the above clearer. If the point of venous collapse (hence zero venous blood pressure) is 7 cm vertical distance above the right atrium, the CVP must be 7 cm of blood (7.4 cmH$_2$O). The atrium cannot be seen but is known to be ~5 cm lower than the manubriosternal angle, which is readily palpated. Thus by measuring the vertical distance between the point of jugular vein collapse and the manubriosternal angle (2 cm in our example), and adding 5 cm, the CVP can be estimated.

Although the accuracy of the inspection method is low, around ±2 cm, it is good enough to detect the grossly elevated CVP that characterizes right

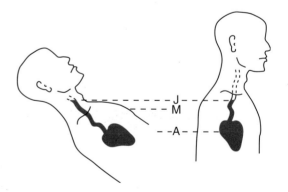

Figure 8.20 Estimation of central venous pressure (CVP) in man. CVP is the pressure at the point where the vena cava enter the right atrium. This is equal to the vertical distance between point of collapse of the jugular vein (J) and the right atrium (A). Since point A cannot be seen, the height of J above the manubriosternal angle (M) is measured instead; M − A is approximately 5 cm. CVP = (J − M) + 5 (cmH$_2$O). In the upright position the jugular vein is normally collapsed.

ventricular failure (Chapter 18). In right ventricular failure the CVP may be so high that the venous pulse is visible in the neck even when the patient is upright. A normal subject has to be semi-supine for the venous pulse to be visible; when upright the transition from collapse to distension is below the clavicle.

Oscillations in CVP are visible in neck veins

The pressure in veins close to the right atrium, including the jugular veins, is pulsatile and mirrors the waveform of the CVP (Section 2.3). Although the jugular pressure pulse is only a few mmHg, it is enough to move the skin. The 'x' and 'y' descents of the wave are normally visible in a tilted subject as inward flickers of the skin. Palpation readily distinguishes a venous pulse (too weak to feel) from an arterial pulse (easily felt).

8.11 Effects of gravity on the venous system

There are marked changes in the human circulation with posture. These are initiated by the effect of gravity on venous blood distribution, and depend on the steep, sigmoidal pressure–volume relation of veins.

Orthostasis distends veins below heart level

The adoption of a standing position, **orthostasis**, increases the pressure in all the blood vessels below heart level, and reduces the pressure in all the vessels above heart level, owing to the drag of gravity on the

vertical column of fluid between the heart and the vessel (Figure 8.2). This is particularly important in veins because their volume is highly sensitive to transmural pressure (Figure 8.19).

Upon tilting a human subject upright there is a transitory closure of the venous valves in the limbs that prevents any substantial venous back-flow. Pressure in the dependent veins then rises steadily over ~30 – 60 s as blood flows in from the arterial system. As venous pressure rises, flow recommences up the limb veins and pushes open the venous valves. This re-establishes an uninterrupted column of blood. The weight of the continuous fluid column between heart and feet raises venous pressure in the feet ninefold, from ~10 mmHg supine to ~90 mmHg in orthostasis (Figures 8.2, 8.21 – 8.23).

There is no counterbalancing rise in extramural pressure during orthostasis (unless the subject is immersed in water), so the dependent veins are greatly distended. This is plainly visible in the back of the hand when the hand is lowered below heart level. In a human adult about 500 ml of blood accumulate in the distended veins below heart level over ~45 s during orthostasis (Figure 8.21). This is widely referred to as venous 'pooling', though the imagery here is misleading; a pool is static whereas the **venous blood flows continuously** in the steady state. Most of the redistributed blood comes ultimately from the intrathoracic compartment, via arterial flow (*not* venous backflow). The loss of blood from the thoracic veins reduces the CVP and impairs the stroke volume through the Frank–Starling mechanism. This causes a transitory arterial hypotension and sometimes dizziness, called **postural hypotension** (Section 17.1). A hand–count among medical students indicates that nearly all healthy individuals

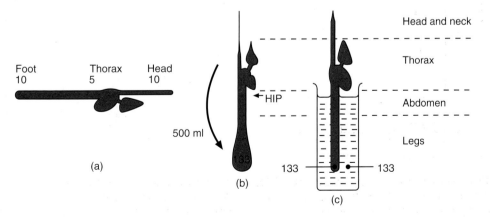

Figure 8.21 Displacement of venous blood volume (red) on moving from supine position (a) to standing (b). The thoracic compartment includes the central veins, heart and pulmonary blood. Numbers are typical pressures in cmH$_2$0. The hydrostatic indifferent point (HIP) is the point where pressure is unaltered by tilting; (c) shows how immersion in water increases central volume and CVP. (After Gauer, O. H. and Thron, H. L. (1963) In *Handbook of Physiology, Circulation*, Vol. 3 (eds Hamilton, W. F. and Dow, P.), American Physiological Society, Bethesda, pp. 2409–2440.)

occasionally experience orthostatic dizziness, especially when warm and venodilated.

Gravity does *not* affect flow in a siphon

This little section deals with a common student misconception, namely that leg venous blood flow must decrease during standing 'because the blood is going uphill against gravity'. This concept is wrong, because it ignores the fact that gravity exerts an equal and opposite 'downhill' pull on the arterial column. Gravity acts equally on the venous and arterial fluid columns, so the pressure difference between the arteries and veins at any level is not affected by orthostasis (Figures 8.2, 11.5). Since pressure **difference** drives flow, blood flow in the steady state is not directly affected by standing. The circulation through the leg or brain in fact resembles flow through a U-tube siphon (Figure 8.22). Flow through a rigid siphon is totally unaffected by the orientation of the siphon;

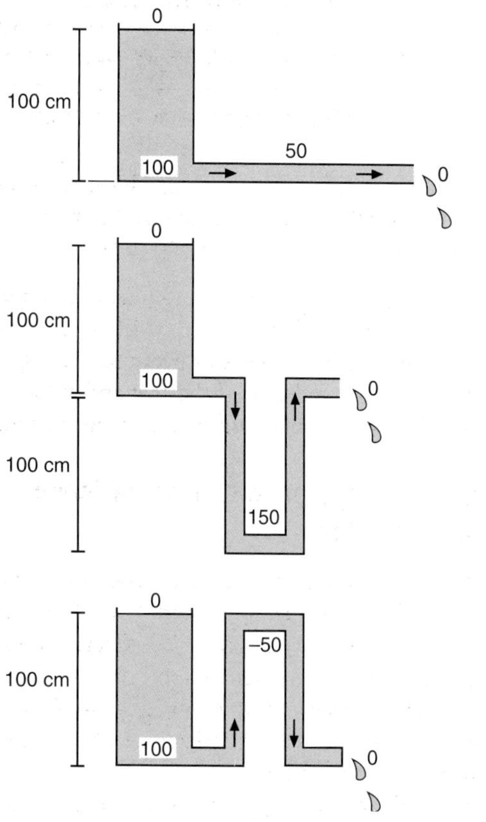

Figure 8.22 The siphon effect in a rigid U-tube. The feed-tank pressure head of 100 cmH$_2$O drives the flow. Flow passes through either a straight tube or a U-tube of equal resistance. The net pressure difference driving flow is the same in each case, so the flow is identical in all three situations (siphon principle). The middle case is equivalent to the legs of a standing man. Numbers refer to pressure in cmH$_2$O at various points

flow is the same whether the siphon is horizontal, vertical, or upside down, for the reasons given above. Similarly, if blood vessels were completely rigid, gravity would have no effect whatsoever on venous or arterial flow in the steady state.

In reality limb blood flow does decline in the steady state during dependency (Figure 8.6), but this is not because 'blood has to go uphill in the veins'. The reduction is caused by an active arteriolar contraction, which is partly a local response to the rise in pressure and partly a baroreceptor reflex.

Veins collapse above heart level

In vessels above heart level, gravity reduces the blood pressure. When the transmural pressure falls to zero or less, the unsupported superficial veins collapse (Figures 8.19–8.21), as is easily observed in the back of one's hand. Deeper veins are better supported and do not collapse completely. Veins within the cranial cavity are a special case. They do not collapse because gravity also reduces the pressure of the cerebrospinal fluid around them, so the **transmural pressure** hardly changes.

Other gravitational effects

Air pilots experience altered *g* forces during aerobatics. A pilot pulling out of a steep dive can experience +3*g* to +4*g* along the body axis. Venous pooling in the lower body is then so severe that the CVP and stroke volume fall rapidly and the pilot experiences a 'blackout' due to cerebral hypoperfusion. To prevent this an anti-gravity suit is worn; bags inflate automatically around the legs to raise extramural pressure and minimize venous distension during turns – rather as in the right panel of Figure 8.21.

Conversely, in an inverted loop-the-loop a high negative *g* force is experienced, i.e. gravity is directed towards the head. This distends the retinal vessels and causes a red-out of vision.

In space travel, the circulation is subjected to zero gravity for long periods. As this is not dissimilar to a supine posture or to floating upright in water (right panel, Figure 8.21), it presents no special problem for the cardiovascular system, until the return to positive gravity.

8.12 Venous flow and accessory pumps

Venous flow is assisted by two accessory pumps, the skeletal muscle pump during exercise and the respiratory pump.

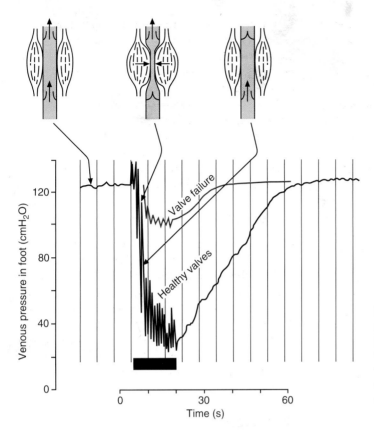

Figure 8.23 The skeletal muscle pump. Pressure in the dorsal vein of the author's foot (solid line) while standing still, interrupted by a short period of rhythmic contraction of the calf muscles (black bar). *Insets* show how the muscle pump operates. The author evidently had competent venous valves in his youth. *Red line* shows effect of failure of venous valves as in varicose veins. (Unpublished results of Levick, J. R. and Michel, C. C.)

The skeletal muscle pump has multiple roles

When a skeletal muscle contracts it compresses the adjacent veins and displaces the blood proximally towards the central veins (Figure 8.23). Venous valves prevent retrograde flow and ensure that the emptied segments refill from the periphery during each relaxation phase. Rhythmic exercise thus has a pumping effect on venous flow. While this is in no way essential for venous flow, it has the following beneficial effects.

- By redistributing venous blood from the periphery into the central veins, the muscle pump prevents CVP from falling during exercise (cf. Figure 6.12). The muscle pump may even increase CVP slightly, shifting the ventricle up the Starling curve.

- Like any other pump, the muscle pump reduces the pressure in its feed line. Venous pressure falls in the foot and ankle because, as the muscle relaxes, blood drains rapidly from the distal veins into the empty muscle veins. At the same time, closure of the proximal valves interrupts the vertical column of blood between limb and heart. The muscle pump thereby reduces the venous pressure in the lower leg from 70–90 mmHg in immobile orthostasis to 20–40 mmHg during

walking, running and cycling. This increases the arterio-venous pressure gradient driving blood through the calf muscle by 50–60%.

- The muscle pump reduces capillary filtration pressure in the feet and ankles, because capillary pressure is close to venous pressure. This greatly reduces the tendency of the feet and ankles to swell with oedema fluid in the upright position.

Valve incompetence causes varicose veins and ulcers

If the venous valves of the leg become incompetent, the muscle pump becomes ineffective. The vertical blood column can no longer be effectively broken up, so the distal leg veins are subjected to a chronically raised pressure load in orthostasis. Over time this leads to a permanent dilatation of the vein, the familiar **varicose vein**.

Chronic venous hypertension in the leg due to valvular incompetence also causes leukocytes to adhere in the dependent microcirculation, through mechanisms that are still being explored. This leads to trophic skin changes, namely discoloration and induration (hardening) followed by skin ulceration – the troublesome **venous ulcer**. Venous ulcers are usually found just above the medial ankle. They are common in the elderly, difficult to treat and a great expense for national health services.

The respiratory pump and effect of coughing

Flow in the vena cava increases during inspiration (Figure 8.24, inset). This is because the fall in intrathoracic pressure expands the intrathoracic veins, and at the same time the descent of the diaphragm compresses the abdominal contents, raises abdominal venous pressure and enhances flow from the abdomen into the thorax.

Conversely, flow in the vena cava slows during expiration. A forced expiration or Valsalva manoeuvre (Chapter 17) markedly impedes central venous flow. Coughing can elevate intrathoracic pressure transiently to 400 mmHg, impeding venous return. **Paroxysmal coughing** can impede venous return to such a degree that fainting ensues.

Flow is pulsatile in the great veins

Flow in the great veins is pulsatile due to the cycle of right atrial pressure changes (Figure 8.24). The flow shows two spurts per cycle. **Peak flow** occurs during the x descent of the atrial pressure wave and is caused by atrial relaxation. Peak inflow is aided by ventricular

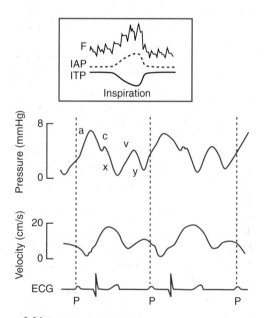

Figure 8.24 Pressure and flow in human superior vena cava over two cycles. *Inset* shows effect of breathing on venous return. F, flow in thoracic inferior vena cava; IAP, intra-abdominal pressure; ITP, intrathoracic pressure. (After Brecher, G. A. (1956) *Venous Return*, Grune and Stratton, New York and Wexler, L., Bergel, D. L., Gabe, T., *et al.* (1968) *Circulation Research*, **23**, 349–359.)

systole, because the ballistic effect of firing out a mass of blood propels the ventricle downwards, like the recoil of a gun (Newton's law of action and reaction). This stretches the atria and helps to suck blood into them. A **second flow-spurt** occurs during the y descent of the atrial pressure wave, due to the opening of the tricuspid valve in diastole. The second spurt is boosted by the elastic recoil of the ventricular walls, especially when end-systolic volume is low during exercise. Thus flow through the great veins is driven primarily by the upstream pressure of ~8 mmHg (pressure from behind or vis a tergo) but is boosted by two transient reductions in downstream pressure due to the motion of the heart (suction from in front or vis a fronte).

SUMMARY

■ The **pattern of blood flow** is laminar in arteries and veins, turbulent in the ventricles and atheromatous arteries, and bolus (single file) in capillaries.

■ **Darcy's law** states that laminar flow $\dot{Q}$ is proportional to the pressure drop along a tube $(P_1 - P_2)$ and is inversely proportional to its resistance R, i.e. $\dot{Q} = (P_1 - P_2)/R$. **Bernoulli's theory** extends this to take account of kinetic energy and gravitational potential energy. **Poiseuille's law** (below) defines the factors responsible for R in a tube.

■ **Blood flow** through major human arteries is measured by the Doppler ultrasound method. Organ blood flow is measured by the Fick principle (e.g. renal blood flow using PAH). Limb blood flow is measured by venous occlusion plethysmography. Microvascular flow is measured by radioisotope clearance.

■ **Human arterial pressure** is usually measured by sphygmomanometry of the brachial artery. The pressure varies with age, exercise, emotional stress, sleep, pregnancy, orthostasis, gravity and many pathological conditions.

■ **Mean pressure** is calculated as diastolic pressure + one-third of the pulse pressure. Mean pressure depends on cardiac output × total peripheral resistance.

■ **Pulse pressure** is systolic pressure minus diastolic pressure. Pulse pressure and systolic pressure depend on stroke volume, arterial stiffness and wave reflection. Wave reflection adds a diastolic wave after the incisura in young subjects but a systolic inflection before the incisura in older subjects, raising systolic pressure.

■ The pressure wave **propagates** rapidly along the arterial tree, with distal systolic augmentation in young subjects. The propagation rate increases with wall stiffness and hence with ageing (arteriosclerosis). Arterial stiffening raises cardiac work and O_2 demand.

■ **Vascular resistance** is located chiefly in terminal arteries and arterioles, across which the pressure falls from ~80 mmHg to ~35 mmHg. Resistance equals $8\eta L/\pi r^4$, where η is blood viscosity, L is length and r is radius (**Poiseuille's law**). Radius is controlled by vascular smooth muscle. Due to the r^4 effect, small increases in vascular tone greatly reduce blood flow, and if widespread increase the total peripheral resistance and mean arterial pressure.

■ In many organs *in vivo*, flow is almost independent of arterial pressure in the physiological range due to active regulation of the resistance by arterioles (**autoregulation**).

■ **Laplace's law** for a tube in mechanical equilibrium shows that wall tension T increases with radius and transmural pressure; $T = \Delta Pr$. Therefore wall tension is least in capillaries and highest in the aorta, which is prone to aneurysm formation.

■ **Blood viscosity** η depends on haematocrit. Viscosity is raised in polycythaemia, leading to hypertension, strokes and heart attacks. Viscosity is reduced in anaemia. Blood viscosity decreases in microvessels, facilitating microvascular perfusion (Fåhraeus–Lindqvist effect). Viscosity increases at low shear rates.

■ **Venous pressure** is ~8–10 mmHg in peripheral veins at heart level. CVP is 0–7 mmHg and can be estimated by inspection of the neck veins.

■ **Peripheral venous volume** is highly variable and influences CVP and stroke volume. It depends on pressure (the steep sigmoidal pressure–volume relation is due to vein profile changes) and smooth muscle tone. Venous tone is controlled by sympathetic nerves, which actively regulate the venous blood volume in the cutaneous, renal and splanchnic circulations.

■ In **orthostasis** gravity raises venous and arterial pressures in the legs (principle of manometry, $\rho g h$). Venous pooling in distended leg veins reduces CVP and stroke volume, leading to transient postural hypotension. The muscle pump counteracts venous pooling during walking. Incompetence of the venous valves leads to chronic venous hypertension, varicose veins and venous ulcers.

FURTHER READING

Reviews and chapters

Blomqvist, C. G. and Stone, H. L. (1983) Cardiovascular adjustments to gravitational stress. In *Handbook of Physiology, Cardiovascular System*, Vol. 3, Part 1, *Peripheral Circulation* (eds Shepherd, J. T. and Abboud, F. M.), American Physiological Society, Bethesda, pp. 1025–1063.

Caro, C. G., Pedley, T. J., Schroter, R. C. and Seed, W. A. (1978) *The Mechanics of the Circulation*, Oxford University Press, Oxford.

Chien, S. (1992) Blood cell deformability and interactions: from molecules to micromechanics and microcirculation (Zweifach Lecture). *Microvascular Research*, **44**, 243–254.

Dormandy, J. A. (1995) Microcirculation in venous disorders: the role of the white blood cells. *International Journal of Microcirculation*, **15**, Supplement 1, 3–8.

Fung, Y. C. (1997) *Biomechanics: Circulation*, 2nd Edition, Springer-Verlag, New York.

Goldsmith, H. L., Cokelet, G. R. and Gaehtgens, P. (1989) Robin Fåhraeus: evolution of his concepts in cardiovascular physiology. *American Journal of Physiology*, **257**, H1005–H1015.

Nichols, W. W. and O'Rourke, M. F. (1998) *McDonald's Blood Flow in Arteries*, 4th Edition, Arnold, London.

Pappenheimer, J. R. (1984) Contributions to microvascular research of Jean Leonard Marie Poiseuille. In *Handbook of Physiology, Cardiovascular System*, Vol. 4, *The Microcirculation* (eds Renkin, E. M. and Michel, C. C.), American Physiological Society, Bethesda, pp. 1–10.

Pickering, T. G. (1990) Physiological aspects of non-invasive ambulatory blood-pressure monitoring. *News in Physiological Sciences*, **5**, 176–179.

Secomb, T. (1995) Mechanics of blood flow in the microcirculation. In *Biological Fluid Dynamics* (eds Ellington, C. P. and Pedley, T. J.), The Company of Biologists, Cambridge, pp. 305–321.

Zweifach, B. W. and Lipowsky, H. H. (1984) Pressure–flow relations in blood and lymph microcirculations. In *Handbook of Physiology, Cardiovascular System*, Vol. 4, *Microcirculation* (eds Renkin, E. M. and Michel, C. C.), American Physiological Society, Bethesda, pp. 251–307.

Research papers

Asgeirsson, B. and Grande, P-O. (1996) Local vascular responses to elevation of an organ above the heart. *Acta Physiologica Scandinavica*, **156**, 9–18.

Fenger-Gron, J., Mulvany, M. J. and Christensen, K. L. (1997) Intestinal blood flow is controlled by both feed arteries and microcirculatory resistance vessels in freely moving rats. *Journal of Physiology*, **498**, 215–224.

Kelly, R. P., Tunin, R. and Kass, D. A. (1992) Effect of reduced aortic compliance on cardiac efficiency and contractile function of in situ canine left ventricle. *Circulation Research*, **71**, 490–502.

Lipowsky, H. H. and Williams, M. E. (1997) Shear rate dependency of red cell sequestration in skin capillaries in sickle cell disease and its variation with vasoocclusive crisis. *Microcirculation*, **4**, 289–301.

Reinke, W., Gaehtgens, P. and Johnson, P. C. (1987) Blood viscosity in small tubes: effect of shear rate, aggregation, and sedimentation. *American Journal of Physiology*, **253**, H540–H547.

Stick, C., Jaeger, H. and Witzleb, E. (1992). Measurements of volume changes and venous pressure in the human leg during walking and running. *Journal of Applied Physiology*, **72**, 2063–2068.

Sutton, D. W. and Schmid-Schönbein, G. W. (1989) Hemodynamics at low flow in resting vasodilated rat skeletal muscle. *American Journal of Physiology*, **257**, H1419–H1427.

Toska, K. and Eriksen, M. (1993) Respiration-synchronous fluctuations in stroke volume, heart rate and arterial pressure in humans. *Journal of Physiology*, **472**, 501–512.

Wilkinson, I. B., MacCallum, H., Hupperetz, P. C., van Thoor, C. J., Cockroft, J. R. and Webb, D. J. (2001) Changes in the derived central pressure waveform and pulse pressure in response to angiotensin II and noradrenaline in man. *Journal of Physiology*, **530**, 541–550.

Yano, M., Kohno, M., Kobayashi, S., Obayashi, M., Seki, K., Ohkusa, T., Miura, T., Fujii, T. and Matsuzaki, M. (2001) Influence of timing and magnitude of arterial wave reflection on left ventricular relaxation. *American Journal of Physiology*, **280**, H1846–H1852.

The endothelial cell

Learning objectives

After reading this chapter you should be able to:

- Outline the structure of the cytoskeleton, intercellular junction, vesicle system and glycocalyx (9.2).
- State the ion channels that influence Ca^{2+} entry and the roles of endothelial Ca^{2+} (9.3).
- List four major vasoactive secretions of endothelium and their actions (9.4–9.5).
- State the main actions of endothelial NO and how its production is regulated (9.4).
- List the actions of endothelium on blood (9.6).
- Outline how circulating leukocytes are captured by endothelium in inflammation (9.8).
- Describe the other roles of endothelium in inflammation (9.8).
- Outline the factors that regulate permeability (9.7).
- State the role of endothelium in angiogenesis, and the main regulatory factors (9.9).
- Describe briefly the significance of NO in atheroma formation (9.10).

Although the activity of endothelium is less obvious than that of cardiac or vascular myocytes, endothelium nevertheless makes numerous active contributions to cardiovascular function. Endothelium is the monolayer of endothelial cells that lines the entire vascular system, with a cumulative weight of several hundred grams in a human. It forms a vast interface between the blood and tissues, with a surface area of $\sim 280\,m^2$ in the skeletal muscles and $\sim 90\,m^2$ in the lungs of a human. This enormous interface facilitates the transfer of nutrients and white cells from blood into the tissue; the transfer of regulatory signals from endothelium to vascular smooth muscle; and numerous effects of endothelium on the circulating blood (Figure 9.1).

9.1 Overview of endothelial functions

- **Endothelium governs blood–tissue exchange.** The primary role of endothelium is to form a semipermeable membrane that retains the plasma and formed elements of blood within the circulation while allowing nutrients to move rapidly between blood and tissue. The structures that govern permeability are an internal coating called the glycocalyx and the intercellular junctions. These structures are permeable to the small solutes, such as glucose, adrenaline and drugs, but impermeable to big

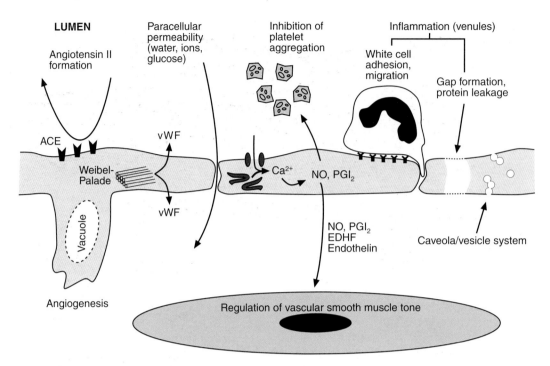

Figure 9.1 Schematic drawing of multiple functions of endothelial cell; lumen is at top. NO, nitric oxide; PGI$_2$, prostacyclin; EDHF, endothelium-derived hyperpolarizing factor; ACE, angiotensin I converting enzyme; vWF, von Willebrand haemostatic factor.

solutes such as the plasma proteins. The intercellular junctions are dynamic structures and can rapidly alter the endothelial permeability. A system of endothelial vesicles mediates a slow but necessary transfer of plasma immunoglobulins, protein-bound minerals and protein-bound hormones into the tissues.

- **Endothelial secretions regulate vascular tone.** Arterial endothelium acts as the middle-man in a number of vascular responses, such as flow-induced vasodilatation. The endothelium senses the shear stress generated by blood flow, and also possesses receptors to agonists such as acetylcholine. Endothelium responds to these signals by secreting vasoactive agents, namely nitric oxide, endothelium-derived hyperpolarizing factor, prostacyclin and endothelin. These agents act on to the adjacent vascular smooth muscle cells to adjust the local blood flow.

- **Surface enzymes transform plasma components.** The luminal surface of endothelium possesses an enzyme, angiotensin-converting enzyme, that chemically modifies several circulating, vasoactive peptides. The large contact area

between plasma and endothelium ensures efficient conversion of the substrate.

- **Endothelium secretes anti-haemostatic agents and a clotting factor.** Nitric oxide and prostacyclin are not only vasodilators but also inhibit the aggregation of platelets, thereby preventing thrombosis (the clotting of circulating blood). Endothelium also secretes von Willebrand factor, which is involved in the clotting cascade.

- **Endothelium is part of the inflammatory defence against pathogens.** During an inflammatory process venular endothelium produces adhesion molecules that capture circulating leukocytes and cause them to migrate into the affected tissue. The venular endothelium also develops large gaps for increased delivery of immunoglobulins to the tissue.

- **Endothelium initiates new blood vessel formation.** The sprouting of capillary endothelial cells is the starting point for the development of all types of new blood vessel (angiogenesis). Angiogenesis is essential for tissue growth, wound repair and cancer growth.

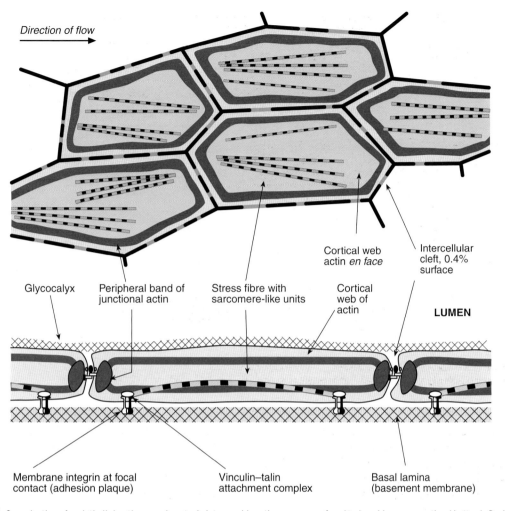

Direction of flow

Glycocalyx

Peripheral band of
junctional actin

Stress fibre with
sarcomere-like units

Cortical
web of
actin

Cortical web
actin *en face*

Intercellular
cleft, 0.4%
surface

LUMEN

Membrane integrin at focal
contact (adhesion plaque)

Vinculin–talin
attachment complex

Basal lamina
(basement membrane)

Figure 9.2 Organization of endothelial actin–myosin cytoskeleton and junctions, seen *en face* (*top*) and in cross-section (*bottom*). Dark inter-cellular lines *en face* represent closed regions of the cleft (~90% of it), lighter lines are open regions due to breaks in junctional strands. (Adapted from Drenckhahn, D. and Ness, W., in Born, G. V. R. and Schwartz, C. J. (eds) (1997); see Further Reading.)

● **Endothelial dysfunction contributes to atheroma.** Disordered endothelial function contributes to the development of arterial atheroma, a major cause of death in Westernized societies. Primary components of the atheromatous plaque include plasma-derived cholesterol and fibrin, which are trapped between the endothelium and tunica media.

The roles of endothelium are thus many and diverse, and differ between different classes of vessel. This chapter is devoted to the cellular biology that underlies these roles. Broader physiological aspects of microvascular solute exchange and fluid balance are covered in Chapters 10 and 11 respectively, and endothelial regulation of vascular tone is integrated with other vascular control processes in Chapter 13.

9.2 Structure of endothelium

Endothelium consists of polygonal, flattened cells, 0.2–0.3 μm thick, arranged in a 'crazy paving' mono-layer (Figures 1.10, 9.2). The cell possesses a unique organelle called the Weibel–Palade body (Section 9.6), as well as the usual organelles. Its endoplasmic reticulum, which contains a small store of Ca^{2+}, approaches to within 8 nm of the cell membrane in arterial endothelium. The following structures are important for membrane formation and permeability.

The actin–myosin cytoskeleton is organized into three systems

The endothelial cytoskeleton consists of numerous thin actin filaments, plus a smaller number of thick

Intro
Also
See
pg 146

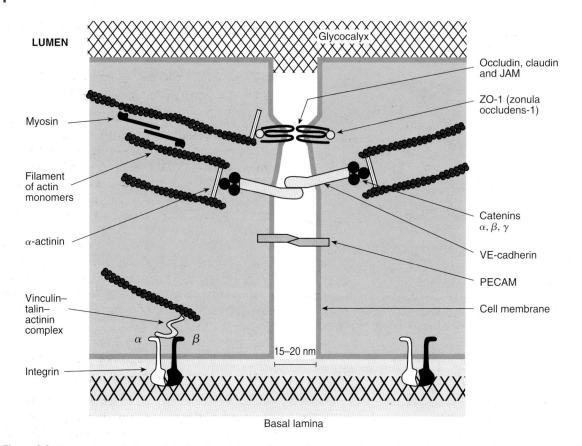

Figure 9.3 The proteins of the intercellular junction, their putative organization and their relation to the actin cytoskeleton. JAM, junctional adhesion molecule; PECAM, platelet–endothelial cell adhesion molecule; VE-cadherin, vascular endothelial cadherin. (Based in part on Drenckhahn, D. and Ness, W., in Born, G. V. R. and Schwartz, C. J. (eds) (1997); see Further Reading.)

myosin filaments, organized into three systems – a thin cortical web, a junctional actin band and stress fibres (Figure 9.2).

The **cortical web** is a thin layer of actin filaments under the luminal and abluminal surfaces, linked to membrane glycoproteins through the protein filamin. The cortical web acts as scaffolding and as an anchor for membrane proteins such as the leukocyte-capturing molecules.

The **junctional actin band** is a prominent ring just inside the cell perimeter (Figure 9.2). The band is attached to the intercellular junction through α-actinin and serves as an anchor for junctional proteins (Figure 9.3). Consequently, disassembly of the actin filaments by the drug cytochalasin causes gaps to develop between the endothelial cells.

Stress fibres on the basal surface of arterial endothelial cells resist the shearing effect of blood flow. They are composed of interdigitating myosin and actin filaments arranged in 2–4 μm long sarcomere-like units, as in muscle myofibrils. The stress fibres are attached through α-actinin, vinculin and talin to the basal cell membrane at **focal contacts** (adhesion plaques), and the membrane is attached to the basal lamina at these points by transmembrane dimers called **integrins** (Figures 9.2, 9.3).

The intercellular cleft is the pathway for water and nutrient transfer

Water and small, lipid-insoluble solutes such as glucose, amino acids and drugs cross the endothelial barrier chiefly through capillary intercellular clefts, which are 20 nm wide and occupy 0.2–0.4% of the capillary surface (Figure 9.2, upper panel).

Junctional strands, which are rows of protein particles in the perimeter membrane, form one to three **tight junctions** across the intercellular cleft, seemingly blocking the pathway (Figures 9.3, 9.4). However the junctional strands do not form a continuous seal around the entire cell perimeter; at intervals there are 150–200 nm long breaks in the strands, providing a continuous, albeit tortuous, pathway across the capillary wall (Figure 9.4). The continuity of the pathway is not apparent in a single cross-section owing to its tortuosity.

Lumen

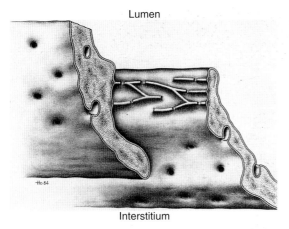

Interstitium

Figure 9.4 Three-dimensional reconstruction of capillary intercellular cleft from serial electron micrographs. The cleft is 500–1000 nm long (top to bottom) and 15–20 nm wide except at the tight junctions. Water and small lipophobic solutes follow the tortuous pathway through the breaks in the junctional strands. (From Bundgaard, M. (1984) *Journal of Ultrastructural Research*, **88**, 1–17, by permission.)

Postcapillary venules have a higher permeability to water than most capillaries because they have fewer junctional strands and wider breaks. Brain endothelium, by contrast, has an extremely low permeability, because it has numerous, complex junctional strands with no breaks.

The junctional protein complex is a dynamic, regulated assembly

In epithelium, which is better understood than endothelium, the formation of a tight or 'occludens' junction depends on the formation of a nearby anchoring or 'adherens' junction. The endothelial junction contains both the proteins associated with occludens junctions, namely occludin, claudin-5, JAM (junctional adhesion molecule) and the linker molecule ZO-1, and also those associated with adherens junctions, namely VE-cadherin and the catenins (Figure 9.3). Vascular endothelial (VE) cadherin is a membrane-spanning glycoprotein whose extracellular domain binds to the VE cadherin of the adjacent cell and whose intracellular domain binds to a complex of α, β and γ catenin. The catenin complex is tethered by α-actinin to the junctional actin band. Another component of the junction, platelet endothelial cell adhesion molecule (PECAM), has a role in leukocyte emigration.

The junctional complex can be altered rapidly via intracellular messengers. Agents that raise endothelial cAMP concentration, such as isoprenaline, increase in the number of junctional strands and junctional protein expression, leading to a fall in permeability. Conversely, a weakening of the junction through the enzymatic phosphorylation of β catenin contributes to inflammatory gap formation.

Arterial endothelium also has gap junctions, which transmit signals

Arterial endothelial cells form numerous gap junctions with their neighbours. See Section 3.1 for an introduction to gap junctions. These **homocellular gap junctions** transmit ions, small chemical messengers (up to ~1000 daltons) and membrane potentials between the endothelial cells and lead to the conduction of vasomotor responses along small arteries ('ascending vasodilatation', Figure 13.10). The endothelium also makes contact with underlying vascular smooth muscle cells through **myoendothelial** or **heterocellular gap junctions**. Conduction of a signal from the endothelium to vascular muscle through the myoendothelial gap junctions is part of the mechanism of ascending vasodilatation (Section 13.7).

The glycocalyx is a negatively charged barrier to macromolecules

The internal or 'luminal' surface of endothelium is coated by a thin layer of negatively charged (anionic) biopolymers, called the glycocalyx (Figures 9.3, 9.5). The structure of the glycocalyx is poorly understood. Its thickness is variously estimated as 60–570 nm, and the constituent biopolymers include the sialoglycoprotein podocalyxin, heparan sulphate proteoglycan, and hyaluronan. The polymer network appears to form a size-selective molecular sieve that retains the plasma proteins within the circulation but allows the passage of water and smaller solutes into the intercellular cleft. The enzymatic removal of the glycocalyx increases the rate of passage of lipoprotein and water across endothelium. The negative charge of the glycocalyx helps to exclude negatively charged plasma proteins such as albumin and the atherogenic low-density lipoproteins.

Caveolae and vesicles mediate transcytosis

Albumin, immunoglobulins and lipoproteins cross the endothelial barrier rather slowly. The main transport mechanism is controversial, but some form of vesicular transcytosis is certainly one mechanism. Up to a quarter of the endothelial cell is occupied by membrane-bound **vesicles** of diameter ~70 nm. At the surface the vesicles make contact with the plasma or interstitial fluid through 20–30 nm wide necks, giving them the appearance of little flasks or **caveolae** (Figures 9.1, 9.5). The cytoplasmic face of a caveola has a striated coat of the protein caveolin. The caveola membrane itself is enriched in cholesterol, sphingomyelin, nitric oxide synthase and receptors for albumin (albondin), insulin, transferrin and caeruloplasmin. The quantitative importance of receptors in trans-endothelial protein transport, however, is uncertain.

Although the cytoplasmic vesicles in tissue section appear to be detached and free-floating, this is an illusion. Serial sections show that 99% of seemingly 'free' vesicles are connected to each other and ultimately to a caveola at one or other surface (Figure 9.6). The caveola/vesicle system is thus a set of racemose invaginations of the cell membrane, resembling bunches of grapes dangling from each surface.

The caveola–vesicle system transports macromolecules into the cell (**endocytosis**; the transfer of receptor-bound materials to endosomes) and across it (**transcytosis**, Section 10.7). When a test protein such as ferritin is injected into the bloodstream, the ferritin appears first in the luminal caveolae, then in the cytoplasmic vesicles and finally, after ~10 s, in the abluminal caveolae and subendothelial space (Figures 9.5, 9.6). The **mechanism of transcytosis** is no longer held to be the diffusion of free-floating vesicles. With the discovery that few vesicles are free, a mechanism based on transient vesicular fusion and transfer of contents was proposed (Figure 9.6). Very occasionally a section reveals a row of fused vesicles and caveolae forming a continuous channel through the cell (Figure 9.6b, left). These rare 'multivesicular transendothelial channels' may contribute to macromolecular permeation.

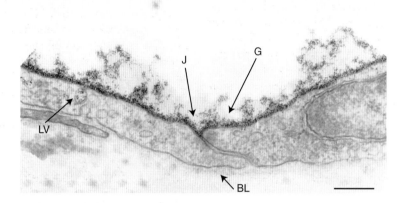

Figure 9.5 Electron micrograph of a continuous capillary after perfusion with cationic ferritin. Each black dot represents one molecule. The cation binds to and reveals the glycocalyx (G). The ferritin fails to permeate the cleft, but does enter the caveolar-vesicular system (arrow; LV, labelled vesicle). The cationized ferritin reduces permeability (see 'The protein effect', Chapter 10), whereas neutral ferritin does not bind to glycocalyx and does not reduce permeability. BL, basal lamina; Bar = 0.2 μm. (From Turner, M. R., Clough, G. and Michel, C. C. (1983) *Microvascular Research*, **25**, 205–222, by permission.)

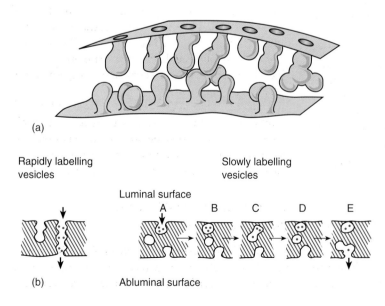

Figure 9.6 The endothelial caveolae–vesicle system. (a) Reconstruction of serial thin sections to show connection of most vesicle, directly or indirectly, with a surface via the caveolae (flask-shaped surface invaginations). Detached vesicles are rare. (b) Frames A–E show how transcytosis of macromolecules (red dots, ferritin) might occur by transient vesicular fusion and mixing of contents. Occasional abluminal vesicles that label unusually rapidly might be part of a multivesicular, transendothelial channel (left frame). ((a) From Frokjaer-Jensen, J. (1983) *Progress in Applied Microcirculation*, **1**, 17–34, by permission; (b) from Clough, G. and Michel, C. C. (1981) *Journal of Physiology*, **315**, 127–142, by permission.)

The basal lamina prevents capillary rupture

The endothelial basal lamina or basement membrane is a 50–100 nm thick layer of extracellular matrix, comprising a lightly staining region next to the cell (**lamina rara**) and an adjacent denser region (**lamina densa**). The basal lamina does not in general prevent the onward passage of plasma proteins that have escaped through the caveola–vesicle system. A criss-cross network of **type IV collagen** molecules gives the membrane great mechanical strength. **Laminin**, an adhesive glycoprotein, and **perlecan**, a negatively charged heparan sulphate proteoglycan, are the other major constituents. The endothelial cell is attached to the collagen and laminin by β_1 **integrins** at the focal contacts (Figures 9.2, 9.3).

Since capillaries lack a tunica media or adventitia, the basal lamina provides most of their mechanical strength and prevents the capillary from being ruptured by the blood pressure. Wall **tension** is actually low due to the small radius of a capillary (see Laplace's law, Section 8.7), but the wall **stress** (tension per unit thickness) is high due to the thinness of the wall. Indeed, capillary wall stress is comparable to that in an artery. In **Goodpasture's syndrome** the basal lamina is weakened by autoantibodies against type IV collagen, and capillary bleeding occurs into the glomerular and alveolar spaces.

Endothelial phenotype varies between vessels

Endothelium shows specialization in different vessels and tissues. In **arterial endothelium** the haemodynamically stressed cells are elongated in the direction of flow and have prominent stress fibres. In the **capillaries of glandular tissues** the endothelium is perforated by circular windows called fenestrations (Section 10.2). In **postcapillary venules** the junctional strand breaks are extensive whereas in **brain microvessels** there are no breaks. Venular endothelium is also enriched in receptors to inflammatory mediators and has a large store of P-selectin (leukocyte 'glue'), so venular endothelium is the primary site of the inflammatory response. In **lymph nodes** the post-capillary venules have unusually tall endothelial cells, called 'high endothelium', through which lymphocytes recycle between blood and the lymphatic system.

9.3 Ion channels and endothelial function

Many endothelial responses are triggered by increased cytosolic Ca^{2+} concentration, e.g. increased nitric oxide production, increased permeability. The basal cytosolic $[Ca^{2+}]$ is only ~0.1 μM, in contrast to 1 mM in extracellular fluid. Increases in cytosolic Ca^{2+} are brought about partly by extracellular Ca^{2+} influx through membrane ion channels and partly by store release (Figure 9.1). In the following account it is assumed that the reader is familiar with the electrophysiological concepts introduced in Chapter 3.

Membrane potential affects endothelial responsiveness

Endothelial cells have a negative intracellular potential of −30 mV to −68 mV. The negative potential is due to **inward rectifier K^+ channels**, along with a variable contribution from K_{Ca} channels (see below) and about −8 mV from the electrogenic $3Na^+–2K^+$-ATPase pump (Figure 9.7). The size of the potential is important because (i) it affects extracellular Ca^{2+} influx and therefore Ca^{2+}-mediated responses (example, Figure 11.27); and (ii) the spread of endothelial hyperpolarization through gap junctions probably contributes to ascending vasodilatation in exercise (Section 13.7). Endothelium cannot generate action potentials because it lacks voltage-gated Na^+ or Ca^{2+} channels. Endothelium does, however, have two other kinds of Ca^{2+}-conducting channel as follows.

Ca^{2+}-conducting channels

Receptor-operated channels (ROCs) are ion channels that are activated by the binding of a pharmacologically active substance or 'agonist' to a specific membrane receptor (Figure 9.7). The receptor is linked to the ion channel by a G-protein. Many of the receptors to histamine, bradykinin, thrombin, serotonin, ATP and acetylcholine have this type of link. The ROCs are poorly selective, transmitting not only Ca^{2+} but also some Na^+ and K^+. The opening of ROCs is followed by a rapid rise in cytosolic $[Ca^{2+}]$ due to the huge electrochemical gradient for extracellular Ca^{2+} entry.

A different kind of Ca^{2+} channel in the endothelial membrane, called the **store-operated channel**, opens in response to depletion of the endoplasmic reticulum store. The ensuing influx of Ca^{2+} is called 'capacitative Ca^{2+} entry' and helps to restock the store.

Calcium-activated K^+ channels hyperpolarize the cell

As well as inward rectifier K^+ channels, endothelium has K^+ channels that are activated by cytosolic Ca^{2+}, called K_{Ca} or calcium-activated potassium channels.

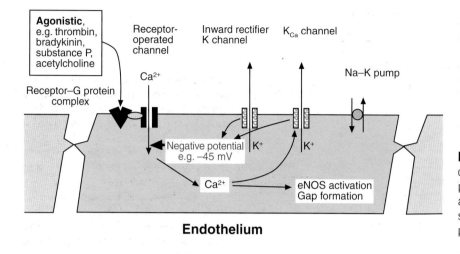

Endothelium

Figure 9.7 Key endothelial ion channels influencing membrane potential and Ca^{2+} entry. The store-activated Ca^{2+} entry channel is not shown here. The store-discharging pathway is shown in Figure 9.9.

Agonists that increase the cytosolic $[Ca^{2+}]$ also indirectly activate K_{Ca} channels (Figure 9.7). The resulting increase in K^+ conductance hyperpolarizes the endothelium (makes it more negative). Hyperpolarization serves two functions. It increase the force driving extracellular Ca^{2+} influx; and it can be transmitted by ionic currents through gap junctions to regulate arteriolar muscle tone (Sections 9.5, 13.7).

9.4 Nitric oxide secretion

Endothelium modulates vascular tone

The role of endothelium as a regulator of vascular tone began to emerge when Vane and colleagues discovered in 1976 that blood vessels secrete a vasodilator substance, **prostacyclin** (PGI$_2$).

A second endothelium-derived vasodilator agent was discovered in 1980, when Furchgott and Zadwadski observed that arterial vasodilatation in response to the acetylcholine analogue carbachol changed into vasoconstriction when the endothelial lining was rubbed away (Figure 9.8). It emerged that acetylcholine stimulates the endothelium to secrete a vasodilator substance, originally called 'endothelium-derived relaxing factor' (EDRF) and now identified as **nitric oxide**. The vasodilator action of the nitric oxide normally overrides the direct vasoconstrictor action of acetylcholine on arterial muscle.

A third endothelial secretion, the vasoconstrictor peptide **endothelin**, was discovered in 1989 by a Japanese group using molecular biology techniques. All three substances, prostacyclin, nitric oxide and endothelin, are secreted as they are produced; they are not stored for later release.

Endothelial NO has multiple functions

Nitric oxide (NO) is generated continuously by endothelium at a low basal rate (Figure 9.9). It is a freely diffusible, soluble, lipophilic (lipid soluble) gas with multiple effects.

- NO inhibits vascular myocyte contraction, leading to vasodilatation (Figure 9.10a). Its main physiological roles are to **modulate basal tone** and to mediate **flow-induced vasodilatation** (Chapter 13). Also some **inflammatory vasodilators**, e.g. bradykinin, act by stimulating endothelium to produce NO.

- NO inhibits vascular myocyte proliferation.

- NO inhibits platelets aggregation and thus protects the vessel against thrombosis.

- NO is a link in the signalling cascade that causes gap formation in venular endothelium during inflammation.

- NO inhibits the nuclear transcription of leukocyte-binding adhesion molecules such as endothelial VCAM.

Loss of the inhibitory effects of NO on smooth muscle proliferation, platelet activation and leukocyte adhesion contributes to the progression of atheroma (Section 9.10).

How NO causes vasodilatation

NO diffuses rapidly from the endothelium into the neighbouring vascular smooth muscle, where it reacts with the haem group of an enzyme, guanylyl cyclase (Figure 9.9). The activated enzyme catalyses the production of cyclic guanosine monophosphate (cGMP).

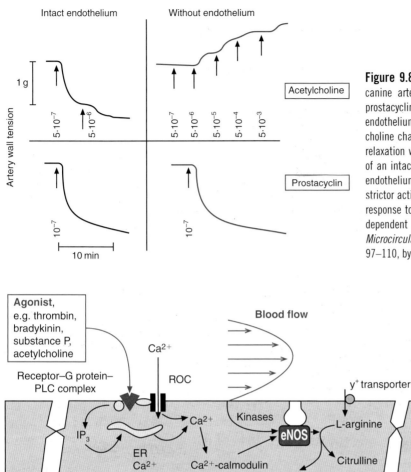

Figure 9.8 Recording of force exerted by a strip of canine artery *in vitro*. Addition of acetylcholine or prostacyclin caused relaxation (*left panels*). When endothelium was rubbed away, the response to acetylcholine changed to contraction (*top right*). Thus, the relaxation was endothelium dependent. The response of an intact vessel depends on the balance between endothelium-mediated relaxation and a direct constrictor action of acetylcholine on smooth muscle. The response to added prostacyclin was not endothelium dependent (*bottom right*). (From Altura, B. (1988) *Microcirculation, Endothelium and Lymphatics*, **4**, 97–110, by permission.)

Figure 9.9 Regulation of nitric oxide production by endothelial nitric oxide synthase (eNOS); ROC, receptor-operated channel; PLC, phospholipase C; IP$_3$, inositol tris-phosphate; ER, endoplasmic reticulum. The shear stress-activated kinases are phosphatidyl inositol-3 kinase and protein kinase B (see text).

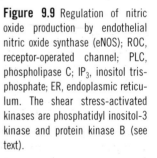

The cGMP activates kinases (enzymes that phosphorylate other proteins to alter their activity), leading to vascular relaxation. In addition, high concentrations of NO can directly activate K_{Ca} channels in the myocyte membrane, leading to vascular relaxation through hyperpolarization (Figure 9.10a).

NO is generated from L-arginine by nitric oxide synthase

Nitric oxide survives only a few seconds in the tissues because it reacts with a metabolic derivative of oxygen, the superoxide anion O_2^- (see Appendix 2, 'Free radicals'). NO must therefore be generated continuously. It is produced by a constitutively expressed enzyme, endothelial nitric oxide synthase (eNOS), which is bound to the inner surface of the cell membrane, particularly the caveolar membrane. eNOS cleaves NO from the amino acid L-arginine (Figure 9.9). NO production can be blocked pharmacologically by inactive analogues, such as *N*-monomethyl-L-arginine or nitroarginine methyl ester (NAME), which compete with normal arginine for eNOS binding sites.

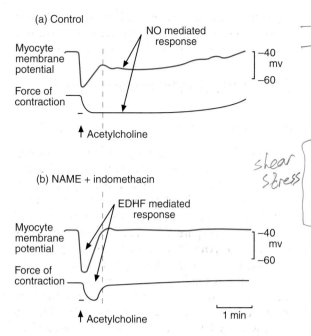

shear stress

Figure 9.10 (a) Endothelium-dependent relaxation of guinea-pig coronary artery (black line) in response to acetylcholine (bar) is mediated partly by hyperpolarization of the vascular smooth muscle (red line). (b) Blockage of production of NO by nitroarginine methyl ester (NAME) and prostacyclin by indomethacin abolishes the late part of the response but leaves an early phase of hyperpolarization and relaxation that is due to EDHF. (From Parkington, H. C., Tona, M. A., Coleman, H. A. and Tare, M. (1995) *Journal of Physiology*, **484**, 469–480, by permission.)

eNOS activity is stimulated by shear stress and agonists

The activity of eNOS (also called isoenzyme NOS-III) is continuously stimulated by the shear stress exerted by flowing blood, and can be increased further by agonists such as inflammatory mediators and acetylcholine. Even greater NO production is achieved in pathological situations through the nuclear transcription of another isoenzyme, inducible nitric oxide synthase (iNOS or NOS-II); this is part of the response to endotoxin and inflammatory cytokines (Section 13.3).

Stimulation by shear stress

Shear stress is the force exerted on the vessel wall by the sliding action of flowing blood, and it is probably the most important stimulus, normally, for the **continuous basal production** of NO. The continuous production of NO has a continuous vasodilator influence on the arterial system, as revealed by constriction when NO production is blocked pharmacologically. During exercise, increased shear stress due to increased flow in the exercising muscle stimulates

further NO production, causing **flow-induced vasodilatation** (Section 13.4).

The shear stress is thought to be transduced (sensed) by the integrins that anchor endothelium to the basal lamina. Transduction leads to the activation of an enzyme, phosphatidyl inositol-3 kinase, which phosphorylates protein kinase B. The latter increases the activity of eNOS through phosphorylation.

One may ask, 'How can the endothelium sense blood flow at all if, as Figure 8.3 shows, the lamina adjoining the wall is stationary?' The answer is that the zero-slip layer is tugging on the endothelium because it is itself being tugged by the adjacent, sliding lamina.

Stimulation of eNOS by agonists

The activity of eNOS is increased by calcium–calmodulin complex. Calmodulin is a Ca^{2+}-binding protein. Agonists that raise intracellular $[Ca^{2+}]$ promote calcium–calmodulin formation and hence increase the eNOS activity and NO production rate (Figure 9.9). Such agonists include bradykinin, thrombin, substance P, ATP, ADP, acetylcholine (via muscarinic M_3 receptors), vasoactive intestinal polypeptide, insulin and in some tissues/species histamine. Several of these agonists are released by inflamed tissues, so NO contributes to the characteristic redness of inflammation (vasodilatation).

Agonists raise endothelial $[Ca^{2+}]$ via two main pathways. Some agonist–receptor complexes activate ROCs (Section 9.3), leading to an influx of extracellular Ca^{2+}. Others trigger a biochemical chain that releases the small Ca^{2+} store in the endoplasmic reticulum (Figure 9.9). The agonist–receptor complex is linked to the membrane-bound enzyme phospholipase C, which catalyses the breakdown of phosphatidyl inositol bisphosphate into inositol trisphosphate (IP_3). The IP_3 activates the store Ca^{2+}-release channels. Activation of store-operated Ca^{2+} channels in the surface membrane then allows a further influx of extracellular Ca^{2+} called the capacitative Ca^{2+} current (Section 9.3).

9.5 Other vasoactive endothelial products

Endothelium-derived hyperpolarizing factor (EDHF)

In small arteries and arterioles, agonists such as acetylcholine or bradykinin can initiate endothelium-dependent hyperpolarization and relaxation of vascular muscle when NO and prostacyclin production have been blocked pharmacologically (Figure 9.10b). Moreover, saline that has been washed over agonist-stimulated, eNOS-blocked endothelium can hyperpolarize and relax isolated vascular muscle. Such experiments showed that endothelium can secrete a soluble, hyperpolarizing chemical that is neither NO nor prostacyclin – an 'endothelium-derived hyperpolarizing factor' or EDHF. EDHF probably contributes more than NO to agonist-induced vasodilatation in small vessels, whereas NO predominates in large arteries. The identity of EDHF is controversial; it may be an epoxide of arachidonic acid, namely EET (epoxyeicosatrienoic acid), which is produced by a cytochrome P450 epoxygenase.

Not all cases of non-NO, endothelium-dependent hyperpolarization involve a released chemical factor. The tunica media of arterioles and feed arteries (diameter ~100 μm) is only a few cells wide, and myoendothelial gap junctions are abundant. Consequently, there is good **electrical coupling** between endothelium and myocytes in small vessels. When the gap junctions are blocked pharmacologically, agonist-induced dilatation fails in some small vessels. It appears that the agonist hyperpolarizes the endothelial cells by activating endothelial K_{Ca} channels, and the hyperpolarization spreads through the myoendothelial gap junctions to the myocytes, causing relaxation. The same process contributes to ascending vasodilatation in active skeletal muscle (Section 13.7). In some small vessels, therefore, no external, soluble EDHF is needed for the hyperpolarization response.

Prostacyclin (PGI₂)

Prostacyclin, like NO, causes vasodilatation and platelet inhibition. It is produced by endothelium in response to agonists such as thrombin. Prostacyclin is generated by the action of the enzyme **cyclooxygenase** on the unsaturated fatty acid **arachidonic acid**. Arachidonic acid is produced from cell membrane phospholipids by **phospholipase A₂**. Unlike the production of NO the production of prostacyclin is not well sustained.

Endothelin

Endothelin is a peptide related to the snake venom sarafotoxin. Endothelin-1, the main isoform secreted by endothelium, causes a powerful, unusually sustained vasoconstriction that lasts 2–3 hours. Over a longer time scale endothelin stimulates vascular and cardiac myocyte proliferation. Endothelial cells have a low basal rate of endothelin synthesis, so endothelin makes a small contribution to the basal vascular tone. Endothelin production can be stimulated by hypoxia, angiotensin II, vasopressin and thrombin. Plasma endothelin levels are raised in pre-eclamptic toxaemia (hypertension of pregnancy) and heart failure.

9.6 Actions of endothelium on blood

ACE catalyses angiotensin II production

Angiotensin I is a relatively inactive circulating decapeptide that is generated in renal plasma (Section 14.8). Angiotensin I is converted into angiotensin II, an octapeptide with strong vasoconstrictor properties, by an enzyme bound to the luminal surface of endothelium (Figure 9.1). The **angiotensin converting enzyme** (ACE) is a zinc carboxypeptidase. Angiotensin II is generated chiefly in the lungs because this is the first large area of endothelium to be encountered by angiotensin I molecules after their production in renal venous plasma. ACE inhibitors such as captopril reduce angiotensin II levels and are widely used to treat hypertension and heart failure.

ACE also rapidly degrades the circulating vasoactive agents bradykinin and serotonin as they pass through the lungs. Since these are pro-inflammatory substances, an occasional side-effect of ACE inhibitors is oedema formation.

Endothelium secretes a haemostatic agent, von Willebrand factor

Endothelial cells contain a unique organelle called the Weibel–Palade body (Figure 9.1). This is a rod-shaped storage organ composed of numerous longitudinal tubules within a membrane. The tubules are made up of stored **von Willebrand factor** (vWF). vWF is an endothelial glycoprotein that is secreted constitutively into the bloodstream. It serves as a carrier for clotting factor VIII, which is part of the clotting cascade that converts plasma prothrombin into active thrombin.

Thrombin, a protease, brings about a crucial event in blood clotting, namely the conversion of soluble fibrinogen into an insoluble fibrin network. Thrombin also cleaves off the ends of endothelial thrombin receptors. The activated receptors trigger the rapid local exocytosis of vWF. The vWF binds to subendothelial collagen and promotes platelet adhesion. In von Willebrand disease, which is a common inherited failure to synthesize vWF, there is prolonged bleeding after injury.

The Weibel–Palade body also contains a store of **P-selectin**, a leukocyte-adhesive protein. When endothelium is activated by an inflammatory agonist, the P-selectin is translocated to the surface and initiates the capture of passing leukocytes (Figure 9.11).

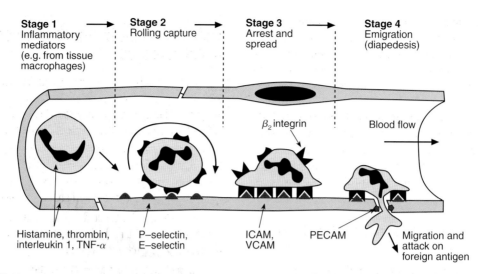

Figure 9.11 Margination, rolling capture, arrest and extravasation of leukocyte in inflammation. TNF-α, tumour necrosis factor α; ICAM, VCAM, PECAM: see text.

NO and prostacyclin inhibit platelet aggregation

NO and prostacyclin both inhibit platelet aggregation. Their anti-haemostatic action counterbalances the effect of vWF. When blood clots, the activated endothelial thrombin receptors cause not only vWF excocytosis, promoting platelet adherence, but also increased endothelial NO and prostacyclin production. The NO and prostacyclin limit the spread of platelet aggregation and thereby prevent uncontrolled vascular thrombosis. The endothelial secretions thus help to achieve a limited, well-regulated haemostatic process rather than a runaway one.

9.7 Endothelial permeability and its regulation

Capillary permeability to solutes and water is covered in Chapters 10 and 11. The endothelial intercellular cleft is the main route for nutrient and water exchange (Figures 9.3, 9.4) and the endothelial cell actively regulates the permeability of the pathway as follows.

An increase in the **plasma velocity** in a capillary causes the endothelium to raise the intercellular permeability. This improves glucose transfer in exercising muscle (Section 10.11). The flow-dependent permeability increase is blocked by inhibitors of eNOS. Microvessel permeability is also increased by **atrial natriuretic peptide**, a hormone involved in the control of plasma volume (Section 14.9). Like NO,

Endothelium forms a permeable membrane with multiple pathways

☐ The *lipid cell membrane* allows the rapid permeation of lipid-soluble molecules (O_2, CO_2, anaesthetics) between blood and tissue.

☐ The *intercellular cleft* is a paracellular pathway that transmits water and small lipophobic solutes (e.g. glucose) – except in brain endothelium, where there are no breaks in the intercellular junctional strands.

☐ Intercellular permeability is *reduced* by the β adrenoceptor–cAMP pathway, which enhances junctional strand formation. Intercellular permeability is *increased* by flow and atrial natriuretic peptide, acting through cGMP.

☐ The *glycocalyx*, a coating of biopolymers on the luminal surface, forms a semipermeable layer that reflects plasma proteins.

☐ *Cytoplasmic vesicles* can transfer plasma proteins slowly across endothelium by a poorly understood process.

☐ In inflammation *wide gaps* form between and through venular endothelial cells. The rapid transfer of plasma proteins and water through the gaps leads to inflammatory swelling.

atrial natriuretic peptide acts by raising endothelial cGMP levels.

Conversely, **β_2-adrenoceptor agonists** such as isoprenaline and terbutaline reduce basal capillary permeability. This effect is mediated through increased cyclic adenosine monophosphate (cAMP). cAMP activates protein kinase A, which enhances junctional strand formation. Thus cAMP is a barrier-enhancing messenger, with the opposite effect to cGMP. It is possible that cGMP acts in part by activating a phosphodiesterase enzyme that degrades cAMP (Section 11.11).

Vascular endothelial growth factor (VEGF) is ubiquitous in growing or healing tissues. Besides stimulating angiogenesis (see below), VEGF causes a chronic increase in endothelial permeability, and was originally named 'vascular permeability factor'.

9.8 Roles in the inflammatory response

Endothelium contributes to the classic signs of inflammation

Inflammation is a set of defensive responses to local infection, burns, mechanical trauma and autoimmune diseases such as rheumatoid arthritis. Celsus (30 BC to AD 38) defined inflammation as a combination of redness (rubor), heat (calor), swelling (tumor) and pain (dolor), to which Galen (AD 130–200) added a fifth criterion, loss of function. This definition remains lucid and valid today. Endothelium has a central role in the generation of the redness, heat and swelling.

The **redness** and **heat** are caused by vasodilatation, which is induced by the chemical mediators of inflammation, namely histamine, bradykinin, prostacyclin, substance P, platelet activating factor, superoxide radicals, cytokines and other factors. Most of these agonists produce vasodilatation by raising endothelial $[Ca^{2+}]$ and thereby stimulating eNOS.

In venules a rise in endothelial $[Ca^{2+}]$ initiates the formation of large **endothelial gaps**. These allow plasma immunoglobulins to gain rapid access to the inflamed tissue. Water too escapes rapidly through the gaps, leading to the characteristic **swelling** of inflammation.

A 6th fundamental feature of inflammation, discovered by Addison and Waller in 1843–1846, is the **emigration of leukocytes**, which in its most gross form leads to pus formation. Endothelium has a crucial role in this process too, as follows.

Endothelium induces circulating leukocytes to emigrate (diapedesis)

Acute inflammation is characterized by the immediate infiltration of polymorphonuclear neutrophils from plasma into the tissue, followed by monocytes and eventually lymphocytes.

Endothelium mediates many aspects of inflammation

☐ Inflammation is characterised by redness, heat, swelling, pain, loss of function and leukocyte emigration. Endothelium plays a key role in the redness, heat, swelling and leukocyte migration.

☐ The *redness* and *heat* are due to vasodilatation. Many vasodilator mediators (e.g. bradykinin, substance P, thrombin and cytokines) act indirectly, by stimulating endothelium to secrete the vasodilator nitric oxide (NO).

☐ The *swelling* is due to the formation of large gaps in venular endothelium. The gaps lead to a rapid efflux of plasma water and immunoglobulins.

☐ *Leukocyte capture* occurs when venular endothelium inserts specific 'glue' molecules (P-selectin, E-selectin, ICAM, VCAM) into its luminal membrane. The arrested leukocytes then emigrate through the intercellular junctions.

Rolling capture. The capture of circulating leukocytes by endothelium (**margination**) begins when inflammatory agonists, such as histamine and thrombin, stimulate venular endothelium to transfer **P-selectin** from the Weibel–Palade body to the surface. P-selectin makes the endothelial surface 'sticky' by interacting loosely with ligands on the leukocyte membrane. The leukocyte adheres only loosely and continues to roll slowly along the vessel wall under the force of the bloodstream. Rolling, marginated leukocytes are seen within minutes of an inflammatory stimulus.

The cytokines interleukin-1, tumour necrosis factor and interferon γ, act more slowly and reinforce rolling capture over several hours. They stimulate endothelium to produce a second leukocyte glue, **E-selectin**, which maintains the rolling margination.

Arrest. Tight-binding proteins are then activated in the endothelium and leukocyte. The endothelial binding proteins are **ICAM** (intercellular adhesion molecule) and **VCAM** (vascular cell adhesion molecule). The ICAM and VCAM bind firmly to ligands that appear on the surface of the slowly rolling leukocyte, namely β_2 integrins. Binding brings the leukocyte to a halt, 'like so many pebbles or marbles over which a stream runs without disturbing them', as Waller graphically described the scene in 1846. In a rare genetic condition called 'leukocyte adhesion deficiency', a lack of β_2 integrins leads to the failure of leukocyte arrest, and hence emigration. This causes a life-threatening susceptibility to bacterial infection.

Emigration. Once arrested the leukocyte inserts a thin foot into the endothelial intercellular junction and squeezes through into the tissue (diapedesis). This process depends on a high local concentration of ICAM-1 and platelet–endothelial cell adhesion molecule (PECAM). In genetic knock-out mice that lack PECAM, leukocytes are trapped at the basal lamina and emigration is greatly reduced. It is inferred, therefore, that PECAM is needed to activate the leukocyte to break through the basal lamina.

The intercellular junction reseals very rapidly, in seconds, after leukocyte migration. Not infrequently leukocytes also migrate through the endothelial cell itself, rather than the intercellular junctions. The transcellular holes quickly reseal.

9.9 Role in angiogenesis

Endothelial cells have a life span of months to years and divide infrequently. However, they can be stimulated to multiply rapidly when there is a need for new vessel formation (angiogenesis). Angiogenesis begins with the growth of a simple endothelial tube, which later differentiates into an artery, vein or capillary. Angiogenesis is essential for tissue growth, tissue adaptation (e.g. increased number of capillaries in trained muscle), wound healing and tumour growth. Endothelium will also grow over the grafts used in vascular surgery.

New vessels originate from capillary sprouts

New vessel formation begins with the degradation of the endothelial basement membrane. This is followed by sprouting of the endothelium from the side of an existing capillary or venules (Figure 9.1). Vacuolation of the cell interior creates a lumen. Division and migration of the cell cause the new tube to extend outwards, until eventually it connects up with another new vessel. The new vessels are hyperpermeable and allow fibrinogen extravasation. This creates an oedematous, fibrin-rich, highly vascular matrix called 'granulation tissue'. The formation of arterioles and venules occurs later by the accretion of connective tissue cells and vascular smooth muscle cells around the endothelial tube.

Angiogenesis is initiated by VEGF and other growth factors

Endothelial growth is initiated by tissue growth factors that induce gene expression in the endothelial cell.

The endothelial growth factors include vascular endothelial growth factor (VEGF) and the acidic and basic fibroblast growth factors (aFGF, bFGF).

VEGF is abundant in tissues that are forming new vessels, such as the placenta, fetal tissue, tumours, psoriatic plaques, rheumatoid pannus, myocardium adjacent to infarcts, and diabetic retina (the leading cause of blindness in the West). The endothelial VEGF receptor is linked to an enzyme, tyrosine kinase, and the receptor–tyrosine kinase complex activates mitogen-activated protein kinase (MAP kinase). The latter activates nuclear transcription factors that switch on gene expression leading to angiogenesis. The new capillaries are at first hyperpermeable, but with maturity their permeability declines, probably due to an increase in the ratio of cAMP to cGMP.

Thrombospondin and angiostatin inhibit angiogenesis

Endothelial growth is normally held in check by anti-angiogenic tissue factors such as thrombospondin and angiostatin. The levels of thrombospondin and angiostatin have to fall for angiogenesis to occur. The discovery of anti-angiogenic factors has led to trials of anti-angiogenic drugs to restrict cancer growth. Once a tumour grows above a millimetre or so in size, its cells are critically dependent on angiogenesis for a supply of nutrients. Anti-angiogenic drugs may therefore be a useful complement to cytotoxic drugs in the treatment of cancer.

9.10 Role in atheroma

Atheroma, also called atherosclerosis, is a patchy, lipid depositional disease of the subendothelial region of large arteries. The bulging atheromatous plaque narrows the arterial lumen, leading to tissue ischaemia and thrombosis. In the heart this results in angina and heart attacks; in the brain, transient ischaemic attacks and strokes; and in the legs, intermittent claudication (ischaemic pain on walking) and gangrenous necrosis (peripheral tissue death, often necessitating amputation). Atheroma is in fact the commonest cause of death and serious morbidity in Westernized societies. The chief predisposing factors are high levels of plasma low-density lipoprotein (LDL) and fibrinogen, smoking, diabetes and hypertension. LDL is a complex of numerous cholesterol molecules bound to a single protein carrier, with a total molecular mass $\sim 3 \times 10^6$ daltons.

The atheromatous plaque is rich in plasma-derived cholesterol

The atheromatous plaque begins as a subendothelial accumulation of LDL (mainly cholesterol) and fibrin derived from the plasma, plus foam cells, which are lipid-laden macrophages derived from migrated plasma monocytes. Later, proliferating vascular smooth muscle cells migrate into the lesion, and platelet aggregation on the surface may trigger thrombosis.

Since atherogenesis involves the transendothelial passage of LDL and fibrinogen, and in the later stages aggregation of platelets to the damaged surface, local dysfunction of arterial endothelium is thought to contribute to the lesion. The nature of the dysfunction is imperfectly understood.

Low NO levels may facilitate plaque development

The idea that low levels of nitric oxide may contribute to atheroma formation stemmed from evidence that NO has several anti-atherogenic actions, as follows:

1 If NO production is stimulated by L-arginine, atheroma formation in hypercholesterolaemic rabbits is reduced. Conversely, inhibitors of

eNOS increase the uptake of LDL and fibrinogen into the artery wall.

2 Low NO levels lead to an increase in endothelial VCAM expression, which promotes monocyte adhesion.

3 NO inhibits vascular smooth muscle growth and migration in cultures.

4 NO strongly inhibits platelet aggregation.

NO thus has four anti-atherogenic actions. Moreover, NO levels are low in smokers (who show impaired NO-dependent vasodilatation) and in diabetics – groups particularly prone to atheroma. Insulin is normally a significant tonic stimulus to NO production, but diabetics either have low insulin levels or are insulin-resistant.

NO reacts with superoxide

Endothelium-dependent vasodilatation is severely impaired in atheromatous arteries. Indeed, atheromatous arteries from patients and monkeys often constrict in response to acetylcholine, in contrast to the usual endothelium-dependent vasodilatation (Figure 9.12). This indicates that NO levels are low;

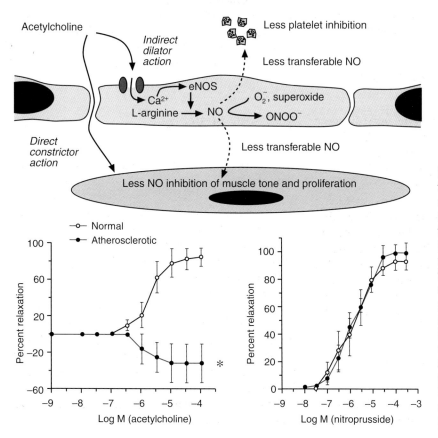

Figure 9.12 Responses of atheromatous iliac artery (filled circles) and normal artery (open circles) of monkey to acetylcholine (*bottom left panel*) and to a direct NO donor, nitroprusside (*bottom right panel*). Atheroma converts normal, NO-dependent vasodilator response to acetylcholine into a constrictor response. Sketch shows proposed explanation; reduced levels of transferable NO in atheroma due to high levels of endothelial superoxide radicals. (Adapted from Munzel, T., Just, H. and Harrison, D. G. The physiology and pathophysiology of the NO/superoxide system. In Born, G. V. R. and Schwartz, C. J. (eds) (1997), pp. 205–217; see Further Reading.)

yet NO generation, as assessed by its degradation product nitrite, is normal or even raised. The low levels of free NO may be the result of increased inactivation of NO by superoxide radicals, (see Appendix 2, 'Free radicals'). NO reacts rapidly with the superoxide radical O_2^- to form peroxynitrite, $ONOO^-$. The latter gives rise to highly reactive hydroxyl radicals that oxidize lipids and damage the cell membrane.

Superoxide is generated by a number of oxidases involved in cellular metabolism. Superoxide generation is increased three-fold in the aorta of cholesterol-fed rabbits, and is also increased in diabetes and by smoking. Moreover superoxide dismutase, an enzyme that scavenges (removes) superoxide radicals, improves the endothelium-dependent vasodilatation in atheromatous vessels. Excessive superoxide production may therefore reduce the level of endothelial NO and the protection it affords against atherogenesis.

SUMMARY

■ Endothelium is a monolayer of flattened cells. Basal actin–myosin stress fibres tether the cell to its basal lamina via integrins, resisting the sheering effect of blood flow. An actin cytoskeleton stabilizes occludens and adherens proteins to form intercellular junctions. The junctional proteins form long, sealing strands, but breaks in the strands allow water and small solutes to permeate the intercellular cleft. A negatively charged surface coat (glycocalyx) acts as a semipermeable membrane and prevents plasma proteins from entering the cleft. A caveola-vesicle system slowly transports some plasma protein into the tissue. The basal lamina prevents capillary rupture by blood pressure.

■ The intracellular potential of -30 to $-60\,mV$ is due chiefly to inward rectifier K^+ channels. When receptor-operated cation channels are activated by inflammatory agonists (e.g. histamine, bradykinin), extracellular Ca^{2+} flows into the cell down the electrochemical gradient. Increased cytosolic $[Ca^{2+}]$ activates K_{Ca} channels, which increases the negative potential and enhances Ca^{2+} entry. Agonists also release a small internal Ca^{2+} store, leading to capacitative Ca^{2+} entry. Increased cytosolic Ca^{2+} triggers the secretion of vasoactive chemicals by arterial endothelium (e.g. NO) and raises permeability in exchange vessels.

■ Endothelium regulates local vascular tone by secreting nitric oxide (NO), endothelium-derived hyperpolarizing factor (EDHF), prostacyclin and endothelin. NO is generated from L-arginine by Ca^{2+}-calmodulin dependent endothelial nitric oxide synthase (eNOS). The normal stimulus to tonic NO production is shear stress, which activates a kinase cascade that phosphorylates eNOS. Increased activation of eNOS mediates (i) flow-induced vasodilatation and (ii) vasodilatation by acetylcholine and many inflammatory agents (e.g. bradykinin).

■ EDHF causes vasodilatation in arterioles. Prostacyclin, like nitric oxide, causes vasodilatation and inhibition of platelet aggregation. Endothelin causes a long-lasting vasoconstriction and is elevated in hypoxia, pre-eclamptic toxaemia and heart failure.

■ Endothelium acts on blood as well as vascular muscle. Angiotensin converting enzyme (ACE) on the endothelial surface catalyses angiotensin II formation. NO and prostacyclin inhibit platelet aggregation to prevent clotting. Von Willebrand factor, released from the endothelial Weibel–Palade body, is a carrier for clotting factor VIII.

■ Venular endothelium contributes to inflammation in two ways. (i) Adhesive proteins are inserted into the luminal membrane (P-selectin, E-selectin, ICAM, VCAM) to capture circulating leukocytes. (ii) Wide gaps form between venular endothelial cells in responses to increased cytosolic $[Ca^{2+}]$. The gaps allow the rapid escape of immunoglobulins and water, leading to inflammatory swelling.

■ Capillary permeability can be modulated without gap formation through changes in the intercellular pathway. Permeability is raised by flow and atrial natriuretic peptide, mediated by cGMP. Conversely, agents that increase endothelial cAMP enhance the intercellular barrier.

■ Vascular endothelial growth factor raises permeability and stimulates capillary sprouting (angiogenesis). Angiogenesis is necessary for tissue and tumour growth. Angiogenesis is inhibited by thrombospondin, angiostatin and angiostatic drugs against cancer.

■ The trapping of plasma low-density lipoprotein and fibrin under arterial endothelium gives rise to atheroma, the biggest killer in Westernized societies. Endothelial NO normally protects against atheroma by reducing LDL and fibrinogen uptake, VCAM expression, smooth muscle proliferation and platelet aggregation. NO levels are low in atheromatous arteries, due in part to its reaction with superoxide.

FURTHER READING

Reviews

Anderson, R. G. W. (1998) The caveolae membrane system. *Annual Review of Biochemistry*, **67**, 199–225.

Born, G. V. R. and Schwartz, C. J. (1997) *Vascular Endothelium: Physiology, Pathology and Therapeutic Opportunities*, Schattauer, Stuttgart. [A goldmine of information!]

Cooke, J. P. and Dzau, V. J. (1997) NO synthase: role in the genesis of vascular disease. *Annual Review of Medicine*, **48**, 489–509.

Curry, F. E. (1998) Regulation of capillary permeability in single perfused microvessels. In *Connective Tissue Biology, Integration and Reductionism* (eds Reed, R. K. and Rubin, K.), Portland Press, London, pp. 195–206.

Davies, P. F. (1995) Flow-mediated endothelial mechanotransduction. *Physiological Reviews*, **75**, 519–560.

Dejana, E., Corada, M. and Lampugnani, M. G. (1995) Endothelial cell-to-cell junctions. *FASEB Journal*, **9**, 910–918.

Fisslthaler, B., Dimmeler, S., Hermann, C., Busse, R. and Fleming, I. (2000) Phosphorylation and activation of the endothelial nitric oxide synthase by fluid shear stress. *Acta Physiologica Scandinavica*, **168**, 81–88.

Folkman, J. (1995) Angiogenesis in cancer, vascular, rheumatoid and other diseases. *Nature Medicine*, **1**, 27–31.

Grossman, J. D. and Morgan, J. P. (1997) Cardiovascular effects of endothelin. *News in Physiological Sciences*, **12**, 113–117.

Hecker, M. (2000) Endothelium-derived hyperpolarizing factor – fact or fiction? *News in Physiological Sciences*, **15**, 1–5.

Klagsbrun, M. and D'Amore, P. A. (1991) Regulators of angiogenesis. *Annual Reviews of Physiology*, **53**, 217–239.

Kvietys, P. R. and Sandig, M. (2001) Neutrophil diapedesis: paracellular or transcellular? *News in Physiological Sciences*, **16**, 15–19.

Nilius, B. and Droogmans, G. (2001) Ion channels and their functional role in vascular endothelium. *Physiological Reviews*, **81**, 1415–1459.

Schini-Kerth, V. B. and Vanhoutte, P. M. (1995) Nitric oxide synthases in vascular cells. *Experimental Physiology*, **80**, 885–905.

Thurston, G., Baluk, P. and McDonald, D. M. (2000) Determinants of endothelial cell phenotype in venules. *Microcirculation*, **7**, 67–80.

van Hinsbergh, V. W. M. (1997) Endothelial permeability for macromolecules. Mechanistic aspects of pathophysiological modulation. *Arteriosclerosis, Thrombosis and Vascular Biology*, **17**, 1018–1023.

Walzog, B. and Gaehtgens, P. (2000) Adhesion molecules: the path to a new understanding of acute inflammation. *News in Physiological Sciences*, **15**, 107–113.

Research papers

Adamson, R. H., Liu, B., Fry, G. N., Rubin, L. L. and Curry, F. E. (1998) Microvascular permeability and number of tight junctions are modulated by cAMP. *American Journal of Physiology*, **274**, H1885–H1894.

Bates, D. O. (1998) The chronic effect of vascular endothelial growth factor on individually perfused frog mesenteric microvessels. *Journal of Physiology*, **513**, 225–233.

Chaytor, A. T., Evans, W. H. and Griffiths, T. M. (1998) Central role of heterocellular gap junctional communication in endothelium-dependent relaxation of rabbit arteries. *Journal of Physiology*, **508**, 561–573.

Corada, M., Mariotti, M., Thurston, G., *et al.* (1999) Vascular endothelial-cadherin is an important determinant of microvascular integrity *in vivo*. *Proceedings of National Academy of Science*, **96**, 9815–9820.

DeFouw, L. M. and DeFouw, D. O. (2001) Differential phosphodiesterase activity contributes to restrictive endothelial barrier function during angiogenesis. *Microvascular Research*, **62**, 263–270.

Dye, J. F., Leach, L., Clark, P. and Firth, J. A. (2001) Cyclic AMP and acidic fibroblast growth factor have opposing effects on tight and adherens junctions in microvascular endothelial cells in vitro. *Microvascular Research*, **62**, 94–113.

Goodwin, A. T., Amrani, M., Gray, C. C., Jayakumar, J. and Yacoub, M. H. (1998) Role of endogenous endothelin in the regulation of basal coronary tone in the rat. *Journal of Physiology*, **511**, 549–557.

Guibert, C. and Beech, D. J. (1999) Positive and negative coupling of the endothelin ET_A receptor to Ca^{2+}-permeable channels in rabbit cerebral cortex arterioles. *Journal of Physiology*, **514**, 843–856.

He, P., Zhang, X. and Curry, F. E. (1996) Calcium entry through conductive pathway modulates receptor-mediated increase in microvessel permeability. *American Journal of Physiology*, **271**, H2377–H2387.

Kevil, C., Okayama, N., Trocha, S. D., Kalogeris, T. J., Coe, L. L., Specian, R. D., Davis, C. P. and Alexander, J. S. (1998) Expression of zonula occludens and adherens junctional proteins in human venous and arterial endothelial cells: role of occludin in endothelial solute barrier. *Microcirculation*, **5**, 197–210.

Meyer, D. J. and Huxley, V. H. (1992) Capillary hydraulic conductivity is elevated by cGMP-dependent vasodilators. *Circulation Research*, **70**, 382–391.

Schnittler, H. J., Wilke, A., Gress, T., Suttorp, N. and Drenckhahn, D. (1990) Role of actin and myosin in the control of paracellular permeability in pig, rat, and human vascular endothelium. *Journal of Physiology*, **431**, 379–401.

Vink, H. and Duling, B. R. (2000) Capillary endothelial surface layer selectively reduces plasma solute distribution volume. *American Journal of Physiology*, **278**, H285–H289.

Voets, T., Droogmans, G. and Nilius, B. (1996) Membrane currents and the resting membrane potential in cultured bovine pulmonary artery endothelial cells. *Journal of Physiology*, **497**, 95–107.

Yamamoto, Y., Imaeda, K. and Suzuki, H. (1999) Endothelium-dependent hyperpolarization and intercellular electrical coupling in guinea-pig mesenteric arterioles. *Journal of Physiology*, **514**, 505–513.

CHAPTER 10

The microcirculation and solute exchange

Learning objectives

After reading this chapter you should be able to:

- Outline how terminal arterioles regulate capillary perfusion (10.1).
- Sketch the ultrastructure of the three main types of capillary (10.2).
- Distinguish between the processes responsible for solute exchange (e.g. glucose, oxygen) and water exchange (10.3).
- State the factors that influence diffusion according to Fick's law (10.3).
- Define 'solute permeability' and explain how it is affected by a porous membrane (10.4).
- Identify the three main categories of solutes with respect to capillary permeation (10.5–10.7).
- Outline the special features of exchange across the blood–brain barrier (10.8).
- Sketch the concentration profile of a metabolized solute (e.g. glucose) along a capillary and use this to define 'the Fick principle' (cf. law), 'extraction' and 'plasma clearance' (10.9).
- Explain the meaning of 'flow-limited' and 'diffusion-limited' exchange (10.10).
- State what is meant by 'capillary recruitment', and list the additional factors that enhance solute exchange in exercising muscle (10.11).

A single, inescapable necessity has driven the evolution of the circulation – the need to deliver metabolic substrates such as oxygen and glucose to the cells of large organisms (Section 1.1). The delivery hatch, so to speak, is the capillary wall. The exchange of materials across the capillary wall thus represents the payload of the entire complex system of cardiovascular pumps, valves and tubes, and is the fundamental reason for its existence.

10.1 Organization and perfusion of exchange vessels

Strictly speaking, the term 'exchange vessel' embraces either side of the capillary bed, because some oxygen diffuses through the walls of the terminal arterioles, and some fluid flows across the walls of pericytic venules. The capillaries, however, account for most of the solute and fluid exchange.

Supply and drainage of the capillary bed

The smallest arteries branch into first-order arterioles, and further divisions give rise to the **terminal arterioles**, which are the last arterial vessels with smooth muscle in their walls. Each terminal arteriole supplies blood to a cluster or **module of capillaries** (Figure 10.1).

Capillary means hair-like. Capillaries are typically $500–1000\,\mu m$ long but only $4–8\,\mu m$ wide, so they are invisible to the naked eye. Their existence was inferred by Harvey from the circulation of blood, and was confirmed by Malpighi in 1661 during his observations of the frog lung through an early microscope.

The venous ends of capillaries unite to form **pericytic venules** (postcapillary venules). These are thin-walled vessels, $\sim 15\,\mu m$ wide, with pericytes but no smooth muscle in the wall. Pericytic venules are highly permeable to water and play a major role in inflammation. Smooth muscle reappears in the walls of venules of width $30–50\,\mu m$.

Arteriovenous anastomoses are muscular microvessels, $20–130\,\mu m$ wide, that directly link arterioles to venules, bypassing the capillary network. They are found chiefly in the skin of the extremities (fingers, nose, lips, earlobes), where they have an important role in temperature regulation (Section 15.3).

Capillary density is adapted to tissue function

The number of capillaries packed into unit volume or cross-section of a tissue is called the capillary density. Skeletal muscle contains $300–1000$ capillaries per mm^2 cross-section, which represents $1–3$ capillaries per muscle fibre. Endurance training causes angiogenesis and can raise the capillary:fibre ratio to $6–8$. In the myocardium and brain, where the metabolic rate is high and sustained, the capillary density is particularly high, namely 3000 per mm^2 cross-section. Capillary density is related to tissue activity for two reasons.

- Capillary density determines the endothelial surface area available for gas and nutrient exchange. The area is $\sim 100\,cm^2$ per gram of skeletal muscle but $\sim 500\,cm^2$ per gram of myocardium or brain.

- Capillary density determines the mean inter-capillary spacing, and therefore the maximum distance from blood to cell. This is important because distance profoundly affects the time needed for diffusional transport (Section 1.1).

The most extreme example of capillary packing is provided by the lungs, which have the staggering capillary surface area of $\sim 3500\,cm^2$ per gram of lung.

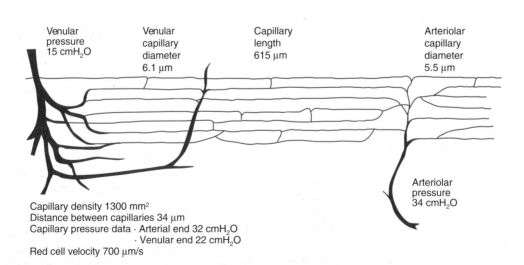

Venular pressure 15 cmH$_2$O
Venular capillary diameter 6.1 µm
Capillary length 615 µm
Arteriolar capillary diameter 5.5 µm
Arteriolar pressure 34 cmH$_2$O

Capillary density 1300 mm^2
Distance between capillaries 34 µm
Capillary pressure data · Arterial end 32 cmH$_2$O
· Venular end 22 cmH$_2$O
Red cell velocity 700 µm/s

Figure 10.1 Capillary bed in relaxed cremaster muscle of a rat, with a terminal arteriole feeding a module of 14 capillaries. Numbers are means of observations. (From Smaje, L. H., Zweifach, B. W. and Intaglietta, M. (1970) *Microvascular Research*, **2**, 96–110, by permission.)

Terminal arterioles regulate the number of perfused capillaries

The contractile state of the terminal arterioles influences the number of capillaries that are well perfused with blood at any one moment, and thus governs the evenness of tissue perfusion. The relaxation of an individual arteriole allows a brisk perfusion of the associated capillary module, and such capillaries are referred to as 'open'. Contraction of a terminal arteriole slows or even stops the blood flow through its associated capillary module, and such capillaries are referred to as 'closed'. In a tissue such as resting skeletal muscle some arterioles are relaxed but others are contracted at any one moment. As a result, a substantial fraction of the capillaries in resting muscle are 'closed' at any one instant.

The task of regulating the number of perfused capillary modules used to be ascribed to largely imaginary 'precapillary sphincters'. In reality there is no discrete sphincteric ring of muscle at the capillary entrance in most tissues. It is the terminal arteriole that regulates the numbers of 'open' and 'closed' capillaries in most tissues.

Capillary blood flow is not constant, owing to vasomotion

An individual terminal arteriole does not usually stay relaxed or contracted for long; its muscle tone changes constantly. This is called **vasomotion**. In some tissues, such as resting skeletal muscle, vasomotion has a regular rhythm with a cycle time of ~15 s, whereas in other tissues, such as skin, vasomotion is less regular. As a result of vasomotion, blood flow in an individual capillary is often inconstant; it may wax and wane every 15 s or so, and can stop for a while in 'closed' capillaries.

Transit time is the time available for exchange

The time that it takes the blood to pass through the capillary bed from entrance to exit is called the **transit time**. Transit time represents the time available for each unit of blood to unload O_2, glucose, etc. and to load up with CO_2, urea etc. Transit times vary due to vasomotion, but in a well-perfused capillary the transit time is typically 0.5–2 s. This corresponds to a blood velocity of 300–1000 μm/s. The transit time can fall to around 0.25 s in exercise as the arterioles dilate and blood velocity increases. In athletes with very high cardiac outputs the transit time through the lung capillaries can become so short during extreme exercise that the blood emerges without achieving full O_2 saturation.

10.2 Three types of capillary

Capillaries are classified into three types according to their ultrastructure: continuous, fenestrated and discontinuous capillaries, in order of increasing permeability to water.

The continuous capillary

Continuous capillaries occur in muscle, skin, lung, fat, connective tissue and the nervous system. The circumference comprises a continuous ring of 1–3 endothelial cells with a continuous basement membrane (Figure 10.2a). The wall is only one cell thick, so the trans-capillary diffusion distance is very short, ~0.3 μm. Pericytes, formerly called Rouget cells, partly envelop the outside of the capillary. Recent

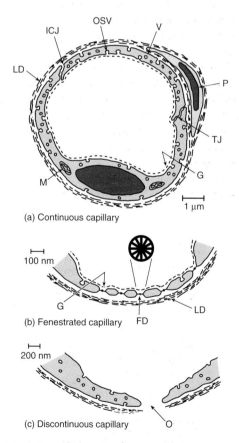

(a) Continuous capillary

(b) Fenestrated capillary

(c) Discontinuous capillary

Figure 10.2 Sketches of capillary wall in transverse section based on electron micrographs. FD, fenestral diaphragm; inset shows diaphragm *en face*; G, glycocalyx; ICJ, intercellular junction; LD, lamina densa of basal lamina; M, mitochondrion; O, open gap; OSV, open surface vesicle or 'caveola'; P, pericyte; TJ, tight part of junction; V, vesicle.

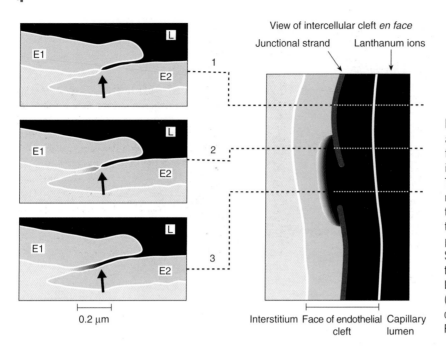

View of intercellular cleft *en face*

Junctional strand   Lanthanum ions

0.2 μm

Interstitium Face of endothelial Capillary
cleft lumen

Figure 10.3 Three sections through an intercellular cleft in a capillary perfused with a solution of lanthanum ions (black) for 10 s before fixation. The cleft is depicted *en face* on the right. The tight junction (arrow) blocks the cleft in Section 1 but a break in the junction strands provides an open pathway in Section 3. The intermediate Section 2 gives the false impression that the tight junction is permeable. L, lumen; E1 and E2, endothelial cells. (Redrawn from electron micrographs of Adamson and Michel (1993); see Research papers.)

genetic knock-out experiments in mice indicate that the pericytes are necessary for the development of capillaries of normal diameter and structure.

The key structures involved in solute exchange are (i) the **intercellular cleft**, where breaks in the junctional strands allow the passage of water and small lipid-insoluble solutes (Figures 9.2–9.4, 10.3); (ii) the **glycocalyx**, which excludes plasma proteins from access to the cleft but is permeable to water and small solute (Figure 9.3); and (iii) the **caveola–vesicle** system, which slowly transfers large molecules across the wall (Figures 9.5, 9.6).

Fenestrated capillaries are specialized for rapid fluid filtration

Fenestrated capillaries are an order of magnitude more permeable than continuous capillaries to water and small lipid-insoluble solutes. They are found in tissues that specialize in fluid exchange (kidney, exocrine glands, intestinal mucosa, synovial lining of joints, choroid plexus, ciliary body of the eye), and also in endocrine glands. The endothelium is perforated by many small circular windows, the fenestrae, of diameter 50–60 nm (Figure 10.2b). In most tissues except the renal glomerulus the fenestra is bridged by an extremely thin membrane or diaphragm of thickness 4–5 nm. The structure of the diaphragm resembles that of a cartwheel, and the wedge-shaped apertures between its spokes allow a very fast transfer of water, nutrients and hormones between the blood and tissue.

Discontinuous capillaries allow blood cell turnover

Discontinuous or sinusoidal capillaries contain endothelial gaps over 100 nm wide and a discontinuity in the underlying basal lamina. As a result, these capillaries are permeable even to plasma proteins. They are found in organs where red cells and/or white cells need to migrate between the blood and tissue, namely in the bone marrow, spleen and liver.

10.3 Basics of diffusion, convection and reflection

Before continuing with the account of solute exchange across the capillary wall, we need to review some basic concepts concerning transport across porous membranes.

Solutes diffuse and water flows

Both solute and water cross the capillary wall by passive transport, i.e. without any energy expenditure by the endothelium; but they do so by entirely different physical processes. Water **flows** across the wall down a **pressure gradient**, whereas solutes **diffuse** across the wall down a **concentration gradient** (Figure 10.4). The Danish physiologist August Krogh established as long ago as 1919 that diffusion gradients alone are enough to account for O_2 transfer from blood to muscle.

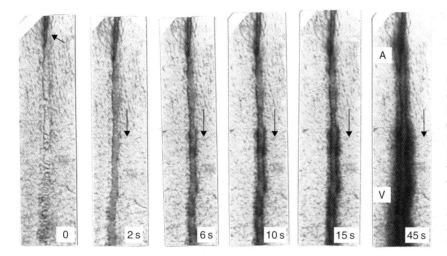

Figure 10.4 Timed sequence showing diffusion of Evans blue (small, lipid-insoluble solute of radius ~1 nm) out of a perfused frog mesenteric capillary. Dye-filled micropipette (arrow) is visible at arterial end of capillary in first frame; other arrows show direction of flow. The arteriovenous gradient of permeability is obvious; venous capillaries are normally more permeable than arterial capillaries. (From Levick, J. R., Doctoral thesis, Oxford.)

It is true that solutes such as glucose are also swept along in the water that is continuously flowing out through the capillary wall – a process called **convective transport**. The flow is so slow, however, that it generally contributes little to the diffusional transport of a metabolite or drug; for a proof see footnote to Table 10.2 later. Conversely, textbooks sometimes state that water molecules can cross the wall quickly by diffusion. This is true in principle; but it is an academic red-herring, because water diffusion is bi-directional and achieves no net transport.

Thus, to understand the trans-capillary movement of glucose, amino acids, drugs and other lipid-insoluble metabolites, we need to focus on diffusion and how it is affected by a porous membrane such as endothelium.

Fick's law describes free diffusional transport in a fluid

The basic law governing diffusional transport was worked out by Adolf Fick, who was Professor of Physiology at Wurzburg in Germany. **Fick's first law of diffusion** (1855) states that the mass of solute transferred by diffusion per unit time, J_s, across a body of liquid depends on four factors (Figure 10.5a).

- J_s is proportional to the **concentration difference** driving diffusion, $C_1 - C_2$, or ΔC (delta means 'a difference in').

- J_s is inversely proportional to **distance**, Δx. The ratio $\Delta C/\Delta x$ is called the concentration **gradient**.

- J_s is proportional to the **surface area**, A.

- J_s is proportional to the **diffusion coefficient**, D.

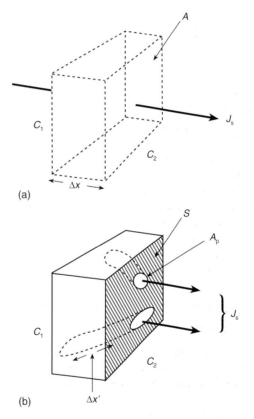

(a)

(b)

Figure 10.5 (a) Free diffusion in bulk solution. The solute diffuses through an unimpeded layer of fluid of thickness Δx and surface area A, driven by concentration difference $C_1 - C_2$. J_s is the diffusion rate (mole/s). (b) Membrane reduces J_s by confining solute to pores of total area A_p. The pathlength through the pore, $\Delta x'$, can exceed the membrane thickness Δx.

The law can thus be summarized as:

$$J_s = -DA\frac{\Delta C}{\Delta x}$$

(10.1)

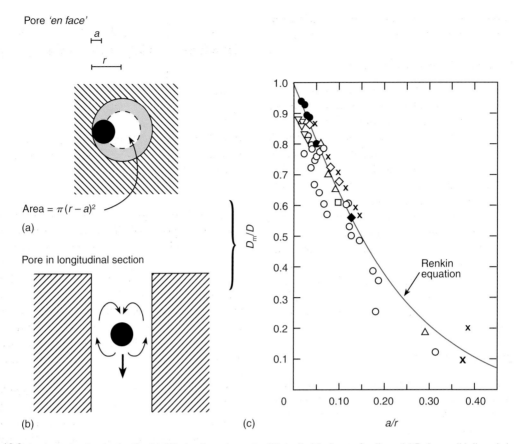

Figure 10.6 A spherical molecule of radius 'a' diffusing through a water-filled cylindrical pore of radius r. (a) End-on or 'bird's eye' view of pore showing steric exclusion of the molecule centre from an annulus of fluid (pink). (b) Longitudinal section through the pore. Arrows indicate how solute movement necessitates solvent flow, giving rise to enhanced hydrodynamic drag within the narrow confines of the pore. (c) Plot of reduced diffusion across a membrane (D_m) relative to the free diffusion coefficient (D) as the ratio of molecular size to pore size increases (a/r). The 'Renkin equation' describes D_m/D as the product of steric exclusion and enhanced hydrodynamic drag or 'restricted diffusion'; see Appendix 2, 'Diffusion'. (From Beck, R. B. and Schultz, J. S. (1972) *Biochimica Biophysica Acta*, **255**, 273–303, by permission.)

The negative sign, which often puzzles students, indicates that the transport is downhill, i.e. down the concentration gradient.

Except for the diffusion coefficient the above factors are self-explanatory. The **diffusion coefficient** is a measure of the ease with which a solute slips through the solvent. Since big molecules encounter more friction than little ones, D is inversely related to solute size. Small molecules such as glucose have a large D and diffuse faster than big molecules such as albumin. See Appendix 2, 'Diffusion' and 'Stokes–Einstein radius' for details.

Porous membranes impede diffusional transport

When a solute diffuses through a large body of solvent, the distant walls of the container do not influence the solute and the process is called free diffusion. However,

when a solute diffuses through narrow pores in a membrane, as with a lipid-insoluble solute crossing the endothelial barrier, the diffusion is slowed by interactions with the pore. Three distinct effects reduce the diffusion rate.

(i) Reduced available area

When solute permeation is confined to aqueous pores, the area available for diffusion is at best the total pore area A_p, which is usually a small percentage of the total surface area of the membrane, S (Figure 10.5b). Transport rate is thus reduced by the factor A_p/S at the very least.

In addition, for a molecule of radius 'a', the centre of the molecule cannot get any closer to the pore rim than distance a. As a result, in a cylindrical pore of radius r the diffusional movements are confined to a central column of fluid of radius $r - a$ (Figure 10.6a).

This geometrical effect is called **steric exclusion**, and it further reduces the diffusional transport rate.

(ii) Restricted diffusion inside a pore

The proximity of the pore wall impedes solute diffusion by a hydrodynamic, frictional effect. In order for a solute molecule to advance along the pore, the water molecules ahead of it have to slip back through the gap between the pore wall and the solute, in order to make space ahead and fill in the space behind (Figure 10.6b). The narrower the gap between the solute and the pore wall, the less easily the water slips past. Put in biophysical terms, the hydrodynamic drag of water on the solute increases as the solute size approaches the pore diameter. As a result, the solute diffusion coefficient within the pore, D_{res}, is smaller than the free diffusion coefficient in bulk solution, D. This is called **restricted diffusion**, and it can be a big effect. For example, D_{res} is half D_{free} when the solute width is 15% of the pore diameter.

(iii) Increased pathlength

Most endothelial junctions run very obliquely through the capillary wall. Consequently the true diffusion distance $\Delta x'$ is greater than the membrane thickness Δx (Figure 10.5b).

Due to the above three effects the diffusional transport of lipid-insoluble solutes such as glucose, lactate, amino acids, peptides, hormones and drugs across unit area of capillary wall is over two orders of magnitude slower than it is across the same area of water. The term **membrane permeability** is a measure of these effects as explained in Section 10.4.

Reflection coefficients can be used to estimate pore size

The reflection coefficient σ (sigma) is a measure of how much difficulty a solute experiences in entering a pore, relative to water, during fluid filtration. Unlike permeability, reflection is unaffected by the number of pores or their length; it just depends on size. The reflection coefficient is chiefly important for understanding osmotic pressure (Chapter 11) but it is introduced here because it arises from the steric exclusion phenomenon described above and enables physiologists to estimate capillary pore size.

If steric exclusion is negligible, as with a small solute in a large pore, the solute enters the pore as freely as water (Figure 10.7c). In this case solute reflection is zero ($\sigma = 0$) and the solute exerts no osmotic pressure across the membrane. If the solute is bigger than the pore, it is totally excluded, its

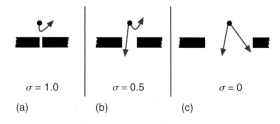

Figure 10.7 The osmotic reflection coefficient (σ) is a measure of the molecular selectivity of a pore, and depends on the ratio of solute width to pore width.

reflection is total ($\sigma = 1$) and the solute exerts its full osmotic potential. If solute molecules are partially excluded, as in Figure 10.6a and Figure 10.7b, they are partially reflected ($\sigma < 1$) and the solution exerts a fraction of its osmotic pressure. This happens when solute width is around $\geqslant$10% of pore width. The reflection coefficient is defined in practice as the osmotic pressure that the solute exerts across the test membrane relative to that which it exerts across a perfect semipermeable membrane of $\sigma = 1$.

As Figure 10.7 indicates, the size of the reflection coefficient depends on the ratio of solute radius to pore radius, a/r. Therefore measurements of reflection coefficient can be used to estimate the endothelial pore radius; for details see Appendix 2, 'Reflection coefficient'. The result is an equivalent cylinder radius of $\sim$4–5 nm for pores in the capillary wall.

10.4 The concept of 'permeability'

The definition of 'permeability'

Because a porous membrane interferes with the diffusion of lipid-insoluble solutes in multiple ways, it is convenient to wrap up all the factors affecting diffusion into one catch-all parameter called permeability. The permeability of a membrane P is defined as the rate of diffusion of solute (J_s) across unit area of membrane per unit concentration difference across the membrane. If we write the definition out in symbols, using S for capillary surface area, we have:

$$P = \frac{J_s}{S\Delta C} \qquad (10.2)$$

This is called the permeability equation. The units of permeability are those of velocity, usually cm/s. The product PS is called the capillary diffusion capacity, and has units of cm^3/s.

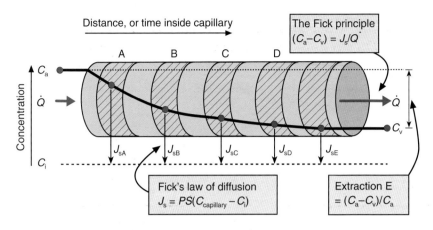

Figure 10.8 Concentration of a rapidly diffusing solute falls nonlinearly along a capillary from arterial concentration C_a to venous concentration C_v. Thin arrows show size of diffusional fluxes (J_s). PS, permeability–surface area product; $\dot{Q}$ is blood flow. The concentration profile is exponential if interstitial concentration C_i is zero or uniform. (For average concentration, see Appendix 2, 'Capillary concentration profile'.)

Permeability and local concentration gradient determine solute flux

The permeability equation can be re-arranged to describe solute transport across the capillary wall, i.e.

$$J_s = PS\Delta C \qquad (10.3)$$

If we divide the capillary into a set of short cylindrical segments (Figure 10.8), eqn 10.3 tells us that the rate of diffusional solute transfer across any one segment depends on three factors, namely:

- the endothelial permeability
- the surface area of the segment
- the concentration difference across the wall.

It is necessary to consider each segment separately rather than the entire capillary, because solute concentration changes nonlinearly along a capillary (Section 10.9).

Permeability depends on pore and solute properties

If we compare the solute diffusion eqn 10.3 with Fick's law of diffusion (eqn 10.1), we can see what determines capillary permeability. The solute diffusion equation is simply a modified form of Fick's law. A comparison shows that the term 'permeability' incorporates the diffusion coefficient, pathlength and available area; for details see Appendix 2, 'Diffusion'. In other words, endothelial permeability to a lipid–insoluble solute depends on:

- the restriction to diffusion, and hence the ratio of solute to pore width;
- the pore area per unit endothelial area, and hence the extent of the breaks in the junctional strands;

- the available, non-excluded fraction of the pore area (again determined by the ratio of solute to pore width);
- the pathlength, and hence the length of the intercellular cleft.

For example, if the junctional strands increase in extent in response to cAMP (Section 9.7), the fractional pore area decreases and the permeability P falls.

As the above considerations show, capillary permeability depends not only on **pore geometry** but also on **solute properties**. The key solute properties are **size**, which influences exclusion from the pore space, and **lipid solubility**. Lipid-soluble solutes access the entire lipid cell membrane, which vastly increases the area available for diffusion. **Solutes thus fall into three main classes**: lipid-soluble molecules (e.g. O_2), small lipid-insoluble molecules (e.g. glucose) and the large lipid-insoluble molecules (e.g. plasma proteins). Capillary permeability to lipid-soluble O_2 is many thousand times greater than to lipid-insoluble glucose; and the permeability to glucose (molecular mass 180 daltons) is nearly 1000 times greater than the permeability to albumin (69000 daltons; Table 10.1).

We must therefore consider these three classes of solute separately.

10.5 Lipid-soluble molecules diffuse rapidly through the cell membrane

The permeability of endothelium to lipophilic ('fat-loving') molecules increases in proportion to their oil-to-water partition coefficient. Since virtually the entire capillary surface is available for diffusion, the permeability is extremely high. Respiratory gases, general anaesthetics and the flow-tracer xenon are

Table 10.1 Capillary permeability to various solutes.

Solute	M	D ($\times 10^{-5}$ cm²/s)	a (nm)	Membrane	Permeability ($\times 10^{-6}$ cm²/s)
Oxygen	32	2.11	0.16	Continuous capillary	~100 000
Urea	60	1.90	0.26	Continuous capillary	26–28
Glucose	180	0.91	0.36	Continuous capillary	9–13
Sucrose	342	0.72	0.47	Continuous capillary	6–9
				Cerebral capillary	0.1
				Fenestrated capillary	>270
Albumin	69 000	0.085	3.55	Continuous capillary	0.03–0.01
				Fenestrated capillary	0.04

M, molecular weight; D, free diffusion coefficient in water at 37°C; a, Stokes–Einstein diffusion radius. (After Renkin, E. M. (1977) *Circulation Research*, **41**, 735–743; Clough, G. E. and Smaje, L. H. (1984) *Journal of Physiology*, **354**, 445–455; Landis, E. M. and Pappenheimer, J. R. (1963) *Handbook of Physiology, Cardiovascular System, Circulation*, Vol. II (eds Hamilton, W. F. and Dow, P.), American Physiological Society, Bethesda, pp. 961–1034.)

examples of lipophilic solutes. The oil:water partition coefficient is ~5 for **oxygen** and 1.6 for **carbon dioxide**. Permeability to O₂ is so high that there is significant O₂ escape from arterioles, reducing the haemoglobin saturation to ~80% at the capillary entrance. However, only part of the deoxygenation is due to O₂ transfer into the tissue. The rest is caused by **diffusional shunting** of O₂ from arterioles into venules, which usually run alongside the arterioles.

10.6 Small lipid-insoluble molecules permeate a small pore system

Lipophobic (fat-hating), hydrophilic (water-loving) solutes include the plasma electrolytes, glucose, lactate, amino acids, vitamins such as B₁₂, hormones such as adrenaline and insulin, and many drugs. These solutes cannot diffuse through the lipid endothelial membrane and are confined to the water-filled pathway through the intercellular junctions, and through fenestrations when present. The intercellular clefts occupy only 0.2–0.4% of the capillary surface, so capillary permeability to small lipophobic solutes is a fraction of that to lipophilic solutes.

How big are the capillary pores? Restricted diffusion provides an answer

In 1951 Pappenheimer, Renkin and Borrero proposed the seminal 'small pore theory' of capillary permeability. Measurements of solute diffusion led them to conclude that endothelium is penetrated by a set of small, aqueous channels that occupy only 0.01–0.04% of the capillary surface area (about one-tenth of the cleft

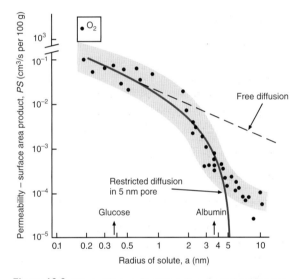

Figure 10.9 Effect of Stokes–Einstein radius of a molecule on capillary permeability. Points refer to lipophobic solutes except for oxygen. Dashed line of slope shows effect of fall in free diffusion coefficient with molecular size. Red line shows decline in permeability in cylindrical pores of radius 5 nm. The permeability to solutes larger than albumin indicates the existence of a few larger pores. Data from mammalian skeletal muscle and skin except for oxygen (lung). (After Renkin, E. M. and Curry, F. E. (1978) In *Membrane Transport in Biology*, Vol. IV (eds Giebisch, G., Tosteson, D. C. and Ussing, H. H.), Springer-Verlag, Berlin, pp. 1–45.)

area), with a width equivalent to a cylinder radius of 3–5 nm.

The estimate of pore size was based on the discovery that, as the size of lipophobic solutes increased, capillary permeability fell faster than the free diffusion coefficient (Figure 10.9). Pappenheimer and colleagues realized that this must be due to steric exclusion and restricted diffusion in narrow pores (Figure 10.6), and from the degree of restriction they calculated the equivalent pore size. For details see Appendix 2, 'Diffusion'. Pore size has also been evaluated from reflection coefficients (Section 10.3). Taking a broad average of the estimates, the channels through cardiac, skeletal muscle and intestinal endothelium have similar restrictive and reflective properties to cylindrical water-filled pores of radius 4–5 nm. It must be emphasized that nobody believes that the small pores are actually cylindrical tubes, only that some of their properties resemble those of tubes.

Physiological differences in permeability are due to differences in pore numbers, not size

Capillary permeability to lipophobic solutes or water spans a range of >100-fold in the various tissues of the body. Fenestrated capillaries are 10–100 times more permeable than continuous capillaries, because each fenestra is a collection of small pores (the gaps between the spokes) of very short pathlength. However, there are also large differences in permeability, up to 10 times, amongst continuous capillaries (e.g. between muscle and mesenteric capillaries) without an immediately obvious anatomical cause.

A clue to the cause is provided by the finding that solute permeability and hydraulic conductance correlate linearly; if one is doubled, so is the other. This proves that differences in permeability are not due to differences in pore radius, since hydraulic flow increases in proportion to r^4 (Poiseuille's law) whereas diffusion is proportional to pore area, πr^2. Differences in normal permeability must therefore be caused by differences in pore **numbers**. It appears that the proportion of the intercellular cleft that is 'open for business', due to breaks in the junctional strands, varies between the capillary beds (Figures 9.2, 9.4, 10.3). The proportion is typically ~10%. More extensive breaks produce vessels of higher permeability (e.g. postcapillary venules), and less extensive breaks vessels of lower permeability (e.g. arterial capillaries). Ultrastructural investigations using markers such as ferrocyanide ions, lanthanum ions and microperoxidase have confirmed that small lipophobic solutes do indeed permeate the intercellular cleft (Figure 10.3).

The glycocalyx is probably responsible for size selectivity

Although the intercellular cleft is the pathway for water and small solute permeation, the cleft itself cannot be the size-limiting structure, i.e. the small pore of width 8–10 nm, because it is 20 nm wide, including at the breaks in the junctional strands. Moreover the small pore is unlikely to have a continuous wall, as indicated by serious discrepancies between estimates of radius based on Poiseuille's law for flow through a walled tube, where conductance is proportional to r^4 and estimates based on diffusion, proportional to r^2. These inconsistencies led Curry and Michel to propose in 1980 that the size-limiting pores are actually the spaces within the glycocalyx, the lattice of biopolymers that coats the internal surface of endothelium and covers the entrance to the intercellular cleft (Figures 9.3, 9.5). This is called the **fibre-matrix theory of capillary permeability**.

The fibre matrix theory (Figure 10.10) proposes that the long biopolymer chains of the glycocalyx form a sufficiently fine network to act as size-selective pores. In support it has been shown that the glycocalyx exclude macromolecules; and that digestion of the glycocalyx by pronase increases the permeability of endothelium. Moreover, the binding of albumin to the glycocalyx (or cationized ferritin, Figure 9.5) greatly reduces endothelial permeability (the **protein effect**), whereas macromolecules that do not bind to the glycocalyx do not reduce permeability. It is thought that the bound albumin influences the size of the pores within the network (Figure 10.10a). The highly anionic plasma protein orosomucoid binds to the glycocalyx, increasing its negative charge density and thereby increasing the reflection of negatively charged solutes.

To summarize, two different structures, the glycocalyx and the breaks in junctional strands, together determine the permeability of continuous endothelium to solutes and water. The **area** available for the passage of water and small solutes (and hence endothelial permeability) depends on the extent of the gaps in the junctional strands. The **size and charge selectivity** of the pathway is determined by the spacing and charge within the glycocalyx polymer network covering the entrance to the clefts. The uniform coating of the junctions and fenestrae by glycocalyx (Figure 10.10b) accounts for the remarkable constancy of the reflection coefficient to plasma proteins (0.8–0.95) in capillary beds that have a 400-fold range in hydraulic permeability.

The concepts of John Pappenheimer and Gene Renkin, the originators of pore theory, and Charles Michel and Roy Curry, the originators of the fibre matrix theory, might be summarized as follows:

The Pappenheimer pore's so small
You cannot make it out at all,

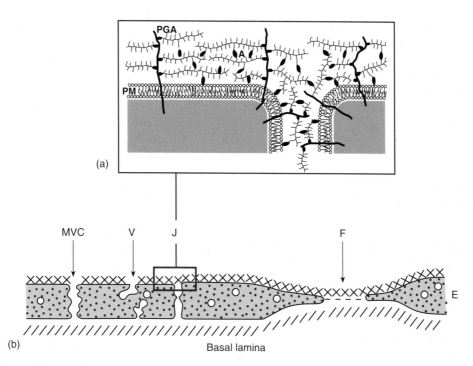

Figure 10.10 Fibre matrix model of capillary permeability. Glycocalyx covers the endothelium (E) and fenestra (F) and intercellular junction (J). The multivesicular transcellular channel (MVC) or vesicles (V) represent the large pore system; these are very few in number. (Inset) Putative details of matrix structure. Proteoglycan fibres (PGA) bind albumin (A) via its positively charged arginine groups. Molecular sieving is governed by the mesh size while the number of channels (J, F) influences total hydraulic and diffusional permeability. PM, plasmalemma membrane. (Adapted from Michel, C. C. (1980) *Journal of Physiology*, **309**, 341–355; and Curry, F. E. (1986) *Circulation Research*, **59**, 367–380, by permission.)

Though many sanguine doctors hope
To see one through the microscope –
Rectangular or round in shape
With many nanometres gape.
Some say the pore contains a fluff
Of glyco-proteinaceous stuff,
Whose fibres subdivide the space
Constructing there a random lace
'Til albumin, a protein, lands
And tidies up those tangled strands,
Through which there flows dilute saline.
All this has never yet been seen,
But Scientists, who ought to know,
Assure us that it must be so.
Oh let us never, never doubt
What nobody is sure about.

(With apologies to Hilaire Belloc)

10.7 Large lipid-insoluble molecules pass through a large pore system

The permeability of continuous and fenestrated endothelium to plasma proteins is around 1 millionth of the permeability to oxygen. Nevertheless there is a small but important flux of plasma proteins into the tissues, as demonstrated by the presence of plasma proteins in lymph at 20–70% of the plasma concentration. Access of plasma proteins to the tissues is necessary for the defence function of immunoglobulins and for the transfer of protein-bound substances such as iron, copper, vitamin A, lipids, thyroxine, testosterone and oestradiol.

The permeability versus molecular size plot identifies a large-diameter transport system

As the red line in Figure 10.9 shows, the permeability of the small pore system declines steeply as solute radius approaches 3.6 nm (albumin), because such solutes are almost as wide as the equivalent small pore, i.e. glycocalyx mesh size. However, for solutes bigger than 4–5 nm there is still a low but finite permeability, and permeability falls off with size only slightly more than the free diffusion coefficient. The permeation of macromolecules that are too big to penetrate the small pores led Grotte, in 1956, to propose the existence of a second transport pathway, that has functional properties equivalent to a small number of large pores of radius 20–30 nm. Measurements of

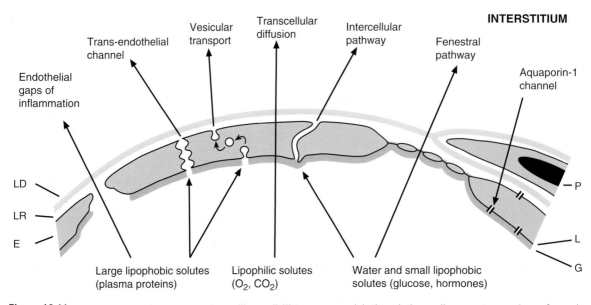

Figure 10.11 Main transport pathways across the capillary wall. Water passes mainly through the small pore system as shown. Some also passes through aquaporin-1 channels in the cell membrane and some through the large pore system. E, endothelium; G, glycocalyx; L, lipid plasma membrane; LR and LD, lamina rara and lamina densa of basement membrane, respectively; P, pericyte.

macromolecular reflection coefficients confirm this; the reflection coefficient does not reach 100% even for molecules as large as fibrinogen (radius 10 nm). Calculations indicate that there is, at most, one large pore per 4000 small pores in continuous capillaries, and there are essentially none in cerebral and renal glomerular capillaries.

Macromolecular permeation depends on charge as well as size

Large plasma proteins such as fibrinogen cross the endothelial layer less readily than smaller proteins such as albumin. In addition, negatively charged macromolecules such as albumin permeate the endothelial barrier less readily than neutral or positively charged ones of similar size. This is attributed to repulsion by the fixed negative charges of the glycocalyx.

Hydraulically continuous channels or vesicular transport?

The large pore system is a functional concept derived from physiological data. There is controversy over whether the system consists of true pores, i.e. hydraulically continuous channels such as the multivesicular channels (Figures 9.6b, 10.10) or whether it is really the caveola–vesicle transport system.

The 'true pore' protagonists point out that macromolecular transfer into the tissue increases in proportion to the pressure driving fluid across the wall,

as would be expected if hydraulically continuous large pores penetrate the wall. Moreover tissue cooling, which should inhibit active vesicular transport, has only a small effect on macromolecular permeation.

Nevertheless, vesicular transport may contribute significantly when filtration rates are low. Macromolecules such as gold-labelled albumin and ferritin (radius 5.5 nm) undoubtedly enter the luminal caveolae and appear soon afterwards in the abluminal caveolae (Figures 9.5, 9.6). What is unclear is how much this contributes to the total protein transport across the capillary wall. It is possible that, at normal, very low capillary filtration rates, both conductive channels and vesicular transport contribute significantly to protein permeation.

Our current understanding of the various parallel pathways for solute movement across the capillary wall is summarized in Figure 10.11.

10.8 Blood–brain barrier and carrier-mediated transport

Specific transporters generally contribute little to transcapillary exchange

As a general rule, transport by integral membrane proteins contributes negligibly to small solute transport across the capillary wall. This is because the transport capacity of ion channels, glucose carriers, amino acid carriers and membrane water channels (aquaporins) is several orders of magnitude lower than that of the intercellular cleft. There are exceptions, however. Carrier-mediated urea transport is important in the descending vasa recta of the kidney (medullary capillaries). Brain endothelium has several specific transporter systems, as follows.

Cerebral capillaries form a blood–brain barrier

Brain capillaries, like all capillaries, are highly permeable to lipophilic solutes such as O_2, CO_2 and general anaesthetics; but they are exceptionally impermeable to lipophobic solutes such as L-glucose, catecholamines and plasma proteins. This is referred to as the blood–brain barrier. The function of the barrier is to protect the neurons from circulating stimulants such as the catecholamines and to prevent the washout of neurotransmitters from the brain parenchyma. The barrier is formed by complex, multiple junctional strands between the endothelial cells, without the usual breaks i.e. the strands form a continuous, unbroken seal. The caveola–vesicle system is also very scanty. Breakdown of the barrier is common in pathological conditions such as local cerebral ischaemia (strokes), cerebral haemorrhage and cerebral inflammation, and leads to cerebral oedema.

Specific endothelial carriers transport solutes into the brain parenchyma

The transport of essential lipid-insoluble solutes across brain endothelium is achieved through specific carrier proteins in the endothelial cell membrane. There are carriers for D-glucose (the natural sugar dextrose), lactate, pyruvate, amino acids and adenosine. This form of transport is transcellular as opposed to paracellular. The transport process is one of facilitated diffusion down concentration gradients, not active transport. In addition cerebral endothelium can actively regulate the K^+ concentration in the cerebral interstitial fluid through a Na^+–K^+-ATPase located in the abluminal membrane (Section 15.4).

10.9 Concentration fall along a capillary, extraction and clearance

The way in which solute concentration decays along a capillary has a direct bearing on how blood flow and exercise affect solute transfer. This section describes the basic concentration profile and the related concepts of extraction and clearance; Sections 10.10 and 10.11 deal with the effects of blood flow and exercise. To understand the concentration profile along a capillary, let us consider the transfer of glucose into an active muscle. The interstitial glucose concentration will be lower than the arterial concentration, owing to glucose consumption by the muscle. For simplicity we will assume that the interstitial glucose concentration is uniform.

Concentration decays non-linearly along a capillary

At the inlet to a capillary the glucose concentration is close to its arterial level (point A in Figure 10.8), so the concentration difference across the capillary wall is high. Due to the operation of Fick's law of diffusion the efflux of solute is rapid at this point (J_{sA} in the figure). As a result the plasma concentration falls off steeply just beyond the inlet, e.g. from A to B in Figure 10.8. Further along the capillary the concentration drop across the wall is smaller (point C), so the solute efflux is slower (flux J_{sC}). As a result the plasma concentration falls off less steeply with axial distance, e.g. from C to D. In the case of lactate or CO_2, where the concentration is higher in the tissue than the capillary, analogous arguments apply but the concentration increases rather than decays along the capillary axis.

The concentration profile along a capillary is thus a curve, and the mean concentration is smaller than the arithmetic average of the arterial and venous concentrations. For mathematical details see Appendix 2, 'Capillary concentration profile'. If the curvature is pronounced, with a steep initial decay, most of the solute exchange occurs near the entrance and relatively little downstream. The curvature depends partly on permeability and partly on blood flow, as explained later.

The Fick *principle* (cf. Fick's law) describes exchange across the whole capillary bed

The net solute exchange across an entire capillary bed is easily worked out from the input arterial concentration C_a and the output (i.e. local venous) concentration C_v, using the Fick *principle*. The Fick principle, described in Section 7.1, is essentially a statement of the law of conservation of mass and must not be confused with Fick's law of diffusion. The Fick principle states that the solute exchange rate equals the arterio-venous concentration difference $C_a - C_v$ multiplied by the blood flow $\dot{Q}$;

$$J_s = \dot{Q}(C_a - C_v) \qquad (10.4)$$

For example, the glucose flux into a muscle can be evaluated by measuring the blood flow, the arterial glucose concentration and the local venous concentrations. Conversely, the Fick principle can be used to work out the concentration drop $C_a - C_v$ that will be produced by any particular combination of solute consumption and blood flow (Figure 10.8).

Extraction (*E*) is the fraction of solute removed from plasma during its transit through the capillary bed

Extraction can be understood by considering an example. If arterial plasma delivers, say, 500 μmoles glucose/min to an active muscle, and 100 μmoles/min diffuses out through the capillary walls into the muscle, the extraction of glucose is 20%. The extraction equals the arteriovenous concentration difference $C_a - C_v$ divided by the arterial concentration C_a (Figure 10.8); for proof see Appendix 2, 'Extraction'. Thus, if glucose enters a capillary bed at a concentration of 5 mM and leaves it at 4 mM, the extraction is $(5-4)/5$ or 20%. For oxygen the extraction is typically 25% at rest and up to 80–90% in exercising muscle.

The dynamics of extraction are illustrated in Figure 10.12, which shows the extraction of a vitamin after a single bolus injection into an artery. The injected solution also contained a non-exchanging or 'reference' solute, namely radiolabelled albumin, as a control for dilution of the sample in the arterial blood. Samples of the venous effluent showed that the concentration of diffusible solute fell below that of the reference solute due to diffusion out of the capillaries. The reference concentration indicates what the test solute concentration would have been if no exchange had taken place. The extracted fraction of the test solute E was calculated for each sample from the difference between the test and reference solute concentrations. The plot in Figure 10.12b shows that the extraction of vitamin B_{12} was initially $\sim$40%, and then declined in obedience to Fick's law of diffusion as the interstitial concentration increased.

Clearance (*Cl*) is the volume of plasma cleared of solute per unit time

Clearance is a measure of how much plasma is emptied of solute per minute as it passes through the

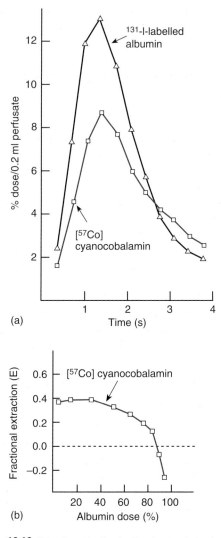

Figure 10.12 Extraction of vitamin B_{12} (cyanocobalamin, radius 0.8 nm) by the microcirculation of cat salivary gland after a brief arterial injection. Albumin (radius 3.6 nm) serves as a non-extracted reference solute (see text). (a) Tracer content in successive venous samples as a percentage of the initial arterial dose. The lines cross at 3 s due to back-diffusion of B_{12} into blood as the plasma concentration falls below the interstitial concentration. (b) Extraction of B_{12} in successive venous samples. Extraction is high at first, then falls as interstitial concentration rises. Permeability can be calculated from the extraction and blood flow (eqn 10.6). (From Mann, G. E., Smaje, L. H. and Yudilevich, D. L. (1979) *Journal of Physiology*, **297**, 335–354, by permission.)

capillary bed. The clearance equals the plasma flow times fractional extraction E;

$$Cl = \text{plasma flow} \times E \qquad (10.5)$$

For example, if the plasma flow through an exercising muscle is 100 ml/min and the glucose extraction is 20%, then 20 ml of plasma are cleared of glucose per minute. Note that the units of clearance are plasma volume/time, not solute mass/time. The latter is clearance $\times$ arterial concentration.

10.10 Effect of blood flow on solute transfer

A rise in blood flow can greatly enhance solute exchange or have virtually no effect at all. To understand this we need to recognize two basic states, one called flow-limited exchange and the other diffusion-limited exchange, each with a characteristic capillary concentration profile. In **flow-limited exchange** the solute flux across the capillary wall is limited by the rate at which blood is delivering solute to the capillary. The associated concentration profile is highly curved, as in the red curves of Figure 10.13. In **diffusion-limited exchange** the solute flux is limited by the rate at which the solute can cross the capillary wall, and the associated concentration profile is relatively flat as in the black curves of Figure 10.13.

In flow-limited exchange, solute transfer rate is proportional to flow

If endothelial permeability is high, solute crosses the capillary wall so quickly that the plasma equilibrates with the pericapillary interstitial fluid before the end of the capillary. This is usually the case for lipophilic solutes such as O_2 and CO_2, and for small lipophobic solutes in fenestrated capillaries. It can also be true for small lipophobic solutes such as urea and glucose in continuous capillaries if a slow blood flow extends the transit time. Curve 1 of Figure 10.13a shows the characteristic concentration profile. The plasma concentration falls steeply near the entrance and is soon equal to the interstitial concentration. Only the first few segments of the capillary contribute to exchange.

If blood flow is increased, as in curves 2 and 3, the time available for exchange shortens but equilibration may still occur before the capillary exit, albeit further downstream. Since the arteriovenous difference ($C_a - C_v$) has not altered, the transcapillary solute flux J_s increases in direct proportion to the blood flow (Fick principle, eqn 10.4). This is illustrated by points 1–3 in panel (b) of Figure 10.13.

Gas exchange in the lungs is a good example of flow-limited exchange. The CO_2 and O_2 in the pulmonary capillary blood equilibrate with the alveolar gas long before the end of the capillary is reached. Consequently, an increase in pulmonary blood flow, i.e. cardiac output, causes a directly proportionate increase in O_2 uptake and CO_2 removal.

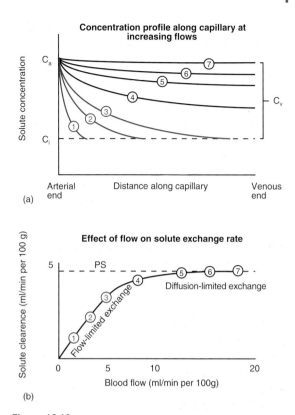

Figure 10.13 Effect of blood flow on diffusional exchange across capillary wall. (a) Decay of plasma concentration at low to high blood flows (curves 1–7) for a constant or zero pericapillary concentration C_i; C_a, C_v, arterial and venous concentrations. Slow transits (curves 1–3) allow sufficient time for equilibration before the capillary exit ($C_v = C_i$, flow-limited exchange); fast transits do not (curves 5–7, $C_v > C_i$, diffusion-limited exchange). (b) Resulting effect of flow on transcapillary exchange expressed as clearance (solute flux/C_a). For details see text. Plateau clearance equals the capillary diffusion capacity PS, in this case for urea in the muscle capillary bed. (Data of Renkin, E. M. (1967) In *International Symposium on Coronary Circulation* (eds Marchetti, G. and Taccardi, B.), Karger, Basel, pp. 18–30.)

In flow-limited exchange the solute clearance rate is a measure of blood flow, not the capillary diffusion capacity PS. This is the basis of the Kety xenon clearance method (Figure 8.6). It is not possible to measure capillary permeability P when exchange is flow-limited, because the fraction of the capillary wall that is contributing to exchange is unknown, i.e. S is unknown.

In diffusion-limited exchange, flow has little effect on solute transfer

In diffusion-limited exchange, solute transfer is limited by endothelial permeability rather than by solute delivery rate, i.e. flow. The plasma solute concentration has not equilibrated with the pericapillary space by the end of the capillary, and the concentration profile is relatively flat, as in curve 5 of Figure 10.13a. Medium-to-large lipophobic solutes such as inulin and cyanocobalamin (vitamin B_{12}) behave in this way. So too do small solutes such as urea and glucose when the transit time is shortened by high blood flows. Diffusion-limited exchange occurs with big molecules at normal flow and with small molecules at high flows.

Raising the blood flow causes relatively little increase in diffusion-limited exchange, because the blood is already spending too little time in the capillary to unload its solute fully. As the transit time shortens, the extraction falls and the venous concentration rises (curves 6 and 7 of Figure 10.13a). The arteriovenous concentration difference $C_a - C_v$ therefore declines. Applying the Fick principle (eqn 10.4), we find that solute exchange J_s increases relatively little with flow, because the rise in $\dot{Q}$ is largely offset by the fall in $C_a - C_v$. Thus points 5–7 in Figure 10.13b show little increase in solute clearance with increasing blood flow.

The ratio of diffusion capacity to blood flow ($PS/\dot{Q}$) determines whether exchange is flow- or diffusion-limited

As indicated above, the degree to which plasma equilibrates with the pericapillary space depends not only on permeability but also on transit time, and hence blood flow. The permeability-surface area product PS, or 'diffusion capacity' of the capillary bed, has the same units as flow $\dot{Q}$, namely cm^3/s, and the dimensionless ratio $PS/\dot{Q}$ determines the nature of the exchange process. If the diffusion capacity exceeds the blood flow, equilibration is reached before the end of the capillary and the exchange is flow-limited. If flow exceeds the diffusion capacity, equilibration is not achieved and the exchange is diffusion-limited.

The exact relation between $PS/\dot{Q}$ and solute exchange was worked out by Renkin and Crone. They considered a simple case where the interstitial concentration is zero – for example, a drug or vitamin has just been injected and is making its first pass through the capillary bed as in Figure 10.12. Renkin and Crone showed that under these conditions the solute extraction is related exponentially to $PS/\dot{Q}$, as follows:

$$E = 1 - \exp(-PS/\dot{Q}) \qquad (10.6)$$

For a derivation, see Appendix 2, 'Capillary concentration profile'. If we substitute some numbers into

Permeability and blood flow influence solute exchange

☐ *Permeability P* (cm/s) is the diffusional solute transfer J_s (g/s) per unit area of membrane S (cm^2) per unit concentration difference ΔC (g/cm^3). Therefore $P = J_s/S\Delta C$.

☐ From the above, *solute transfer rate* depends on the diffusion capacity of the capillary bed PS (cm^3/s) and mean concentration difference between plasma and tissue, i. e. $J_s = PS\Delta C$. This is *Fick's law of diffusion* applied to a membrane.

☐ Capillary permeability depends on *solute properties* (lipid solubility, molecular size) and *membrane porosity*. Porosity is determined by breaks in the intercellular junctional strands, fenestrae, and size-selective small pores in the glycocalyx.

☐ If diffusion capacity PS (cm^3/s) exceeds blood flow (cm^3/s) by $\geq 5\times$, solute *equilibrates* with the pericapillary space before the capillary exit (*flow-limited exchange*). Raising flow increases the solute transfer rate, e.g. pulmonary gas exchange.

☐ If PS is less than the blood flow ($PS/\dot{Q} \leq 1$), the solute does not equilibrate with the pericapillary space (*diffusion-limited exchange*). Extraction is low and solute exchange is not appreciably limited by flow.

the Renkin–Crone equation, we see that the extraction is >99% when $PS/\dot{Q}$ is 5 or more. This corresponds to virtual equilibration with the interstitial fluid, and hence flow-limited exchange. If $PS/\dot{Q}$ is 1 or less, the extraction is 63% or less, so there is no equilibration with the interstitial space and exchange is diffusion limited. As a rule-of-thumb, exchange is flow-limited at $PS/\dot{Q} \geq 5$ and becomes increasingly diffusion-limited at $PS/\dot{Q} < 1$. For glucose in skeletal muscle capillaries, $PS/\dot{Q}$ is ~5 at rest due to the low resting blood flow and ~1 during exercise due to the increased blood flow (diffusion-limited exchange).

There are intermediate states between flow-limited and diffusion-limited exchange

The concepts of flow-limited exchange and diffusion-limited exchange are actually the extremes of a continuous spectrum. At intermediate $PS/\dot{Q}$ values of 1 to 5, the end-capillary solute concentration has not quite equilibrated with the tissue but has fallen well below the arterial level, as in curve 4 of Figure 10.13. An increase in blood flow in this intermediate regime shortens the transit time and thus raises the end-capillary concentration. Because the mean capillary concentration increases significantly, the transcapillary solute flux also increases significantly, in accordance with Fick's law of diffusion. The solute flux does not, however, increase as much as it would for purely flow-limited exchange, as can be seen by comparing points 4 to 5 in Figure 10.13b (intermediate regime) with points 2 to 3 (flow-limited regime).

Increased blood flow can also trigger active increases in permeability

We have been concerned above with the passive, biophysical effect of blood flow on solute exchange. Recent work indicates, however, that blood flow can also induce active increases in endothelial permeability. This is considered further in the next section, which describes how several factors combine to achieve a match between solute transfer and demand when demand is increased, for example during exercise.

10.11 Physiological regulation of solute transfer

The transfer of O_2 and nutrients across the capillary wall should, ideally, keep pace with their consumption by the tissue. In exercising muscle the O_2 consumption can increase up to 20–40 fold. A corresponding increase in transcapillary transport is achieved by three main mechanisms:

- a more uniform perfusion of the capillary bed through capillary recruitment

- a steeper concentration gradient from plasma to tissue

- increased blood flow.

Additional factors include an increase in the O_2 diffusion velocity through muscle myoglobin as intracellular P_{O_2} falls; and, in the case of small lipophobic solutes such as glucose, probably an increase in capillary permeability with flow.

Capillary recruitment improves exchange in exercising muscle

In skeletal muscle each capillary supplies a cylindrical envelope of muscle called a Krogh cylinder (Figure 10.14). The radius of the Krogh cylinder depends on the capillary density and the fraction of the capillaries

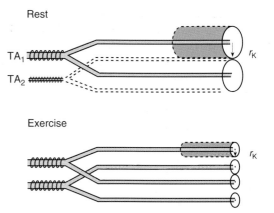

Figure 10.14 The Krogh cylinder concept and capillary recruitment in exercising skeletal muscle. At rest, contraction of terminal arteriole 2 (TA$_2$) stops the perfusion of one capillary module (dashed lines), so the Krogh cylinder radius is large (r_K). Metabolic vasodilatation during exercise dilates terminal arteriole 2, increasing the perfused capillary area and reducing the maximum diffusion distance r_K.

that is well perfused at any moment in time. In resting skeletal muscle, half to three-quarters of the capillaries are either not perfused or are perfused only sluggishly at any one moment, because the terminal arterioles supplying them are in the constricted phase of their vasomotion cycle (Section 10.1). As a result the Krogh cylinder has a large radius in resting muscle.

During exercise the terminal arterioles dilate, which increases the number of well-perfused capillaries. This is called capillary recruitment. Recruitment not only increases the **surface area** for exchange but also reduces the **diffusion distance**, i.e. the radius of the Krogh cylinder (Figure 10.14) and makes the oxygen supply more uniform.

Steeper concentration gradients develop as metabolic rate increases

An increase in cellular metabolic rate lowers the intracellular concentration of glucose, oxygen, etc., and therefore increases the concentration difference between the plasma and the active cell. For glucose, for example, the mean concentration difference across the capillary wall increases from ~0.3 mM in resting muscle to ~3 mM during heavy exercise (Table 10.2). The increased concentration difference and reduced diffusion distance (due to capillary recruitment) greatly increase the concentration gradient $\Delta C / \Delta x$.

Blood flow increases with metabolic rate

Blood flow increases in direct proportion to metabolic rate in most organs, including muscle (Figure 10.15).

Table 10.2 Transport of glucose from blood to 100 g skeletal muscle *in vivo*.

	Rest	Heavy exercise	Fractional change (exercise/rest)
Glucose consumption rate (J_s)[†]	1.4 μmol/min	60 μmol/min	43 ×
Arterial concentration (C_a)	5 mM	5 mM	–
Venous concentration (C_v)	4.44 mM	4 mM	0.9 ×
Extraction (E)	11.2%	20%	1.8 ×
Blood flow	2.5 ml/min	60 ml/min	24 ×
Perfused capillary density	250/mm^2	1000/mm^2 ⎫	4 ×
Diffusion capacity (PS)[‡]	5 cm^3/min	20 cm^3/min ⎭	
Mean concentration difference across capillary wall (ΔC)*	0.3 mM	3 mM	10 ×
Mean pericapillary concentration (C_i)	4.7 mM	2 mM	0.4 ×
Krogh cylinder radius	36 μm	18 μm	0.5 ×

* ΔC is calculated as J_s/PS – see eqn 10.3.

[†] Diffusion, and not fluid filtration, is the dominant transcapillary transport process for glucose and other small solutes. This is clear from a simple calculation based on the consumption by resting skeletal muscle (1.4 μmol/min 100 g^{-1}). Net transcapillary fluid flow is 0.005 ml/min 100 g^{-1} and since plasma contains 5 μmol glucose per ml, the maximum convective transport of glucose is 0.025 μmol/min. This is a mere 2% of the total glucose transfer. (After Crone, C. and Levitt, D. G. (1984) In *Handbook of Physiology, Cardiovascular System*, Vol. IV, *Microcirculation* (eds Renkin, E. M. and Michel, C. C.), American Physiological Society, Bethesda, p. 431.)

[‡] It now seems possible that part of the increase in PS could be due to increased permeability to glucose, P, as flow increases (see text).

This is necessary to increase the delivery of O_2 and glucose and to prevent the exchange from becoming flow-limited. Metabolites such as glucose are diffusion-limited at the high flows that occur during exercise, so solute transfer is not limited by solute delivery rate.

Endothelial permeability increases in response to flow

Recent measurements of K^+, Na^+, urea and fluorescein exchange indicate that an increase in blood flow not only increases solute delivery but also triggers a rapid increase in capillary permeability. Flow-mediated increases in permeability are blocked by inhibitors of nitric oxide production, so they are attributed to active increases in endothelial porosity. This would help to explain the large increase in transcapillary glucose flux in exercising muscle.

To draw the various threads together, let us finish this chapter with two specific examples of how solute flux is adjusted to demand, namely the transport of glucose and O_2 in exercising skeletal muscle.

Glucose transport in exercising muscle

The various factors that increase glucose delivery to exercising muscle fibres are brought together in Table 10.2 and Figure 10.15. Capillary recruitment reduces the radius of the Krogh cylinder and hence diffusion distance Δx. Recruitment also enhances the diffusional surface area S, and PS may be raised

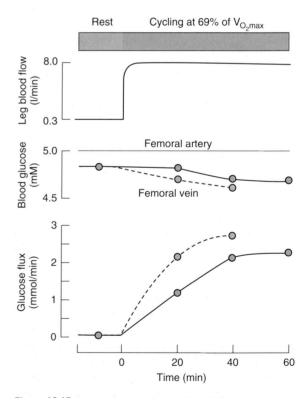

Figure 10.15 Increased glucose flux from blood to leg muscles during cycling, calculated by Fick principle (flux = blood flow × arteriovenous concentration difference). At first the muscle burns extracted glucose and stored glycogen. As the glycogen store is depleted, blood glucose extraction increases. Grey circles with dashed lines show greater glucose extraction when muscle glycogen was depleted prior to exercise. (From data of Blomstrand, E. and Saltin, B. (1999) *Journal of Physiology*, **514**, 293–302.)

further by an effect of flow on P. A fall in tissue glucose concentration raises the gradient across the capillary wall, and the resulting increase in diffusional flux raises the fractional extraction and arteriovenous concentration difference $C_a - C_v$ (Figure 10.15). Increased blood flow delivers glucose faster to the capillary and prevents a major fall in the mean intracapillary plasma concentration, thereby avoiding a flow-limitation of exchange. The new transcapillary glucose flux equals the increased blood flow times increased $C_a - C_v$ (Figure 10.15).

Oxygen transport in exercising muscle

Oxygen permeates endothelium so rapidly that the capillary wall offers a negligible resistance to its transport. The main diffusional resistance to O_2 transport in muscle resides in the extravascular pathway, because it is >20 μm long (cf. 0.3 μm across the capillary wall). The main fall in O_2 concentration thus occurs between the pericapillary space and muscle mitochondria, rather than between the plasma and pericapillary space. The O_2 transfer from blood to muscle mitochondria is in the intermediate regime between flow- and diffusion-limited exchange. That is to say, the end-capillary P_{O_2} (partial pressure of O_2, 40 mmHg at rest) is well below the arterial P_{O_2} of 100 mmHg but has not achieved equilibrium with the mitochondrial P_{O_2}, ~20 mmHg in resting muscle (Figure 10.16, top panel).

During exercise the mitochondrial P_{O_2} is estimated to fall to <5 mmHg, increasing the gradient between arterial blood and muscle. Consequently the oxygen extraction increases and the end-capillary P_{O_2} can fall as low as ~15 mmHg. Increased blood flow is essential to deliver O_2 faster. Even a moderately exercising muscle consumes more O_2 per minute than its total resting arterial supply, so exchange would become flow-limited if there were no increase in flow. These changes are summarized in Figure 10.16 (bottom panel).

An extra mechanism that aids O_2 transport in exercising muscle is the presence of partly deoxygenated **myoglobin** in the muscle sarcoplasm. Although there is a large drop in P_{O_2} from the blood to a point just inside the sarcoplasm, the P_{O_2} appears to be surprisingly uniform across the muscle fibre itself, despite its considerable size. This is due to the presence of myoglobin, which is present in red muscle at up to 7 g/kg. As P_{O_2} falls, the partially deoxygenated myoglobin greatly speeds up the rate of diffusion of O_2 because oxygen can 'hop' from one unoccupied binding site to the next. This is called facilitated diffusion.

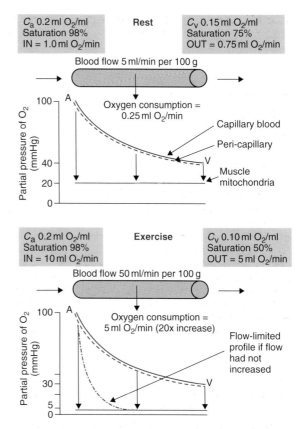

Figure 10.16 Oxygen exchange along the capillary in resting and exercising skeletal muscle. Mitochondrial P_{O_2} is a rough estimate based on myoglobin saturation. Note that the O_2 demand of exercising muscle exceeds the total resting arterial supply. If blood flow did not increase, the oxygen content of the blood would approach zero soon after entering the capillary. A, arterial end of exchange microvessels (strictly, the terminal arteriole); V, venous end of exchange system.

SUMMARY

■ A dense network of fine, thin-walled capillaries subserves nutrient and water exchange between blood and tissue.

■ **Solutes** such as O_2 and glucose **diffuse** across the capillary wall down **concentration gradients**. **Water**, by contrast, **flows** across the wall down a **pressure gradient**.

■ **Fick's law of diffusion** states that diffusional solute transfer (mass per unit time) in free solution is proportional to concentration gradient (concentration difference/distance), area and free diffusion coefficient. For diffusion through porous membranes the concept of **permeability** is employed to incorporate the effect of reduced available area, restricted intrapore diffusion coefficient and increased pathlength. Diffusional transport equals permeability

$P \times$ membrane area $S \times$ concentration drop across the membrane ΔC.

■ **Permeability** depends on **capillary ultra-structure** and on **solute properties**. The three types of capillary, namely continuous, fenestrated and discontinuous, form a hierarchy of increasing permeability. Solutes fall into three classes as follows.

(i) **Lipid-soluble molecules** such as O_2, CO_2 and anaesthetics diffuse across the entire endothelial cell membrane, so they permeate the wall extremely rapidly.

(ii) **Small, lipid-insoluble molecules** such as glucose, amino acids and many drugs diffuse via an aqueous pathway through the intercellular cleft and fenestrations. The pathway occupies only a fraction of the capillary surface so permeation is slower than for lipid-soluble molecules. The entrance to the pathway is guarded by small pores (equivalent radius 4–5 nm) that exclude and reflect the plasma proteins. The pores are probably the tiny spaces between the biopolymer molecules of the endocapillary coat (glycocalyx). **Blood–brain barrier capillaries** have exceptionally tight intercellular junctions, so glucose and amino acid transfer is mediated by specific carrier proteins and facilitated diffusion.

(iii) **Large, lipid-insoluble molecules** such as plasma proteins (radius $\geqslant 4$ nm) cross the endothelium slowly through a limited large pore system, the identity of which is controversial. Both vesicular transport and multivesicular channels may contribute.

■ **Solute transfer rate** can be increased hugely, e.g. in exercising muscle, through a combination of (i) **increased concentration difference** due to increased tissue metabolic rate; (ii) **recruitment** of under-perfused capillaries through arteriolar dilatation (increasing S, reducing the diffusion distance across the Krogh cylinder, and improving perfusion homogeneity); and (iii) **increased capillary blood flow**.

■ **The effect of blood flow** depends on whether solute exchange is **flow-limited**, **diffusion-limited** or **intermediate**. If the diffusion capacity PS exceeds flow $\dot{Q}$ by five times or more, plasma equilibrates with pericapillary fluid before the capillary exit. Such exchange is flow-limited and raising flow increases the exchange rate proportionately (e.g. pulmonary O_2 uptake). If $PS/\dot{Q}$ is <1, equilibration is not achieved during the capillary transit and exchange is diffusion-limited (e.g. glucose in exercising muscle); transfer is no longer limited by solute delivery rate.

FURTHER READING

Reviews and chapters

Abbott, N. J. (2000) Inflammatory mediators and modulation of blood–brain barrier permeability. *Cellular and Molecular Neurobiology*, **20**, 131–147.

Duelli, R. and Kuschinsky, W. (2001) Brain glucose transporters: relationship to local energy demand. *News in Physiological Sciences*, **16**, 71–76.

Ellsworth, M. L., Ellis, C. G., Popel, A. S. and Pittman, R. N. (1994) Role of microvessels in oxygen supply to tissue. *News in Physiological Sciences*, **9**, 119–123.

Hudlicka, O., Egginton, S. and Brown, M. D. (1988) Capillary diffusion distances – their importance for cardiac and skeletal muscle performance. *News in Physiological Sciences*, **3**, 134–138.

Intaglietta, M. and Johnson, P. C. (eds) (1995) Functional capillary density: active and passive determinants. *International Journal of Microcirculation*, **15**, 213–276.

Jürgens, K. D., Papadopoulos, S., Peters, T. and Gros, G. (2000) Myoglobin: just an oxygen store or also an oxygen transporter? *News in Physiological Sciences*, **15**, 269–274.

Michel, C. C. (1996) Transport of macromolecules through microvascular walls. *Cardiovascular Research*, **32**, 644–653.

Michel, C. C. (1998) Capillaries, caveolae, calcium and cyclic nucleotides: a new look at microvascular permeability. *Journal of Molecular and Cellular Cardiology*, **30**, 2541–2546.

Rippe, B. (1998) Transport of solutes and water across the microvasculature: the three-pore model. In *Connective Tissue Biology. Integration and Reductionism* (eds Reed, R. K. and Rubin, K.), Portland Press, London, pp. 221–239.

Wissig, S. L. and Charonis, A. S. (1984) Capillary ultrastructure. In *Edema* (eds Staub, N. C. and Taylor, A. E.), Raven Press, New York, pp. 117–142.

Wittenberg, B. A. and Wittenberg, J. B. (1989) Transport of oxygen in muscle. *Annual Reviews of Physiology*, **51**, 857–878.

Research papers

Adamson, R. H. and Michel, C. C. (1993) Pathways through the intercellular clefts of frog mesenteric capillaries. *Journal of Physiology*, **466**, 303–327.

Fischer, S., Wobben, M., Marti, H. H., Renz, D. and Schaper, W. (2002) Hypoxia-induced hyperpermeability in brain microvessel endothelial cells involves VEGF-mediated changes in the expression of zonnula occludens-1. *Microvascular Research*, **63**, 70−80.

He, P. and Curry, F. E. (1993) Albumin modulation of capillary permeability: role of endothelial cell [Ca^{2+}]. *American Journal of Physiology*, **265**, H74−H82.

Montermini, D., Winlove, C. P. and Michel, C. C. (2002) Effects of perfusion rate on permeability of frog and rat mesenteric microvessels to sodium fluorescein. *Journal of Physiology*, **543**, 959−975.

Predescu, D. and Palade, G. E. (1993) Plasma-lemmal vesicles represent the large pore system of continuous microvascular endothelium. *American Journal of Physiology*, **265**, H725−H733.

Turner, M. R. and Pallone, T. L. (1997) Hydraulic and diffusional permeability of isolated outer medullary descending vasa recta from the rat. *American Journal of Physiology*, **272**, H392−H400.

Vink, H. and Duling, B. R. (2000) Capillary endothelial surface layer selectively reduces plasma solute distribution volume. *American Journal of Physiology*, **278**, H285−H289.

Wagner, R. C. and Chen, S. C. (1991) Trans-capillary transport of solute by the endothelial vesicular system: evidence from thin serial section analysis. *Microvascular Research*, **42**, 139−150.

Watson, P. D. (1995) Permeability of cat skeletal muscle capillaries to small solutes. *American Journal of Physiology*, **268**, H184−H193.

CHAPTER 11

Circulation of fluid between plasma, interstitium and lymph

Learning objectives

After reading this chapter you should be able to:

● State the forces governing microvascular fluid exchange and the Starling equation (11.1).

● Define 'osmotic reflection coefficient' and state its importance (11.1, 11.3, 11.11).

● Outline the factors determining capillary pressure (11.2).

● Give typical values for human capillary pressure and plasma colloid osmotic pressure (11.2, 11.3).

● Sketch how interstitial protein concentration alters with filtration rate and explain its importance (11.4).

● Sketch how the Starling pressures and fluid exchange alter along the capillary axis (11.6).

● State the circumstances under which capillaries absorb interstitial fluid (11.6).

● Explain why normal tissue does not 'pit' but oedematous tissue does (11.7).

● Draw an interstitial pressure–volume relation, marking the normal and oedematous zones (11.7).

● List the functions of the lymphatic system and state how lymph is moved (11.8).

● Categorize the causes of oedema and explain the 'safety margin' (11.10).

● List the changes that lead to inflammatory swelling (11.11).

The pressure inside capillaries causes fluid to filter slowly out into the interstitial space, from where it is returned to the bloodstream by the lymphatic system. Although the capillary filtration rate is low, the cumulative volume filtered over many hours is substantial. Indeed, **the entire plasma volume completes an extravascular circulation in under one day**, except for the plasma proteins. Consequently, the distribution of fluid between the plasma and interstitial compartment is greatly influenced by capillary and lymphatic function. Increased capillary filtration reduces the plasma volume by as much as 20% during prolonged standing or exercise. In cardiac failure and many other diseases increased capillary filtration causes oedema, which is an excess of water in the tissue spaces. To understand oedema formation we must begin with the forces that govern fluid exchange.

11.1 Starling principle of fluid exchange

Flow across the capillary wall is a process of **plasma ultrafiltration across a semipermeable membrane**. That is to say, water and electrolytes pass through the wall more easily than plasma proteins, so the filtrate has a reduced protein content. The filtrate becomes interstitial fluid. The process of ultrafiltration probably takes place at the entrance to the intercellular cleft, which is guarded by the protein-reflecting, water-conducting small pore system (glycocalyx, Chapter 9). The intercellular clefts, along with fenestrations when present, are the chief pathways for fluid exchange.

Blood pressure drives filtration; plasma colloid osmotic pressure opposes it

The primary force driving ultrafiltration is the **capillary blood pressure**, as Carl Ludwig recognized in 1850. Filtration is opposed by the **osmotic pressure of the plasma proteins**, which tends to suck fluid into the capillary, as discovered by Ernest Starling in 1896. Starling injected isotonic saline into the tissues of a dog hindlimb and found it was absorbed directly into the bloodstream, as revealed by haemodilution. He concluded that the plasma proteins, or 'colloids', exert an absorptive force, which he called colloid osmotic pressure. Colloid osmotic pressure (COP) and oncotic pressure are synonyms for the osmotic pressure of the plasma proteins. Students unfamiliar with osmosis should note that osmotic pressure is a **suction** force, not a pushing force (Section 11.3). Its importance is that **plasma COP is the sole force retaining water within the plasma compartment**. Starling's discovery led to the use of solutions of artificial colloids to replace lost plasma in wounded soldiers during World War I, and more recently to the development of plasma substitutes such as urea-linked gelatin solution – a good example of a practical benefit arising from 'pure' research.

Rate and direction of fluid exchange are governed by four pressures

The **Starling principle of fluid exchange** (not to be confused with Starling's law, Section 6.4) states that the rate and direction of fluid movement across any particular segment of capillary wall depends on the local hydraulic pressure difference across the wall minus the opposing colloid osmotic pressure difference (Figure 11.1). In other words:

Capillary filtration rate ∝
[Hydraulic drive − Osmotic suction]

If the hydraulic drive exceeds the osmotic suction, fluid filters from the plasma into the interstitium. If the osmotic suction exceeds the hydraulic drive, the filtration rate is negative, i.e. fluid is absorbed from the interstitium into the plasma.

If the above statement is written out in symbols, using J_v for volume filtered per unit time, we get a simple but powerful equation that enables us to understand fluid exchange quantitatively. The hydraulic drive is the capillary blood pressure P_c minus the interstitial fluid pressure P_i. The osmotic suction is the plasma colloid osmotic pressure π_p minus the colloid osmotic pressure of the surrounding or 'pericapillary' interstitial fluid, π_i. So, replacing words with symbols:

$$J_v \propto [(P_c - P_i) - (\pi_p - \pi_i)]$$

The proportionality factor in this relation depends on the surface area of the wall S and its hydraulic

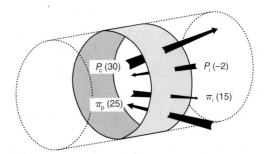

Figure 11.1 Four Starling pressures govern fluid exchange: P_c, capillary blood pressure; P_i, interstitial fluid pressure; π_p, plasma colloid osmotic pressure (COP); and π_i, interstitial fluid COP. Hydraulic pressures are expressed relative to atmospheric pressure (760 mmHg); an interstitial pressure of '−2 mmHg' is an absolute pressure of 758 mmHg, so the force arrow is directed into the capillary. Values in mmHg for warm human skin at heart level. (From Levick, J. R. and Michel, C. C. (1978) *Journal of Physiology*, **274**, 97–109; and Bates, D. O., *et al.* (1994); see Research papers.)

conductance L_p. Writing in these proportionality factors, we get:

$$J_v = L_pS[(P_c - P_i) - (\pi_p - \pi_i)] \qquad (11.1)$$

This equation still lacks one crucial term, however. As written above, it neglects the fact that endothelium is as an **imperfect** semipermeable membrane, that is to say, it is slightly leaky to plasma proteins. The effect of the imperfection is dealt with by introducing the reflection coefficient, as follows.

The reflection coefficient accounts for imperfect semipermeability

When a membrane is leaky to a solute, the osmotic pressure of the solute is not fully exerted (Figure 10.7). The ratio of the osmotic pressure exerted across the leaky membrane ($\Delta\pi_{effective}$) to the full osmotic pressure across a perfect semipermeable membrane ($\Delta\pi_{ideal}$) is called the reflection coefficient σ

$$\sigma = \frac{\Delta\pi_{effective}}{\Delta\pi_{ideal}} \qquad (11.2)$$

For plasma proteins and endothelium σ is typically $0.80-0.95$. In other words, only 80–95% of the plasma colloidal osmotic pressure is exerted in practice. (NB: The reduction is unrelated to the presence of protein outside the membrane; the effective osmotic pressure of the latter is likewise reduced by a factor σ.) Thus the osmotic pressures in eqn 11.1 are reduced by a factor σ and the true expression for fluid movement becomes:

$$J_v = L_pS[(P_c - P_i) - \sigma(\pi_p - \pi_i)] \qquad (11.3)$$

This is called the **Starling equation**. As we shall see below, the Starling equation is central to understanding both normal fluid exchange and clinical disorders such as oedema, inflammatory swelling and posthaemorrhagic fluid absorption.

The Starling equation applies to each short segment of the capillary wall, where P_c etc. can be regarded as virtually uniform. For the whole vessel, however, the pressure falls from the arterial end to the venous end, so filtration rate falls too (Section 11.6).

The Starling principle has been proved in single capillaries

Fluid movement across the wall of a single capillary can be measured using a technique invented by an American medical student, Eugene Landis, in 1926. The capillary is cannulated with a micropipette and then blocked downstream by a glass rod (Figure 11.2a). If ultrafiltration occurs out of the blocked segment, the trapped red cells creep towards the blocker and the lost fluid is replaced from the pipette. Conversely, if there is an absorption of interstitial fluid, the red cells are pushed back towards the pipette. The transcapillary flow is calculated from the red cell velocity, and capillary pressure is measured through the micropipette.

The above approach established that the capillary filtration rate increases linearly with pressure, as the Starling equation predicts (Figure 11.2b). The slope of the relation represents the endothelial hydraulic conductance L_p. The plot also proves that the capillary wall is a semipermeable membrane, because the filtration rate falls to zero when capillary pressure is close to the plasma colloid osmotic pressure, and reverses

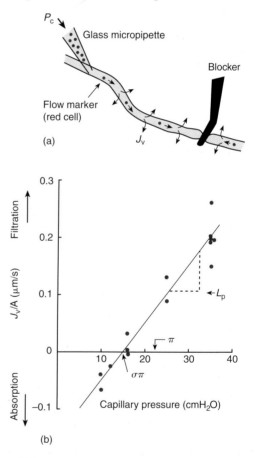

Figure 11.2 (a) Modified Landis red cell method for measuring fluid exchange in a single capillary. Filtration rate is red cell velocity × cross-sectional area of capillary. Measurements are made at several capillary pressures. (b) Initial filtration rate per unit wall area (J_v/A) is a function of capillary pressure. Intercept at zero filtration equals effective osmotic pressure ($\sigma\pi$, 15 cmH$_2$O) exerted *in vivo* by an infused albumin solution, whose COP *in vitro* (π) was 22 cmH$_2$O. The slope equals hydraulic conductance (L_p). (From Michel, C. C. (1980) *Journal of Physiology*, **309**, 341–355, by permission.)

direction to absorption when capillary pressure is lowered further. The transient nature of the fluid absorption is described later (Section 11.6).

In human limbs the filtration rate increases with venous pressure

In human limbs or isolated perfused organs, changes in the volume or weight are used to assess filtration rate. Capillary pressure in a human limb can be raised by congesting the venous outflow, using a proximal sphygmomanometer cuff inflated to ~40 mmHg. After the vascular volume has stabilized, the limb swells slowly due to increased capillary filtration (Figure 11.3a). In the same way a **deep venous thrombosis**

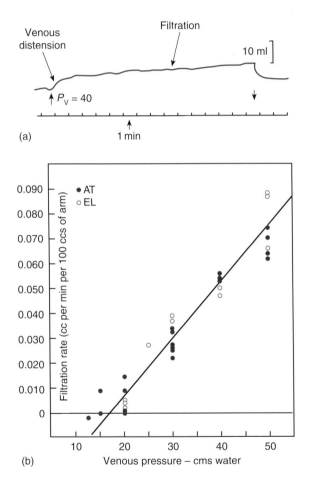

Figure 11.3 Capillary filtration in the human forearm. (a) Forearm volume measured by plethysmography (see Figure 8.5). First arrow marks inflation of a venous congesting cuff around upper arm to 40 cmH₂0, and second arrow deflation. After venous distension has stabilized, the slow swelling is due to capillary filtration. (b) Filtration rate (swelling rate after >2 min) at a series of venous pressures. The slope, 0.003 ml/min/mmHg venous pressure per 100 ml forearm, depends on the aggregate capillary filtration capacity. (From the classic work of Krogh, A., Landis, E. M. and Turner, A. H. (1932) *Journal of Clinical Investigations*, **11**, 63–95.)

of the leg leads to leg oedema. The swelling rate increases linearly with venous pressure (Figure 11.3b) and the slope of the relation is called the tissue **capillary filtration capacity**. The capillary filtration capacity is the sum of the capillary area × conductance values, $\Sigma(L_pS)$, in unit tissue volume.

The increased filtration into human limbs in response to venous congestion raises the question of what determines capillary pressure.

11.2 Capillary pressure and its control

Capillary blood pressure is the most variable of the four Starling pressures and is the only one under nervous control. The pressure depends on distance along the capillary axis, arterial and venous pressures, vascular resistance and gravity.

Pressure decays along a capillary

Pressure falls along a capillary owing to its resistance to blood flow. In human skin at heart level the capillary pressure falls from ~32–36 mmHg at the arterial end to 12–25 mmHg at the venous end. Capillary pressure is lower in the lungs (~10 mmHg) and in portal circulations (renal tubular capillaries ~14 mmHg, hepatic sinusoids ~6–7 mmHg).

The pre- to postcapillary resistance ratio R_A/R_V regulates capillary pressure

Capillary pressure must lie between arterial and venous pressures, and it is usually closer to the venous than arterial pressure. How closely the capillary pressure approaches the arterial or venous pressure depends on the ratio of precapillary, arteriolar resistance R_A to postcapillary, venular resistance R_V. If R_A/R_V is high, the pressure drop across the arterioles is large and only an attenuated pressure 'gets through' to the capillary. As a result the capillary pressure is close to venular pressure (Figure 11.4, right side). Conversely, if R_A/R_V is low as in inflammation, capillary pressure is high (Figure 11.4, left side). R_A/R_V is normally quite high, ~4. Consequently, capillary pressure is normally low, and is four times more sensitive to venous pressure than to arterial pressure. This is why venous hypertension causes oedema but arterial hypertension does not.

Due to the dependence of capillary pressure on R_A/R_V, **the sympathetic vasomotor nerves can influence fluid exchange**. After a haemorrhage sympathetic-mediated arteriolar vasoconstriction

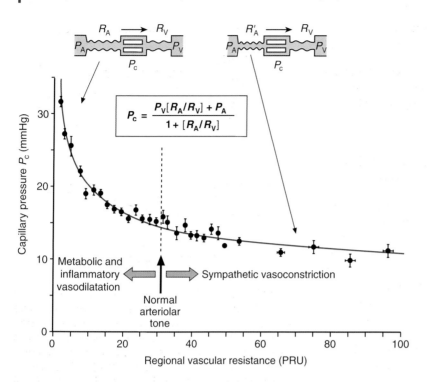

Figure 11.4 Control of capillary pressure by resistance vessel tone in cat skeletal muscle. Pressure was measured towards the venous end of the capillary bed at a fixed venous pressure of 7 mmHg (P_V) and arterial pressure 100 mmHg (P_A). The peripheral resistance unit (PRU) reflects mainly precapillary resistance. Inset shows how precapillary resistance (R_A) affects capillary pressure (P_c). Blood flow from artery to midcapillary equals $(P_A - P_c)/R_A$. Flow from midcapillary to vein equals $(P_c - P_V)/R_V$. Since the two flows are virtually equal, $(P_A - P_c)/R_A = (P_c - P_V)/R_V$. This gives the Pappenheimer–Soto Rivera equation defining capillary pressure: see the box. (Data from Maspers, M., Björnberg, J. and Mellander, S. (1990) *Acta Physiologica Scandinavica*, **140**, 73–83, by permission.)

raises R_A/R_V and thus reduces the capillary pressure. Plasma colloid osmotic pressure now predominates over capillary pressure, so interstitial fluid is absorbed and tops up the depleted circulation (Section 18.2).

A daily example of the active regulation of R_A/R_V occurs in the human foot during standing, as described next.

The attenuation of increased capillary pressure below heart level

Arterial and venous pressures increase linearly with vertical distance below heart level due to the operation of gravity (Figure 8.2). Arterial and venous pressures reach ∼180 mmHg and ∼90 mmHg respectively in the feet of a standing human. Capillary pressure increases too, to ∼95 mmHg in the motionless dependent foot (Figure 11.5, graph). This is why oedema is common in the feet and ankles, or in the sacral region of bed-ridden patients. Capillary pressure does not increase as much, however, as the arterial and venous pressures. The increase in capillary pressure is attenuated by a local, arteriolar vasoconstriction called the **veni-arteriolar response**, which raises R_A/R_V to 20–30 (Figure 11.5, top right). The raised precapillary resistance shifts the capillary pressure towards the lower, venous limit of its range, and thus helps to limit the rate of fluid filtration.

We should next consider the major factor opposing capillary pressure, namely plasma colloid osmotic pressure.

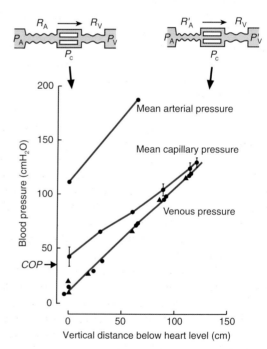

Figure 11.5 Pressure in nailfold skin capillaries of the human foot measured by direct micropuncture with the foot at various distances below heart level. Popliteal artery pressure and dorsal foot vein pressure increase with distance below heart level in the expected fashion, but capillary pressure increases relatively less. Top insets illustrate how a vasoconstrictor response attenuates the rise in capillary pressure. This '*veni-arteriolar response*' may be mediated by the Bayliss myogenic response but also requires an intact sympathetic innervation. (From Levick, J. R. and Michel, C. C. (1978) *Journal of Physiology*, **274**, 97–109, by permission.)

11.3 Osmosis across capillaries

As Figure 11.2 shows, the capillary can absorb fluid from the interstitium by osmosis under suitable conditions. What exactly is osmosis, and what does osmotic pressure mean?

Osmosis is the flow of water molecules from a dilute to a stronger solution

Consider a plane, such as the entrance to a pore, within a solution such as plasma (Figure 11.6). The total pressure on the plane arises from its bombardment by solvent molecules and solute molecules, both of which are in continuous thermal motion. If the solution is at, say, atmospheric pressure, the sum of the solvent and solute bombardments equals one atmosphere. The solvent itself, therefore, must exert less than one atmosphere pressure (just as in a mixture of gases under 1 atmosphere pressure each gas has a partial pressure of less than one atmosphere). In other words, the solute lowers the free energy level of the solvent (Figure 11.6). If the opposite side of the membrane is exposed to pure solvent (or a less concentrated solution) at atmospheric pressure, there is a difference in solvent energy level across the membrane. This drives a flow of solvent through the pore, called the osmotic flow.

An osmotic flow can be halted by applying enough pressure (e.g. capillary blood pressure) to the concentrated solution to raise the energy level of its solvent to equal that of solvent on the other side of the membrane. **The hydrostatic pressure that is required to halt an osmotic flow from pure solvent into a solution is called the 'osmotic pressure' of the solution**. This is the formal definition of an osmotic pressure, and is why a suction effect became known as a pressure.

It should be noted that during osmosis water flows hydraulically through the pore. Contrary to popular belief, water does **not** move along the pore by diffusion. Experimental work has proved that osmotic flow obeys Poiseuille's law of hydraulic flow (Section 8.7), not Fick's law of diffusion (Section 10.3).

Albumin contributes disproportionately to colloid osmotic pressure

As a rule-of-thumb, plasma colloid osmotic pressure (COP) is approximately the same as the mid-capillary blood pressure. The COP of human plasma is $21-29$ mmHg, corresponding to a protein concentration of $65-80$ g/l (Figure 11.7).

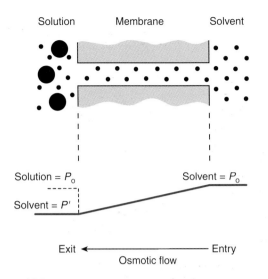

Figure 11.6 Osmotic flow between a solution (left) and solvent (right) exposed to equal pressure, P_0 (atmospheric pressure). Owing to the presence of solute, the 'partial pressure' P' of solvent within the solution (i.e. its free energy level) is less than P_0. This sets up a hydraulic pressure gradient within the pore, which produces an osmotic flow of solvent into the solution. (After Mauro, A. (1981) In *Water Transport Across Epithelia* (eds Ussing, H. H., Bindslev, N., Lassen, L. A. and Sten-Knudsen, D.), Munksgaard, Copenhagen, pp. 107–110.)

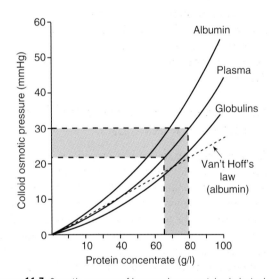

Figure 11.7 Osmotic pressure of human plasma proteins in isotonic saline (pH 7.4, 37°C). Pink region shows the normal range for human plasma. Dashed line is the van't Hoff law prediction for albumin. The actual COP deviates from this, and is given, in mmHg, by polynominal equations:

albumin $\pi = 0.28C + 1.8.10^{-3}C^2 + 1.2.10^{-5}C^3$,
plasma $\pi = 0.21C + 1.6.10^{-3}C^2 + 0.9.10^{-5}C^3$,
globulins $\pi = 0.16C + 1.5.10^{-3}C^2 + 0.6.10^{-5}C^3$,

where concentration C is g/l. (From Scatchard, G., *et al.*, summarized by Landis, E. M. and Pappenheimer, J. R. (1963) In *Handbook of Physiology 2, Circulation III* (eds Hamilton, W. F. and Dow, P.), American Physiological Society, Washington, pp. 961–1034.)

Albumin accounts for about two-thirds of human COP, though it is only half the plasma protein mass. Albumin COP is non-ideal; that is to say, it exceeds the COP predicted by the van't Hoff's law of osmosis; for details see Appendix 2, van't Hoff's law. The excess COP is due chiefly to the fact that each albumin molecule carries 17 negative charges at physiological pH, and therefore attracts extra Na^+ ions into the solution (**the Gibbs−Donnan effect**). The associated Na^+ ions account for roughly a third of the albumin osmotic pressure.

Colloid osmotic pressure differs greatly from crystalloid osmotic pressure

The total osmotic pressure of plasma is extremely high, ~5800 mmHg, but 99.6% of this is due to the presence of 300 mmoles of 'crystalloids' per litre, chiefly sodium chloride and bicarbonate. The crystalloid osmotic pressure, though huge, has no effect on capillary fluid exchange under most circumstances, because it is almost identical in the interstitial fluid and plasma, and because the endothelial reflection coefficient to crystalloids is only ~0.1. The plasma proteins, though present at only ~1 mmol/l, exert a sustained osmotic pressure of ~25 mmHg and supply the chief fluid-retaining force. There are a few circumstances, however, in which crystalloid osmotic pressure affects fluid exchange, as described next.

Aquaporins provide a water-only, transcellular pathway of low conductance

In addition to the high-conductance intercellular clefts that transmit water and crystalloids, there is a low-conductance pathway through the endothelial cell membrane that conducts water but not crystalloids. The specific water-only channels are formed by the glycoprotein aquaporin-1. Their chief role is probably cell volume regulation as in other cells. The contribution of aquaporin channels to transcapillary flow is generally small because their hydraulic conductance is low and there is usually no significant gradient in crystalloid concentration. If a crystalloid osmotic gradient develops, however, the aquaporin pathway becomes important. Since crystalloids are 100% reflected by the water-only channels, their full osmotic pressure is exerted across the channels. This is relevant in the following situations.

During **peritoneal dialysis**, which is a procedure used to treat patients with renal failure, a concentrated glucose solution is infused into the peritoneal cavity. The glucose (a crystalloid) sucks fluid osmotically from the plasma into the peritoneal cavity, enabling the physician to control the plasma volume.

Mercuric chloride, which blocks aquaporin-1 channels, blocks this fluid transfer.

In the **renal outer medulla**, long capillaries called the descending vasa recta are particularly rich in aquaporin-1 channels. A sodium chloride gradient created by the renal tubules draws water through these channels.

In **exercising muscle**, lactate and K^+ ions are released by the contracting fibres and accumulate in the interstitium. Their crystalloid osmotic pressure draws water out of the plasma compartment through the aquaporin channels, to the detriment of the plasma volume (Section 11.9).

Having considered the COP inside the capillary, we should next consider that outside.

11.4 Magnitude and dynamics of interstitial COP

Interstitial protein concentration and COP are substantial

There is widespread misconception that the protein content and COP of interstitial fluid are insignificant. This is untrue for most tissues. Indeed, more than half of the entire plasma protein mass is located in the interstitial fluid compartment (16% of the body by weight) rather than the plasma compartment (4%), and the average concentration of interstitial plasma protein is ~20−30 g/l. The composition of interstitial fluid has been assessed by the analysis of pre-nodal lymph and implanted wicks. Human leg lymph contains 15−35 g/l of plasma protein, intestinal lymph 30−40 g/l and lung lymph 40−50 g/l. These protein levels represent between 23% (leg) and 70% (lung) of the plasma concentration. Interstitial COP is thus far from negligible (Table 11.1), and it substantially reduces the difference in COP, $\pi_p - \pi_i$, across the capillary wall.

Interstitial protein concentration and COP are a dynamic function of filtration rate

Plasma proteins escape continuously from the bloodstream into the interstitium through the large pore system (Section 10.7), and water filters continuously into the interstitium through the small pore system (Figure 11.8, top panel). What, then, determines the protein concentration and hence COP of the interstitial fluid? If protein mass m enters the interstitium in time t (flux J_s), and water volume V enters the interstitium over the same time interval

Table 11.1 Starling pressures in human subcutaneous tissue (mmHg).

	Normal subjects	Congestive cardiac failure
Chest		
Plasma COP	26.8	23.3
Interstitial fluid COP	15.6	10.5
Interstitial fluid pressure	−1.5	−1.4
Ankle		
Plasma COP (arterial)	26.8	23.3 ⎱ mild
Interstitial fluid COP	10.7	3.4 ⎰
Interstitial fluid pressure	0.1	0.4 ⎰ oedema

COP, colloid osmotic pressure. Interstitial fluid from a soaked wick. Interstitial pressure by a wick-in-needle method. (From Noddeland, H., Omvik, P., Lund-Johansen, P, *et al.* (1984) *Clinical Physiology*, **4**, 283–297.)

(flow J_v), the interstitial protein concentration C_i is given by the **interstitial dilution relation:**

$$C_i = \frac{m/t}{V/t} = \frac{J_s}{J_v} \qquad (11.4)$$

In other words, interstitial protein concentration in the steady state equals the rate of arrival of protein divided by the rate of arrival of water. Interstitial protein concentration is thus not a static quantity but a dynamic variable governed by two continuous influxes.

As a result of the interstitial dilution relation **there is an inverse relation between interstitial protein concentration and capillary filtration rate**, which is sometimes called 'washdown' (Figure 11.8, lower panel). When capillary pressure is raised, the water transfer rate increases more than the protein transfer rate, because the small pore system sieves out the plasma proteins (Section 10.6). Consequently, the concentration of protein around the capillary falls. Conversely, if water filtration rate were reduced to zero, the interstitial protein concentration would eventually equilibrate with the plasma level due to protein permeation through the large pore system.

Thus, pericapillary COP (that immediately outside the membrane) is not only a **determinant** of filtration rate according to the Starling principle (eqn 11.3), but is also a **function** of filtration rate, i.e. dependent on it, as stated by the interstitial dilution relation (eqn 11.4). The dependence of filtration rate and pericapillary COP on each other has important physiological consequences, which we will return to in Section 11.6. Before that, however, we

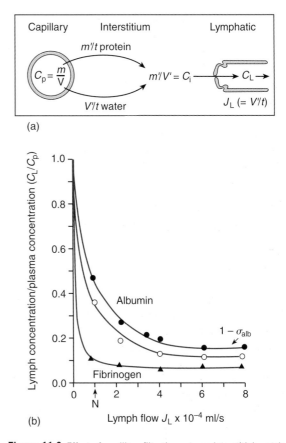

(a)

(b)

Figure 11.8 Effect of capillary filtration rate on interstitial protein concentration. (a) Mass of protein entering the interstitium in a given time (m'/t or J_s) is diluted by the volume of filtrate over the same period (V'/t or J_v) to form interstitial fluid (concentration C_i). This drains away as lymph. (b) Effect of net filtration rate (equal to lymph flow, J_L) on lymph/plasma concentration ratio (C_L/C_p) in dog paw. Filtration rate was varied by venous congestion. N is normal value. Curves are for albumin (●, radius 3.55 nm), γ-globulin (○, radius 5.6 nm) and fibrinogen (▲, radius 10 nm). At high flows C_L/C_p falls to a limit, namely $1 − \sigma$. (From Renkin, E. M., *et al.* (1977), plotted by Curry, F. E. (1984) In *Handbook of Physiology, Cardiovascular System*, Vol. IV, Part II, *Microcirculation* (eds Renkin, E. M. and Michel, C. C.), American Physiological Society, Bethesda, pp. 309–374, by permission.)

need to consider the fourth Starling pressure, the interstitial fluid pressure.

11.5 Interstitial matrix and interstitial fluid pressure

Interstitium is a biphasic porous material composed of fluid and biopolymers

Interstitium, the substance that occupies the spaces between parenchymal cells, is a complex

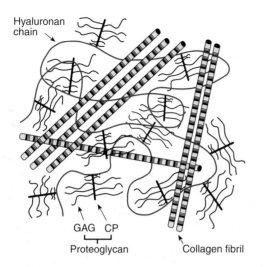

Hyaluronan chain

GAG CP
Proteoglycan
Collagen fibril

Figure 11.9 String-of-pearls model of interstitial matrix organization. The hyaluronan chain is the 'string' to which proteoglycan 'pearls' are anchored. Interstitial fluid occupies the inter-chain spaces. GAG, sulphated glycosaminoglycan chain (long, chondroitin sulphate; short, keratan sulphate); CP, core protein. Microfibrils and glycoproteins, such as fibronectin, not shown.

biochemical material; it is not simply a pool of liquid bathing the cells (Figure 11.9). The interstitial space is transected by **collagen fibrils and microfibrils**, and the space between the fibrils is subdivided further by **glycosaminoglycan chains** (GAGs), which are long polymers of amino sugars. Most GAGs are sulphated (chondroitin, keratan, dermatan and heparan sulphates) and the chains are up to 40 nm long. The non-sulphated GAG, **hyaluronan**, is extraordinarily long, ~5000 nm, and has a molecular mass of 2−6 million dalton. Multiple sulphated GAG chains are anchored to a linear core protein to form a large, brush-shaped molecule called a **proteoglycan**, and multiple proteoglycans are anchored to each hyaluronan chain. **Glycoproteins** such as the cell-binding 'glue' fibronectin form further structural elements. The interstitium thus comprises a three-dimensional network of biopolymers, the solid phase, and a space–filling solution of electrolytes and escaped plasma proteins, the fluid phase.

GAGs expand the interstitial compartment

The various interstitial components have specific functions. The collagen fibrils serve as **tensile elements**. The GAGs have two functions; they serve as **water-attracting, expansion elements**, and they determine the **hydraulic conductivity** of interstitium.

GAG chains endow the interstitium with a tendency to attract water and swell, and are responsible for its large volume and hydrated state. If a slice of connective tissue or Wharton's jelly from the umbilical cord (interstitium of low cellularity) is brought into contact with saline, the interstitial matrix imbibes the saline and swells. The swelling can be halted by lowering the saline pressure to a subatmospheric values. The subatmospheric pressure that exactly counteracts the suction effect of the GAGs is called **gel swelling pressure**. (As with osmosis, this kind of 'pressure' represents a suction force, not a pushing force.) The gel swelling pressure is caused by the osmotic activity of the GAGs, which is due chiefly to Na^+ ions attracted by their fixed negative charges (the **Gibbs−Donnan** effect).

The interstitial matrix *in vivo* is usually undersaturated, i.e. it still has a swelling tendency despite the continuous input of water by capillary filtration. The unsaturated state is preserved by the lymphatic system, which pumps water away from the interstitium, leaving the interstitial fluid at a subatmospheric pressure.

In some tissues, such as skin, the swelling tendency of the interstitial matrix is partially counteracted by fibroblasts. The fibroblasts exert tension on the collagen fibrils through $\alpha_2\beta_1$-integrins at membrane focal contact points, and the tensed collagen fibrils help to prevent the matrix from swelling.

GAGs reduce hydraulic conductivity, so interstitial fluid is not easily displaced

Interstitial water occupies the minute spaces inside the GAG matrix. The average effective radius of these spaces or 'mean hydraulic radius' ranges from a mere 3 nm in cartilage, which has the highest GAG concentration, to 300 nm in the vitreous body of the eye. Because the spaces are tiny, their resistance to flow is high. As a result, interstitium has a gel-like consistency, as exemplified by Wharton's jelly (mean hydraulic radius 30 nm). The low mobility of interstitial water stabilizes shape, prevents shifts in interstitial fluid under the drag of gravity and impedes bacterial spread.

Interstitial fluid pressure is commonly subatmospheric

Interstitial fluid pressure is difficult to measure owing to the low mobility of the fluid. This problem was first overcome by the American physiologist Arthur Guyton in 1960, who implanted a hollow perforated capsule under the skin of dogs (Figure 11.10). After several weeks the **Guyton capsule** had filled with interstitial fluid, and the pressure of the fluid proved to be subatmospheric, around −5 mmHg. This

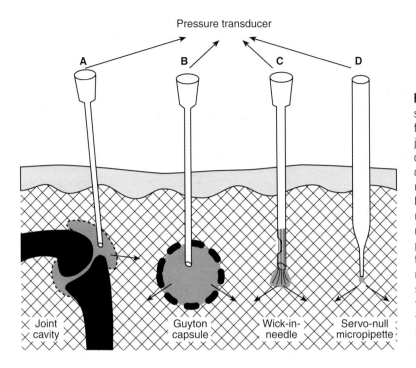

Pressure transducer

A   B   C   D

Joint cavity

Guyton capsule

Wick-in-needle

Servo-null micropipette

Figure 11.10 Methods for measuring interstitial fluid pressure. (A) Cannulation of a free fluid space in contact with interstitium, e.g. joint cavity, epidural space. (B) Guyton's chronic capsule method. (C) Acute wick method of Fadnes, Reed and Aukland; fine cotton filaments conduct interstitial pressure into a hypodermic needle. (D) Acute micropipette method. A 1 M NaCl-filled micropipette is connected to a motorized pump that varies the pressure until fluid neither enters nor leaves the tip (null flow) as indicated by its electrical resistance. All methods rely on equilibrating a small volume of free fluid (pink) to interstitial fluid pressure; arrows show how the linking fluid is absorbed by the interstitial matrix until its subatmospheric pressure equals that in the matrix.

evoked considerable controversy, since interstitial fluid pressure was previously thought to be positive.

More recent, acute techniques such as the **wick-in-needle** and **servo-null micropipette** methods (Figure 11.10) confirm that interstitial fluid pressure is indeed slightly subatmospheric in many tissues, including the skin and subcutis, relaxed muscle, joint spaces and epidural space (-1 to -3 mmHg). Pressure is above atmospheric in the kidney ($+1$ to $+10$ mmHg), myocardium, bone marrow and flexed joints.

11.6 Fluid balance: filtration versus absorption

Having covered the four pressures that influence fluid exchange, we can now address the problem of tissue volume homeostasis. In other words, how is an accumulation of capillary filtrate in the interstitium avoided? A major factor in volume homeostasis is undoubtedly lymphatic drainage. A second possibility, long believed in but now contradicted by a substantial body of evidence, is that venous capillaries are continuously reabsorbing most of the filtrate generated by arterial capillaries.

Lymph drains away the filtration fraction

Virtually all tissues form lymph. Even the lungs generate lymph, despite the capillary pressures being smaller than the plasma COP. The continuous formation of lymph proves that there is normally a net filtration of fluid out of the microcirculation, and thus a net imbalance of the Starling pressures along the capillary. The ratio of lymph flow to plasma flow gives the fraction of plasma water that escapes during transit through the capillary (the **filtration fraction**). The filtration fraction is only $\sim$0.2–0.3% in most tissues. However, since $\sim$4000 l of plasma pass through the human microcirculation over the course of a day, a small filtration fraction generates a large volume of lymph, namely $\sim$4–8 l/day. In certain circumstance (fenestrated vessels in the renal glomerulus and salivary gland; high filtration pressures in the feet) the filtration fraction can be a hundred times higher, e.g. 20% in glomerular capillaries.

Filtration rate decays as blood passes along the capillary

Blood pressure falls from $\sim$35 mmHg in arterial capillaries to $\sim$15 mmHg in venous capillaries and venules. As a result, the filtration rate dwindles progressively along the capillary axis. Since the inlet and outlet pressures straddle the plasma COP of 25 mmHg (Figure 11.11, top left), it was traditionally held that arterial capillaries filter fluid and venous capillaries continuously reabsorb most of it, thus preserving tissue volume. This view is

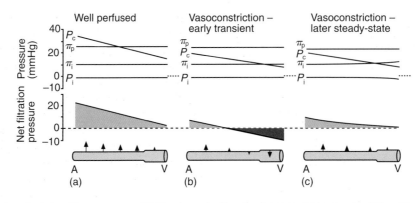

Figure 11.11 Axial gradient of capillary pressure and fluid exchange in skin, muscle or mesenteric microcirculation at heart level. Shaded area is sum of Starling pressures, $(P_c - P_i) - \sigma(\pi_p - \pi_i)$. Arrows indicate transcapillary flow; A, arterial end of capillary; V, venules. (a) Filtration along entire length of a well-perfused capillary. (Data from Levick, J. R. (1991) *Experimental Physiology*, **76**, 825–857.) (b) Transient absorption immediately after arteriolar constriction or haemorrhage, due to fall in P_c. (c) Loss of absorption with time due to rise in π_i and fall in P_i. See text for symbols.

not supported by modern evidence. Figure 11.11 shows the measured Starling pressures along a capillary in muscle, mesentery or warm skin at heart level. Blood pressure in venous capillaries does indeed fall below plasma COP, but plasma COP is not the net absorption pressure; the latter depends also on the COP and fluid pressure outside the capillary (Starling principle, eqn 11.3). When interstitial COP and pressure are taken into account, the venous capillaries have a net filtration pressure (Figure 11.11, bottom left).

The Starling equation, eqn 11.3, predicts that the capillary filtration rate will be zero when the blood pressure P_c equals the net opposing pressure, namely $\sigma(\pi_p - \pi_i) + P_i$. The net opposing pressure is 12.5 mmHg in Figure 11.11a (ignoring for the moment any gradients at the pore exits). The blood pressure in the venous capillaries and venules is greater than 12.5 mmHg, so the venous exchange vessels are in a state of slight filtration, not absorption. Figure 11.12, which shows data from 12 tissues, confirms that venular blood pressure generally exceeds the net opposing pressure $\sigma(\pi_p - \pi_i) + P_i$. This indicates that **well-perfused capillaries are normally in a state of filtration along their entire length**, with the filtration rate dwindling to close to zero at the venular end.

The traditional textbook dogma that venous capillaries are normally in a state of sustained absorption is not supported by direct measurements of the Starling pressures (Figure 11.12), nor by direct observations of fluid exchange (next section), nor by theory, and must be abandoned for most tissues.

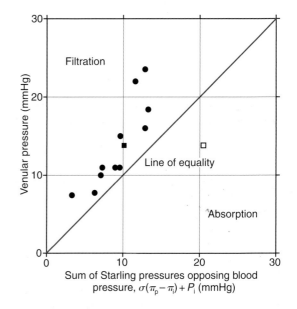

Figure 11.12 Comparison of venular pressure and the opposing pro-absorption Starling pressures in 12 tissues, including muscle, skin and joints (filled symbols). Dog lung is the lowest, left point; cat mesentery the highest, right point. The filled square represents fasting rat intestinal mucosa. The unfilled square shows the switch to absorption in mucosal capillaries, due to a fall in π_i and rise in P_i, after the rat drank some water. (Data from many laboratories summarized by Levick, J. R. and Mortimer, P. S. (1999); see Further Reading.)

Venous capillaries absorb fluid transiently when pressure falls

The exchange vessels can absorb fluid for a while if the normal Starling pressures are disturbed, as Starling showed in his seminal experiment (Section 11.1).

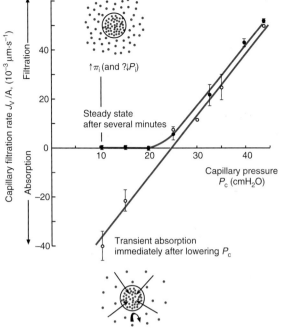

Figure 11.13 Demonstration that capillary pressures below plasma COP (32 cmH$_2$O here) generate a transient but not sustained absorption. Method as in Figure 11.2. Upon lowering capillary pressure to venular levels, there was transient fluid absorption (open circles) but after several minutes of capillary perfusion at low pressure the absorption ceased (closed circles). *Inset sketch, bottom, shows peri-capillary protein (red dots) being reflected (curved arrow) during water absorption (long arrows), leading to a rise in pericapillary protein concentration (upper sketch).* (Adapted from Michel, C. C. and Phillips, M. E. (1987) *Journal of Physiology*, **388**, 421–435, by permission.)

Precapillary vasoconstriction or, in a clinical setting **haemorrhage**, can reduce the capillary pressure sufficiently for absorption to develop transiently (Figure 11.11b). Absorption is not well maintained, however, because the selective absorption of interstitial water raises the protein concentration in the pericapillary space and endothelial clefts, raising π_i. Absorption also makes P_i more subatmospheric. The changing interstitial forces gradually abolish the net absorptive force, so absorption fades away with time and a state of slight filtration is restored, as in Figure 11.11c.

The experiment in Figure 11.13 shows that absorption is not sustained at capillary pressures below the plasma COP. Capillary pressure was deliberately lowered to venular levels and held there. At first there was a transient absorption of fluid, in agreement with the Starling principle. Within a few minutes, however, absorption ceased. There is a sound **theoretical reason** for this, namely that the protein concentration and COP around a leaky semipermeable membrane depend on filtration rate (the interstitial dilution relation, Figure 11.8). If filtration rate declines or stops, plasma proteins accumulate outside the membrane. This reduces the difference in COP across the membrane. As a result absorption at low capillary pressure should in theory dwindle and eventually cease, as was indeed observed.

Fluid exchange in the lung. The lung generates lymph. This is an example of filtration out of capillaries at a pressure ($\sim$10 mmHg) that is well below plasma COP (25 mmHg). Filtration occurs because the interstitial protein concentration is $\sim$70% of that in plasma, with an interstitial COP of 16–20 mmHg. The difference in COP across the capillary wall (5–9 mmHg) is smaller than the capillary pressure. Fluid exchange in the lung is on the flat part of the steady-state line of Figure 11.13.

How is the net filtration rate kept low?

In most tissues the rate of production of lymph (a measure of net filtration rate) is low. For example, the human foot in the supine position overnight produces only 0.22 ml lymph per 100 g per hour. To account for this, the sum of the four Starling pressures averaged over time and distance must be small, around 1 mmHg or less. This may be due to two factors, pore exit microgradients and vasomotion.

Pore exit microgradients. The emerging stream of ultrafiltrate at the exits of the small pores dilutes the interstitial protein very locally, i.e. inside the intercellular cleft and in the immediate pericapillary region. This reduces the COP acting on the small pore exits and so reduces the filtration rate. It is becoming increasingly clear that it is the properties of the space close to the small pore exit, rather than the properties of the entire interstitium, that govern fluid movement.

Vasomotion is the cycling of arterioles between a dilated state and constricted state. This occurs several times per minute in a regular cycle in some tissues, such as skeletal muscle. Since capillary pressure is influenced by precapillary resistance (Figure 11.4), each constrictor phase reduces the capillary pressure, which may cause a transient absorption of fluid. Such a microcirculation will alternate between states (a) and (b) in Figure 11.11, reducing the time-averaged filtration force and lymph formation rate.

Tissues with an independent fluid input can sustain fluid absorption

Sustained absorption of fluid into the microcirculation is a normal feature of **intestinal mucosal**

The Starling principle of fluid exchange

■ Capillary filtration rate per unit area depends on four Starling pressures: *capillary blood pressure* minus *interstitial fluid pressure*, which is opposed by *plasma colloid osmotic pressure* (COP) minus *interstitial COP*.

■ Filtration rate also depends on the *hydraulic conductance* and *osmotic reflection coefficient* of the endothelium.

■ In most tissues the Starling pressures add up to a *net filtration force*, even in venous capillaries or lungs. This generates interstitial fluid and lymph.

■ *Osmotic absorption* occurs transiently when capillary pressure is reduced by precapillary vasoconstriction and/or hypovolaemia. Absorption is transient because absorption raises the abluminal COP and reduces interstitial pressure.

■ Oedema is caused by ↑ capillary pressure (e.g. heart failure), or ↓ plasma COP (e.g. malnutrition), or ↑ endothelial conductance and ↓ reflection coefficient (inflammation), or ↓ lymphatic drainage (e.g. postmastectomy oedema).

capillaries after drinking water, as indicated by the unfilled square in Figure 11.12. It also occurs in **peritubular capillaries** as part of normal renal function, and in **lymph node capillaries** (see later). Sustained absorption is possible when the interstitial space has an independent input of fluid, such as water from the gut lumen or from renal tubules or from afferent lymphatics. Part of the fluid serves to flush the interstitial space and prevent the accumulation of interstitial plasma protein, thus abolishing the inverse link between interstitial protein concentration and capillary filtration rate of Figure 11.8. (This was essentially what Starling did in his seminal demonstration of fluid absorption; Section 11.1.) In the intestine 80% of the water transferred into the tissue from the gut lumen is absorbed into the microcirculation, while the other 20% acts as a flushing solution that lowers π_i and raises P_i to maintain the net absorptive force. The flushing solution drains into the lymphatic system.

11.7 Interstitial compliance and conductivity: effects of oedema

There are 10–12 l of fluid in the human interstitial compartment, which serves as a reservoir for the plasma compartment (3 l). If the plasma volume is reduced by a haemorrhage, there is a transient absorption of fluid from the interstitial compartment to top up the plasma compartment. Conversely, if plasma volume is increased by over-infusion or renal retention of fluid, excess fluid spills over into the interstitium, increasing the interstitial volume. The effect of the fluid transfer on interstitial fluid pressure depends on the shape of the interstitial pressure–volume relation, or compliance curve.

The interstitial compliance curve flattens out in the oedema zone

Normal range. Figure 11.14 shows the non-linear relation between interstitial fluid volume and pressure in subcutaneous interstitium, which is a common site for clinical oedema. In normally hydrated tissue the interstitial pressure is subatmospheric, and a small change in volume alters the pressure markedly. The pressure–volume relation is steep and the interstitial compliance (volume change per unit pressure change) is small. This is because a change in the water content alters the GAG concentration and hence the gel swelling pressure (Section 11.5).

Oedematous range. If sufficient fluid is added, the glycosaminoglycans become so dilute that the swelling pressure becomes negligible. The interstitial fluid pressure is close to atmospheric pressure at this point. The further addition of fluid cannot lower the swelling pressure any more. Consequently, the interstitium can now accommodate increasing volumes of fluid with relatively little change in pressure; the pressure–volume relation is flat and the interstitial compliance is ~20 times higher than normal. This is the situation in an oedematous limb. The slight rise in pressure with volume is due to the distension of the loose collagen and elastin network. In an oedematous leg about 98% of the excess fluid is found in the subcutaneous plane and the pressure is just above atmospheric (Table 11.1). In tissues that are confined within an inelastic fibrous capsule, such as the anterolateral muscle compartment of the leg, the pressure–volume curve is steeper and interstitial fluid pressure can reach higher levels.

The pitting test reveals increased interstitial hydraulic conductivity in oedema

Water normally makes up 65–99% of the interstitium by weight, depending on the tissue. Even so, it is not easily displaced because interstitial GAGs at a physiological concentration create a low hydraulic

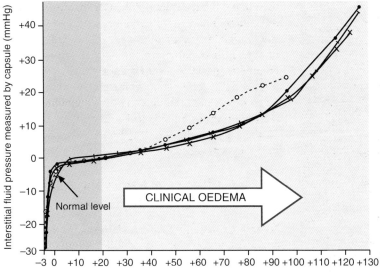

Figure 11.14 The interstitial compliance curve. Pressure was recorded in a subcutaneous capsule in four dog hindlimbs (mean −6 mmHg). Changes in interstitial volume were assessed by changes in leg weight. Absorption was induced by hyperosmotic dextran solution i.v. and oedema by perfusing with saline at raised venous pressure. Clinical oedema was detected at +20% leg weight, corresponding to an estimated 300% rise in subcutaneous fluid volume. (From Guyton, A. C. (1965) *Circulation Research*, **16**, 452, by permission.)

conductivity (Section 11.5). The hydraulic conductivity depends on the water content expressed as a volume fraction or 'porosity' ε, and the surface area of the fixed biopolymers S, which is the source of hydraulic resistance. The ratio ε/S is called the mean hydraulic radius, and as noted earlier it ranges from 3 nm in articular cartilage to 300 nm in the vitreous body of the eye.

Interstitial conductivity rises sharply as the ratio ε/S is increased by hydration. Conductivity is very large when pools of free fluid are present, as in clinical oedema. Increased conductivity is the basis of a clinical test for subcutaneous oedema called the **pitting test**. When finger pressure is applied to normal skin for a minute, no impression is made because the interstitial fluid mobility is very low and little fluid is displaced. In an oedematous tissue, by contrast, the conductivity is high and fluid is rapidly displaced, creating a distinct pit in the tissue (Figure 11.15).

Solute transport and exclusion in interstitium

Small solutes such as O_2 and glucose diffuse freely through the spaces between the interstitial proteoglycans. Macromolecules such as albumin experience restricted diffusion and steric exclusion in the interstitial matrix. See Section 10.3 for an explanation of these terms. Albumin is sterically excluded from 20–50% of the water in subcutaneous and muscle interstitium. As a result the effective interstitial protein concentration, namely the mass of protein divided by the available water volume, is higher than the apparent concentration (mass

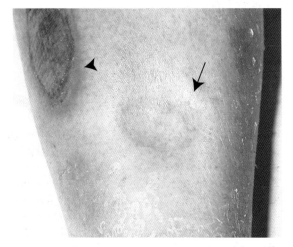

Figure 11.15 Photograph of back of calf (the ankle is off lower edge of picture) to show pitting oedema (arrow), in a patient with cardiac failure. The oedema was exacerbated by dependency. Note the skin damage (arrowhead, *top left*) caused by an oedema blister. (Courtesy of Professor P. Mortimer, Department of Dermatology, St. George's Hospital, London.)

divided by total water volume). Protein is transported through the interstitial space to the lymphatic system by convection, i.e. wash-along in the stream of capillary filtrate.

11.8 Lymph and the lymphatic system

The lymphatic system was explored in the 1650s by Rudbeckius, Bartholin and others. Its three main functions are as follows.

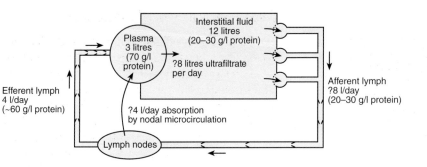

Figure 11.16 Estimate of extra-vascular circulation of fluid and plasma protein in a 65 kg human. (After Renkin, E. M. (1986) *American Journal of Physiology*, **250**, H706–H710.)

- **Preservation of fluid balance.** Lymph vessels return the capillary ultrafiltrate and escaped plasma proteins to the bloodstream by draining into the neck veins. This completes the extravascular circulation of fluid and protein (Figure 11.16) and maintains tissue volume homeostasis. If lymphatic function is impaired, the tissue develops a severe, protein-rich form of oedema called **lymphoedema**.

- **Nutritional function.** Intestinal lymph vessels called lacteals absorb and transport tiny globules of digested fat called chylomicra (Figure 11.17).

- **Defence function.** As fluid drains from the interstitium, it carries foreign materials such as antigens, viruses, bacteria, carbon particles, etc. to the lymph nodes (Figure 11.17). Lymph drainage thus provides an effective and economical method for immuno-surveillance of the tissues. The lymph nodes filter out and phagocytose particulate matter, giving rise to blackened lung nodes of smokers and coal miners. Bacterial and viral antigens activate lymphocytes in the node and stimulate their release into the efferent (postnodal) lymph for transport to the bloodstream. Efferent lymph thus has a higher white cell content than afferent (prenodal) lymph.

Structure of lymphatic vessels

Lymphatic capillaries

The lymphatic system begins as microscopic lymphatic capillaries, which form an initial lymphatic network. This can take the form of an anastomosing set of tubes of diameter 10–50 μm, as in the skin, or blind-ended sacs as in the intestinal villi (Figure 11.17). The wall comprises a single layer of endothelial cells and incomplete basement membrane. Some

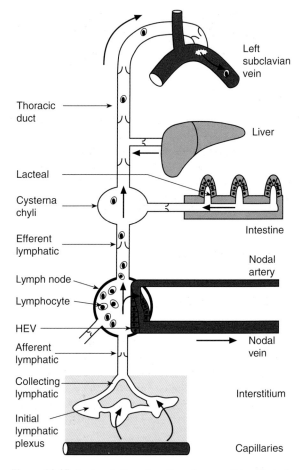

Figure 11.17 The lymphatic system. Curved arrow within node indicates absorption of some water by nodal capillaries. HEV, high endothelial venule where circulating lymphocytes re-enter the node.

of the endothelial intercellular clefts are 14 nm or more wide, so interstitial proteins and fine particles readily enter the lymphatic capillaries. Due to its oblique orientation the intercellular cleft may act as flap valve, allowing fluid into the lumen when lymph pressure is low but closing when lymph pressure rises above interstitial pressure (Figure 11.18). The outer surface of the wall is tethered to the surrounding tissues by radiating fibrils, the **anchoring**

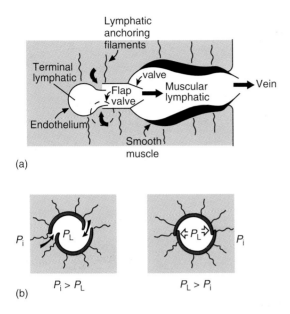

Figure 11.18 Simplified model for lymphatic transport. (a) Interstitial fluid enters the initial lymphatic down a pressure gradient. Each muscular segment pumps lymph into the next one and ultimately into the venous system. (b) Proposed operation of endothelial junctions in the initial lymphatics as flap valves. P_i, interstitial pressure; P_L, lymph pressure. (From Granger, H. J., *et al.* (1984) In *Edema* (eds Staub, N. C. and Taylor, A. E.), pp. 189–228, see Further Reading, by permission.)

filaments, which help to dilate the vessels in oedematous tissues.

Collecting and afferent lymphatics

The initial lymphatic network drains into collecting vessels. These feed into afferent lymph trunks that run alongside major blood vessels. **Semilunar valves** direct the lymph centrally. From the collecting vessel onwards the lymphatic wall acquires a coat of smooth muscle. Such vessels are actively contractile. The smooth muscle is abundant in man and ruminants but scanty in dogs and rabbits.

Lymph nodes

Multiple afferent vessels enter the hilum of a lymph node. The node is a highly cellular mass of lymphocytes and phagocytic cells permeated by a network of sinuses that carry the lymph flow. The sinuses are endothelial tubes with gaps that allow lymphocytes to enter the lymph. The node is supplied with nutrients by continuous capillaries. The nodal capillaries drain into special **high-endothelial venules**. Lymphocytes in the blood penetrate the intercellular junctions of the high-endothelial venules to re-enter the node, thus completing their own unique circulation.

Efferent lymphatics and the thoracic duct

Lymphocyte-rich efferent lymph from the legs and viscera is pumped into a large lymphatic trunk on the posterior abdominal wall. This possesses a saccular dilatation called the **cisterna chyli**, which acts as a temporary receptacle for chyle; chyle is the fatty lymph formed in intestinal lacteals after a fatty meal. The ultimate lymphatic trunk, the thoracic duct, receives around three-quarters of the body's efferent lymph. The thoracic duct empties into the left subclavian vein at its junction with the jugular vein. Smaller cervical and right lymphatic trunks carry a smaller flow from the head and neck.

The initial lymphatics may fill by a squeeze-and-recoil mechanism

Prenodal lymph is simply interstitial fluid that has entered the lymphatic capillary. The filling mechanism is unclear, but may resemble that of a Pasteur pipette, where one first squeezes the rubber bulb empty (phase 1) and then allows its recoil to suck up fluid (phase 2). According to this lymphatic suction theory, the initial lymphatic plexus is first emptied by compression caused by tissue movement, and then re-expands due to the tension in the tethering filaments. The elastic recoil of the filaments and wall reduce the intra-lymphatic pressure below interstitial fluid pressure and the pressure gradient drives interstitial fluid into the lymphatic system (Figure 11.19).

Lymph flow is coupled to capillary filtration rate

The rate of lymph formation is coupled to interstitial fluid pressure and volume (Figure 11.20). The higher the interstitial fluid pressure and volume, the greater is the lymph flow, up to a limit. Since interstitial pressure and volume are influenced by capillary filtration rate, they provide the vital link between capillary filtration rate and lymph flow. A link is essential in order to match lymph drainage rate to capillary filtration rate and thus avoid oedema.

Extrinsic and intrinsic mechanisms contribute to lymph flow

Lymph has to be pumped along the lymphatic system. It will not flow spontaneously because the pressure at the venous outlet is higher than in the initial lymphatics. In the collecting lymphatics and more proximal vessels, smooth muscle pumps the lymph along. The initial lymphatics generally lack smooth

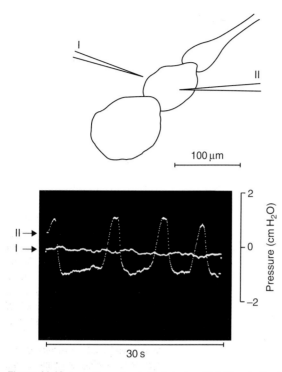

Figure 11.19 Lympatic suction in the bat wing. (*Top*) Micropipettes in the interstitium and a contractile lymphatic recorded the interstitium-to-lymph pressure gradient. (*Bottom*) Interstitial pressure (I) exceeded lymph pressure (II) for 43% of the time, because lymph pressure fell to subatmospheric levels during relaxation. (From Hogan, R. D. (1981) In *Interstitial Fluid Pressure and Composition* (ed. Hargens, A. R.), Williams and Wikins, Baltimore, pp. 155–163, by permission.)

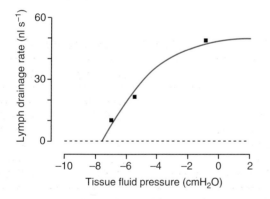

Figure 11.20 Effect of increasing tissue fluid pressure upon lymphatic drainage rate from pleural and peritoneal spaces in rabbits. The relation is crucial to preventing fluid accumulation in extravascular compartments. (Based on Miserocchi, G., Negrini, D., Mukenge, P., Turconi, P. and Del Fabbro, M. (1989) *Journal of Applied Physiology*, **66**, 1579–1585; and Miserocchi, G. and Negrini, D. (1997) In *The Lung* (eds Crystal, R. G., West, J. B., *et al.*), Lippincott–Raven, Philadelphia.)

muscle, however, and extrinsic pumping is important here. Since the initial lymphatics are in series with the muscular lymphatics, both extrinsic and intrinsic propulsion are necessary overall.

Extrinsic propulsion

Lymph flow in non-contractile vessels is brought about by intermittent compression of the lymphatics by tissue movements – for example, by the contraction of skeletal muscle, or peristalsis in the intestine, or the pulsation of adjacent arteries in connective tissue. The flow of lymph from the leg of an anaesthetized dog is greatly increased by passive movements of the leg, demonstrating the power of extrinsic propulsion.

Intrinsic propulsion

Lymphatic vessels with abundant smooth muscle, as in the human leg, show spontaneous, rhythmic contractions at ~8–15 cycles per minute (Figure 11.21a). Successive segments of the vessel behave like mini-hearts linked in series, and the pumping cycle has striking similarities to the cardiac cycle. Each segment has pacemaker cells that trigger local action potentials leading to contraction. The action potentials are generated by L-type Ca^{2+} channels and fast Na^+ channels. Contraction is preceded by a diastolic filling phase, with the distal valve open and the proximal valve closed. This is followed by an isovolumetric contraction phase (all valves closed), an ejection phase (proximal valve open; ejection fraction ~25%) and an isovolumetric relaxation phase (all valves closed). Thus the segment traces out a pressure–volume loop analogous to that of the heart (Figure 11.21b).

Human leg lymphatic vessels can pump to at least 40–50 mmHg. This is an important snippet of information when dealing with **envenomation**, for example a snake bite. A tourniquet pressure of 40–70 mmHg is required to prevent the transmission of venom up the human lymphatic system.

Lymphatic contractions are regulated by filling pressure and catecholamines

The frequency of contraction, and to a limited degree stroke volume, increase with **distension**. This enables a given lymphatic segment to increase its output in response to an increased input from a more distal segment. The maximal output of isolated lymphatics is reached at a diastolic distending pressure of ~4–8 cmH2O, beyond which the stroke volume and output begin to fall.

The larger lymphatic vessels are innervated by **sympathetic noradrenergic nerves**. Sympathetic nerve activity and circulating adrenaline both increase the frequency of lymphatic contraction. After a haemorrhage, lymphatic frequency and

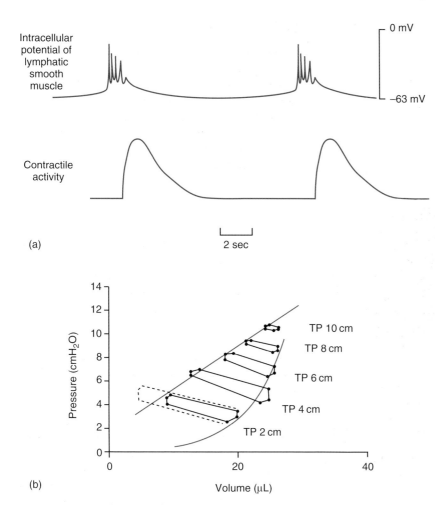

(a)

2 sec

(b)

Figure 11.21 Electrical and contractile properties of lymphatic smooth muscle. (a) Periodic bursts of action potentials and contractions in an isolated bovine lymphatic trunk. (Redrawn from work of McHale, N. and colleagues (1977) *Journal of Physiology*, **272**, 33P–34P; and (1991) *Journal of Physiology*, **438**, 168P, by permission.) (b) Pressure–volume cycle of contracting sheep mesenteric lymphatic vessels at various diastolic distensions (TP, transmural pressure). Dashed loop shows increased contractility and ejection fraction after a haemorrhage. (Adapted from Li, B., Silver, I., Szalai, J. P. and Johnston, M. G. (1998) *Microvascular Research*, **56**, 127–138, by permission.)

contractility are increased, the ejection fraction rises to around 40% and the transfer of interstitial fluid into the depleted circulation is enhanced (Figure 11.21b, dashed loop).

Lymph nodes absorb some of the lymph

The concentration of plasma protein in postnodal lymph from the legs of dogs and sheep is up to twice as great as in the prenodal lymph. This is chiefly due to the absorption of water by blood capillaries in the node. Postnodal lymph is unrepresentative, therefore, of interstitial fluid composition or filtration rate. Estimates of fluid turnover in humans, which were formerly based on thoracic duct lymph flow, have been revised upwards in light of this. A plausible estimate of the extravascular circulation in humans is presented in Figure 11.16. However, the exact proportion of human afferent lymph that is absorbed by nodes is unknown, and probably depends on posture, since nodal capillary pressure must increase with dependency.

Table 11.2 Postnodal lymph flow and composition in man.

	Flow * (%)	L/P †
Thoracic duct	(1–3 l/day)	0.66–0.69
Liver	30–49%	0.66–0.89
Gastrointestinal	~37%	0.50–0.62
Kidney	6–11%	0.47
Lungs	3–15%	0.66–0.69
Limbs and cervical trunks	<10%	0.23–0.58

* Expressed as percentage of total thoracic duct flow.
† Concentration of protein in postnodal lymph relative to plasma.
(From Joffey, J. M. and Courtice, F. C. (1970) *Lymphatics, Lymph and the Lymphomyeloid Complex*, Academic Press, London.)

The flow and composition of lymph shows regional variations

Postnodal lymph flow in the human thoracic duct averages 1–3 l per day. Of this, the liver contributes 30–50% (Table 11.2). Hepatic lymph is particularly

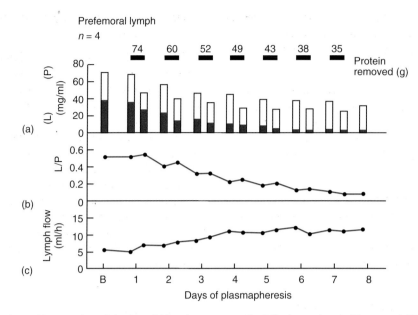

Figure 11.22 Experimental hypoproteinaemia in sheep. (a) Protein was removed by daily plasmapheresis (the removal of blood and replacement of only the cells, water and electrolytes). This caused protein concentration in the plasma to fall (P, top of white bars). (b) The concentration of protein fell relatively further in postnodal leg lymph (L, red bars), so the L/P ratio fell. (c) Lymph flow, an indication of capillary filtration rate, more than doubled. These data illustrate the operation of two **safety factors against oedema formation**, namely dilution of interstitial protein (lowering the pericapillary COP) and increased lymphatic drainage. (From Kramer, G., *et al.* In Renkin, E. M. (1986) *American Journal of Physiology*, **250**, H706–H710, by permission.)

rich in plasma protein due to the discontinuities in hepatic capillaries. Intestinal lymph flow is abundant after a meal and makes the second greatest contribution to thoracic duct flow. Lung and renal lymph flows are substantial too. The limbs contribute a variable quantity of lymph depending on exercise intensity. The concentration of plasma protein in lymph varies from region to region and depends on the permeability and reflection coefficient of the capillaries, the molecular size and charge of the individual protein and the capillary filtration rate (Figures 11.8, 11.22).

11.9 Challenges to fluid balance: orthostasis and exercise

Two physiological events can increase the capillary filtration rate sufficiently to cause a fall in plasma volume. They are orthostasis, which is the adoption of an upright position (sitting or standing) and physical exercise.

Orthostasis causes dependent swelling and plasma volume reduction

During orthostasis the increase in capillary pressure below heart level raises the filtration rate into dependent tissues. Swelling of the feet is a common experience during long-haul flights or in the cinema, and people often unlace their shoes on this account. The foot swells initially at ~30 ml/h. Over the course of 15–40 min of standing the increased plasma ultrafiltration into dependent tissues reduces the plasma volume by 6–20%, with a concomitant haemoconcentration. For example, the plasma COP of university students increases from 25 mmHg to 29 mmHg over the course of an 8-h period of sitting in lectures, reading, etc.

Dependent swelling and the decline in plasma volume would be considerably worse were it not for the following compensatory mechanisms.

- **Postural vasoconstriction.** Precapillary vasoconstriction in the dependent tissue raises R_A/R_V and thus attenuates the rise in dependent capillary pressure (Figure 11.5). This is a local reaction mediated by the myogenic response (Section 13.2) and veni-arteriolar response (Section 15.3).

- **Local haemoconcentration.** Postural vasoconstriction reduces the local blood flow (Figure 8.6). The low plasma flow, in conjunction with the increased filtration pressure, increases the filtration fraction. The latter can be as high as 20–27% in the foot during standing.

The ensuing local haemoconcentration raises the plasma COP in the venous capillaries to 35–44 mmHg, which attenuates the raised filtration rate.

- **Reduced capillary filtration capacity.** The contraction of some terminal arterioles may stop flow completely through capillary modules for short periods, thereby reducing the capillary filtration capacity. The evidence for this is conflicting in limbs.

- **The skeletal muscle pump.** Dynamic exercise in the upright position reduces venous pressure in the active limbs (Figure 8.23), which in turn reduces capillary pressure. The movement also enhances **lymph transport**.

Exercise causes muscle swelling and plasma volume reduction

People working out on weights at the gym notice that skeletal muscle swells rapidly and dramatically during intense exercise. Likewise rock-climbers, for reasons not unconnected with their well-being, become keenly aware of swollen, pumped forearm muscles during steep, fingery climbs. A 20% increase in muscle volume over 15 min is not uncommon. The causes of swelling are as follows:

- **Local dilatation of the resistance vessels** in active skeletal muscle raises the blood flow, but by reducing R_A/R_V it also raises the capillary pressure and filtration rate (Figure 11.4).

- **Capillary recruitment** in exercising muscle enhances O_2 transport, but it raises the capillary filtration capacity too (Figure 10.14). The above two changes account for only a small part, however, of the swelling.

- **Increased interstitial osmolarity** is the chief cause. The release of small solutes such as lactate and K^+ into the interstitial space by the contracting muscle fibres raises the interstitial fluid osmolarity by 20–30 mmol/l, i.e. by 7–10%. This corresponds to an increased crystalloid osmotic pressure of 380–580 mmHg (see van't Hoff's law, Appendix 2). This osmotic pressure is exerted across the **water-only aquaporin channels** of the endothelial cell. Although the conductance of these channels is low, the osmotic force is so large that the net filtration rate increases substantially. Since the aquaporin reflection coefficient is 1, the venous

effluent from active muscle has a raised Na^+ concentration.

The osmolarity of the sarcoplasm too increases during muscle contraction, due to the breakdown of creatine phosphate and the formation of lactate. Consequently, intracellular swelling contributes to the muscle swelling.

During hard exercise involving numerous large muscle groups, for example strenuous cycling, human muscle volume can expand by up to 1100 ml, and the plasma volume falls by as much as 600 ml (20%). The relative preservation of plasma volume is brought about by a compensatory absorption of interstitial fluid from non-exercising tissues into the plasma compartment, which minimizes the fall in blood volume during exercise.

11.10 Oedema

Oedema is an excess of interstitial fluid. In clinical practice common sites for oedema are subcutaneous tissue (peripheral oedema), the lungs (pulmonary oedema), the abdominal cavity (ascites) and other body cavities (synovial, pericardial and pleural effusions). Inflammation can cause oedema in almost any tissue.

In **subcutaneous oedema** the tissue is on the flat part of the compliance curve of Figure 11.14, so increased filtration evokes little opposing rise in interstitial fluid pressure. The oedema is not usually detected until the interstitial volume has doubled, which corresponds to about a 10% swelling of the limb. Peripheral oedema impairs cell nutrition due to increased diffusion distance, causes deformity, discomfort and impaired limb usage, and may cause skin ulceration and blistering (Figure 11.15).

Pulmonary oedema is commonly caused by left ventricular failure, which elevates the left ventricular filling pressure and therefore pulmonary venous pressure. The stiff oedematous lung is difficult to inflate, causing the symptom dyspnoea (difficulty in breathing). In extreme cases the interstitial oedema spills over into the alveolar spaces, with fatal results.

Causes of oedema

Oedema inevitably develops if the capillary filtration rate exceeds the lymphatic drainage rate for a sufficient period, as shown by the relation:

Tissue swelling rate =
(Capillary filtration rate − Lymphatic drainage rate)

Oedema can thus arise from a high filtration rate or a low lymph flow. Since filtration is governed by the Starling equation, eqn 11.3, the latter provides a logical scheme for classifying oedema, as follows.

Raised capillary pressure, P_c

Capillary pressure increases when venous pressure is raised. This happens chronically in:

- right ventricular failure
- over-transfusion
- deep venous thrombosis
- dependent tissues (ankles, sacral region).

Pressures of 20–40 mmHg can develop in the venous limbs of skin capillaries during right ventricular failure. The resulting oedema fluid has a low protein concentration, 1–10 g/l, due to the interstitial dilution relation of Figure 11.8.

Reduced plasma COP, π_p

Clinical oedema develops when the plasma protein concentration falls below ~30 g/l. The fall in plasma COP raises the capillary filtration rate, as indicated by increased lymph flow (Figure 11.22). The interstitial protein concentration falls to 1–6 g/l. The reduced interstitial COP and increased lymph flow both help to attenuate the oedema. Hypoproteinaemia can arise from:

- malnutrition (inadequate protein intake);
- intestinal disease (malabsorption and protein loss);
- nephrotic syndrome (leakage of albumin into urine, often at >20 g/day, due to glomerular membrane breakdown);
- hepatic failure (failure to synthesize albumin, fibrinogen, α-globulin and β-globulin).

Hepatic failure often results from cirrhosis. Hepatic cirrhosis is a fibrotic condition in which the oedema is typically intra-abdominal (ascites) because there is a rise in portal vein pressure as well as a fall in plasma COP.

Increased capillary permeability ($\uparrow L_p$, $\downarrow \sigma$, $\uparrow P_{protein}$)

Inflammation involves the breakdown of the endothelial barrier. The hydraulic conductance and protein permeability increase and the reflection coefficient decreases. This causes a severe form of oedema with a high protein content, >30 g/l (Section 11.11).

Lymphatic insufficiency

Impaired lymphatic drainage causes the accumulation of plasma proteins as well as fluid in the tissue spaces, because lymph is the sole means of returning escaped plasma proteins to the circulation. Consequently lymphoedema is characterized by a protein content of >30 g/l. Chronic lymphoedema is associated with the deposition of a fibrous adipose tissue in the interstitium, as a result of which chronic lymphoedema may not pit easily ('brawny' non-pitting oedema). In Western countries lymphatic insufficiency is usually due either to the poor development of limb lymph trunks (**idiopathic lymphoedema**) or to damage to the lymph nodes by surgery and radiotherapy during **cancer treatment** (Figure 11.23). The commonest cause world-wide, however, is **filariasis**, a nematode worm infestation transmitted by mosquitoes. The

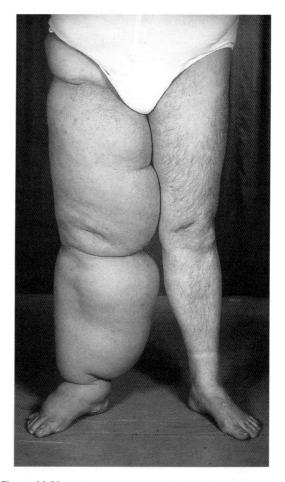

Figure 11.23 Lymphoedema caused by surgery to treat testicular cancer. (Courtesy of Professor P. Mortimer, Department of Dermatology, St. George's Hospital, London.)

nematodes impair lymphatic function in the limbs and scrotum, causing a gross lymphoedema associated with hyperkeratotic elephant-like skin (elephantiasis).

Oedema does not develop until a pressure 'safety margin' is exceeded

Clinicians have long recognized that oedema does not become apparent clinically unless the plasma COP or venous pressure have changed by about 15 mmHg. There is thus a margin of safety against oedema of ~15 mmHg. The margin of safety is thought to be due to the operation of three factors that 'buffer' the capillary filtration rate, namely the elevation of interstitial fluid pressure, the reduction of interstitial COP, and the elevation of lymph flow (Figure 11.24).

- **Elevation of interstitial fluid pressure (P_i).** Over the normal part of the interstitial compliance curve, a small increase in interstitial volume causes a relatively large increase in interstitial pressure (Figure 11.14). This reduces the filtration pressure $P_c - P_i$. If P_i is normally -2 mmHg and clinical oedema appears at about $+1$ mmHg, the change in P_i gives a safety margin of 3 mmHg. On the oedema part of the compliance curve, by contrast, large volumes of fluid can accumulate with little increase in pressure.

- **Fall in interstitial COP (π_i).** An increase in capillary ultrafiltration rate reduces the interstitial protein concentration and COP (Figure 11.8). This increases the difference in COP across the capillary wall (Figure 11.24a), which attenuates the capillary filtration rate. This process is most effective as a buffer mechanism if the interstitial protein concentration is normally high, as it is in the lung.

- **Increased lymph flow.** The increase in lymphatic drainage rate with interstitial volume and pressure (Figures 11.20, 11.24) helps to prevent oedema formation. For example, lymph flow increases 20-fold in response to a 30 mmHg elevation of venous pressure in the cat intestine. Clearly, however, there comes at point at which lymph flow cannot keep up with capillary filtration rate, and oedema then develops.

11.11 The swelling of inflammation

The cardinal features of inflammation are swelling, redness, heat, pain, leukocyte emigration and loss of function (Section 9.8). The swelling is caused by a protein-rich oedema that can form very rapidly, causing blisters, rashes, swollen joints, pleural, pericardial and peritoneal effusions, cerebral oedema and the swelling of other organs.

Chemical mediators initiate gap formation in venules

Swelling is triggered by local chemical mediators of inflammation, which are released from a variety of

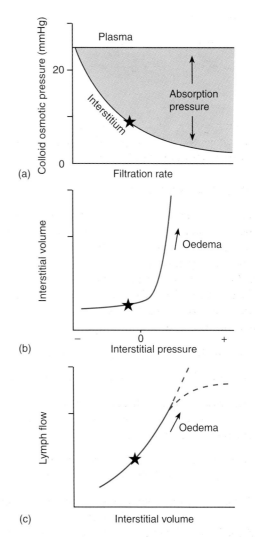

Figure 11.24 Three safety factors against oedema. Stars indicate normal state. (a) When capillary filtration rate increases, the COP difference opposing filtration (absorption pressure) increases too, because interstitial protein concentration falls. (b) Change in interstitial pressure with volume in subcutaneous space. Compliance is very large above atmospheric pressure, so there is little further rise in pressure. This is Figure 11.14 turned on its side. (c) Lymph flow increases with interstitial hydration, opposing oedema formation. Dashed lines indicate that lymph flow reaches a limit in stationary tissue but may not do so in moving flexed limbs. (After Taylor, A. E. and Townsley, M. I. (1987) *News in Physiological Science*, **2**, 48–52.)

tissue cells in response to the primary stimulus, e.g. infection, physical trauma. Mediators include histamine, bradykinin, serotonin, thrombin, substance P and platelet activating factor, all of which are also vasoactive. Superoxide radicals, leukotrienes and cytokines (interleukins, tumour necrosing factor) also trigger inflammation. Cytokines are pro-inflammatory agents secreted by monocytes, fibroblasts and endothelial cells. Severe hypoxia and hypoglycaemia in ischaemic myocardium likewise produce inflammatory changes.

The chemical mediators act primarily on the **postcapillary venule** to cause **endothelial gap formation** (Figures 11.25, 11.26). The gaps greatly increase the venular permeability to water and plasma proteins, leading to an outpouring of protein-rich fluid into the tissue. If fluorescein-labelled macromolecules are injected into the circulation, the leakage sites are seen as 'hot-spots' of extravasated fluorescein around the venules. The greater the inflammatory stimulus, the greater the number of the hot-spots.

In pharmacology the **blueing test** in rat skin is widely used in screening for inflammatory agents. The dye Evans blue is injected into the plasma. Since it binds to albumin, little escapes into normal tissues. If inflammation is present, the dye-albumin complex leaks out rapidly and colours the inflamed region blue.

The inflammatory response to a natural stimulus often shows two phases. Over the first 10–30 min there is a large but transient rise in permeability which then decays (Figure 11.25). This is followed by a second, more sustained increase lasting many hours. Histamine, serotonin and bradykinin cause only a transient increase in permeability whereas thrombin and VEGF can cause a longer-lasting increase.

The extravasated fluid has a high fibrinogen content

The extravasated fluid has a high plasma protein concentration and is often called an **exudate** to distinguish it from the low protein oedema or **transudate** that forms in cardiac failure, venous thrombosis and hypoproteinaemia. Around 30 g/l is considered to be the boundary between transudates and exudates. Inflammatory exudates contain much more fibrinogen than normal due to the lack of molecular size-selectivity at endothelial gaps. The fibrinogen content is clinically important because its conversion into insoluble fibrin clots can cause serious complications, e.g. intestinal adhesions following peritonitis.

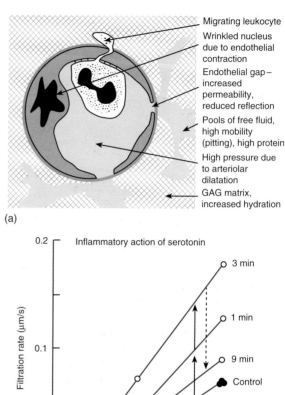

(a)

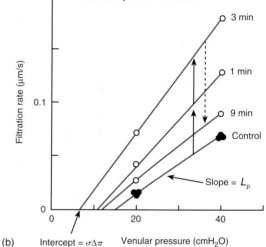

(b)

Figure 11.25 (a) Structural changes during acute inflammation. (b) Effect of a chemical mediator of inflammation, serotonin, on permeability of a single rat venule. Hydraulic permeability increases (slope of relation, L_p) and osmotic reflection coefficient decreases (intercept at zero filtration, $\sigma\Delta\pi$). Although serotonin was infused continuously, the increased permeability was transient, returning towards baseline by 9 min. (Adapted from Michel, C. C. and Kendall, S. (1997) *Journal of Physiology*, **501**, 657–662, by permission.)

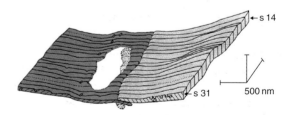

Figure 11.26 Three-dimensional reconstruction of an inflammatory gap in frog endothelium caused by brief heat injury. The gap is transcellular; it passes through the cell on the left, close to but separate from the intercellular junction. The process of an underlying, third cell can be seen through the gap (stippled grey). (Based on electron-micrographs of 18 serial sections by Neale, C. R. and Michel, C. C., by permission.)

Net filtration force and permeability both increase

Exudation is rapid and severe because the chemical mediators of inflammation affect almost every term in the Starling equation (eqn 11.3).

- **Capillary pressure.** The chemical mediators cause arteriolar vasodilatation, which reduces R_A/R_V and thus increases the capillary filtration pressure (Figure 11.4). The vasodilatation also causes the characteristic **reddening** and **heat** of inflammation.

- **Interstitial fluid pressure, P_i.** In established swelling P_i is increased to ~ 2 mmHg above atmospheric pressure and acts as a minor check on filtration. However, in skin and submucosal inflammation P_i falls transiently at the onset of the inflammation, by several mmHg, to a more subatmospheric value, before rising gradually as fluid accumulates. The initial fall in P_i is caused by the release of bonds between fibroblast $\alpha_2\beta_1$-integrins and collagen fibrils. This eliminates the gel-compressing action of the fibroblasts and allows a fuller expression of the glycosaminoglycan swelling pressure. The latter enhances the initial swelling rate.

  In the case of **burns** the fall in P_i at the onset is dramatic and contributes to the remarkably rapid fluid accumulation. Immediately after a burn P_i can fall transiently to -30 mmHg. If fluid extravasation is prevented by circulatory arrest the P_i can fall to around -100 mmHg. The large suction force is attributed to the denaturation of collagen by heat. The resulting gelatin is water-soluble and exerts a gel swelling pressure.

- **Interstitial osmotic pressure.** The interstitial COP increases as plasma proteins leak through the endothelial gaps into the interstitial fluid. This reduces the difference in COP across the wall and thus increases the filtration rate.

- **Osmotic reflection coefficient, σ.** The effectiveness of the residual difference in COP across the endothelium is reduced by a fall in σ, which can decline to ~ 0.4 due to gap formation. The fall in σ is manifested as a leftward shift of the intercept in Figure 11.25.

- **Hydraulic conductance of the wall, L_p.** The above changes greatly increase the net filtration force across the venules, i.e. the term inside the square brackets in eqn 11.3. The effect of the increased filtration force is amplified many fold by an increase in the hydraulic conductance of the wall due to gap formation. L_p can increase two- to seven-fold. The increase in L_p is seen as an increase in slope in Figure 11.25.

The net result of the above five changes is an increase in fluid extravasation rate by up to $50-100$ times. The rapid leakage of plasma, combined with the obstruction of flow by marginating leukocytes (Section 9.8), can cause plugging of the microcirculation by packed columns of red cells (**stasis**).

Endothelial gaps can be intercellular and/or transcellular

The increased hydraulic conductance and protein permeability are caused by the development of gaps up to 1 μm wide in the endothelial lining of postcapillary venules. Figure 11.26 shows one such gap reconstructed from serial electron micrographs. The gap can be **intercellular**, resulting from a separation of the junctions between endothelial cells; or it can be **transcellular** i.e. pass directly through the endothelial cell, close to but not through the intercellular junction. Histamine, serotonin and substance P produce predominantly intercellular gaps, whereas vascular endothelial growth factor, heat injury, excessive pressure, psoriasis and encephalomyelitis produce more transendothelial gaps.

A biochemical cascade transduces the inflammatory stimulus into gap formation

Inflammatory stimuli such as histamine, bradykinin, serotonin and thrombin trigger multiple signalling pathways in the endothelial cell. At present the initial stages are better understood than the final stages.

Increased cytosolic Ca^{2+} is an early step in the cascade

The binding of an agonist to its cognate endothelial receptor activates receptor-operated Ca^{2+} channels (ROCs) and, indirectly, store-operated Ca^{2+} channels (Section 9.3 and below), leading to an influx of extracellular Ca^{2+}. If the force driving extracellular Ca^{2+} influx is reduced by depolarizing the venule with KCl, the rise in cytosolic Ca^{2+} and the rise in hydraulic conductance are reduced in parallel (Figure 11.27). Such observations indicate that extracellular Ca^{2+} is the main source of the elevated cytosolic Ca^{2+}.

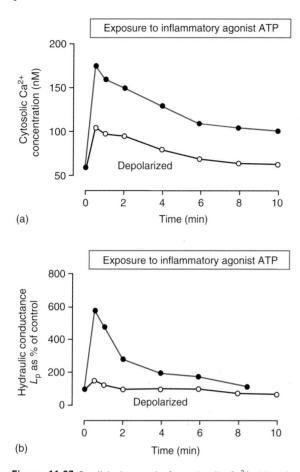

(a)

(b)

Figure 11.27 Parallel changes in free cytosolic Ca^{2+} (a) and hydraulic permeability (b) during the inflammatory response of frog venular endothelium to an inflammatory agonist. ATP was used because frogs do not respond to common mammalian agonists, such as histamine. Depolarization of cells with a high potassium solution (open symbols) greatly reduced the Ca^{2+} transient and the conductance change (see text). (Redrawn from work of He, P., Zhang, X. and Curry, F. E. (1996) *American Journal of Physiology*, **271**, H2377–H2387.)

The agonist–receptor complex activates not only ROCs but also membrane-bound phospholipase C (Figure 11.28). The phospholipase C catalyses the breakdown of phosphatidyl inositol bisphosphate into two cytosolic messengers, inositol trisphosphate (IP_3) and diacylglycerol (DAG). The IP_3 triggers the release of stored Ca^{2+} from the endoplasmic reticulum, and store depletion activates the store-operated Ca^{2+} entry channels of the surface membrane. The DAG activates protein kinase C, a phosphorylating enzyme implicated in some inflammatory responses.

The above mechanisms raise the cytosolic free Ca^{2+} concentration by ~four-fold within a minute. Although this is necessary for the permeability increases, as shown by the experiment in Figure 11.27, it is not sufficient by itself; it is merely a link in a

chain, as shown by the following observation. When the production of nitric oxide is blocked pharmacologically, an inflammatory agonist will still increase the cytosolic Ca^{2+} but this no longer increases the permeability. The cytosolic Ca^{2+} must act, therefore, by triggering nitric oxide formation.

Increased nitric oxide and cyclic GMP are further steps in the cascade

The rise in cytosolic Ca^{2+}, and hence Ca^{2+}-calmodulin complex, activates endothelial nitric oxide synthase. The increased NO production activates guanylyl cyclase, leading to a rise in cyclic guanosine monophosphate, cGMP (Section 9.4). cGMP is a permeability-enhancing messenger in venules, and activates the enzymes phosphodiesterase 2 and protein kinase G.

Phosphodiesterase 2 is more abundant in venular than arterial endothelium, which may help to explain the localization of the inflammatory response to venules. Phosphodiesterase 2 degrades cAMP, a permeability-reducing agent (Section 9.7). cAMP activates protein kinase A, which promotes junctional strand formation and inhibits actin–myosin contraction. Agents that raise the intracellular cAMP concentration, such as the β-adrenoceptor agonists isoprenaline and terbutaline, attenuate inflammatory increases in permeability and reduce endothelial gap formation. Conversely, a fall in cAMP raises the permeability.

Exactly how the changes in protein kinase A, C and G activity lead to gap formation is still under investigation, but both a loosening of the intercellular junctions and endothelial cell contraction are implicated, as follows.

Redistribution of junctional proteins loosens the junctions

Intercellular gap formation is associated with a re-distribution of the key junctional protein VE-cadherin away from the junction, following the phosphorylation of tyrosine groups on the cadherin and associated β-catenin by tyrosine phosphatase (Figure 9.3). There are also changes in the peripheral actin band to which the junctional proteins are attached.

Endothelial cell contraction probably contributes to gap formation

Endothelial contraction was first suspected from the rounding up of cells and nuclear wrinkling in

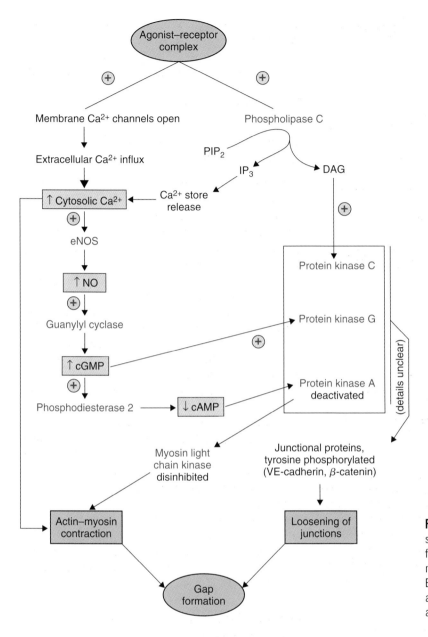

Figure 11.28 Current understanding of the signal transduction cascade leading to gap formation in inflammation. Major second messengers are highlighted in grey boxes. Enzymes are in red. Plus signs denote an activation step. Changes in the peripheral actin band and focal adhesions not shown.

inflamed venules. The raised cytosolic free Ca^{2+} induces contraction by forming Ca^{2+}–calmodulin complex, which activates myosin light chain kinase. The latter activates actin–myosin contraction as in vascular smooth muscle (Section 12.2). Inhibitors of myosin light chain kinase attenuate the hyperpermeability response to agonists. Moreover, myosin light chain kinase is inhibited by cAMP-activated protein kinase A. Therefore, a fall in cAMP during the inflammatory response may facilitate the endothelial contractile response to the increased cytosolic Ca^{2+}.

Transcellular gaps may arise from a thinning of the cell due to actin–myosin contraction. As the cell thins, vacuoles and vesicles may fuse across the cell, forming fenestrations and gaps.

Long-term increases in permeability involve cytokines, VEGF and leukocytes

In chronic inflammation the microvascular permeability is raised for long periods – months or even years – often due to the continuous production of cytokines, for example in rheumatoid arthritis. The chronic hyperpermeability of psoriasis and tumours is associated with high levels of **vascular endothelial growth factor** (VEGF), which was originally identified not as a growth factor but as 'vascular permeability factor'. VEGF causes arteriolar vasodilatation, a chronic increase in endothelial permeability and angiogenesis (Section 9.9).

Leukocytes have an important role in chronic inflammation. The penetration of leukocytes through endothelium (Section 9.8) does not in itself raise the permeability, because the endothelium reseals quickly behind the migrating leukocytes. Activated leukocytes can increase permeability, however, through the release of pro-inflammatory products. These include the potent leukotrienes and the confusingly named 'platelet activating factor' (Section 13.5). Other leukocyte products such as superoxide anions, hydrogen peroxide and elastase (a potent protease) can damage the endothelium directly and increase its permeability.

Steroids (glucocorticoids) are often used to suppress chronic inflammatory states such as rheumatoid arthritis. Steroids suppress the leukocyte migration, cytokine production, gap formation and vasodilatation.

SUMMARY

■ Capillary filtration affects fluid partitioning between the plasma and interstitial compartments, and washes proteins and antigens into the lymphatic system. The filtration fraction is low in continuous capillaries (0.2–0.3%) but high in fenestrated capillaries (20% in renal glomerular capillaries). In humans the net fluid turnover is ~4–8 l/day.

■ The capillary wall is an **imperfect semipermeable membrane** across which plasma proteins exert 80–95% of their potential colloid osmotic pressure (COP). The protein reflection coefficient σ is 0.80–0.95. The **Starling principle** states that the filtration rate per unit area of endothelium is proportional to the hydraulic conductance and the sum of the Starling pressures. The latter is the hydraulic pressure difference across the wall, [capillary pressure − interstitial fluid pressure], minus the effective colloid osmotic pressure difference, $\sigma \times$ [plasma COP − interstitial COP].

■ **Capillary pressure** at heart level falls from ~35 mmHg at the inlet to ~12 mmHg at the outlet. It depends on arterial and venous pressures and is actively regulated through the precapillary, arteriolar resistance, which is under sympathetic nervous control. Capillary pressure is raised in dependent tissues due to the effect of gravity, so dependent tissues (ankles, sacral region) are prone to oedema.

■ **Human plasma COP** is 21–29 mmHg, to which albumin contributes disproportionately.

■ **Interstitial COP** is typically one-third or more of the plasma COP due to escaped plasma proteins, but its magnitude is dynamic. Interstitial COP falls as filtration rate increases, and this buffers the filtration rate. Conversely, when fluid is transiently absorbed by capillaries, interstitial COP rises and terminates the absorption after a while.

■ **Interstitial fluid pressure** is slightly subatmospheric in many tissues, and increases to around +2 mmHg in oedema. Fluid mobility is normally low due to the resistance of interstitial glycosaminoglycan chains. Mobility is high in oedema (pitting test) due to glycosaminoglycan dilution. The pressure−versus−hydration curve (compliance curve) is steep in the physiological range but flat in the oedematous range.

■ The sum of the Starling pressures generally favours **filtration**, even in postcapillary venules. Fluid **absorption** occurs transiently when capillary pressure is reduced by precapillary vasoconstriction or hypovolaemia. The transience of absorption is due to the ensuing rise in pericapillary COP and fall in interstitial fluid pressure. Absorption is only sustained in tissues where the interstitium is continuously flushed by an independent stream of liquid, e.g. intestinal mucosa during water absorption, renal peritubular capillaries, lymph node microcirculation.

■ **The lymphatic system** returns the escaped plasma proteins and fluid to the circulation. Lymph flow is coupled to microvascular filtration rate. Flow in the initial lymphatics is driven by extrinsic compression, whereas the main lymphatic vessels have smooth muscle and valves and pump lymph actively. Pumping is enhanced by distension and sympathetic activity. Some fluid can be reabsorbed by the microcirculation of lymph nodes and the rest drains via efferent lymph trunks into neck veins. Impairment of lymph transport, whether idiopathic, post-surgical or infective (filariasis) results in high-protein **lymphoedema**.

■ During **orthostasis** capillary pressure rises in the dependent tissues, so filtration rate increases and plasma volume falls. **Exercising muscle** swells because crystalloids such as lactate and K^+ ions released by the active muscle fibres exert osmotic pressure across water-only, aquaporin channels in endothelium. Plasma volume falls as a result.

■ **Clinical oedema** develops when the sum of the Starling pressures increases sufficiently to exceed the 'safety margin' against oedema, ~15 mmHg. The safety margin is due to the fall in interstitial COP, rise in interstitial fluid pressure and increased lymph flow as filtration rate increases. Low-protein oedema results from a rise in capillary pressure (dependent oedema, cardiac failure, deep venous thrombosis) or a fall in plasma COP (malnutrition, intestinal disease, hepatic failure, nephrotic syndrome).

■ **Inflammatory swelling** is a high-protein oedema (exudate) caused by an increase in endothelial permeability to water and proteins as well as an increased net filtration force. The filtration force is increased by vasodilatation, by an initial dip in interstitial pressure (especially in burns) and by a rise in interstitial COP due to protein leakage.

■ The increase in permeability is due to the formation of intercellular and transcellular gaps in venular endothelium. Inflammatory mediators such as histamine and thrombin raise the endothelial cytosolic Ca^{2+} concentration, which triggers a biochemical cascade involving nitric oxide, cGMP, cAMP and protein kinases. This causes gap formation through a loosening of intercellular junctions and cell contraction. In addition leukocytes marginate and emigrate, and activated leukocytes release endothelium-damaging factors such as free oxygen radicals and proteases.

FURTHER READING

Reviews and chapters

Aukland, K. (1994) Why don't our feet swell in the upright position? *News in Physiological Sciences*, **9**, 214–219.

Aukland, K. and Reed, R. K. (1993) Interstitial–lymphatic mechanisms in the control of extracellular volume. *Physiological Reviews*, **73**, 1–78.

Comper, W. D. (1996) *Extracellular Matrix* (2 volumes), Harwood, Academic Publishers, Amsterdam.

Laurent, T. C. (1987) Structure, function and turnover of the extracellular matrix. *Advances in Microcirculation*, Vol. 13 (eds Altura, B. M. and Davis, E.), Karger, Basle, pp. 15–34.

Levick, J. R. and Mortimer, P. S. (1999) Fluid balance between microcirculation and interstitium in skin and other tissues; revision of classical filtration–reabsorption scheme. In *Progress in Applied Microcirculation*, Vol. 23 (ed. Messmer, K.), Karger, Basle, pp. 42–62.

McHale, N. G. and Levick, J. R. (2002) Physiology of lymph production and propulsion. In *Diseases of the Lymphatics*, Chapter 3 (eds Brouse, N. J.,

Burnand, K. G. and Mortimer, P. S.), Arnold, London.

Michel, C. C. (1997) Starling: the formulation of his hypothesis of microvascular fluid exchange and its significance after 100 years. *Experimental Physiology*, **82**, 1–30.

Michel, C. C. and Curry, F. E. (1999) Microvascular permeability. *Physiological Reviews*, **79**, 703–761.

Reed, R. K., Berg, A. and Rubin, K. (1998) β_1-integrins and control of interstitial fluid pressure. In *Connective Tissue Biology, Integration and Reductionism* (eds Reed, R. K. and Rubin, K.), Portland Press, London, pp. 27–40.

Sabolic, I. and Brown, D. (1995) Water channels in renal and nonrenal tissues. *News in Physiological Sciences*, **10**, 12–17.

Staub, N. C. and Taylor, A. E. (1984) *Edema*, Raven Press, New York.

Varani, J. and Ward, P. A. (1994) Mechanisms of neutrophil-dependent and neutrophil-independent endothelial cell injury. *Biological Signals*, **3**, 1–14

Yuan, S. Y. (2000) Signal transduction pathways in enhanced microvascular permeability. *Microcirculation*, **7**, 395–403.

Research papers

Bates, D. O., Levick, J. R. and Mortimer, P. S. (1994) Starling pressure imbalance in the human arm and alteration in postmastectomy oedema. *Journal of Physiology*, **477**, 355–363.

Bjerkhoel, P., Lindgren, P. and Lundvall, J. (1995) Protein loss and capillary protein permeability in dependent regions upon quiet standing. *Acta Physiologica Scandinavica*, **154**, 311–320.

Carlsson, O., Nielsen, S., Zakaria, E. R. and Rippe, B. (1996) In vivo inhibition of transcellular water channels (aquaporin 1) during acute peritoneal dialysis. *American Journal of Physiology*, **271**, H2254–H2262.

Feng, D., Nagy, J. A., Pyne, K., Haramel, I., Dvorak, H. F. and Dvorak, A. M. (1999) Pathways of macromolecular extravasation across microvascular endothelium in response to VPF/VEGF and other vasoactive mediators. [Gap formation.] *Microcirculation*, **6**, 23–44.

Harris, N. R., Benoit, J. N. and Granger, D. N. (1993) Capillary filtration during acute inflammation: role of adherent neutrophils. *American Journal of Physiology*, **265**, H1623–H1628.

Hayes, P. M., Lucas, J. C. and Shi, X. (2000) Importance of post-exercise hypotension in plasma volume restoration. *Acta Physiologica Scandinavica*, **169**, 115–124.

He, P., Zeng, M. and Curry, F. E. (2000) Dominant role of cAMP in regulation of microvessel permeability. *American Journal of Physiology*, **278**, H1124–H1133.

Howarth, D. M., Southee, A. E. and Whyte, I. M. (1994) Lymphatic flow rates and first aid in simulated peripheral snake or spider envenomation. *Medical Journal of Australia*, **161**, 695–700.

Hu, X., Adamson, R. H., Liu, B., Curry, F. E. and Weinbaum, S. (2000). Starling forces that oppose filtration after tissue oncotic pressure is increased. [Pore exit microgradients.] *American Journal of Physiology*, **279**, H1724–H1736.

Lim, M. J., Chiang, E. T., Hechtman, H. B. and Shepro, D. (2001) Inflammation-induced subcellular redistribution of VE-cadherin, actin and γ-catenin in cultured human lung microvessel endothelial cells. *Microvascular Research*, **62**, 366–382.

McDonald, D. M., Thurston, G. and Baluk, P. (1999) Endothelial gaps as sites for plasma leakage in inflammation. *Microcirculation*, **6**, 7–22.

Park, J. H., Okayama, N., Gute, D., Krsmanovic A., Battarbee, H. and Alexander, J. S. (1999) Hypoxia/aglycemia increases endothelial permeability: role of second messengers and cytoskeleton. *American Journal of Physiology*, **277**, C1066–C1074.

Rumbaut, R. E., McKay, M. K. and Huxley, V. H. (1995) Capillary hydraulic conductivity is decreased by nitric oxide synthase inhibition. *American Journal of Physiology*, **268**, H1856–H1861.

Watson, P. D., Garner, R. P. and Ward, D. S. (1993) Water uptake in stimulated cat skeletal muscle. *American Journal of Physiology*, **264**, R790–R796.

CHAPTER 12

Vascular smooth muscle: excitation, contraction and relaxation

Learning objectives

After reading this chapter you should be able to:

● Outline the ultrastructural features underlying vascular contraction (12.2).

● List the differences between the contractile process in vascular and cardiac myocytes (12.1, 12.3).

● Give the roles of K_{ATP} and K_{IR} channels, voltage-sensitive Ca^{2+} channels, receptor-operated channels and Cl^{-} channels (12.4).

● Outline the significance of the following agents for vascular tone: Ca^{2+}-calmodulin; myosin light chain kinase; myosin light chain phosphatase; inositol trisphosphate: diacylglycerol; protein kinases (12.5).

● Give the meaning of 'electromechanical coupling' and 'pharmacomechanical coupling' (12.5, 12.7).

● Explain how sympathetic activity triggers contraction in an action-potential generating myocyte (12.6).

● Outline three mechanisms for the induction of vascular relaxation (12.7).

12.1 Overview

The middle layer, or tunica media, of the arteries, arterioles, venules and veins is composed chiefly of vascular smooth muscle cells (VSM, vascular myocytes). The vascular myocytes are spindle-shaped cells, $20-60\,\mu m$ long by $\sim4\,\mu m$ wide at the centre. They are wrapped in a helical pattern around the vessel axis so that their contractile tension (tone) regulates the vessel diameter. Unfortunately, VSM physiology varies considerably between different blood vessels; not all vascular myocytes behave alike, making the subject tricky for teacher and student alike! Contraction is governed primarily by cytosolic Ca^{2+} concentration, but in a more complex way than in the heart. The chief differences are as follows.

● **Role of membrane potential.** Action potentials are not essential for the contraction of vascular muscle, unlike cardiac or skeletal muscle. Three activation patterns can be discerned, depending on the vessel. (i) Many vascular myocytes develop graded, sustained depolarizations that elicit graded, sustained contractions; no action potentials are generated (Figure 12.1). (ii) Some myocytes fire action potentials on top of an underlying depolarized state. This evokes twitch increments of the underlying contractile tension (Figures 12.2a, 12.2b). (iii) Some myocytes, particularly in large vessels, contract via pathways unrelated to membrane potential (Figure 12.2c). Patterns (i) and (ii) are called **electromechanical coupling**, and pattern (iii) is called **pharmacomechanical coupling**.

- **Myosin rather than actin is activated.** Whereas cardiac contraction is brought about by the activation of actin filaments (through the effect of Ca^{2+} on troponin), VSM contraction is brought about primarily by activation of the **myosin** filaments. The myosin is activated enzymatically by phosphorylation following a rise in cytosolic Ca^{2+}.

- **Force is regulated via sensitivity to Ca^{2+} as well as Ca^{2+} concentration.** Agonists increase cardiac contractile force through increased cytosolic $[Ca^{2+}]$. Agonists increase vascular tone both through increased $[Ca^{2+}]$ *and* increased sensitivity to Ca^{2+}.

- **Duration of contraction.** A cardiac contraction lasts $\sim$300 ms whereas many blood vessels maintain a tonic, partially contracted state (**basal tone**) from birth to death. VSM contraction must therefore be viewed as a process of increased tone rather than contraction *de novo*, and dilatation as a process of tone reduction.

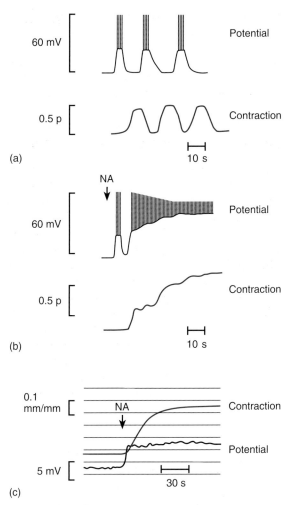

(a)

(b)

(c)

Figure 12.2 Diverse characteristics of vascular smooth muscle. (a) Upper trace shows membrane potential in a spontaneously active vessel *in vitro* (guinea pig portal vein), illustrating automaticity. Regular spontaneous slow depolarizations trigger bursts of action potentials, followed after some delay by contraction (lower trace; p is tension). (b) Response of same preparation to addition of noradrenaline (NA, 10^{-6} g/ml) illustrating electromechanical coupling. (c) By contrast, response of sheep carotid artery to superfused noradrenaline demonstrates pharmacomechanical coupling. There is only a small depolarization and no action potentials, yet a sustained contraction occurs. ((a) and (b) From Golenhofen, K., Hermstein, N. and Lammel, E. (1973) *Microvascular Research*, **5**, 73–80. (c) From Keatinge, W. R. and Harman, C. M. (1980) *Local Mechanisms Controlling Blood Vessels*, Academic Press, London, by permission.)

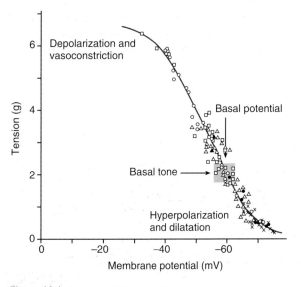

Figure 12.1 Dependence of contractile tension on membrane potential in an artery (electromechanical coupling). Membrane potential varied with the extracellular concentration of H^+ ($\triangle$), K^+ ($\square$), Ca^{2+} ($\bullet$), noradrenaline ($\circ$) and oxygen tension ($\times$). The highlighted box indicates membrane potential and force under control conditions. (After Siegel, G., *et al.* (1991) *Journal of Vascular Medicine and Biology*, **3**, 140–149.)

To understand the remarkable properties outlined above, we need to consider the cell structure, the mix of membrane ion channels, the biochemistry of myosin activation, and the signal transduction pathways that modulate the tonic contractile state. To avoid undue repetition it is assumed that the reader is familiar with the basic concepts of electrophysiology covered in Chapter 3.

12.2 Structure of the vascular myocyte

Structures of particular importance for vascular contraction include the contractile units, the Ca^{2+} store and the intercellular junctions (Figure 12.3).

The contractile machinery comprises sarcomere-like units of actin and myosin

The basic contractile unit is a sarcomere-like unit composed of actin and myosin filaments. Thick filaments of myosin (2.2 μm × 315 nm) interdigitate with thin filaments of actin (1.5 μm × 37 nm). The filaments are longer than in cardiac sarcomeres, so VSM is capable of a greater degree of shortening. The myosin isotype differs from that in the heart and only participates in contraction when it is **phosphorylated**, i.e. when phosphate groups are added to it by a kinase enzyme, so contractile force is regulated through thick-filament activation rather than thin-filament activation. As in cardiac muscle the actin molecules form a double helical filament, the groove of which is occupied by tropomyosin; but troponin, the calcium-sensitive regulatory protein of cardiac

myocytes, is absent. Its place is taken by the inhibitory proteins **caldesmon** and **calponin**.

VSM lacks the Z lines found in cardiac myocytes. Instead, the actin filaments are rooted in 'dense bands' on the inner surface of the cell and in 'dense bodies' in the cytoplasm. These are composed of α-actinin, the same material as Z lines. The dense bodies are not aligned in register across the cell so VSM is not striated. A third kind of filament, the intermediate filament (intermediate in thickness) acts as a cytoskeleton and links up the various dense bodies and dense bands so that the cell contracts as a whole. Vascular intermediate filaments consist chiefly of the proteins desmin and vimentin.

Smooth endoplasmic reticulum holds a releasable store of Ca^{2+}

The smooth endoplasmic reticulum of VSM (sarcoplasmic reticulum, SR) contains a releasable store of Ca^{2+} ions. The SR is, however, relatively poorly developed, especially in resistance vessels, and accounts for only 1– 4% of the cell by volume. Consequently, the Ca^{2+} store is not very big. For this reason resistance vessels depend on an influx of extracellular Ca^{2+} ions, as well as SR store release, for a stimulated contraction. Resistance vessels are therefore very sensitive to calcium-channel blockers such as nifedipine.

The subsarcolemmal SR approaches to within 12–20 nm of the surface membrane (sarcolemma) in places. Here, periodic dark-staining bands extend from the SR to the surface membrane. These may be channels involved in calcium-induced calcium release, as in cardiac myocytes.

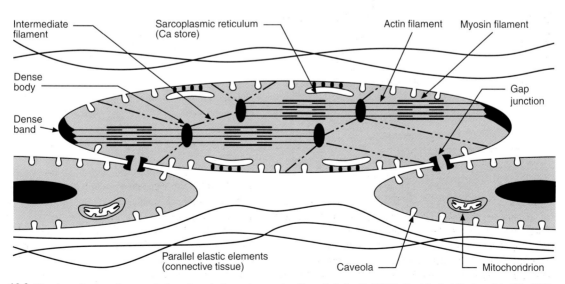

Figure 12.3 Structure of a vascular myocyte based on electron micrographs. (From Gabella, G. (1984) *Physiological Reviews*, **64**, 455–477.)

Gap junctions transmit potentials

Adjacent vascular myocytes are connected by electrically conductive gap junctions. The gap junction, or nexus, is formed by the protein connexin as in the cardiac myocyte. Six connexins combine to form a narrow, hollow tube that connects the cytoplasm of one myocyte with the next. This allows ionic currents to transmit depolarization from cell to cell. The spread is decremental, however, and extends for only 1 mm or so along the longitudinal axis of the vessel.

In arterioles and small feed arteries there are also gap junctions between the innermost vascular myocytes and the endothelial cells. These **myoendothelial junctions** transmit regulatory, hyperpolarizing signals from the endothelium to the vascular myocytes; see 'Endothelium-derived hyperpolarizing factor', Section 9.5.

Caveolae

The myocyte surface is heavily invaginated with pits called caveolae. The caveolae are so numerous that they increase the total membrane area by up to 75%. Their internal surface is lined by the protein caveolin and is often in close proximity to the SR. Although the functions of caveolae are still speculative, there is evidence that they are sites where membrane proteins such as receptors, exchangers and kinase are concentrated and interact.

12.3 Contractile properties

Resistance vessels and arteries are normally in a state of continuous, partial contraction called **basal tone**. Mechanisms exist to increase the tone (vasoconstriction) or reduce it (vasodilatation). Contraction can be increased by the sympathetic vasomotor nerves, which release noradrenaline: by circulating hormones such as adrenaline (acting on α-adrenoreceptors), angiotensin II (AT_1 receptors) and vasopressin, and by paracrine substances such as endothelin (ET_A and ET_B receptors), serotonin ($5HT_2$ receptors), histamine (H_1 receptors) and thromboxane. It is necessary to specify the receptor because some 'vasoconstrictors' cause vasodilatation when bound to different receptors, e.g. adrenaline and β_2-adrenoreceptors, histamine and H_2 receptors. In the laboratory contraction is often induced by isotonic KCl, which depolarizes the cell (Figure 12.4).

Vascular contraction is illustrated in Figures 12.2, 12.4 and 12.9, and displays the following characteristics.

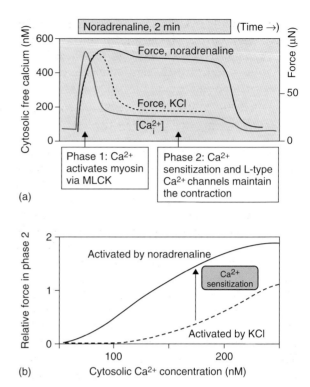

(a)

(b)

Figure 12.4 Response of rabbit mesenteric artery to 2 min exposure to noradrenaline or a depolarizing solution of concentrated KCl. (a) Changes in cyotosolic free Ca^{2+} concentration (red line) and contractile force (solid black line) in response to noradrenaline. In phase 2, force is well maintained despite a fall in $[Ca^{2+}]$. Force is not well sustained in phase 2 after KCl depolarization (dashed line, no noradrenaline); it simply mirrors free $[Ca^{2+}]$, with a time lag. (b) Dependence of force on free $[Ca^{2+}]$ in phase 2. Noradrenaline steepens the relation and shifts it upwards, compared with KCl depolarization. This is called Ca^{2+} sensitization. (Redrawn from Ito, T., Kajikuri, J. and Kurigama, H. (1992) *Journal of Physiology*, **457**, 297–314.)

Vascular contraction is slow but sustained

- **Speed.** Vascular myocytes contract very slowly (Figure 12.4a). The shortening velocity is about 1/10th that of skeletal muscle because the myosin crossbridges make and break much more slowly than those of skeletal muscle.

- **Shortening.** The degree of shortening can be substantial due to the length of the contractile filaments. Vascular myocytes can shorten to less than one half of their relaxed length.

- **Force.** The force of contraction is regulated chiefly by external chemical stimuli ('agonists') such as noradrenaline released from sympathetic terminals.

- **Duration.** The sustained nature of VSM contraction is remarkable. Many arterioles and arteries maintain a state of partial contraction throughout life. This sustained tone is a crucially important property because dilatation, and with it the ability to raise blood flow, is achieved entirely through a reduction in the tone.

Long-lasting 'latch' crossbridges maintain vascular tension economically

The energy cost of maintaining vascular contraction throughout the body would be great were it not for the ability of VSM to maintain a contraction using just 1/300th of the energy required by striated muscle for a similar contraction. This is due to a fundamental difference in the operation of the contractile machinery. In a skeletal muscle fibre, the crossbridges last a very short time, so tension can only be maintained by a continuous, rapid making and breaking of crossbridges, which consumes much ATP. In VSM a special type of long-lasting crossbridge is formed, that recycles either infrequently or not at all, and thus consumes little ATP. This is called the **latch state**. The muscle is in effect locked into the contracted, crossbridged state, as in the latch muscles that keep the shells of bivalves closed. In this way the VSM avoids fatigue.

Vasomotion (automaticity) is the rhythmic contraction of certain vessels

Arteries and veins generally have a stable vascular tone, membrane potential and cytosolic Ca^{2+} level unless stimulated. By contrast many arterioles (e.g. in skeletal muscle), the terminal pial arteries and the portal vein (Figure 12.2a) undergo regular rhythmic contractions that are independent of external stimulation and occur several times per minute. This is called vasomotion. Vasomotion is due to a co-ordinated oscillation in cytosolic $[Ca^{2+}]$, which causes the myocytes to contract synchronously. Co-ordination is probably mediated by the gap junctions. In large vessels such as the portal vein, spontaneous depolarization triggers action potentials which cause the Ca^{2+} oscillations. In arterioles it may be the other way round; a cyclical release of Ca^{2+} from the IP_3-sensitive SR store activates surface ion channels ($i_{Cl(Ca)}$, see below) that cause rhythmic depolarization.

Cytosolic free Ca^{2+} is the primary factor governing contraction

Vascular contractile force is regulated primarily by cytosolic free Ca^{2+} concentration, as shown in Figure 12.4b. The cytosolic Ca^{2+} concentration is determined by the balance between three processes (Figure 12.5), namely:

1 The entry of extracellular Ca^{2+} through **voltage-sensitive Ca^{2+} channels** and/or **receptor-operated channels** in the surface membrane.

2 The release of **stored Ca^{2+}** from the SR.

3 The removal of cytosolic Ca^{2+} by **Ca^{2+}–ATPase pumps** in the surface membrane (termed Ca^{2+} expulsion) and in the SR membrane (termed Ca^{2+} sequestration). Ca^{2+} expulsion is aided by $Na^+–Ca^{2+}$ exchangers but Ca^{2+}–ATPase pumps predominate in VSM, unlike the heart. Because the voltage-sensitive Ca^{2+} channels have a low but finite open state probability under basal conditions, the sarcolemmal Ca^{2+}–ATPase pumps have to expel Ca^{2+} continuously to avoid Ca^{2+} accumulation.

When sympathetic nerve activity or circulating agonists tip the balance in favour of an increase in cytosolic Ca^{2+}, myocyte tension increases and the vessel contracts. Conversely, when agonists tip the balance in favour of a fall in Ca^{2+} concentration, tension falls and the vessel dilates. A major factor influencing the open state of Ca^{2+} channels is the membrane potential, so we turn our attention next to the ion channels that govern membrane potential.

12.4 The ion channels

The membrane potential in a pressurized arterial vessel with basal tone is around $-50\,mV$ to $-60\,mV$ (Figure 12.1). This is a relatively depolarized state compared with a cardiac myocyte. The main kinds of sarcolemmal ion channel are (Figure 12.5):

- inward rectifier K^+ channels (K_{IR})
- ATP-dependent K^+ channels (K_{ATP})
- calcium-dependent K^+ channels (K_{Ca}) and voltage-dependent K^+ channels (K_v)
- voltage-sensitive Ca^{2+} channels (VSCC)
- receptor-operated cation (Ca^{2+}) channels (ROCs)
- other non-selective cation channels (i_{cat})
- calcium-activated chloride channels ($Cl_{(Ca)}$).

Differences in the channel population between vessels account for their electrical diversity (Figure 12.2). The roles of the various ion channels are as follows.

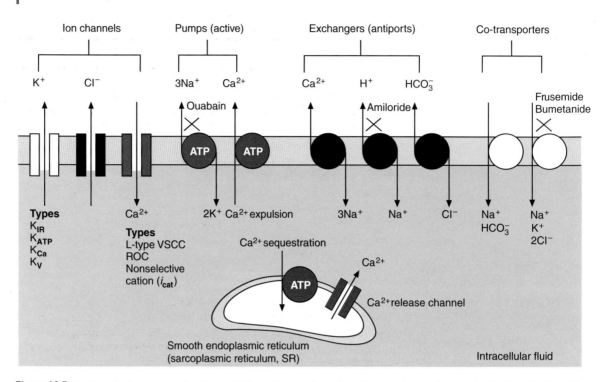

Figure 12.5 Ion channels, ion pumps and exchangers in the surface membrane (sarcolemma) of a vascular myocyte. For channel abbreviations, see text. Crosses denote transport blockers. The Na^+–HCO_3^- cotransporter and Na^+–H^+ exchanger combat intracellular acidosis during sustained contraction. The HCO_3^-–Cl^- exchanger contributes to the high chloride concentration in vascular myocytes.

K^+ channels generate the negative membrane potential

A myocyte has ~50 000 K^+ channels, of which a substantial fraction is open at any one moment. A small outward current of K^+ flows through these channels down the electrochemical gradient for K^+ (Table 12.1), leaving behind a net negative charge. Similarly, K^+ efflux restores the negative potential after an action potential, if the myocytes can generate one.

The Nernst equilibrium potential for K^+, E_K, is −90 mV, so a basal potential of −50 mV is much smaller than expected for a membrane permeable solely to K^+ (Section 3.3). This is because the membrane is permeable not only to K^+ but also to chloride and calcium ions, in a ratio of ~10:4:2 at −50 mV. A small efflux of Cl^- and influx of Ca^{2+} reduce the membrane potential.

The high intracellular $[K^+]$ is preserved by the Na^+–K^+–ATPase pumps of the surface membrane (Figure 12.5). The pump expels three Na^+ ions for every two K^+ ions that enter the cell, so it is electrogenic. Blockage by ouabain shows that the pump usually contributes no more than −11 mV to the potential.

The myocyte membrane potential is important because it controls the voltage-sensitive Ca^{2+} channels.

Table 12.1 Ionic composition of vascular smooth muscle.

Ion	Intracellular (mM)	Extracellular (mM)	Nernst equilibrium potential[§] (mV)
K^+	165	5	−89
Na^+	9	137	+69
Ca^{2+}	0.0001[†]	1.2[‡]	+124
*Cl^-	54	134	−23
HCO_3^-	7.3	15.5	−19
pH	7.06	7.40	−20

* Chloride ion concentration is unusually high is VSM.
[†] Relaxed state.
[‡] Plasma calcium is ~2.5 mM but only 1.2 mM is in the ionic form.
[§] See Chapter 3.

Consequently the K^+ channels influence vascular tone. For example, hypoxia increases the fraction of open K^+ channels, leading to hyperpolarization (a more negative potential), closure of voltage-sensitive Ca^{2+} channels, reduced Ca^{2+} influx and thus vascular relaxation. Moreover, the relatively depolarized basal potential contributes to the sustained basal tone, because voltage-sensitive Ca^{2+} channels have a significant open probability at −50 mV to −60 mV, and the attendant small influx of Ca^{2+} maintains basal tone.

Table 12.2 Ion channels present in vascular smooth muscle membrane.

Channel	Properties	Role
Potassium		
Inward rectifying (K_{IR})	Mainly in arterioles. Open at resting potential. Blocked by Ba^{2+}. Open state increased by K_o^+, up to 25 mM	Supplies part of outward current for membrane potential. Contributes to vasodilator response to interstitial K^+ e.g. in exercise
Delayed rectifying, voltage-dependent (K_V)	Opens slowly on depolarization beyond -30 mV. Outward rectifying. Blocked by 4-aminopyridine (4-AP)	Contributes repolarization current after action potential
ATP-dependent (K_{ATP}, K_{NDP})	Closed by normal [ATP] (5–10 mM). Opens at low ATP, raised ADP, GDP, adenosine A_1 receptors and [H^+]. Blocked by glibenclamide, $\rightarrow$ vasoconstriction. Activated by cromakalim, pinacidil, CGRP and VIP, $\rightarrow$ vasodilatation	Links vascular tone to metabolic state of tissue during exercise and hypoxia. Low basal activity maintained by protein kinase A, and increased in cAMP-PKA mediated vasodilatation
Calcium-activated (K_{Ca})	Open state promoted by Ca_i^{2+} and depolarization. A big conductance (BK) subtype is often strongly expressed. Blocked by tetraethyl ammonium (TEA) and iberiotoxin	Contributes to membrane potential and repolarization. Can suppress a.p. if abundant. Acts as a negative feedback 'brake', e.g. on myogenic contraction. Implicated in action of NO
Calcium-conducting		
Voltage-sensitive (VSCC)	L-type = large conductance and long opening. Abundant in small arteries. Blocked by dihydropryidines, e.g. nifedipine	Inward current for action potential, electromechanical coupling and Bayliss myogenic response. Modulates resting potential.
	T-type = tiny conductance and transient opening	Little importance
Receptor-operated (ROC)	Non-selective cation channel (Ca^{2+}, Na^+, K^+) linked to a receptor, e.g. α_1-adrenoceptor, ATP receptor. Not sensitive to nifedipine	Mediates pharmacomechanical coupling for NAd, angiotensin, vasopressin, 5HT, histamine
Chloride		
Calcium-activated (Cl_{Ca})	Open state promoted by Ca_i^{2+} (>0.2 μM)	Contributes 'inward' current $i_{Cl(Ca)}$ (actually an efflux of negative ions) for slow EJP. Also modulates basal membrane potential
Other channels		
Non-selective cation channel	Permeable to Ca^{2+}, Na^+, K^+. Activated indirectly by second messenger diacylglycerol. (Called a ROC if directly coupled to a receptor)	Contributes depolarizing current i_{cat} for fast and slow EJPs (excitatory junction potentials)
Stretch-sensitive cation channels	Activated by physical stretch. Conducts Na^+ and Ca^{2+}, $\rightarrow$ depolarization and VSCC activation	Contractile response of smooth muscle to stretch, i.e. Bayliss myogenic response and autoregulation of blood flow

The types of K^+ channels present in VSM include the inward-rectifier channel K_{IR}, the voltage-dependent channel K_V, the ATP-dependent K^+ channel K_{ATP} and the calcium-dependent K^+ channel K_{Ca} (Table 12.2). The different properties of these channels affect vascular responsiveness as follows.

Inward-rectifier channels (K_{IR}) mediate K^+-induced vasodilatation in exercise

The K_{IR} channel is the only K^+ channel that is opened by an increase in extracellular [K^+], in the range 5–25 mM. The increased K^+ permeability shifts the potential towards E_K. As a result, moderate increases in extracellular $[K^+]$, such as occur in exercising muscle, cause vascular hyperpolarization and vasodilatation. Larger, pharmacological levels of extracellular K^+ depolarize the myocyte (because E_K becomes negligible) and therefore cause contraction.

ATP-dependent K^+ channels (K_{ATP}) respond to metabolic status

The ATP-dependent K^+ channel, K_{ATP}, links vascular tone to tissue metabolic state. The open probability of the K_{ATP} channel increases when intracellular ATP falls to a very low level, as in severe ischaemia, and when ADP, GDP, adenosine and H^+ concentrations increase, as they do during moderate hypoxia. The channel's alternative name, nucleotide diphosphate-dependent channel or K_{NDP}, emphasizes the response to ADP during hypoxia. Hypoxic hyperpolarization and vasodilatation are shown in Figure 12.1 (crosses). The K_{ATP}-activating drug **cromakalim** similarly causes hyperpolarization and vasodilatation.

Under normal conditions many K_{ATP} channels are closed, but a fraction are open, as demonstrated using **glibenclamide**. Glibenclamide is a K_{ATP}-blocker, and it causes partial depolarization and vasoconstriction. The K_{ATP} channels are partially active in the basal state due to their phosphorylation by background levels of active protein kinase A (Section 12.7).

Ca-dependent K^+ channels (K_{Ca}) stabilize the membrane potential

Calcium-dependent K^+ channels of big conductance (K_{Ca}, BK) influence the electrical excitability of the myocyte. K_{Ca} channels are activated by intracellular Ca^{2+} and by depolarization. They are partially active under basal conditions and can be blocked by **iberiotoxin**. Increased activation leads to hyperpolarization and therefore closure of voltage-sensitive Ca^{2+} channels. These effects counteract the K_{Ca} activating stimuli, namely depolarization and intracellular Ca^{2+}. Due to this negative feedback, K_{Ca} channels have a stabilizing effect on the membrane potential. When present in large numbers the K_{Ca} channels prevent a myocyte from generating an action potential. Action potentials can often be generated in previously inexcitable myocytes if the K_{Ca} channels are blocked pharmacologically.

Voltage-activated K^+ channels (K_v) likewise show increased open probability with depolarization and help to stabilize the membrane potential.

Voltage-sensitive Ca^{2+} channels (VSCCs) mediate contraction in electromechanical coupling

Voltage-sensitive calcium channels (also called voltage-operated, voltage-gated or voltage-dependent) are characterized by a selective permeability to divalent cations (Ca^{2+}, Ba^{2+}) and an increased open probability in response to depolarization. As a result, **vascular tension is graded function of membrane depolarization in many vessels** (Figure 12.1). The predominant type of VSCC is the L-type Ca^{2+} channel, the characteristics of which were illustrated in Figure 4.3.

Unlike the fast Na^+ channels responsible for nerve action potentials, VSCCs do not activate at a sharp threshold; their open probability is a continuous function of membrane potential. Consequently VSCCs have a low but finite open state probability at the basal potential of $-50\,mV$ to $-60\,mV$. This allows a small but finite flux of extracellular Ca^{2+} into the myocyte. The resulting cytosolic Ca^{2+} concentration, though low, is sufficient to activate the myosin motor partially and generate basal tone.

Arterioles and terminal arteries have ~ 1000 VSCCs per myocyte; large arteries generally have smaller numbers. In many arterioles and small arteries the L-type Ca^{2+} channels are sufficiently abundant to generate **action potentials** in response to a depolarizing stimulus, for example in response to noradrenaline at sympathetic nerve endings (Figure 12.6a). The upstroke of the VSM action potential is due to the calcium current i_{Ca-L}. The L-type Ca^{2+} channel is blocked by the dihydropyridine **nifedipine**, which therefore acts as a vasodilator and is used to treat hypertension.

Receptor-operated non-selective cation channels (ROCs) mediate contraction in pharmacomechanical coupling

Receptor-operated channels were discovered during experiments on VSM that had been experimentally depolarized using isotonic K^+ solution. When noradrenaline was applied, the contractile tension increased even though no change in membrane potential was possible. Contraction only occurred when extracellular Ca^{2+} was present. Thus the existence of channels permeable to Ca^{2+}, insensitive to membrane potential and activated by an agonist receptor was inferred.

Receptor-operated channels (ROCs) are nonselective cation channels; they are impermeable to

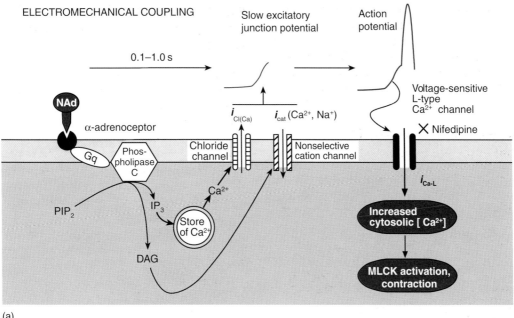

Figure 12.6 Comparison of electromechanical and pharmacomechanical coupling evoked by noradrenaline. Similar coupling can be evoked through histamine H_1 receptors, serotonin and angiotensin II receptors. (a) Electrical responses leading to L-type Ca^{2+} channel mediated contraction in arterioles and portal vein. (b) Contraction is independent of potential during pharmacomechanical coupling. PIP_2, phosphatidyl inositol bisphosphate; IP_3, inositol trisphosphate; DAG, diacylglycerol; i, current; MLCK, myosin light chain kinase.

anions but permeable to Ca^{2+}, Na^+ and K^+ ions. The Ca^{2+} permeability is generally three to five times bigger than the Na^+ permeability. The channel is activated by a receptor–agonist complex coupled to the channel (Figure 12.6b). In the case of noradrenaline the α-adrenoceptor is linked to the ROC by a G protein. In the case of ATP (a co-transmitter of sympathetic nerves, Section 12.6), the receptor is part of the ion channel itself (a **ligand-gated channel**).

ROCs mediate pharmacomechanical coupling, which is the induction of contraction by an agonist without the necessity of a change in membrane potential. There can be a small but essentially irrelevant depolarization in such cases due to the cation current through the ROC (Figure 12.2c).

Non-selective cation channels contribute to electromechanical coupling

Some non-selective cation channels, particularly in arterioles, are not coupled to a receptor but are activated indirectly through a short biochemical chain of latency 0.1–1.0 s (Figure 12.6a). The α-adrenoceptor activates a membrane-bound enzyme, phospholipase C, which generates inositol trisphosphate (IP$_3$) and diacylglycerol (DAG). The DAG activates the non-selective cation channels. The activated channels conduct an inward current of Ca^{2+} and Na^+, called i_{cat}. The current i_{cat}, aided by the chloride current described next, produces a small depolarization called an excitatory junction potential, which mediates electromechanical coupling (see later).

Chloride channels too contribute to electromechanical coupling

The membrane of an electrically excitable myocyte contains chloride-conducting channels that are activated by cytosolic Ca^{2+} (Figure 12.6a). These channels transmit a chloride current, $i_{Cl(Ca)}$, which along with i_{cat} depolarizes arterioles following α-adrenoceptor activation. The α-adrenoceptor activation leads to IP$_3$ formation: the IP$_3$ triggers Ca^{2+} release from the subsarcolemmal SR store and the Ca^{2+} activates the $Cl_{(Ca)}$ channels.

The opening of chloride channels causes an efflux of Cl^- because cytosolic Cl^- concentration is unusually high in vascular myocytes, ~54 mM (Table 12.1). This is probably due to the operation of the chloride–bicarbonate exchanger (Figure 12.5). Since the chloride equilibrium potential is around −20 mV (Table 12.1) and the membrane potential is −50 mV, a current of Cl^- ions is driven out of the cell when the Cl^- channels open. The loss of negative ions depolarizes the cell, shifting it towards the chloride equilibrium potential.

It is clear from the above survey that vascular myocytes have a diverse armoury of ion-conducting channels, and the channels are activated in diverse ways. The next section explains how the channels link receptor activation to myocyte contraction (excitation–contraction coupling).

12.5 Mechanisms linking receptor activation and contraction

One of the most important physiological drives to vascular contraction is the activation of α-adrenoceptors (synonym, α-adrenoreceptor) by noradrenaline released from sympathetic fibres. This paradigm (example) is described below. Other vasoconstrictor agents such as angiotensin II, serotonin, thromboxane and endothelin act through similar pathways but with different weightings of the various components.

α-adrenoceptors sometimes act through membrane depolarization

Contractile tension depends primarily on cytosolic free $[Ca^{2+}]$, which can be increased by both depolarization-dependent and depolarization-independent pathways.

- **Contraction induced by graded, sustained depolarization.** Many arteries show a graded, sustained depolarization upon stimulation with noradrenaline. This activates VSCCs, leading to sustained contraction (electromechanical coupling, Figure 12.1). The depolarization is brought about by $i_{Cl(Ca)}$ and i_{cat}, which are activated through the PLC–IP$_3$–DAG cascade (Figure 12.6a and below). The hormone angiotensin II evokes a third depolarizing mechanism, K^+ channel inhibition.

- **Contraction induced by action potentials.** Some arterioles, small arteries and certain veins fire VSCC-based action potentials in response to strong sympathetic stimulation. This too induces electromechanical coupling (Figures 12.2a, 12.2b).

- **Contraction unrelated to membrane potential.** In large arteries noradrenaline can initiate a rise in cytosolic Ca^{2+} by activating ROCs and by triggering the release of stored Ca^{2+} via IP$_3$. This is not dependent on membrane depolarization and is called pharmacomechanical coupling (Figures 12.2c, 12.6b).

α-adrenoceptors activate the phospholipase C–IP$_3$–DAG pathway

The α-adrenoceptor is coupled to a trimeric membrane GTPase, G_q, which activates the membrane-bound enzyme **phospholipase C** (Figure 12.7). Phospholipase C (PLC) catalyses the breakdown of a membrane phospholipid, phosphatidyl inositol bisphosphate (PIP$_2$) into the second messengers **inositol trisphosphate** (IP$_3$) and **diacylglycerol** (DAG).

The IP$_3$ activates the Ca^{2+}-release channels of the sarcoplasmic reticulum (SR) store. The effect of store release depends on the extent and arrangement of the SR. If the SR is scanty and close to the surface membrane, the increase in subsarcolemmal Ca^{2+} may

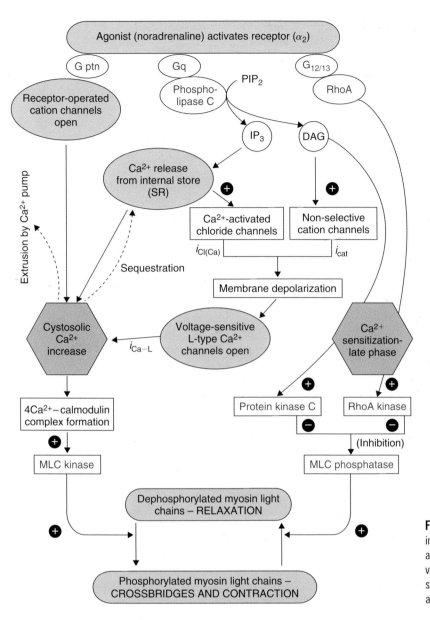

Figure 12.7 Flow chart for noradrenaline-induced vasoconstriction. Relative importance of various pathways varies with vessel, tissue and agonist. +, activation step; −, inactivation step. Other symbols as in legend for Figure 12.6.

act purely locally to activate adjacent chloride channels and elicit the depolarizing current $i_{Cl(Ca)}$. If the SR is extensive, as in large arteries, store discharge raises the general cytosolic pool of free Ca^{2+}.

The other second messenger, DAG, activates the depolarizing current i_{cat}. Also, DAG and Ca^{2+} together activate protein kinase C, which contributes to Ca^{2+} sensitization (see below). The isoform protein kinase C−ε also inhibits K_{ATP} channels, promoting depolarization and contraction.

The contractile response has two phases

The activation of α-adrenoceptors triggers a contractile process with two distinct phases (Figure 12.4).

In the **initial phase** there is a rapid, large increase in cytosolic $[Ca^{2+}]$, leading to contraction. In the **second phase**, which starts $30-60$ s later, the cytosolic $[Ca^{2+}]$ retreats to a lower but still elevated level as Ca^{2+} is pumped back into the SR store; yet the force of contraction is well maintained. The signal transduction pathways for the two phases are as follows.

The initial phase is mediated by high cytosolic [Ca²⁺]

Cytosolic free $[Ca^{2+}]$ increases from $\sim 0.1\,\mu M$ to $\sim 1\,\mu M$ within seconds of exposure to noradrenaline, as observed in myocytes loaded with Ca^{2+}-sensitive fluorescent dye. This is quickly followed by a rise in tension (Figure 12.4a). The Ca^{2+} comes from both the extracellular fluid and the internal store (Figure 12.7).

Store release is important in large arteries

In large arteries the SR is well developed and contributes substantially to the cytosolic Ca^{2+} transient, whereas in resistance vessels it is less developed and contributes less. Store discharge is triggered chiefly by the receptor–G_q–PLC–IP_3 cascade. Calcium-induced calcium release analogous to that in cardiac myocytes (Section 3.7) has been reported but seems less important. Store replenishment is brought about by an influx of extracellular Ca^{2+} called 'capacitive Ca^{2+} entry' through special **store-operated channels** in the surface membrane.

Extracellular Ca^{2+} influx is important in resistance vessels

The influx of Ca^{2+} from the extracellular fluid makes a big contribution to cytosolic $[Ca^{2+}]$ in resistance vessels, which tend to have abundant VSCCs and scanty SR. The VSCCs are activated by the agonist-evoked depolarizing currents $i_{Cl(Ca)}$ and i_{cat}. Extracellular Ca^{2+} also passes through the receptor-operated channels. In both cases influx is driven by the enormous electrochemical gradient for Ca^{2+} (Table 12.1).

Ca^{2+} leads to myosin light chain kinase activation

The rise in cytosolic Ca^{2+} does not activate the actin filament, as in the heart; instead it activates an enzyme, myosin light chain kinase, that acts on the myosin filament (Figure 12.7).

Myosin light chain kinase activates the myosin motor

The myosin light chain is part of the mobile head that forms the crossbridge with actin. Vascular myosin, unlike striated muscle myosin, only forms crossbridges when the light chains are phosphorylated. Phosphorylation is brought about by myosin light chain kinase (MLCK), with ATP supplying the phosphate. MLCK is itself activated by Ca^{2+}-calmodulin complex. Calmodulin is a cytoplasmic regulatory protein related to troponin C. When calmodulin has bound four Ca^{2+} ions, it activates the MLCK. The phosphorylated myosin heads then form crossbridges

with actin, and use ATP as the energy source for tension generation.

Myosin light chain phosphatase causes relaxation

The extent to which myosin heads are phosphorylated depends on the balance between MLCK activity and myosin light chain phosphatase activity. Myosin light chain phosphatase is an enzyme that dephosphorylates the myosin (Figure 12.7). When Ca^{2+} concentration falls, MLCK activity declines and the phosphatase reduces the level of myosin phosphorylation. This turns off the myosin motor and causes relaxation.

Summary of initial phase

The initial $30-60\,s$ activation sequence begins with the binding of an agonist such as noradrenaline to its receptor. The activated receptor evokes a rise in cytosolic Ca^{2+} concentration by multiple mechanism (whose relative importance varies between vessels), namely the release of stored Ca^{2+} via the second messenger IP_3, depolarization of the membrane by $i_{Cl(Ca)}$ and i_{cat}, and the opening of Ca^{2+}-conducting channels in the surface membrane, namely VSCCs and ROCs. Calmodulin binds four Ca^{2+} ions and the Ca^{2+}-calmodulin complex activates MLCK. The latter phosphorylates the myosin light chain. The phosphorylated myosin heads form crossbridges with the actin filament, and the crossbridges row the myosin filament into the spaces between the actin filaments to generate shortening and tension. Myosin light chain phosphatase reverses the effect of MLCK when cytosolic $[Ca^{2+}]$ falls, leading to relaxation.

In the sustained phase, myosin light chain phosphatase inhibition causes Ca^{2+} sensitization

During the sustained response the cytosolic Ca^{2+} concentration falls back from its peak value (Figure 12.4). Some depolarization persists, so the VSCCs continue to transmit extracellular Ca^{2+} into the cell, maintaining the cytosolic $[Ca^{2+}]$ above baseline. The fact that VSCCs contribute to the sustained phase is supported by the observation that nifedipine partially inhibits the sustained contraction. However, some additional mechanism clearly comes into play, because the contraction is well maintained despite a substantial fall in cytosolic $[Ca^{2+}]$ (Figure 12.4).

Regulation of vascular myocyte tone

■ Active vascular tension (tone) is well sustained and is regulated by sympathetic noradrenaline, the hormones adrenaline, angiotensin II and vasopressin, and paracrine agonists such as NO, endothelin, hypoxia, histamine, etc.

■ Tone is raised primarily through cytosolic $[Ca^{2+}]$. Ca^{2+}-calmodulin complex activates myosin light chain (MLC) kinase, which phosphorylates myosin heads to cause crossbridge formation. Dephosphorylation by MLC phosphatase causes relaxation.

■ Agonists raise cytosolic $[Ca^{2+}]$ through (i) depolarization, which activates voltage-sensitive Ca^{2+} channels; (ii) receptor-operated Ca^{2+} channels; (iii) IP_3 generation leading to Ca^{2+} store release.

■ Tone is also regulated through Ca^{2+} sensitization, due to MLC phosphatase inhibition by rhoA kinase and protein kinase C.

■ Relaxation is induced by hyperpolarization, by cAMP-activated protein kinase A, and by cGMP-activated protein kinase G. These pathways reduce cytosolic $[Ca^{2+}]$.

actin filament, reducing its inhibitory effect on cross-bridge formation. This may explain how tone is often maintained in large arteries despite a falling level of myosin light chain phosphorylation.

Vascular contraction is thus regulated through changes in cytosolic Ca^{2+} concentration *and* changes in Ca^{2+} sensitivity.

12.6 Response to sympathetic stimulation

Sympathetic vasoconstrictor fibres innervate nearly all arteries and arterioles and mediate many vascular reflexes. Sympathetic neurotransmission is described below, while transmitter release modulation and reuptake are covered in Chapter 14.

Junctional varicosities occur at the neuromuscular junction

The terminal part of a sympathetic axon runs along the adventitia–media border and bears a string of swellings, around a 1000 per fibre, called **junctional varicosities** (Figures 1.10, 14.2). The gap between the varicosity and closest myocyte is only ~75 nm and there are up to six varicosities per myocyte. Each varicosity contains about 500 small, dense-cored vesicles grouped close to the prejunctional membrane, plus a smaller number of large vesicles. The vesicles contain a variable mixture of ATP and noradrenaline.

Neurotransmitter release is quantal

When a sympathetic action potential reaches a varicosity, N-type calcium channels in the varicosity membrane open, causing a rise in intraneural $[Ca^{2+}]$. This leads to the discharge of a single vesicle into the junctional cleft. Neurotransmitter is thus released as a discrete, uniform-sized packet or quantum. Probably only ~1 in every 100 action potentials succeeds in releasing a quantum from any one varicosity. The released neurotransmitters diffuse rapidly across the short neuromuscular gap and binds to receptors on the vascular myocyte.

Noradrenaline evokes a slow excitatory junction potential

Both noradrenaline and ATP are released *in vivo*, leading to complex electrical and mechanical responses. It is helpful to look first at the effect of a brief pulse of noradrenaline alone, delivered through

The additional mechanism is the sensitization of the contractile process to Ca^{2+}.

Ca^{2+} sensitization is brought about by kinases (Figure 12.7). Kinases are a large family of enzymes that phosphorylate other proteins and thereby alter their activity. The kinase chiefly responsible for Ca^{2+} sensitization is **rhoA kinase**, which inhibits myosin light chain phosphatase, the enzyme that turns off the myosin motor. This allows a greater level of myosin phosphorylation for a given level of MLCK and Ca^{2+}, and hence a greater activation of the contractile machinery. RhoA kinase is activated by rhoA, a monomeric GTPase that is itself activated by vasoconstrictor receptors.

In addition **protein kinase C-α** is activated by DAG following α-adrenoceptors activation (Figure 12.6b) and contributes variably to Ca^{2+} sensitization, depending on the vessel. Pharmacological activators of protein kinase C cause a slow, sustained vasoconstriction with little or no rise in Ca^{2+}, and inhibitors of protein kinase C impair noradrenaline-evoked contractions to a variable degree. Protein kinase C activates a protein, CPI–17, that inhibits myosin light chain phosphatase.

There is also evidence that protein kinases phosphorylate **caldesmon**, a regulatory protein on the a micropipette in the laboratory. The response of a spike-forming myocyte is illustrated in Figure 12.8. Activation of the myocyte α-adrenoceptors is followed by a delay of ~0.1–1.0 seconds as the PLC–G_q–DAG/IP$_3$–Ca^{2+} chain grinds into action (Figure 12.7). A slow depolarization then develops, called the **slow excitatory junction potential** (slow EJP,

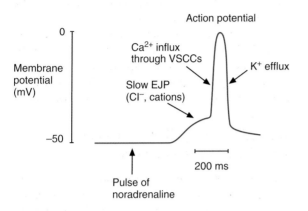

Figure 12.8). The slow EJP is generated by two currents, namely i_{cat}, the cation current through DAG-activated non-selective cation channels, and $i_{Cl(Ca)}$, the chloride current through Ca^{2+}-activated chloride channels (Figure 12.6a).

If the EJP is big enough and the VSCCs numerous enough, the activation of VSCCs results in positive feedback and generates an action potential (Figure 12.8). The action potential is a spike of variable amplitude lasting 10–100 ms, generated by the inward current i_{Ca-L}. The ensuing transient increase in cytosolic [Ca^{2+}] elicits a twitch contraction. Repolarization is brought about by an efflux of K$^+$ ions through K$_{IR}$ and K$_{Ca}$ channels.

Figure 12.8 Response of an action potential-generating vascular myocyte to a brief pulse of noradrenaline from a micropipette (cf. sympathetic vesicle, Figure 12.9). VSCC, voltage-sensitive channel permeable to Ca^{2+}. (Courtesy of Professor W. A. Large, Department of Pharmacology, St. George's Hospital Medical School, London.)

Sympathetic stimulation evokes both fast and slow EJPs, and both pharmaco- and electromechanical coupling

Let us next consider the more complex response to sympathetic stimulation. Figure 12.9 shows the electrical and mechanical responses to nerve stimulation in a small arterial vessel. When the perivascular sympathetic fibres are stimulated briefly and at low intensity, an electrical response with two components is evoked (Figure 12.9a). After a latency of only ~15 ms there is a small, rapidly rising depolarization of ~10 mV that is short-lived (1 s). This is called a **fast excitatory junction potential** (fast EJP). It is followed by a slower-rising, longer-lasting depolarization that resembles the slow EJP evoked by noradrenaline in Figure 12.8.

The **fast EJP** is evoked by ATP released from the sympathetic vesicle, as demonstrated by the abolition of fast EJPs by inhibitors of purinergic (ATP) receptors (Figure 14.3). Purinergic receptors are directly linked to ROCs, rather as the acetylcholine receptor is linked to Na$^+$ channels in skeletal neuromuscular junctions. As a result, the ATP-gated ROCs activate rapidly. They conduct a small depolarizing current of cations into the cell.

The **slow EJP** is evoked by noradrenaline, as proved by its abolition by the α-adrenoceptor blocker prazosin (Figure 12.9, top right). The slow EJP is generated by i_{cat} and $i_{Cl(Ca)}$ following activation of the slow PLC–G_q–DAG/IP$_3$–Ca^{2+} pathway (Figure 12.6a).

The mechanical response, a slow contraction, is at first sight puzzling. Contraction precedes the slow EJP, so it cannot be caused by the slow EJP. Nor can the contraction be a response to the fast EJP, because prazosin abolishes the contraction but not the fast EJP (Figure 12.9, top right). The electrical events are

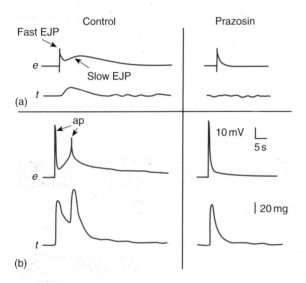

Figure 12.9 Simultaneous records of membrane potential recorded by an intracellular microelectrode (*e*) and tension (*t*) in a rat tail artery. The perivascular nerves were stimulated by a single external pulse in each frame in the absence (*left*) or presence (*right*) of the α-adrenoreceptor blocker, prazosin. (a) Medium intensity stimulation produced a fast excitory junction potential (EJP) and a slower one. Only the latter was blocked by prazosin. Note that contraction precedes the slow EJP. (b) Higher intensity of stimulation evoked larger fast and slow EJPs, each of which triggered an action potential (ap) and associated twitch contraction. (From Cheung, D. W. (1984) *Pfluger's Archiv*, **400**, 335–337, by permission.)

thus not the cause of the contraction. The slow contraction is in fact an example of **pharmacomechanical coupling**, due to the activation of ROCs by α-adrenoceptors.

If the stimulation strength is increased, the fast EJP becomes larger. This opens more VSCCs and triggers an action potential, which elicits a twitch contraction (Figure 12.9, bottom left). The slow depolarization becomes larger too and triggers another action potential. The latter produces a second twitch superimposed on the underlying slow contraction. The twitches are examples of **electromechanical coupling**, while the underlying slow contraction reflects pharmacomechanical coupling.

It must be stressed that the response to sympathetic stimulation varies greatly from vessel to vessel; not all vessels respond as above, although the pattern is a common one.

12.7 Vasodilator mechanisms

Vasodilatation is brought about by a reduction of the tonic contractile tension of myocytes, i.e. relaxation. Relaxation can be produced by three different routes, which converge on the lowering of cytosolic $[Ca^{2+}]$ and thus a reduction in MLKC activation. This allows myosin light chain phosphatase to predominate and deactivate the myosin motor.

Hyperpolarization mediates the vasodilator responses to hypoxia and K_o^+ (exercise)

Hyperpolarization-mediated vasodilatation is illustrated in Figure 12.1. Hyperpolarization reduces the open state probability of the VSCCs, leading to a fall in cytosolic free $[Ca^{2+}]$ and relaxation. Hyperpolarization-mediated vasodilatation occurs during hypoxia, due to K_{ATP} activation; and during exercise due to K_{IR} activation (Section 12.4). Hyperpolarization-mediated vasodilatation is also evoked by the sensory nerve neuropeptides **calcitonin-gene related peptide** and **vasoactive intestinal polypeptide**, and by K_{ATP}-activating drugs such as cromakalim, pinacidil and diazoxide.

The cAMP–PKA pathway mediates vasodilatation to adrenaline

The circulating hormone adrenaline causes vasodilatation in arterioles that possess abundant β_2-adrenoceptors, notably those in skeletal muscle and myocardium. This is because the biochemical linkage of the β_2-adrenoceptor differs from that of the α-adrenoceptors (Figure 12.10). The β_2-adrenoceptor, like the β_1-receptor in the heart, is linked to the trimeric membrane GTPase G_s, which stimulates the membrane-bound enzyme **adenylate cyclase**. Adenylate (or adenylyl) cyclase catalyses the conversion of ATP to cyclic adenosine monophosphate,

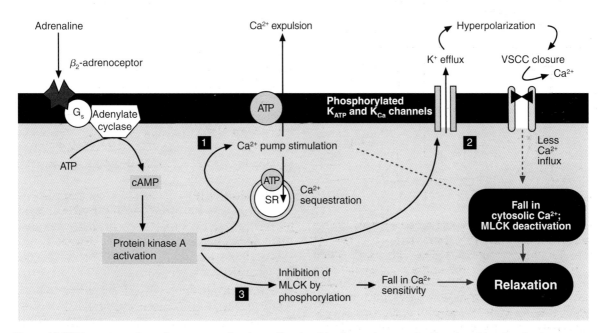

Figure 12.10 Mechanisms of β_2-adrenoceptor mediated vasodilatation. Adenylate cyclase can also be activated by adenosine A_{2A} receptors, histamine H_2 receptors, VIP and CGRP receptors. It can also be activated experimentally by the drug *forskolin*. (After Ushio-Fukai, M., *et al.* (1993), see Research papers, and Siegel, G. (1996), see Reviews and chapters.)

cAMP. cAMP activates a phosphorylating enzyme, **protein kinase A**. The protein kinase A (PKA) induces vascular relaxation through the following pathways (Figure 12.10).

- PKA acts on the pump regulator, phospholamban, to disinhibits the **Ca^{2+}–ATPase pumps** in the SR and surface membrane. This leads to Ca^{2+} sequestration and Ca^{2+} expulsion respectively, reducing the cytosolic free Ca^{2+}.

- PKA phosphorylates **K$_{ATP}$ and K$_{Ca}$ channels**, increasing their open state probability. The resulting hyperpolarization reduces the open probability of VSCCs and thus reduces Ca^{2+} influx.

- PKA phosphorylates **MLCK**, which inhibits it and thereby reduces Ca^{2+} sensitivity.

Many agonists besides adrenaline produce vasodilatation through the cAMP pathway. They include prostacyclin, adenosine (the A$_{2A}$ receptor), histamine (the H$_2$ receptor), vasoactive intestinal polypeptide and calcitonin-gene related peptide.

The cGMP–PKG pathway mediates vasodilatation to nitric oxide

The vasodilator nitric oxide (NO), NO-releasing drugs such as glyceryl trinitrate (used to relieve angina), and the hormone atrial natriuretic peptide all produce vasodilatation by raising the level of intracellular **cyclic guanosine monophosphate** (cGMP). NO reacts with the haem group of the enzyme guanylate (guanylyl) cyclase. The activated guanylate cyclase catalyses the production of cGMP from guanosine trisphosphate, and the cGMP activates **protein kinase G** (PKG); see Section 9.4 and Figure 9.9. Protein kinase G phosphorylates phospholamban to disinhibit the Ca^{2+}–ATPase pumps of the SR and surface membrane, leading to Ca^{2+} sequestration and Ca^{2+} expulsion respectively. Protein kinase G also reduces Ca^{2+} sensitization.

SUMMARY

■ Vascular smooth muscle (VSM) comprises spindle-shaped cells joined by gap junctions that allow a decremental cell-to-cell spread of electrical excitation.

■ The contractile machinery comprises long inter-digitating thin (actin) and thick (myosin) filaments. The actin filaments are attached to cytoplasmic dense bodies and to the cell membrane at dense bands.

■ Contractile tension is related to cytosolic [Ca^{2+}] which, through Ca^{2+}–calmodulin formation, activates **myosin light chain kinase** (MLCK). MLCK catalyses the phosphorylation of myosin heads, which leads to myosin–actin crossbridge formation and contraction. Long-lasting crossbridges maintain tension with little energy expenditure (the **latch state**), enabling arterioles and arteries to maintain a basal tone throughout life without fatigue. Relaxation is brought about by **myosin light chain phosphatase**, which dephosphorylates the myosin.

■ **Membrane K$^+$ channels** generate the basal potential of around −50 mV. ATP-sensitive channels (K$_{ATP}$), Ca-activated channels (K$_{Ca}$) and inward-rectifier channels (K$_{IR}$) all contribute.

■ **Voltage-sensitive L-type Ca^{2+} channels** (VSCCs) have a low but finite open probability at −50 mV, leading to basal tone generation. Their open probability increases steeply with depolarization, leading to Ca^{2+} influx and contraction (**electromechanical coupling**). This is prominent in resistance vessels, which have abundant VSCCs.

■ Cytosolic Ca^{2+} can also be raised independently of depolarization (**pharmacomechanical coupling**) through the activation of **receptor-operated cation channels** (ROCs) and through the release of Ca^{2+} from the **sarcoplasmic reticulum (SR) store** by the second messenger IP$_3$. The IP$_3$, along with diacylglycerol (DAG), is generated from phosphatidyl inositol bisphosphate by phospholipase C (PLC). PLC is linked by G$_q$ protein to α-adrenoceptors and histamine H$_1$ receptors.

■ The Ca^{2+} inputs from activated VSCCs, ROCs and the SR store are counterbalanced in the steady state by Ca^{2+}–ATPase pumps in the surface membrane (Ca^{2+} expulsion) and SR store (Ca^{2+} sequestration).

■ An **agonist-induced contraction** (e.g. by α-adrenoceptors) has two phases. In the initial phase there is a high cytosolic [Ca^{2+}] due to VSCC activation, ROC activation and SR store release. This is followed by a sustained phase of lower but still elevated [Ca^{2+}], during which an increased Ca^{2+} sensitivity helps to maintain the contraction. **Ca^{2+} sensitization** is due to the inhibition of myosin light chain phosphatase by rhoA kinase and protein kinase C, which are activated indirectly by vasoconstrictor agonists.

■ **Sympathetic nerve activity** is a major regulator of vasoconstriction *in vivo*. Axon varicosities release noradrenaline and ATP. Low concentrations of noradrenaline elicit contraction through ROC activation (**pharmacomechanical coupling**). In resistance vessels there is also a depolarization-mediated vasoconstriction, initiated by fast EJPs due to ATP and slow EJPs due to noradrenaline. The noradrenaline triggers the $PLC-IP_3-DAG$ pathway, which activates Cl_{Ca} and non-selective cation channels. The depolarizing currents $i_{Cl(Ca)}$ and i_{cat} produce the slow EJP. If the EJPs are large enough and VSCCs numerous enough, as in arterioles, positive feedback produces a Ca^{2+}-mediated action potential and twitch (**electromechanical coupling**).

■ In some arterioles regular spontaneous waves of Ca^{2+} store discharge and membrane depolarization lead to rhythmic contractions called **vasomotion**.

■ **Vasodilatation** is brought about by a fall in cytosolic $[Ca^{2+}]$, which deactivates MLCK and allows myosin light chain phosphatase to turn off the myosin motor. Cytosolic $[Ca^{2+}]$ can be reduced by three processes:

(i) **Hyperpolarization** reduces the VSCC open probability. Examples include K_{ATP}-mediated hyperpolarization during hypoxia and K_{IR}-mediated hyperpolarization as interstitial K^+ rises in exercising muscle.

(ii) **cAMP.** Activation of β_2-adrenoceptors, adenosine A_{2A} receptors and histamine H_2 receptors activates adenylate cyclase via G_s protein. Adenylate cyclase catalyses cAMP production, which activates protein kinase A. Protein kinase A stimulates $Ca^{2+}-ATPase$ pumps to reduce cytosolic $[Ca^{2+}]$:phosphorylates K^+ channels to cause hyperpolarization and VSCC closure: and inactivates MLCK by phosphorylation.

(iii) **cGMP.** NO and atrial natriuretic peptide activate guanylate cyclase, leading to a rise in cGMP and protein kinase G activation. This produces relaxation by similar actions to protein kinase A.

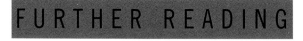

FURTHER READING

Reviews and chapters

Bolton, T. B. and Large, W. A. (1986) Are junction potentials essential? Dual mechanism of smooth muscle activation by transmitter release from autonomic nerves. *Quarterly Journal of Experimental Physiology*, **71**, 1–28.

Bolton, T. B. and Tomita, T. (eds) (1996) *Smooth Muscle Excitation*, Academic Press, London.

Brock, J. A. and Cunnane, T. C. (1993) Neurotransmitter release mechanisms at the sympathetic neuroeffector junction. *Experimental Physiology*, **78**, 591–614.

Edvinsson, L. and Uddman, R. (eds) (1993) *Vascular Innervation and Receptor Mechanisms*, Academic Press, New York. [Chapters on adrenergic transmission, ATP, NO.]

Folkow, B. and Nilsson, H. (1997) Transmitter release at adrenergic nerve endings: total exocytosis or fractional release? *News in Physiological Sciences*, **12**, 32–36.

Hirst, G. D. S. and Edwards, F. R. (1989) Sympathetic neuroeffector transmission in arteries and arterioles. *Physiological Reviews*, **69**, 546–604.

Horowitz, A., Menice, C. B., LaPorte, R. and Morgan, K. G. (1996) Mechanisms of smooth muscle contraction. *Physiological Reviews*, **76**, 967–1003.

Jackson, W. F. (1998) Potassium channels and regulation of the microcirculation. *Microcirculation*, **5**, 85–90.

McDaniel, N. L., Rembold, C. M. and Murphy, R. A. (1994) Cyclic nucleotide dependent relaxation in vascular smooth muscle. *Canadian Journal of Physiology and Pharmacology*, **72**, 1380–1385.

Mulvaney, M. J. and Aalkjaer, C. (1990) Structure and function of small arteries. *Physiological Reviews*, **70**, 922–961.

Mulvany, M. J., Alkjaer, C., Arner, A. and Hellstrand, P. (1998) Vascular Smooth Muscle (Symposium). *Acta Physiologica Scandinavica*, **164**, 339–644.

O'Donnell, M. E. and Owen, N. E. (1994) Regulation of ion pumps and carriers in vascular smooth muscle. *Physiological Reviews*, **74**, 683–722.

Quayle, J. M., Nelson, M. T. and Standen, N. B. (1997) ATP-sensitive and inwardly rectifying potassium channels in smooth muscle. *Physiological Reviews*, **77**, 1165–1216.

Siegel, G. (1996) Vascular smooth muscle. In *Comprehensive Human Physiology*, Vol. 2 (eds Greger, R. and Windhorst, U.), Springer-Verlag, Berlin, pp. 1941–1964.

Somlyo, A. P. (1985) Excitation–contraction coupling and the ultrastructure of smooth muscle. *Circulation Research*, **57**, 497–507.

Somlyo, A. P. and Somlyo, A. V. (2000) Signal transduction by G-proteins, Rho-kinase and protein phosphatases to smooth muscle and non-muscle myosin II. *Journal of Physiology*, **522**, 177–185.

Taggart, M. J. (2001) Smooth muscle excitation–contraction coupling: a role for caveolae and caveolins? *News in Physiological Science*, **16**, 61–65.

Research papers

Amédée, T., Benham, C. D., Bolton, T. B., Byrne, N. G. and Large, W. A. (1990) Potassium, chloride and non-selective cation conductances opened by noradrenaline in rabbit ear artery cells. *Journal of Physiology*, **423**, 551–568.

Bae, Y. M., Park, M. K., Lee, S. H., Ho, W-K. and Earm, Y. E. (1999) Contribution of Ca^{2+}-activated K^+ channels and nonselective cation channels to membrane potential of pulmonary arterial smooth muscle cells of the rabbit. *Journal of Physiology*, **514**, 747–758.

Draeger, A., Amos, W. B., Ikebe, M. and Small, J. V. (1990) The cytoskeletal and contractile apparatus of smooth muscle: contraction bands and segmentation of the contractile elements. *Journal of Cell Biology*, **111**, 2463–2473.

Haddock, R. E., Hirst, G. D. S. and Hill, C. E. (2002) Voltage-independence of vasomotion in isolated irideal arterioles. *Journal of Physiology*, **540**, 219–229.

Hayabuchi, Y., Davies, N. W. and Standen, N. B. (2001) Angiotensin II inhibits rat arterial K_{ATP} channels by inhibiting steady-state protein kinase A activity and activating protein kinase Cϵ. *Journal of Physiology*, **530**, 193–205.

Helliwell, R. M. and Large, W. A. (1997) α_1-adrenoceptor activation of a non-selective cation current in rabbit portal vein by 1,2-diacyl-sn-glycerol. *Journal of Physiology*, **499**, 417–428.

Loeb, A. L., Godeny, I. and Longnecker, D. E. (2000) Functional evidence for inward-rectifier potassium channels in rat cremaster muscle arterioles. *Microvascular Research*, **59**, 1–6.

Nobe, K. and Paul, R. J. (2001) Distinct pathways of Ca^{2+} sensitization in porcine coronary artery: effect of Rho-related kinase and protein kinase C inhibition on force and intracellular Ca^{2+}. *Circulation Research*, **88**, 1283–1290.

Smirnov, S. V. and Aaronson, P. I. (1992) Ca^{2+} currents in single myocytes from human mesenteric arteries: evidence for a physiological role of L-type channels. *Journal of Physiology*, **457**, 455–475.

Woodsome, T. P., Eto, M., Everett, A., Brautigan, D. L. and Kitazawa, T. (2001) Expression of CPI-17 and myosin phosphatase correlates with Ca^{2+} sensitivity of protein kinase C-induced contraction in rabbit smooth muscle. *Journal of Physiology*, **535**, 553–564.

Ushio-Fukai, M., Abe, S., Kobayashi, S., Nishimura, J. and Kanaide, H. (1993) Effects of isoprenaline on cytosolic calcium concentrations and on tension in the porcine coronary artery (action of cAMP). *Journal of Physiology*, **462**, 679–696.

CHAPTER 13

Control of blood vessels I: intrinsic control

Learning objectives

After reading this chapter you should be able to:

- Sketch how arteriolar diameter responds to a rise in pressure (the myogenic response) (13.2).
- List the principle physiological roles of nitric oxide in the circulation (13.3).
- State the role of functional (metabolic) hyperaemia and list four putative mediators (13.4).
- Give thumbnail sketches of the autacoids histamine, bradykinin, serotonin, prostacyclin and thromboxane (13.5).
- Illustrate the meaning of 'autoregulation' by drawing a plot of blood flow as a function of blood pressure. Draw a second curve to show how autoregulation is affected by functional hyperaemia (13.6).
- Explain how dilatation is co-ordinating along the arterial system (13.7).
- Give the meaning of 'reactive hyperaemia' and outline the key mechanisms (13.8).
- State the meaning of ischaemia–reperfusion injury and its basic mechanisms (13.9).

13.1 Overview of vascular control and its roles

The active tension of smooth muscle in the tunica media, the vascular tone, controls the width of a blood vessel. An increase in tone causes vasoconstriction. Conversely, a reduction in tone causes vasodilatation, because the wall is distended by the internal blood pressure as the media relaxes (Section 8.7). A high vascular tone is an essential pre-requirement for vascular dilatation (reduced tone), and tissues capable of major hyperaemia (increased blood flow) have a high vascular tone at rest, e.g. skeletal muscle.

Even after blockage of the sympathetic vasoconstrictor nerves, arterioles and arteries maintain some vascular tone, called **basal tone**. In veins, by contrast, the basal tone is generally low. Basal tone is the result of a continuous interplay between vasoconstrictor influences, such as the myogenic response and endothelin, and vasodilator influences, such as nitric oxide. Vascular tone in vivo is generally higher than basal tone due to the tonic activity of sympathetic vasoconstrictor nerves. Before delving into the regulatory processes, however, let us summarize the functional importance of vascular tone, drawing together some key points from earlier chapters.

Vascular tone regulates local blood flow, arterial pressure, capillary filtration and central venous pressure

- **Local blood flow** within a tissue is controlled by the width of the resistance vessels, namely the arterioles and terminal arteries. A small change in radius r causes a big change in the resistance due to the r^4 term in Poiseuille's law of flow (Section 8.7). Consequently, moderate changes in vascular tone can alter the blood flow over a huge range (Figure 13.1). In skin, skeletal muscle and exocrine glands the flow is regulated over a $20\times$ range to meet the demands of temperature regulation, exercise and liquid secretion respectively.

- **Arterial pressure** is the product of total peripheral resistance and cardiac output (Section 8.5). Arterial pressure is continuously regulated during normal, daily activities by the adjustment of resistance vessel tone. During hypovolaemic emergencies such as haemorrhage, peripheral vasoconstriction helps to maintain the blood pressure.

- **Capillary recruitment** and **capillary pressure** are regulated by local arteriolar tone (Figures 10.14, 11.4). As a result, arteriolar tone influences perfusion homogeneity, local fluid filtration rate and, through the latter, plasma volume.

- **Central venous pressure** is affected by the distribution of blood between the peripheral and central veins. Contraction of the peripheral veins and venules displaces a considerable volume of blood into the central veins, thus raising the cardiac filling pressure and, through Starling's law of the heart, the stroke volume (Section 6.6).

From the above résumé we see that changes in vascular tone act both at a **local** level to regulate tissue perfusion, nutrient exchange and water exchange; and at the level of the **whole animal** to regulate arterial blood pressure, plasma volume, central venous pressure and stroke volume.

Vascular tone is controlled by intrinsic and extrinsic mechanisms

The mechanisms regulating vascular tone fall into two classes, namely intrinsic and extrinsic (Figure 13.2). **Intrinsic regulation** is the regulation of tone by local factors sited entirely within an organ or tissue. The main intrinsic regulatory mechanisms are:

- **the Bayliss myogenic response** to arterial pressure changes;
- **endothelial secretions** (nitric oxide, EDHF, prostacyclin, endothelin);
- **vasoactive metabolites** generated by active tissues (e.g. adenosine in exercising muscle);
- **autacoids** (local vasoactive paracrine secretions such as histamine); and
- **temperature**, which is chiefly important in the skin and is covered in Chapter 15.

Important physiological responses mediated entirely by intrinsic regulation include the **autoregulation** of flow, **functional hyperaemia** and **reactive hyperaemia**. Intrinsic regulation also contributes to pathological responses such as **inflammation** and **arterial vasospasm**.

Extrinsic regulation is brought about by factors originating outside the organ, namely:

- the **vasomotor nerves** (sympathetic, parasympathetic and others); and
- circulating **hormones** such as adrenaline, angiotensin, vasopressin and insulin.

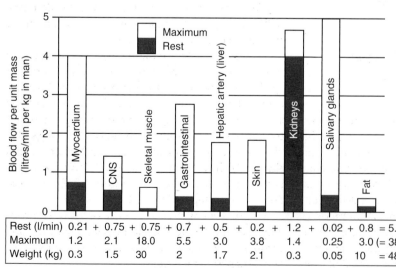

Figure 13.1 Range of blood flow between rest and maximal function in various tissues of a 70 kg human. Maximal flow through all organs simultaneously, 38 l/min, would exceed the output capacity of the heart. (Redrawn from Mellander, S. and Johansson, B. (1968) *Pharmacological Reviews*, **20**, 117–196, by permission.)

	Myocardium	CNS	Skeletal muscle	Gastrointestinal	Hepatic artery (liver)	Skin	Kidneys	Salivary glands	Fat	
Rest (l/min)	0.21 +	0.75 +	0.75 +	0.7 +	0.5 +	0.2 +	1.2 +	0.02 +	0.8	= 5.1
Maximum	1.2	2.1	18.0	5.5	3.0	3.8	1.4	0.25	3.0	(= 38!)
Weight (kg)	0.3	1.5	30	2	1.7	2.1	0.3	0.05	10	= 48

Local control   **Extrinsic control**

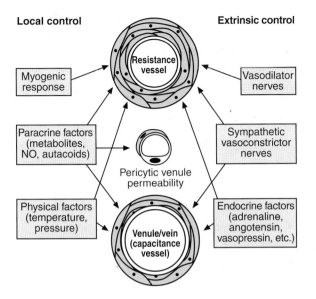

Figure 13.2 Overview of vascular control in resistance vessels, exchange vessels and capacitance vessels.

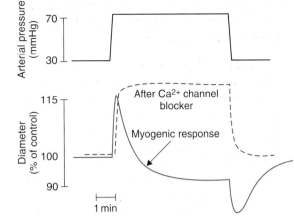

Figure 13.3 Change in diameter of an isolated rat cerebral artery upon raising the luminal pressure. Initial passive stretch is followed by active contraction – the Bayliss myogenic response. This is abolished by blocking the L-type Ca^{2+} channels with nimodipine. (Based on McCarron, J. G., Crichton, C. A., Langton, P. D., MacKenzie, A. and Smith, G. L. (1997) *Journal of Physiology*, **498**, 371–379.)

It is useful to think of vascular regulation as a **hierarchy of control processes**. The lower level is the intrinsic regulatory system, which provides for the local needs of an individual organ. The higher level is the extrinsic regulatory system, which can modify or override the intrinsic controls to meet the needs of the whole animal – for example the sympathetic-mediated peripheral vasoconstriction that follows a haemorrhage. Intrinsic control is described in this chapter and extrinsic control in Chapter 14.

13.2 The myogenic response to blood pressure

Arterial vessels respond actively to changes in blood pressure, and can be compressed by external pressure.

Arterial vessels contract when blood pressure is raised – the Bayliss myogenic response

The myogenic response was discovered by Sir William Bayliss, brother-in-law of Ernest Starling, in 1902. When blood pressure is raised acutely in an artery or arteriole, the increased pressure immediately distends the vessel mechanically. Most systemic arterioles and arteries then react to the distension within seconds with a well-sustained contraction, the myogenic response (Figure 13.3). Conversely, a fall in pressure elicits a fall in vascular tone. The myogenic response is important because it contributes to

basal tone, and because it stabilizes local blood flow and capillary filtration pressure in the face of changes in arterial blood pressure (Section 13.6, Autoregulation).

The myogenic response is mediated by depolarization and Ca^{2+}

The mechanisms behind the myogenic response are only partly worked out but may be as follows. When a myocyte is stretched, it becomes partially depolarized, probably due to the activation of volume-regulated chloride channels and stretch-sensitive non-selective cation channels. Depolarization increases the open probability of the L-type Ca^{2+} channels and raises cytosolic $[Ca^{2+}]$, which activates the contractile machinery. In support it is found that the myogenic response is impaired by the Ca^{2+} channel blocker nifedipine (Figure 13.3), by chloride channel blockers, and by gadolinium ions, which block stretch-activated cation channels.

The maintenance of the myogenic response over long periods appears to involve a vasoconstrictor agent, 20-HETE (20-hydroxy-eicosa-tetra-enoic acid). The 20-HETE is produced from arachidonic acid by the enzyme P450 ω-hydroxylase. Its action is to reduce the open-state probability of myocyte K_{Ca} channels, thereby maintaining depolarization and the Ca^{2+}-channel open state. Ca^{2+} sensitization by activated protein kinase C (Figure 12.7) may also contribute to the maintained response.

Increased shear stress in the narrowed vessel probably acts as a 'brake' on the myogenic constriction through increased endothelial production of vasodilators such as nitric oxide.

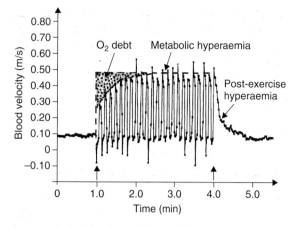

Figure 13.4 Metabolic hyperaemia recorded in human femoral artery during rhythmic quadriceps muscle exercise. Flow was measured by the Doppler ultrasound method. Note the slow build-up to maximum response, creating a nutritional debt; the post-exercise period of hyperaemia repays the nutritional debt. (From Walloe, L. and Wesche, J. (1988) *Journal of Physiology*, **405**, 257–273, by permission.)

Stretch is the stimulus – but what is stretched?

A puzzling feature of the myogenic response is that the wall is only stretched temporarily, when the pressure is first raised, yet the response is well maintained. During the maintained contraction the vessel width and myocyte length are actually smaller than at the outset (Figure 13.3). A speculative explanation is that microscopic regions of the myocyte membrane are under increased stress due to the evoked contraction, and that the stretch-sensitive ion channels are located in these microscopically stressed regions.

External pressure leads to skin pressure ulcers

A high pressure applied to the outside of a blood vessel compresses it mechanically and thus impairs the blood flow. This occurs within myocardium and skeletal muscle (Figure 13.4) during their contraction phase. In the skin vascular compression during sitting, kneeling and lying impairs blood flow. If a patient is bedridden by age or paralysis, the prolonged impairment of skin nutrition through vascular compression frequently causes horrific ulcers over the buttocks and heels called bed sores.

13.3 Regulation by endothelial NO and endothelin

Endothelium synthesizes and releases the vasodilator agents nitric oxide (NO), endothelium-derived

hyperpolarizing factor (EDHF) and prostacyclin (PGI_2), and also the vasoconstrictor agent endothelin. These agents act in a paracrine fashion on the adjacent myocytes. The reader is referred to Sections 9.4 and 9.5 for an account of the production, biochemistry and diverse roles of each agent. The present section concentrates on the roles of NO and endothelin in vascular control.

The chief roles of NO in vascular control are as follows:

- the continuous modulation of **basal tone**
- basal tone reduction during **pregnancy**
- **flow-induced vasodilatation** in conduit arteries during exercise
- the vasodilatation responsible for **sexual erection**
- vasodilatation during **inflammation**
- vasodilatation during **endotoxic shock**.

Continuous, shear-stimulated NO production modulates basal tone

The chief stimulus to endothelial NO production is normally the shear stress resulting from blood flow. This accounts, typically, for 60–80% of NO formation. Shear stress, not the flow itself, is the stimulus, as demonstrated by the observation that an increase in blood viscosity (and hence shear stress) will evoke vasodilatation at a fixed flow. Shear stress activates protein kinase B which activates endothelial NO synthase, eNOS (Figure 9.9). The NO causes local vasodilatation, which reduces shear stress. NO production thus provides a negative feedback that stabilizes endothelial shear stress. Lesser drives to NO production include circulating **insulin** and **oestrogen**.

In humans tonic NO production was demonstrated by the finding that L-NMMA, a blocker of NO synthesis, causes forearm vasoconstriction when infused into the brachial artery (Figure 13.5). Vascular tone is thus the result of a balance between NO-mediated relaxation and vasoconstriction driven by the myogenic response, endothelin, sympathetic nerve activity and circulating hormones.

During **pregnancy** high oestrogen levels stimulate NO production, leading to a generalized reduction in vascular tone. This causes a fall in blood pressure despite a 50% increase in cardiac output.

Flow-induced arterial dilatation supports exercise hyperaemia

If an increased flow is driven through an isolated artery, it causes dilatation and a fall in resistance. As a result, hardly any increase in pressure gradient is

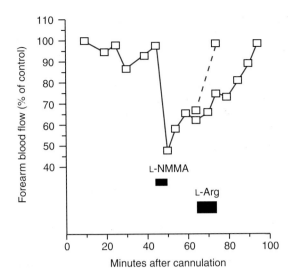

Figure 13.5 Role of NO in regulating vascular resistance in human forearm. N-monomethyl-L-arginine (L-NMMA), an inhibitor of nitric oxide production, was infused into the brachial artery. The 50% reduction in flow indicated that there is normally a tonic production of the vasodilator NO. Inhibition was reversed by the NO substrate, L-arginine (broken line). (After Vallance, P., Collier, J. and Moncada, S. (1989) *The Lancet*, **ii**, 997–1000.)

needed to maintain the higher flow. The flow-induced dilatation is caused by shear-induced endothelial NO secretion.

Flow-induced vasodilatation occurs in large, conduit arteries *in vivo* during exercise. For example, the diameter of the human brachial artery increases by 10% or more during forearm exercise. At the onset of the exercise the small resistance vessels within the active muscle dilate due to the release of vasodilator metabolites by the active muscle (Section 13.4). The fall in net vascular resistance increases the blood flow through the conduit artery supplying the muscle, raising its wall shear stress. This stimulates NO secretion. As a result the conduit artery supplying an active muscle group dilates despite being far beyond the reach of vasodilator metabolites.

Arterial resistance is a tiny fraction of the total vascular resistance at rest, but flow-induced arterial vasodilatation is nevertheless important. Without it the arterial resistance would limit the hyperaemia once the downstream resistance has fallen. Endothelial NO thus **couples conduit artery resistance to arteriolar resistance**.

Sexual erection is mediated by neural NO

Penile erection is brought about by the vasodilatation of resistance vessels in the corpus cavernosum. The vasodilatation is induced by NO-producing or 'nitridergic' parasympathetic nerves (Section 14.2). The vasodilator effect of NO is mediated through raised cGMP (Figure 9.9). The new drug for the treatment of male impotence, sildenafil (Viagra), is a selective inhibitor of the cGMP-degrading enzyme **phosphodiesterase type 5**. By raising vascular cGMP, sildenafil mimics the action of the nitridergic nerves.

Inflammation is characterized by endothelium-mediated vasodilatation

The local heat and redness of an inflamed tissue are caused by vasodilatation. The vasodilatation is partly due to increased NO production. Several inflammatory autacoids, including bradykinin, thrombin and substance P, produce vasodilatation by activating eNOS. In addition the inflammatory cytokines induce the synthesis of 'inducible nitric oxide synthase' (see below).

Inducible NOS contributes to endotoxin shock

Endotoxin shock is a severe, intractable form of hypotension caused by bacterial infection. Endotoxin is a bacterial lipopolysaccharide that stimulates monocytes to secrete cytokines. Over several hours the cytokines induce the nuclear transcription of a form of NOS called inducible nitric oxide synthase (iNOS or NOS-II). The expression of iNOS in vascular myocytes, macrophages and endothelial cells contributes to a generalized vasodilatation and hence hypotension. iNOS differs from the constitutive eNOS in that it is a cytosol enzyme: it does not require activation by Ca^{2+}-calmodulin complex: and it produces NO at a greater, more sustained rate than eNOS.

Nitrate drugs act through NO release

Drugs such as glyceryl trinitrate, sodium nitroprusside and isosorbide dinitrate have long been used as vasodilators to treat cardiac angina. It is now appreciated that the nitrodilators act by mimicking the endothelial release of NO. They are very effective as venodilators as well as arterial dilators, and part of their therapeutic effect is through the reduction of central venous pressure, which reduces stroke work and hence O_2 demand.

Endothelin contributes to basal tone and some pathological states

The endothelium-secreted peptide endothelin undergoes prolonged binding to ET_A and ET_B receptors on arterial and venous myocytes. The receptors activate receptor-operated Ca^{2+} channels and the phospholipase $C-IP_3-DAG$ pathway (Figure 12.7), which raise the cytosolic $[Ca^{2+}]$. The ensuing vaso- and venoconstriction last 2–3 hours.

Physiological role

Although plasma endothelin levels are low, the inhibition of endothelin production by phospharamidon causes dilatation in the human forearm and rat coronary artery. Similarly the ET-receptor antagonist bosentan causes a slight fall in blood pressure. Such observations indicate that endothelin contributes a little to the basal tone of resistance vessels.

Pathological roles

Endothelin production is stimulated by hypoxia, leading to raised plasma levels at **high altitude**. This may contribute to high-altitude pulmonary hypertension. Endothelin levels are also high in a form of acute hypertension associated with pregnancy, called **pre-eclamptic toxaemia**. Endothelin has no clear role in other forms of hypertension.

Plasma endothelin is increased in **heart failure** and contributes to the characteristic renal and peripheral vasoconstriction. In support of this, bosentan increases peripheral blood flow, dilates veins and reduces blood pressure in patients with heart failure.

Endothelin levels are also raised in the cerebrospinal fluid following a subarachnoid haemorrhage, ischaemic stroke or brain injury. The endothelin is thought to contribute to the associated **cerebral vasospasm**, since the vasospasm is ameliorated by ET_A receptor antagonists.

13.4 Regulation by metabolic vasoactive factors

Whenever the metabolic rate of skeletal muscle, myocardium or a region of the brain increases, the blood flow to the active region increases (Figures 13.4, 13.6, 15.14). The vascular response is finely graded so that O_2 delivery increases in proportion to O_2 demand (Figure 15.4). Such metabolism-driven increases in blood flow are called **functional hyperaemia** or **metabolic hyperaemia**. The hyperaemia is brought about by the release of vasodilator substances from the active parenchyma into the interstitial fluid, from which they diffuse into the tunica media of the local resistance vessels. The resistance vessels show a gradient of sensitivity to metabolic vasodilators, distal arterioles being the most sensitive and larger vessels less sensitive (Figure 13.7).

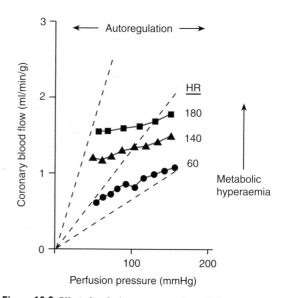

Figure 13.6 Effect of perfusion pressure and metabolic rate on coronary blood flow in dog. Dashed lines are theoretical pressure–flow lines at constant conductance (steepest line, highest conductance). At any given metabolic rate (heart rate, HR), blood flow increases relatively little with pressure and shifts to lower conductance lines as pressure is raised (*autoregulation*). At any given perfusion pressure, flow increases with metabolic rate (heart rate); this is *functional or metabolic hyperaemia*. (Data from Laird (1983), In *Cardiac Metabolism* (eds Holland, A. and Noble, M.), Chichester, Wiley, pp. 257–278.)

It is still not certain which chemical agents account for metabolic hyperaemia. Acidosis, hypoxia, adenosine, K^+ ions, phosphate ions and hyperosmolarity all increase in the active tissue and each has a vasodilator effect. Their relative importance is contentious and varies between tissues. Cerebral vessels, for example, are particularly sensitive to CO_2 and K^+, while adenosine is particularly important in striated muscle.

Acidosis

An increase in metabolic rate raises the rate of production of CO_2 (which forms carbonic acid in solution) and lactic acid, leading to local tissue acidosis. Acidosis causes vasodilatation (Figures 12.1, 13.8 and Appendix 2), as discovered by W. H. Gaskell in 1880. **Cerebral blood vessels** are particularly sensitive to CO_2, and arterial CO_2 is an important regulator of cerebral blood flow (Section 15.4). By contrast the vessels in skeletal muscle and myocardium respond only weakly to CO_2 or lactic acid, so acidosis probably contributes relatively little to exercise hyperaemia.

Hypoxia

Hypoxia acts both locally on the vasculature (see below) and reflexly (Chapter 18). Since hypoxia has opposite effects on the systemic and pulmonary circulations, we need to consider them separately.

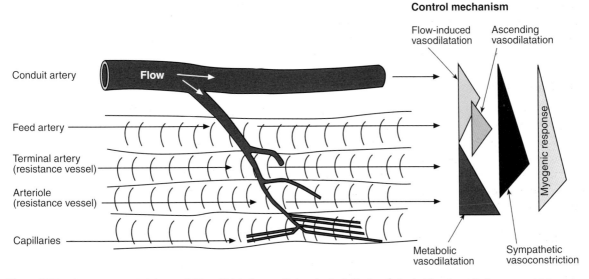

Figure 13.7 Differential control of the arterial tree. Metabolic vasodilators dominate the terminal arterioles. Sympathetic vasoconstrictor nerves dominate the more proximal resistance vessels. Ascending vasodilatation involves electrical transmission up the arterial tree to the feeding arteries. Flow-induced vasodilatation is important in the feeding and conduit arteries. (Adapted from Brown, M. D. (1995) In *Cardiovascular Regulation* (eds Jordan, D. and Marshall, J.), Portland Press, London, pp. 113–126.)

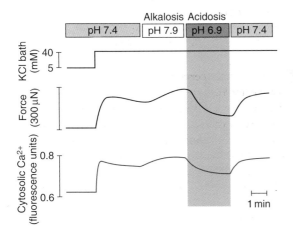

Figure 13.8 Effect of extracellular pH on vascular tone in strips of rat mesenteric artery. To increase the starting level of tone, the tissue was depolarized by KCl solution, but similar responses occur in non-depolarized tissue. The effect of acidity was similar whether CO_2 or HCl was used. (Adapted from Austin, C. and Wray, S. (1995); see Research papers.)

Hypoxia dilates systemic resistance vessels

The partial pressure of O_2 in arterial blood, PaO_2, is normally 100 mmHg or 13 kPa. If blood with a PaO_2 of <40 mmHg or 5 kPa is perfused through skeletal muscle, myocardium or the brain, the arterioles dilate. Systemic hypoxia thus has a vasodilator effect, and the resulting increase in tissue perfusion helps to restore the O_2 supply. Hypoxic relaxation can be produced in isolated vascular myocytes and is mediated by hyperpolarization (Figure 12.1). The

hyperpolarization is partly due to K_{ATP} activation; (see Appendix 2, 'Hypoxia').

The situation during exercise differs from systemic hypoxia (perfusion with hypoxic arterial blood). During normal exercise the arterioles are perfused with blood of normal PaO_2. Since O_2 freely permeates the arteriole wall, the tunica media is unlikely to be hypoxic. The skeletal muscle fibres, by contrast, become increasingly hypoxic as their O_2 consumption increases. This local tissue hypoxia leads to the parenchymal formation of the vasodilator agent **adenosine** (see below). Studies with blockers indicate that adenosine formation contributes substantially to metabolic hyperaemia.

Hypoxia constricts pulmonary vessels and large systemic arteries

Although hypoxia dilates systemic arterioles, it constricts pulmonary blood vessels. Pulmonary hypoxic vasoconstriction can cause serious illness at high altitude and is considered further in Section 15.5. Hypoxia can also trigger the contraction of large systemic arteries (see Appendix 2, 'Hypoxia').

Adenosine

Adenosine causes vasodilatation, partly through the receptor–adenylate cyclase–cAMP pathway (Figure 12.10 and Appendix 2). Adenosine is formed in the interstitial fluid of skeletal muscle and myocardium by the dephosphorylation of interstitial adenosine monophosphate (AMP) by AMP 5′-nucleotidase, an ecto-enzyme (outward facing enzyme) on the cell membranes. AMP is a breakdown product of ATP and is released into the interstitial fluid in increasing amounts during exercise or systemic hypoxia.

In the myocardium during exercise there is a good correlation between metabolic rate, the adenosine content of coronary venous blood, and the coronary blood flow. Experimental degradation of the myocardial adenosine by the infusion of adenosine deaminase approximately halves the metabolic hyperaemia. Similarly, the metabolic hyperaemia of skeletal muscle or brain is substantially attenuated by perfusion with the adenosine receptor blocker phenyltheophylline. Some hyperaemia always persists however, indicating that adenosine is not the sole factor responsible for metabolic hyperaemia.

Interstitial K$^+$

During muscle contraction or brain neuronal activity, K$^+$ ions are transferred from the intracellular to extracellular compartment by the repolarizing, outward K$^+$ current after each action potential. In the early stages of exercise the interstitial [K$^+$] in the active muscle can rise from 4 mM to 9 mM. Increases in interstitial [K$^+$] in this range cause myocyte hyperpolarization, leading to vasodilatation. The hyperpolarization is due to K$_{IR}$ channel activation and Na$^+$–K$^+$ pump stimulation.

The rise in interstitial [K$^+$] is most pronounced in the early stages of exercise or neuronal activity. Interstitial [K$^+$] then decays, especially in the brain, as the tissue reaches a new steady state. It is thought, therefore, that interstitial [K$^+$] contributes more to the initial stage of metabolic hyperaemia than to the later stage.

Phosphate ions and hyperosmolarity

Both interstitial phosphate and increased interstitial osmolarity elicit vasodilatation, and may contribute to exercise hyperaemia. **Inorganic phosphate ions** are released into the interstitial fluid of active muscle following the breakdown of creatine phosphate and ATP. Along with the accumulation of K$^+$ ions and lactate (30 mM in intense exercise, cf. 0.6 mM normally) this raises the **osmolarity** of the interstitial fluid in the early stages of exercise. The osmolarity of the venous blood draining active muscle increases by 4–40 mmol/l.

To summarize, none of the identified metabolic factors can by themselves explain the rapid onset and sustained nature of metabolic hyperaemia, but all appear to play some role. A full 'accountancy' of the factors in metabolic hyperaemia still eludes us.

Mechanisms of action of individual vasodilators

Some readers will wish to know how each metabolic agent induces vascular muscle relaxation – which ion channels are activated etc. Others may feel that their heads are spinning enough already! The mechanisms have been largely omitted from the main text because multiple pathways are generally involved. Short accounts are provided in the Appendix under the same headings as above.

13.5 Regulation by autacoids

Autacoids are vasoactive organic chemicals that act in a paracrine fashion, i. e. they are produced locally, released locally and act on nearby cells. Autacoids are chiefly involved in pathological events such as inflammation and bleeding. They include histamine, bradykinin, serotonin (5-hydroxytryptamine), prostaglandins, thromboxane, leukotrienes and PAF (platelet activating factor). The following 'thumbnail sketches' describe the principal autacoids.

Histamine

Histamine is produced by the decarboxylation of the amino acid histidine and is stored in granules in mast cells and basophilic leukocytes. It is one of the chemical mediators of **inflammation**, being released in response to trauma and allergic reactions such as urticaria, anaphylaxis and asthma. Histamine dilates arterioles, constricts veins and increases venular permeability. Its effect depends on whether the target vessel has H$_1$ or H$_2$ receptors. H$_1$ receptors activate the phospholipase C–IP$_3$ pathway leading to vasoconstriction (Figure 12.6) and increased venular permeability (Figure 11.28). H$_2$ receptors activate the adenylate cyclase–cAMP pathway leading to vascular relaxation (Figure 12.10). Histamine also contributes to the itching, prickly sensation of mild inflammation.

Bradykinin

Bradykinin is a nonapeptide that causes vasodilatation of resistance vessels and increased venular permeability. It is generated by an enzyme, kallikrein, that is activated during inflammation. Kallikrein cleaves bradykinin from a plasma protein precursor, kininogen. Bradykinin contributes to the hyperaemia, swelling and pain of **inflammation**, and is the most potent pain-producing autacoid. Its vasodilator effect is mediated by endothelial NO production in some tissues, possibly EDHF in human skin, and prostacyclin in other tissues.

Serotonin (5-hydroxytryptamine, 5-HT)

Serotonin is produced from the amino acid tryptophan in platelets, argentaffin cells of the intestine, some central neurons, and stinging nettles. Serotonin causes vasoconstriction and increased venular permeability leading to inflammatory swelling. It also contributes to the pain of inflammation.

- **Platelet serotonin.** Platelets normally release serotonin during blood clotting. The serotonin-mediated vasoconstriction helps to arrest the bleeding. In atheromatous coronary arteries, however, platelets can be activated inappropriately, and the released serotonin, thromboxane and PAF (see below) cause **coronary vasospasm**.

- **Argentaffin cell serotonin.** In the intestinal tract serotonin may contribute to the regulation of local blood flow and intestinal smooth muscle. Argentaffin cells occasionally give rise to **carcinoid tumour**, which releases large quantities of serotonin into the circulation and causes attacks of hypertension and diarrhoea.

- **Central neuron serotonin.** Serotonin is a central neurotransmitter, and the hallucinogenic drug lysergic acid diamine (LSD) is a serotonin antagonist. Serotonin is common in neurons close to cerebral blood vessels. The release of perivascular serotonin probably contributes to **cerebral artery vasospasm** in the initial phase of migraine and in subarachnoid haemorrhages.

Prostaglandins and thromboxane

The prostaglandins and thromboxane are vasoactive agents produced from the fatty acid arachidonic acid through the action of cyclo-oxygenase (COX). A collective term for COX products is 'eicosanoid'. Eicosanoid synthesis can be reduced therapeutically by COX inhibitors such as aspirin, ibuprofen and indomethacin ('non-steroidal anti-inflammatory drugs').

Prostaglandins are produced by many kinds of cell – endothelium, leukocytes, fibroblasts and macrophages. Different prostaglandins have different actions. The F series (PGF) are mainly vasoconstrictor agents, while the E series (PGE) and prostacyclin (PGI$_2$) are vasodilators (Figure 9.8). The vasodilator prostaglandins contribute to **inflammatory vasodilatation** and **reactive hyperaemia** (see later).

Thromboxane A$_2$ is a powerful vasoconstrictor and **thrombotic agent**. It is synthesized via COX within platelets. When released during blood clotting, the powerful vasoconstrictor action of thromboxane helps to stop the bleeding. Like serotonin it is released inappropriately by atheroma-activated platelets and contributes to **vasospasm** in atheromatous coronary arteries.

Thrombosis is the formation of an organized blood clot inside a vessel. The first stage of thrombosis is the aggregation of platelets, which is mediated by released thromboxane. Low doses of **aspirin** inhibit the platelet COX and reduce the platelet thromboxane content, without much affecting endothelial COX and the production of endothelial prostacyclin, which is an anti-aggregation factor. Low doses of aspirin thus provide protection against thrombosis, and are widely prescribed as a prophylaxis against thrombosis in patients with coronary atheroma.

Leukotrienes

Leukotrienes are vasoactive agents produced by leukocytes from arachidonic acid via the enzyme lipoxygenase (LOX). They are important mediators of the **inflammatory response**. Leukotrienes cause leukocyte margination and emigration, gap formation in the walls of venules, and vasoconstriction. Their gap-inducing action is 1000 times more potent than that of histamine.

Platelet activating factor (PAF)

PAF is a vasoactive lipid produced by activated inflammatory cells such as polymorphonuclear leukocytes and macrophages. Despite its name PAF exerts many of its major effects on smooth muscle. PAF contributes to the increased venular permeability of **inflammation**. It is particularly important as a mediator of bronchoconstriction in asthmatics. PAF may also contribute to vasospasm in atheromatous coronary arteries.

13.6 The autoregulation of blood flow

The intrinsic mechanisms described above – the myogenic response, endothelial secretions, vasodilator metabolites and autacoids – account for several major circulatory responses without any help from extrinsic nerves or hormones. The most important of these responses are the **autoregulation** of flow, **functional hyperaemia** and **reactive hyperaemia**.

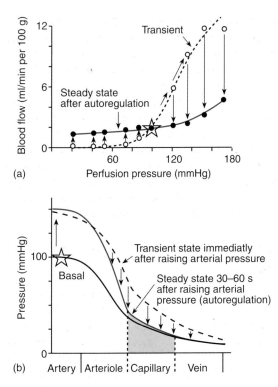

Figure 13.9 Autoregulation of (a) blood flow and of (b) capillary pressure in isolated, perfused skeletal muscle. The dashed lines show the transient flow or pressure immediately after changing perfusion pressure from its control level of 100 mmHg (star), before autoregulation has had time to 'kick in'. Over the next 30–60 s arteriolar contraction/dilatation (arrows) adjusts the flow and capillary pressure to a steady-state value (solid curve) that is only slightly different from the control value. ((a) From Jones, R. D. and Berne, R. M. (1964) *Circulation Research*, **14**, 126, by permission.)

Autoregulation keeps blood flow almost constant when pressure changes

The relation between perfusion pressure and the blood flow in myocardium, brain, kidney, skeletal muscle and intestine is truly remarkable, because changes in perfusion pressure over a wide range have little effect on the steady state blood flow. The plot of flow versus pressure is almost flat (Figures 13.6, 13.9a, 8.18). This phenomenon is called autoregulation.

At first sight the flat autoregulation line appears to defy the laws of flow, which state that flow increases with perfusion pressure. The relative constancy of tissue blood flow is due to the active response of resistance vessels. A rise in pressure initially raises the flow (Figure 13.9a, dashed line) but within 30–60 seconds the arterioles respond by contracting. This increases the vascular resistance and reduces the flow almost to its former level (Figure 13.9a, solid line). Conversely, a fall in pressure evokes vasodilatation, which reduces the resistance and restores the flow.

Active changes in vascular calibre thus hold flow almost constant in the steady-state. The pressure range for autoregulation has upper and lower limits, and during severe hypotension the cerebral blood flow, renal function etc. do decline.

The usefulness of autoregulation is that it preserves the blood flow to an organ when arterial pressure is fluctuating or falling. In the **brain** autoregulation will maintain blood flow during spinal anaesthesia even though spinal anaesthesia causes hypotension. In the **myocardium** autoregulation helps to maintain blood flow downstream of a stenosed coronary artery, where pressure is reduced. In the **kidney** autoregulation maintains a constant renal perfusion and glomerular capillary pressure, thus stabilizing the glomerular filtration rate. This leads us to the second major function of autoregulation, namely the regulation of capillary pressure.

Autoregulation stabilizes capillary pressure

As well as stabilizing tissue perfusion, autoregulation stabilizes the capillary blood pressure and hence fluid turnover (Figure 13.9b). In a study where skeletal muscle was perfused from an artificial pump, the capillary pressure increased by only 2 mmHg as the arterial pressure was raised from 30 to 170 mmHg. This is because capillary pressure depends on the pre- to postcapillary resistance ratio (Section 11.2), and the resistance ratio is increased by the autoregulatory contraction of arterioles as arterial pressure is raised. Due to the increased resistance and pressure drop across the arterioles, capillary blood pressure hardly increases.

Capillary pressure autoregulation helps to protect tissues against oedema formation when arterial pressure rises. Capillary pressure autoregulation is particularly important in the kidney, where it ensures a virtually constant glomerular filtration rate.

Autoregulation is chiefly due to the myogenic response

Two mechanisms have been proposed for autoregulation, namely the myogenic response (Section 13.2) and vasodilator washout, i.e. a reduction in the tissue concentration of vasodilator metabolites by a transiently increased blood flow following increased arterial pressure. Indirect evidence indicates that the myogenic mechanism predominates in the brain, kidney, intestine, liver and spleen. For example the blockage of 20-HETE formation (the vasoconstrictor agent involved in sustained myogenic responses) severely impairs autoregulation in the brain and kidney.

The hierarchy of vascular control

■ The regulation of vascular tone can be viewed as a three tier hierarchy.

■ *Bottom tier.* The most basic form of regulation is *autoregulation*. Resistance vessels react to changes in blood pressure so that blood flow varies little with pressure. Autoregulation is due chiefly to the Bayliss myogenic response.

■ *Middle tier.* The autoregulated flow is increased or decreased by *intrinsic regulatory chemicals* produced within the tissue. The chief ones are the vasodilators of functional hyperaemia (CO_2, lactate, adenosine, K^+, phosphate and hyperosmolarity), endothelial secretions (NO, EDHF, prostacyclin, endothelin) and autacoids (histamine, bradykinin, serotonin, thromboxane, PAF).

■ *Top tier.* The highest level of control is *extrinsic regulation* from outside the tissue by vasomotor nerves and hormones. This brings vascular regulation under the control of the brain.

An autoregulated flow can be changed by metabolic factors and sympathetic activity

Autoregulation does not mean that blood flow is unchangeable, only that it is insensitive to arterial pressure. Changes in metabolic or sympathetic activity can still alter the blood flow, by resetting autoregulation to operate at a different level. Figure 13.6 illustrates how autoregulation and changes in blood flow can co-exist. Increasing the myocardial metabolic rate raised the blood flow (metabolic hyperaemia), but the pressure–flow relation remained relatively flat and autoregulated at each work rate. Autoregulation is reset by vasodilator metabolites to operate at a higher but still autoregulated flow.

13.7 Metabolic (functional) hyperaemia

In skeletal muscle, heart and brain the blood flow increases almost linearly with metabolic rate (Figures 13.6, 15.4). This linkage is called metabolic, functional or active hyperaemia. Metabolic hyperaemia is caused by the accumulation of the metabolic vasodilators described in Section 13.4, namely CO_2 and lactic acid, adenosine, K^+, phosphate and osmolarity. As well as acting directly on the vessel, most of these agents also inhibit the release of noradrenaline from sympathetic fibres (neuromodulation, Figure 14.2). Studies using eNOS inhibitors indicate that NO contributes little (~20%) or insignificantly to exercise hyperaemia. Autacoids do not contribute to normal metabolic hyperaemia, though bradykinin makes a contribution in limbs with ischaemic arterial disease.

It is worth repeating that functional hyperaemia is due entirely to intrinsic regulation, not to vasodilator nerves. Although functional hyperaemia might be called automatic, it should not be called autoregulation, because autoregulation is by definition a **constancy** of flow in the face of pressure changes. The co-existence of functional hyperaemia and autoregulation is illustrated in Figure 13.6.

Blood flow oscillates during rhythmic exercise

In rhythmically exercising skeletal muscle the mean blood flow is increased but the flow oscillates. The flow falls during each contraction phase because the vessels within the contracting muscle are compressed (Figure 13.4). The same is also true of myocardium (Figure 15.5). In both skeletal muscle and myocardium most of the hyperaemia occurs during the relaxation phases. Myoglobin within the muscle fibres holds a small O_2 reserve for use during the poorly perfused contraction phase.

An O_2 debt develops at the onset of exercise

The hyperaemic response to exercise is not instantaneous; as Figure 13.4 shows, the hyperaemia takes a minute or so to develop fully. As a result there is relative deficit of perfusion during the first minute, which builds up an 'O_2 debt'. The store of high-energy creatine phosphate in the muscle fibres is drawn on during this period. The O_2 debt ceases to grow any bigger once the increasing blood flow matches O_2 supply to demand. When the exercise stops, the hyperaemia does not cease instantly but decays gradually over many minutes (Figure 13.11). This period is called **post-exercise hyperaemia**. The post-exercise hyperaemia quickly repays the metabolic debt.

Hyperaemia is impaired during static exercise

Metabolic hyperaemia during static exercise is less pronounced than during dynamic exercise because the sustained rise in intra-muscle pressure limits the dilatation of resistance vessels. Consequently an O_2 debt builds up rapidly and progressively. This leads to the anaerobic production of lactic acid and rapid fatigue of the muscle.

The arterial tree undergoes a co-ordinated dilatation

The structure of the arterial supply to a skeletal muscle is shown in Figure 13.7. Under resting conditions the resistance of the conduit and feed arteries is relatively small (≤30%) compared with that of the resistance vessels. During functional hyperaemia, however, the resistance of resistance vessels can fall to 1/20th of normal. Under these conditions the resistance of the conduit and feed arteries would seriously limit the blood flow unless these arteries dilated as well, which they do. The arterioles and terminal arteries within the active tissue dilate first, through metabolic vasodilatation, and this induces the subsequent dilatation of the local conduit and feed arteries. Thus exercise hyperaemia is achieved through the co-ordinated dilatation of arterioles, terminal arteries, feed arteries and conduit arteries.

The mechanisms responsible for the co-ordinated vasodilatation are:

- **metabolic vasodilatation** of the terminal arteries and arterioles, i.e. resistance vessels;
- **ascending vasodilatation** of the smaller, feed arteries;
- **flow-induced vasodilatation** of the large, conduit arteries.

The conduit and feed arteries are often located outside the active muscle, beyond the reach of vasodilator metabolites, so large-vessel dilatation cannot be attributed directly to vasodilator metabolites. The relative importance of each mechanism in the different classes of vessel is graded as shown in Figure 13.7.

Ascending (conducted) vasodilatation occurs in feed arteries

Feed arteries are vessels of diameter up to 0.5 mm located between the conduit artery and terminal arteries, and they show the strange property of ascending or conducted vasodilatation. That is to say, when a vasodilatation is initiated distally in the intra-muscle arteriolar network by metabolites (or by acetylcholine in a laboratory experiment), the dilatation spreads rapidly up the arterial system in a proximal direction and within 30–60 s dilates the feed arteries several mm away, including those located outside the tissue (Figure 13.10).

Ascending vasodilatation is caused by the conduction of a signal (possibly hyperpolarization, possibly a chemical) along the arterial tree. Since ascending vasodilatation halts when it reaches a ring of damaged

endothelium, it is inferred that the signal is transmitted by the gap junctions of arterial endothelial cells. From the endothelial cells the signal is transmitted to the media through the myoendothelial gap junctions.

Flow-induced dilatation occurs in large, conduit arteries

Widening of the main conduit artery to an exercising muscle group is an automatic sequel to the metabolic dilatation of resistance vessels. The increased blood flow raises the artery wall shear stress, which stimulates an increase in endothelial NO production (Figure 9.9).

Summary of functional hyperaemia

Increased tissue activity elicits a co-ordinated dilatation of the arterial system supplying that tissue. The metabolic hyperaemia is due primarily to metabolite-induced dilatation of local arterioles, but

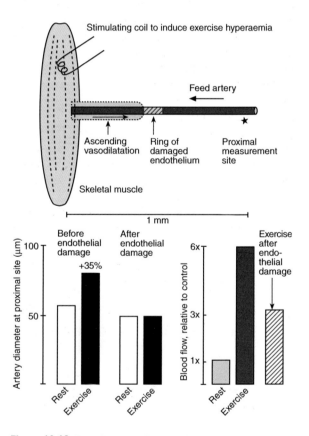

Figure 13.10 Ascending vasodilatation of a feed artery in response to contractions of a hamster muscle. Metabolic hyperaemia caused a 6× increase in blood flow. After destruction of a ring of endothelium the ascending dilatation halted at the ring and the metabolic hyperaemia was reduced by 47%. (Adapted from Segal, S. S. and Jacobs, T. L. (2001); see Research papers.)

ascending vasodilatation of feed arteries and flow-induced vasodilatation of conduit arteries are necessary for the full expression of the hyperaemia. Without ascending vasodilatation, the resistance of the feed arteries can seriously limit the exercise hyperaemia. In one study it was found that blocking the ascending vasodilatation reduced the exercise hyperaemia by 50%.

13.8 Reactive (post-ischaemic) hyperaemia

If a conduit artery is compressed to arrest the blood flow to a tissue, or to reduce flow to a point where it cannot meet the tissue O_2 requirement (a state called ischaemia), the blood flow upon releasing the compression is many times higher than normal (Figure 13.11). This is called reactive or post-ischaemic hyperaemia. It is particularly obvious in the skin, which flushes a bright pink after a period of compression. The reactive hyperaemia then decays exponentially with time. The value of reactive hyperaemia lies in optimizing the supply of O_2 and nutrients to ischaemic tissue.

The **myogenic response** probably contributes significantly to the hyperaemia that follows a brief arterial occlusion ($<30\,s$). The arterioles dilate myogenically in response to the fall in transmural pressure. With longer occlusions **vasodilator metabolites** accumulate, and after 3 min of occlusion the vasodilatation is near-maximal in human limbs. Since reactive hyperaemia is reduced (but not abolished) by indomethacin, **prostaglandins** too must contribute to the vasodilatation. A minor contribution by **nitric**

oxide has also been reported for some tissues. The longer the ischaemic period, the greater is the accumulation of vasodilator substances and the greater the total cumulative blood flow afterwards. Long occlusions are followed by a hyperaemic plateau before the exponential decay towards normal commences.

13.9 Ischaemia–reperfusion injury

Surgeons may have to arrest the blood supply to a region for a long period – hours, for example, during an aortic aneurysm repair, or during organ transplant surgery (kidney, heart–lung, liver). When the clamped artery is subsequently released it is often found that, instead of the brisk reactive hyperaemia that follows a few minutes of occlusion, the hyperaemia is weak and flow falls to abnormally low levels within minutes ('no-reflow' phenomenon). Moreover the tissues show biochemical and structural signs of cellular damage soon after the flow is restarted. This is called ischaemia–reperfusion injury. Ischaemia–reperfusion injury occurs in the intestine, liver, heart and limbs, and may also affect the rim of tissue around a myocardial or cerebral infarct.

The tissue injury is caused, paradoxically, by the restored blood supply rather than by the ischaemia itself. For example, three hours of ischaemia followed by an hour of reperfusion produces more tissue injury than does 4 hours of ischaemia. Both the O_2 content and white cell content of the reperfused blood appear to contribute to the injury, since (i) reperfusion with leukocyte-free blood attenuates reperfusion injury; and (ii) reperfusion with hypoxic blood likewise attenuates reperfusion injury. A third factor contributing to reperfusion injury, particularly in the heart, is cytosolic Ca^{2+} overload (Section 6.12).

Leukocyte adhesion and activation contribute to reperfusion damage

Ischaemic endothelial cells express selectins and other adhesion molecules at their surface. As leukocytes in the reperfusing blood reach the microvessels, the leukocytes adhere to the endothelium (see Section 9.8). Leukocytes are ~100 times stiffer than red cells, and their adhesion within microvessels, coupled with ischaemic swelling of the endothelium, impedes microvascular perfusion. At the same time the activated, adherent leukocytes cause inflammation by releasing leukotrienes and PAF, and

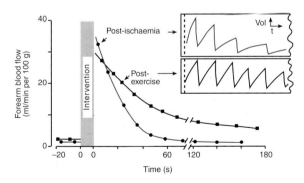

Figure 13.11 Forearm blood flow in a medical student measured by venous occlusion plethysmography (see Section 8.3) after 120 s of ischaemia (brachial artery occlusion) or after 30 s of strenuous forearm exercise. Note that blood flow remains elevated for a longer period after exercise. Insets show typical forearm volume traces during plethysmographic measurements.

cause tissue damage through the formation of super-oxide anions and hydrogen peroxide, and through the release of leukocyte elastase, a potent protease. In laboratory experiments antibodies against the leukocyte−endothelial adhesion molecules attenuate ischaemia−reperfusion injury.

Free oxygen radicals are an important cause of reperfusion injury

The presence of oxygen in the reperfusing blood contributes strongly to reperfusion injury. The oxygen gives rise to free radicals such as the superoxide radical $O_2^-\bullet$ and hydroxyl radical $OH\bullet$. These are highly reactive particles because they have an unpaired electron in their outer shell. They react readily with membrane lipids and proteins to cause cellular damage.

There are two generators of free oxygen radicals during reperfusion. Activated, adherent leukocytes are one source. The enzyme **NADPH oxidase in leukocytes** generates superoxide radicals.

The tissue itself is the second generator of radicals in myocardium and intestinal mucosa, due to the presence of an enzyme, **xanthine dehydrogenase**. Intestinal villi in particular have a high concentration of xanthine dehydrogenase and are very sensitive to reperfusion injury. During the ischaemic period xanthine dehydrogenase is converted to xanthine oxidase by a Ca^{2+}-triggered protease, which is present in the heart and viscera but not skeletal muscle. At the same time the enzyme substrate, hypoxanthine, accumulates owing to the breakdown of ATP via adenosine. When O_2 is reperfused, xanthine oxidase oxidizes the hypoxanthine to xanthine, and in the course of this reaction harmless molecular O_2 is converted into superoxide and hydroxyl radicals. Reperfusion thus generates a burst of toxic radicals.

Reperfusion injury in many tissues is attenuated by allopurinol, an inhibitor of xanthine oxidase. Reperfusion injury is also attenuated by scavengers of free oxygen radicals such as superoxide dismutase and dimethyl sulphoxide, confirming the role of free oxygen radicals in reperfusion injury.

Cytosolic Ca^{2+} overload contributes to myocardial reperfusion injury

Reperfusion injury in myocardium is also caused in part by overloading of the cytosol with Ca^{2+} during the ischaemic period. This was described under 'The paradox of myocardial ischaemia−reperfusion injury' in Section 6.12.

SUMMARY

■ Although complex in detail, the control of blood vessels can be conceptualized fairly simply as a hierarchy of three control systems, each of which can override and modify the lower one.

■ The **lowest level of control** is the **Bayliss myogenic response**, namely vascular contraction in response to an increase in blood pressure. This helps to generates basal tone in resistance vessels. The myogenic response also keeps blood flow and capillary pressure almost constant when arterial pressure changes (**autoregulation**).

■ A **second level of control** is exerted by **local chemical factors**. Vasodilator agents related to the local metabolic activity of the tissue (adenosine, CO_2, lactate, K^+, phosphate, osmolarity) act on the arterioles and raise the blood flow to match the tissue metabolic requirement (**functional** or **metabolic hyperaemia**). This process is well developed in myocardium, brain and skeletal muscle. **Ascending (conducted) vasodilatation** ensures that feed arteries do not limit the hyperaemia, while **shear-induced vasodilatation** dilates the conduit artery.

■ A period of reduced perfusion evokes **post-ischaemic** or **reactive hyperaemia**, which is due to the myogenic response and metabolite accumulation. Longer periods of ischaemia can be followed by **reperfusion injury**, due to adherent leukocytes and free oxygen radical generation by leukocyte NADPH oxidase and tissue xanthine oxidase.

■ **Endothelial nitric oxide** has a tonic vasodilator influence on basal tone, especially in pregnancy. Increased NO mediates flow-induced vasodilatation in conduit arteries, and the vasodilator action of bradykinin, substance P and acetylcholine. Inducible NO synthase contributes to endotoxin hypotension. Nitridergic parasympathetic fibres induce the dilatation that drives genital erection.

■ **Autacoids** are paracrine vasoactive agents such as histamine, bradykinin, serotonin, prostaglandins, leukotrienes and PAF. Autacoids modify local vascular tone, generally in pathological situations such as inflammation and bleeding.

■ The **third level of control** is the **neuro-endocrine system**, which brings the vasculature under central and reflex control for the benefit of the organism as a whole (next chapter).

FURTHER READING

Reviews and chapters

Calver, A., Collier, J. and Vallance, P. (1993) Nitric oxide and cardiovascular control. *Experimental Physiology*, **78**, 303–326.

Delph, M. D. and Laughlin, M. H. (1998) Regulation of skeletal muscle perfusion during exercise. *Acta Physiologica Scandinavica*, **162**, 411–419.

Granger, D. N. and Korthuis, R. J. (1995) Physiological mechanisms of postischemic tissue injury. *Annual Review of Physiology*, **57**, 311–332.

Gustafsson, F. and Holstein-Rathlou, N-H. (1999) Conducted vasomotor responses in arterioles: characteristics, mechanisms and physiological significance. *Acta Physiologica Scandinavica*, **167**, 11–21.

Hill, S. J. (1990) Distribution, properties and functional characteristics of 3 classes of histamine receptor. *Pharmacological Reviews*, **42**, 45–83.

Marshall, J. M. (1999) The integrated response to hypoxia: from circulation to cells. *Experimental Physiology*, **84**, 449–470.

Meininger, G. A. and Davis, M. J. (1992) Cellular mechanisms involved in the vascular myogenic response. *American Journal of Physiology*, **263**, H647–H659.

Melkumyants, A. M., Balashov, S. A. and Khayutin, V. M. (1995) Control of arterial lumen by shear stress on endothelium. *News in Physiological Sciences*, **10**, 204–210.

Moncada, S. (1992) The L-arginine:nitric oxide pathway. *Acta Physiologica Scandinavica*, **145**, 201–227.

Roman, R. J. (2002) P-450 metabolites of arachidonic acid in the control of cardiovascular function. *Physiological Reviews*, **82**, 131–185.

Segal, S. S. (1992) Communication among endothelial and smooth muscle cells coordinates blood flow control during exercise. *News in Physiological Sciences*, **7**, 152–156.

Soloviev, A. I. and Braquet, P. (1992) Platelet-activating factor – a potent endogenous mediator responsible for coronary vasospasm. *News in Physiological Sciences*, **7**, 166–172.

Research papers

Austin, C. and Wray, S. (1995) The effects of extracellular pH and calcium change on force and intracellular calcium in rat vascular smooth muscle. *Journal of Physiology*, **488**, 281–291.

Carr, P., Graves, J. and Poston, L. (1993) Carbon dioxide induced relaxation in rat mesenteric arteries precontracted with noradrenaline is endothelium dependent and mediated by nitric oxide. *Pflüger's Archives*, **423**, 343–345.

Dart, C. and Standen, N. B. (1995) Activation of ATP-dependent K^+ channels by hypoxia in smooth muscle cells isolated from the pig coronary artery. *Journal of Physiology*, **483**, 29–39.

Doughty, J. M. and Langton, P. D. (2001) Measurement of chloride flux associated with the myogenic response in rat cerebral arteries. *Journal of Physiology*, **534**, 753–761.

Edmunds, N. J. and Marshall, J. M. (2001) Oxygen delivery and oxygen consumption in rat hindlimb during systemic hypoxia: role of adenosine. *Journal of Physiology*, **536**, 927–935.

Fisslthaler, B., Dimmeler, S., Hermann, C., Busse, R. and Fleming, I. (2000) Phosphorylation and activation of the endothelial nitric oxide synthase by fluid shear stress. *Acta Physiologica Scandinavica*, **168**, 81–88.

Hussain, S. T., Smith, R. E., Medbak, S., Wood, R. F. M. and Whipp, B. J. (1996) Haemodynamics and metabolic responses of the lower limb after high intensity exercise in humans. *Experimental Physiology*, **81**, 173–187.

Kanwar, S., Smith, C. W. and Kubes, P. (1998) An absolute requirement for P-selectin in ischemia/reperfusion-induced leukocyte recruitment in cremaster muscle. *Microcirculation*, **5**, 281–287.

Karim, F. and Goonewardene, I. P. (1996) The role of adenosine in functional hyperaemia in the coronary circulation of anaesthetized dogs. *Journal of Physiology*, **490**, 793–803.

Knot, H. J. and Nelson, M. T. (1998) Regulation of arterial diameter and wall [Ca^{2+}] in cerebral arteries of rat by membrane potential and intravascular pressure. *Journal of Physiology*, **508**, 199–209.

Lynge, J., Juel, C. and Hellsten, Y. (2001) Extracellular formation and uptake of adenosine during skeletal muscle contraction in the rat: role of adenosine transporters. *Journal of Physiology*, **537**, 597–605.

McCarron, J. G. and Halpern, W. (1990) Potassium dilates rat cerebral arteries by two independent mechanisms. *American Journal of Physiology*, **259**, H902–H908.

Segal, S. S. and Jacobs, T. L. (2001) Role for endothelial cell conduction in ascending vasodilatation and exercise hyperaemia in hamster skeletal muscle. *Journal of Physiology*, **536**, 937–946.

Siegel, G., Schnalke, F., Schaarschmidt, J., Müller, J. and Hetzer, R. (1991) Hypoxia and vascular muscle tone in normal and arteriosclerotic human coronary arteries. *Journal of Vascular Medicine and Biology*, **3**, 140–149.

Wennmalm, D. and Sandgren, G. (1991) Metabolic and myogenic components of reactive hyperaemia in the human calf. *Acta Physiologica Scandinavica*, **142**, 529–530.

Control of blood vessels II: extrinsic control

Learning objectives

After reading this chapter you should be able to:

• Sketch the sympathetic pathway from brain to a blood vessel and the adrenal medulla (14.1).

• Name the neurotransmitters and receptors involved in sympathetic vasomotor neurotransmission (14.1).

• List the chief functions of sympathetic vasoconstrictor nerves (14.1).

• State the distribution, main neurotransmitters and roles of (i) parasympathetic vasodilator nerves (14.2) and (ii) sympathetic vasodilator nerves (14.3).

• Explain the meaning of 'sensory axon reflex' (14.4).

• List the similarities and differences between the cardiovascular effects of adrenaline and noradrenaline (14.6).

• Outline the formation, action and regulation of angiotensin II, vasopressin and atrial natriuretic peptide (14.7–14.9).

• State the importance and main mechanisms of venous control (14.10).

The previous chapter focussed on the intrinsic regulation of vascular tone by mechanisms originating within the tissue. Local mechanisms, however, serve only local needs. To serve the more general needs of the whole organism, such as the homeostasis of blood pressure, the central nervous system superimposes a sentient control system over the entire peripheral vasculature by means of autonomic vasomotor nerves and endocrine secretions. Since control is imposed from outside the tissue, this is called extrinsic regulation. Extrinsic regulation is in general the efferent limb of a vascular reflex. The afferent or sensory limb of the reflex is described in Chapter 16.

There are three kinds of autonomic vasomotor nerve:

• sympathetic vasoconstrictor nerves
• parasympathetic vasodilator nerves
• sympathetic vasodilator nerves.

The labels 'vasoconstrictor' and 'vasodilator' refer to the effect of an increase in nerve activity, but it is important to remember that a reduction in nerve activity has the reverse effect. Vasodilatation is often induced not by vasodilator fibres but by reduced activity in sympathetic vasoconstrictor fibres. The flushed skin of warm extremities is an example.

Of the various classes of vasomotor nerve the
sympathetic vasoconstrictor fibres are the most
widespread and the most important physiologically.
Students accustomed to associating sympathetic
activity with alarm and dilatation should note that
**the vast majority of sympathetic vasomotor
fibres are vasoconstrictor fibres**.

14.1 Sympathetic vasoconstrictor nerves

The sympathetic system comprises bulbospinal, pre- and postganglionic fibres

The pathway controlling the sympathetic vasoconstrictor fibres begins in the medulla of the brainstem.
From here descending excitatory and inhibitory fibres

called bulbospinal fibres pass down the spinal cord.
The bulbospinal fibres synapse with sympathetic preganglionic neurons in the intermediolateral columns
of grey matter, in the thoracicolumbar segments T1
to L3 (Figure 14.1).

Cholinergic preganglionic fibres act on nicotinic receptors in sympathetic ganglia

The activity of spinal preganglionic neurons depends
on the interplay of excitatory and inhibitory inputs
from the bulbospinal fibres and from local spinal
inputs. The axons of the preganglionic neurons
travel through the ventral roots of the spinal nerves
and white rami communicantes into the sympathetic chain. The axons may travel up or down the
chain for several segments before synapsing with

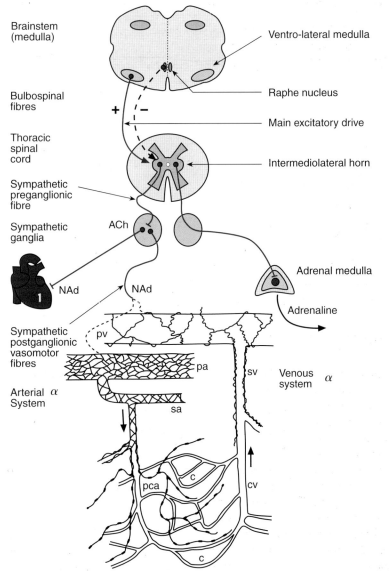

Figure 14.1 Sympathetic innervation of cardiovascular system. α and β refer to predominant
adrenoceptors on the end-organs. NAd, noradrenaline; ACh, acetylcholine. One descending tract
(bulbospinal tract) excites the sympathetic IML
cells; other bulbospinal fibres inhibit the cell. pa
and pv, primary artery and vein to an organ,
respectively; sa and sv, small artery and vein,
respectively; pca, precapillary arteriole; c, capillary; cv, collecting venule. (Adapted from Furness,
J. B. and Marshall, J. M. (1974) *Journal of
Physiology*, **239**, 75–88, by permission.)

Smoking and the vascular system

■ Smoking induces vasoconstriction. This reduces cutaneous and coronary blood flow and raises blood pressure.

■ The vasoconstriction is due to increased sympathetic vasoconstrictor nerve activity, increased circulating adrenaline and reduced nitric oxide. The first two effects are caused by the stimulation of nicotinic receptors on the postganglionic cells.

■ NO levels are low because NO reacts with free oxygen radicals, which are increased by smoking. Smoking-activated leukocytes generate free radicals in oxidative bursts.

■ Low levels of NO and prostacyclin facilitate platelet aggregation, thrombosis and atheroma.

■ The walls of arterioles are thickened, probably due to the hypertension and the loss of the inhibitory effect of NO on myocyte proliferation.

postganglionic neurons in the sympathetic ganglia. Some preganglionic axons do not synapse until they reach the adrenal medulla or a distant ganglion (the coeliac or hypogastric ganglion). The preganglionic fibres are mostly cholinergic and the **postganglionic receptors are nicotinic**, being blocked by hexamethonium. The nicotinic receptors contribute to the vascular effects of smoking. Smoking causes vasoconstriction and an increase in blood pressure because it stimulates postganglionic cells, which increases the sympathetic vasoconstrictor fibre activity and adrenaline secretion. Smoking also impairs NO-mediated vasodilatation (Concept Box 18).

Noradrenergic postganglionic fibres innervate the tunica media

The postganglionic neurons send non-myelinated axons from the sympathetic chain through the grey rami communicantes for distribution in the mixed peripheral nerves. Some fibres also course directly over the major vessels. At their terminations the fibres run along the outer border of the tunica media. Except in veins the fibres do not penetrate the inner media, perhaps due to the higher pressure there. Most small arteries and terminal resistance arteries are richly innervated but the smallest arterioles are poorly innervated. Small arterioles are controlled chiefly by local tissue metabolites (Figure 13.7). The venous system shows a similar pattern of innervation but it is generally less dense, and skeletal muscle veins have almost no sympathetic innervation.

Noradrenaline from sympathetic varicosities excites α-adrenoceptors

The terminal sympathetic axon resembles a string of beads (Figure 1.10). Each bead, or varicosity, contains dense-cored vesicles packed with the neurotransmitter noradrenaline (norepinephrine in the American literature). The passage of an action potential along a sympathetic axon releases only a small fraction of its noradrenaline, because only a few out of the hundreds of varicosities succeed in releasing a vesicle.

The released noradrenaline diffuses quickly across the junctional gap and binds to α-adrenoceptors on the vascular myocyte membrane (Figure 14.2). There are two kinds of α receptor. The α_1-receptor is found on most blood vessels. The α_2-receptor occurs as a pre-junctional receptor on the sympathetic varicosities and also post-junctionally on resistance vessels in human limbs, along with the α_1-receptors (Table 14.1). Post-junctional α_1- and α_2-receptors contribute roughly equally to sympathetic-mediated resistance in resting human limbs. The α-adrenoceptors elicit vasoconstriction through electromechanical and pharmacomechanical coupling (Section 12.6). The response of a small artery to sympathetic stimulation is shown in Figure 12.9.

About 80% of the noradrenaline is then transported back into the axon, terminating its action and restocking the axon. Transmitter action is terminated to a lesser extent by degradation by the post-junctional enzymes catechol-O-methyltransferase and monoamine oxidase, and by diffusion into nearby capillaries (Figure 14.2). Much of the circulating plasma noradrenaline is a 'spillover' from sympathetic terminals.

Noradrenaline release is modulated by local metabolites and agonists

The amount of neurotransmitter released by the axon increases with impulse frequency. Transmitter release is also influenced by the chemical environment of the varicosity, a process known as **neuromodulation** (Figure 14.2). Many vasodilator metabolites, such as H^+, K^+ and adenosine, act on the varicosity to depress noradrenaline release and thus enhance metabolic hyperaemia. Most vasodilator autacoids have a similar effect. Noradrenaline itself binds to pre-junctional α_2-receptors (autoreceptors) which inhibit the further release of noradrenaline. By contrast, the vasoconstrictor hormone **angiotensin II facilitates transmitter release** and thereby amplifies its own direct vasoconstrictor effect.

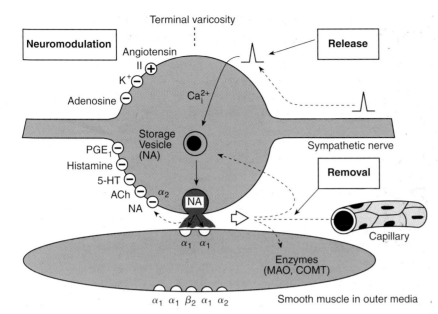

Figure 14.2 Neurotransmission at the junctional varicosity of a sympathetic vasoconstrictor nerve. Not to scale (the varicosity is 2 μm long × 1 μm wide, the axon 0.1–0.5 μm wide and the smooth muscle cell 4 μm wide at the centre). NA, noradrenaline; for other abbreviations see text. ATP and neuropeptide Y, which act as co-transmitters with NA in some fibres, are not shown.

Table 14.1 Adrenergic receptors in the cardiovascular system.

Receptor	Subtype	Principal location and effect	Agonist	Antagonist	Medical use of antagonist
α		Vascular smooth muscle: vasoconstriction	Noradrenaline (NA) Adrenaline (Ad)	Ergotamine Phentolamine Phenoxybenzamine	Migraine Raynaud's vasospasm Acute hypertension (phaeochromocytoma)
	α_1	Postjunctional receptor of vascular smooth muscle: vasoconstriction	Specific agonist = phenylephrine Also NA and Ad	Prazosin	Anti-hypertension drug
	α_2	Prejunctional receptors of nerve varicosity: inhibition of NA release. Also vascular smooth muscle in human limbs	NA (and Ad) Clonidine	Yohimbine Rauwolscine	–
β		SA node, myocardium and arterioles of coronary, skeletal muscle and liver Increased heart rate, contractility and vasodilatation	Specific agonist = isoprenaline Also NA and Ad	Propranolol Oxprenolol	Relief of angina by reducing cardiac work Hypertension
	β_1	Subtype found in pacemaker and myocardium	NA Ad	Practolol (toxic) Atenolol Metroprolol	Angina relief Hypertension Arrhythmia control
	β_2	Arterioles of skeletal muscle, heart and liver: also bronchiole smooth muscle	Ad		

ATP and neuropeptide Y contribute to sympathetic neuromuscular transmission

The α-adrenoceptor blockers phentolamine and phenoxybenzamine completely abolish the vasoconstrictor response of most veins and the pulmonary artery to sympathetic stimulation. In many systemic arteries, however, α-blockers only partially block the vasoconstrictor response. This led to the discovery of additional neurotransmitters or 'co-transmitters' in the sympathetic varicosities, namely the purine ATP and the peptide neuropeptide Y (Table 14.2). The contribution of the co-transmitters varies from tissue to tissue.

Table 14.2 Main transmitter agents coexisting in perivascular nerves.*

Sympathetic vasoconstrictor fibre	Noradrenaline (NA)
	Adenosine triphosphate (ATP)
	Neuropeptide Y (NPY)
Parasympathetic dilator fibre	Acetylcholine (ACh)
	Vasoactive intestinal polypeptide (VIP)
	Nitric oxide (NO)
Sensory-dilator axons (C-fibre)	Substance P (SP)
	Calcitonon-gene related peptide (CGRP)
	ATP

* The ratio of transmitter substances within the fibre varies from tissue to tissue.
(From Burnstock, G. (1988) *Acta Physiologica Scandinavica*, **133**(Suppl. 571), 53–57.)

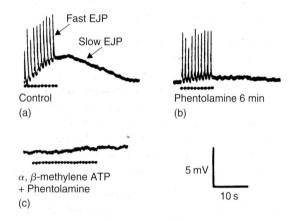

Figure 14.3 Evidence for co-transmission by noradrenaline and ATP in sympathetic vasoconstrictor nerves to the rat tail artery. (a) Intracellular potential during sympathetic nerve stimulation at each dot. Each stimulus produces a fast excitatory junction potential (fast EJP) (spike) plus a slower depolarization (baseline under the spike, slow EJP). The spikes are not action potentials (see voltage scale). (b) Phentolamine, an α-adrenoceptor blocker, abolishes the slow response. (c) α, β-methylene ATP, a desensitizer of purinergic receptors, abolishes the fast EJPs. (After Sneddon, P. and Burnstock, G. (1984) *European Journal of Pharmaology*, **106**, 149–152.)

ATP is synthesized locally and released with noradrenaline from the varicosities in some large arteries and small mesenteric arteries. The ATP stimulates post-junctional P_{2X} purinergic receptors, which activate non-selective cation channels. The cation current causes a fast, brief depolarization of the myocyte called a fast excitatory junction potential (Figures 14.3, 12.9).

Neuropeptide Y is synthesized in the postganglionic cell body and transported slowly along the axon to the sympathetic terminals, where it may be stored in the large dense-cored vesicles along with noradrenaline. Neuropeptide Y has been identified in the vasomotor nerves innervating skeletal muscle, kidney, salivary gland, spleen and nasal mucosa. It is released

chiefly in response to high frequency stimulation, which occurs under conditions of stress. Neuropeptide Y produces a slower, more prolonged depolarization than ATP and sensitizes the post-junctional membrane to noradrenaline. Some workers consider the latter, neuromodulatory effect to be its chief action.

Sympathetic fibres are tonically active

Sympathetic vasoconstrictor fibres are continuously active, with an average impulse frequency of 0.5–1/second in resting subjects and a highest mean frequency of 8–10/second. The discharge rate is not even, however. In skin the activity is irregular, whereas in muscle it occurs in pulsed bursts. The tonic sympathetic activity contributes substantially to vascular tone. Consequently, a reduction in sympathetic activity or pharmacological blockade causes vasodilatation. For example, in resting skeletal muscle interruption of the tonic sympathetic drive increases the blood flow from $2-5\,\mathrm{ml\,min^{-1}\,100\,g^{-1}}$ to $6-9\,\mathrm{ml\,min^{-1}\,100\,g^{-1}}$. The latter flow is far from maximal, however, due to the persistence of basal tone.

Sympathetic drive to different tissues is independently regulated

Students sometimes have the false notion that the entire sympathetic nervous system behaves like a single entity, i.e. when activity increases in one tissue, it does so in all tissues. Although this can happen, for example during a haemorrhage, it is generally not the case. The sympathetic vasoconstrictor activity to the skin is regulated independently of that to muscle, which in turn is regulated independently of that to the gastrointestinal tract – just as motor-neuron activity to the leg is independent of that to an arm. This is because each tissue is represented separately by a specific region within the ventrolateral brainstem. As a result, the sympathetic nerve activity to skin can be raised at the same time as the sympathetic nerve activity to muscle is reduced, as happens during the human *alerting response* to stress. Activation of the sympathetic system is not an 'all-or-none' affair but is finely graded and adjusted regionally according to circumstances.

Reduced sympathetic activity elicits vasodilatation

Although it is natural to think of vasoconstriction as the primary role of vasoconstrictor nerves, vasodilatation in response to reduced sympathetic activity is important too. Indeed, the observation that a rabbit ear flushes upon cutting the cervical sympathetic nerve led to the discovery of the vasoconstrictor nerves by

Claude Bernard in 1851. Two examples of vasodilatation through reduced sympathetic activity are as follows.

- If blood pressure rises, the baroreceptor reflex evokes a widespread fall in sympathetic activity (Section 16.2). The resulting vasodilatation helps to bring blood pressure back towards normal.

- If body temperature rises, the hypothalamic temperature-regulating centre evokes a fall in vasoconstrictor nerve activity to skin, and the ensuing cutaneous vasodilatation helps to bring the temperature back down (Section 15.3).

Increased sympathetic activity raises peripheral resistance and reduces local blood flow and volume

The effects of increased sympathetic activity are illustrated in Figure 14.4.

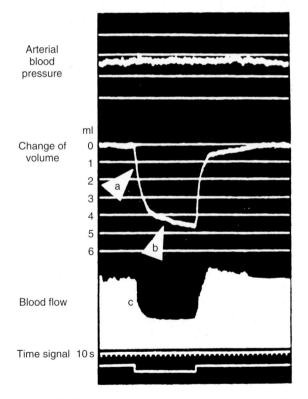

Figure 14.4 Three effects of sympathetic stimulation at just 2 impulses/s in cat hindquarters (signal). Arrow (a) indicates the decrease in volume due to reduction in capacitance vessel size. This is mostly secondary to a fall in venous pressure induced by arteriolar contraction; skeletal muscle veins have little direct innervation. Arrow (b) indicates the slow fall in volume due to capillary absorption of interstitial fluid, secondary to fall in capillary pressure induced by arteriolar contraction. Arrow (c) shows reduced blood flow due to contraction of resistance vessels. (From Mellander, S. (1960) *Acta Physiologica Scandinavica*, **50**(Suppl.), 176, by permission.)

- **Local blood flow** is reduced. This action can be sustained for long periods in some tissues, e.g. skin. In the intestine the arterioles quickly 'escape' from the vasoconstriction, but the veins do not.

- **The volume of blood** in an organ is reduced through venoconstriction (Figure 14.5). This can displace 28 ml blood/kg in the intestinal tract and liver, and 15 ml/kg in skin. In skeletal muscle the venous system lacks an effective innervation, but up to 7.5 ml/kg can be expelled passively because venous pressure falls secondary to arteriolar contraction (Figure 14.4, arrow a).

- **Capillary pressure** is reduced by the arteriolar constriction (Figure 11.4). This can lead to the osmotic absorption of interstitial fluid into the plasma compartment (Figure 14.4, arrow b).

- **Total peripheral resistance** is raised when there is a generalized increase in sympathetic outflow. This increases the arterial blood pressure. The **regulation of blood pressure** is one of the major functions of the sympathetic vasomotor system, both normally and in pathophysiological situations. To this end, sympathetic activity is controlled reflexly by information from pressure receptors (Chapter 16).

Increased sympathetic outflow is an important part of the body's defence against hypovolaemia (low blood volume, e.g. after a haemorrhage). Under these

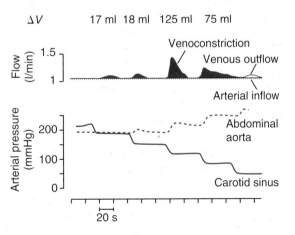

Figure 14.5 Active splanchnic venoconstriction in response to the sympathetic activity in a dog. Step reductions in carotid sinus pressure (isolated) elicit a reflex increase in sympathetic outflow. Arterial inflow and the outflow from the inferior vena cava were measured. Each transient excess of outflow over inflow marks an episode of venoconstriction. ΔV is the total volume of blood displaced by each venoconstriction. Aortic pressure increases due to a sympathetically mediated arteriolar constriction. (After Hainsworth, R. and Karim, F. (1976) *Journal of Physiology*, **262**, 659–677, by permission.)

circumstances the reduced peripheral flow, central displacement of peripheral venous blood, interstitial fluid absorption and increased total peripheral resistance constitute a life-preserving package of responses to support cardiac output and arterial pressure (Section 18.2).

Sympathetic activity and mean blood pressure show regular oscillations

The sympathetic discharge to skeletal muscle and the gastrointestinal system waxes and wanes with the respiratory cycle. Cardiac output too oscillates with respiration owing to a fall in left ventricular stroke volume during inspiration (Section 2.5, 'splitting of second sound'), which is not fully counteracted by the concomitant sinus tachycardia (Section 5.8). The oscillations in cardiac output and sympathetic activity cause oscillations of blood pressure in phase with respiration, called **Traube–Hering waves** (Section 8.4).

Human blood pressure may also oscillate at ~6 cycles/min, i.e. a lower frequency than the respiratory cycle. These oscillations are called **Mayer waves**. Mayer waves are attributed to cyclic changes in sympathetic vasomotor tone driven by a resonance in the baroreceptor reflex.

14.2 Parasympathetic vasodilator nerves

In a limited number of tissues the arteries and resistance vessels are innervated by vasodilator fibres as well as by the ubiquitous sympathetic vasoconstrictor fibres. Vasodilator fibres occur in the parasympathetic, sympathetic and sensory systems.

The parasympathetic system comprises long preganglionic and short postganglionic fibres

Parasympathetic fibres have a more restricted distribution than sympathetic fibres. Moreover the fibres are not tonically active, unlike sympathetic fibres. Parasympathetic fibres fire only when organ function demands a rise in blood flow.

The **preganglionic fibres** are much longer than their sympathetic counterparts and extend all the way to the innervated tissue. The preganglionic fibres emerge from the central nervous system in two 'outflows', one carried by the **cranial nerves** (e.g. the vagus) and the other by the **sacral spinal nerves**.

The cranial outflow innervates the cerebral and coronary arteries, salivary glands, exocrine pancreas and gastrointestinal mucosa. The sacral outflow innervates the genitalia, bladder and colon. Skin and muscle do not have a parasympathetic innervation.

Within the end-organ the long preganglionic fibres synapse with **postganglionic neurons**. Short postganglionic axons innervate the resistance vessels.

Parasympathetic vasodilatation is mediated by acetylcholine and NANC

The postganglionic axon terminals release the classic neurotransmitter **acetylcholine**. This elicits hyperpolarization and relaxation of the myocytes after a second or so (Figure 14.6). The relaxation is due partly to cholinergic stimulation of endothelial nitric oxide synthase, at least in some vessels. The direct effect of acetylcholine on myocytes is to cause vasoconstriction through M_3 muscarinic receptor activation (Figure 9.8).

Parasympathetic vasodilatation is often only partly inhibited by atropine, a muscarinic receptor blocker, because the fibres also release a **non-adrenergic, non-cholinergic (NANC) transmitter** (Figure 14.6). The predominant NANC transmitter is the neuropeptide **vasoactive intestinal polypeptide** (VIP).

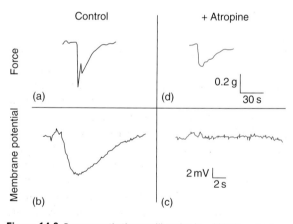

Figure 14.6 Parasympathetic vasodilatation in rabbit lingual artery. Noradrenergic fibres were blocked by guanethidine, so perivascular stimulation excited only parasympathetic responses. (a) Mechanical response showing dilatation. (b) Membrane potential showing slow hyperpolarization (baseline −51 mV). (c) Total abolition of electrical response by atropine, i.e. electrical response is purely cholinergic. (d) Dilatation, however, is only partially blocked by atropine, revealing the existence of non-cholinergic dilator transmitter − possibly vasoactive intestinal polypeptide. Removal of the arterial endothelium by rubbing did *not* abolish these responses. (From Brayden, J. E. and Large, W. A. (1986) *British Journal of Pharmacology*, **89**, 163–171, by permission.)

The neuropeptide **substance P** also contributes in some tissues. In other tissues parasympathetic terminals generate **nitric oxide** as a neurotransmitter. Nitridergic nerves may exist around cerebral, temporal, mesenteric and possibly coronary arteries, as well as in the genitalia (see later).

Parasympathetic dilatation in the salivary glands and pancreas subserves fluid secretion

Blood flow to the submandibular **salivary gland** increases ten-fold upon stimulation of the parasympathetic fibres of the chorda tympani nerve. The increased blood flow is needed to supply the water for salivation; a salivary gland can secrete its own weight in fluid in just 1 minute. The vasodilatation is mediated partly by acetylcholine (being partly blocked by atropine) and partly by VIP and substance P.

In the **pancreas** VIP rather than acetylcholine seems to be the main parasympathetic transmitter, so these fibres are called 'peptidergic'.

In the **intestinal submucosa** the postganglionic fibres release mainly acetylcholine. The vasodilatation is largely blocked by L–NMMA, indicating that it is mediated by acetylcholine-stimulated production of nitric oxide.

Parasympathetic dilatation in genitalia subserves erection

The sacral parasympathetic nerves innervate the blood vessels of erectile tissue, rendering these vasomotor nerves truly essential to the continuation of the species! Stimulation of the parasympathetic pelvic nerve in a dog causes a profound vasodilatation of the arterioles feeding the corpus cavernosum of the penis. This reverses the usual balance of resistances, so that the resistance to inflow becomes smaller than the resistance to outflow. The sinuses of the corpus therefore fill with blood at a high pressure, creating distension and erection. Withdrawal of sympathetic vasoconstrictor tone may be a supplementary factor.

Parasympathetic-induced erection in rats and rabbits is blocked by inhibitors of nitric oxide synthase but not by atropine, indicating that the parasympathetic fibres are chiefly **nitridergic** rather than cholinergic. The axons contain nitric oxide synthase and secrete NO upon electrical stimulation. Enhancement of the NO-triggered biochemical pathway by **sildenafil (Viagra)** is a successful treatment for human erectile dysfunction. The vasodilator action of NO is mediated by myocyte cGMP (Figure 9.9), which is normally degraded by an enzyme, phosphodiesterase.

Inhibition of the particular isoform present in the corpus vessels, namely phosphodiesterase type 5 (PDE5), by sildenafil raises the cGMP level and promotes erection.

Parasympathetic **VIP** may contribute to vasodilatation and erection. Immunocytochemistry reveals VIP in the parasympathetic nerves of the penile artery, and venous blood analysis shows that VIP is released on pelvic nerve stimulation.

14.3 Sympathetic vasodilator nerves

Most sympathetic vasomotor fibres are noradrenergic and cause vasoconstriction. In certain species and tissues, however, there is a limited distribution of sympathetic cholinergic fibres that cause vasodilatation.

In non-primates sympathetic cholinergic fibres to muscle mediate vasodilatation during the 'alerting response'

In cat, dog, goat and sheep, but not primates, the small arteries of skeletal muscle are innervated by sympathetic vasodilator nerves whose neurotransmitter is acetylcholine, as well as by sympathetic vasoconstrictor nerves. Selective excitation of the sympathetic cholinergic nerves causes vascular relaxation and increased muscle blood flow.

Unlike the sympathetic vasoconstrictor system, the sympathetic cholinergic system is controlled by the forebrain and is activated solely as part of the **alerting response** (Table 14.3). The alerting response is a co-ordinated set of cardiac and vascular changes evoked by mental stress, fear, danger or anticipation of exercise (Section 16.8). The vasodilatation is transient and the system plays no part in the reflex control of blood pressure.

Although sympathetic cholinergic fibres increase the muscle blood flow, they do not increase the microvascular permeability−surface area product, probably because they act chiefly on small arteries of diameter 0.1−0.2 mm rather than on arterioles. Metabolic hyperaemia, by contrast, has its greatest effect on arterioles (Figure 13.7), as a result of which it causes capillary recruitment and a rise in permeability−surface area product. It cannot be emphasized too strongly that **local metabolic factors cause the functional hyperaemia associated with normal, non-emotional exercise**, not sympathetic vasodilator nerves.

Table 14.3 Comparison of sympathetic vasoconstrictor and vasodilator nerves.

Feature	Sympathetic constrictor nerve	Sympathetic dilator nerve
Main neurotransmitter	Noradrenaline (and ATP)	Acetylcholine (and VIP)
Distribution	Most organs and tissue	Restricted; e.g., skeletal muscle of some species, and sweat glands
Tonically active?	Yes	No
Central control	Brainstem	Forebrain
Involvement in baroreceptor reflex	Major factor governing activity	Negligible
Role in blood pressure homeostasis	Very important	Little
Duration of effect	Mostly well sustained	Transient

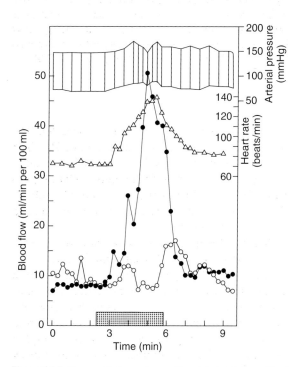

Figure 14.7 Human altering response. Closed circles, forearm blood flow, chiefly to skeletal muscle; open circles, hand blood flow, chiefly to skin; triangles, heart rate. During the time represented by the rectangle the experimenters told the subject that a leak in the apparatus was causing severe haemorrhage (!). The increase in forearm flow is comparable with that in severe exercise, and greatly exceeds the maximum flow that withdrawal of sympathetic vasoconstrictor tone can produce. (From Blair, D. A., Glover, W. E., Greenfield, A. D. M. and Roddie, L. C. (1959) *Journal of Physiology*, **148**, 633–647, by permission.)

In human muscle the alerting response vasodilatation is due to other mechanisms

Acute mental stress, such as mental arithmetic, causes vasodilatation in human forearm muscles (Figure 14.7), though not in the calf muscles. This was at one time attributed to a sympathetic cholinergic innervation, but such an innervation now seems unlikely in humans for the following reasons. (i) Primates as a group lack a sympathetic cholinergic innervation of skeletal muscle vessels (but have one to the skin, see below). (ii) Electrode recordings show that sympathetic activity to human muscle is reduced, not increased, by stress. (iii) Axillary nerve block does not prevent the human forearm vasodilator response to stress.

The causes of the vasodilatation are only partly understood. One factor is a doubling of plasma **adrenaline** concentration, which is brought about by sympathetic stimulation of the adrenal medulla. In support it is found that β-adrenoceptor blockers impair the vasodilator response to stress. A second factor is the **reduction in sympathetic vasoconstrictor activity to the muscle**, though this alone is insufficient to explain the large increase in flow. The finding in some but not all studies that atropine, a blocker of acetylcholine muscarinic receptors, attenuates stress-induced vasodilatation remains a puzzle.

Sympathetic cholinergic fibres mediate sweating and vasodilatation in proximal human skin

Human sweat glands are innervated by sympathetic cholinergic nerves. Their stimulation causes sweating and a marked cutaneous vasodilatation. Since sweating and vasodilatation usually occur together, a system of sudomotor–vasodilator cholinergic fibres is probably responsible. The vasodilatation is only partly blocked by atropine. The additional neurotransmitter may be VIP, which can be demonstrated by immunohistology in vasomotor fibres close to the sweat glands.

14.4 Vasodilatation by nociceptive C-fibres

Antidromic stimulation of sensory fibres causes vasodilatation

The strange ability of sensory nerves to cause cutaneous vasodilatation was discovered by Bayliss early in the 20th century. He stimulated the dorsal root of a spinal nerve antidromically, sending action potentials in the 'wrong' direction down the sensory nerves, and found that this caused cutaneous vasodilatation. Antidromic activity may explain how the infection of a dorsal root by herpes zoster virus causes the characteristic segmental cutaneous hyperaemia of shingles.

The Lewis triple response involves nociceptor-mediated vasodilatation

Our understanding of the motor function of a sensory fibre has been advanced by studying the Lewis triple response. In 1927 Sir Thomas Lewis noted that the reaction of human skin to a mild trauma such as a scratch involves three responses. They are:

- **Local redness** caused by vasodilatation along the line of the scratch, probably through the release of K^+ and inflammatory autacoids from activated cells.

- **Local swelling** around the scratch (a wheal) caused by inflammatory oedema.

- **A spreading flare.** The flare is an area of redness that gradually extends laterally from the line of trauma for 2–3 cm. Remarkably, the flare is mediated by sensory nerves, since it is abolished by local anaesthetics such as lignocaine, and by sensory denervation (Figure 14.8). A flare is present in some species (e.g. man, rat) but not all.

The flare is caused by a 'sensory axon reflex'

The flare is mediated by nociceptive (harm-sensing) C-fibres. To explain the lateral spread of the flare, which occurs too rapidly to be due to autacoid diffusion, Lewis proposed the **axon reflex**. The action potential elicited by the trauma not only propagates centrally along the C-fibre but also passes antidromically down an axon side branch to reach blood vessels up to a centimetre away (Figure 14.9). The arrival of the action potential in the axon branch terminal

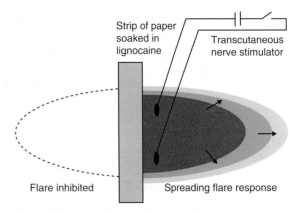

Figure 14.8 Sensory fibre-mediated vasodilatation in skin, viewed *en face*. The nociceptive C-fibres were stimulated by transcutaneous electrical stimulation. The spreading flare was recorded by a laser Doppler imager. The flare is abolished by the sensory anaesthetic lignocaine. (After the work of Schmelz, M. and Petersen, L. J. (2001); see Further Reading.)

causes it to release vasodilator neuropeptides. The released neuropeptides include **substance P**, which stimulates endothelial NK_1 receptors to stimulate NO synthesis, and **calcitonin-gene related peptide** (CGRP), which activates the cAMP pathway (Figure 12.10). CGRP is extremely potent and its effect lasts many hours.

Mast cell histamine is also implicated, at least in rat skin. Many substance P-containing fibres terminate on mast cells, which possess NK_1 receptors. Receptor activation by substance P causes the mast cell to release granules of histamine, which causes further vasodilatation. Since histamine also stimulates the local C-fibres, a chain reaction might occur, which could explain why the flare sometimes spreads 2–3 cm. In humans, however, mast cell histamine is probably not involved in the spreading flare (though it is involved in the local wheal), because histamine levels are not raised in fluid sampled from the flare region.

Antidromic C-fibre activity can cause neurogenic inflammation

Antidromic stimulation of C-fibres causes not only vasodilatation but also a pathological rise in microvascular permeability through substance P and histamine release. This leads to plasma exudation and high-protein oedema, and is called neurogenic inflammation. Neurogenic inflammation is readily elicited in rat skin and joints. Healthy human skin is not very susceptible to neurogenic inflammation, but becomes more susceptible in the presence of dermatological disorders.

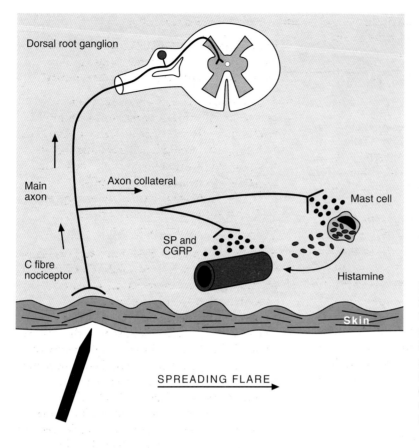

Dorsal root ganglion

Main axon

Axon collateral

Mast cell

SP and CGRP

C fibre nociceptor

Histamine

Skin

SPREADING FLARE

Figure 14.9 A sensory axon reflex causes the lateral flare response to a scratch. Vasodilatation is due to the release of substance P (SP) and CGRP from nociceptive C-fibre axon branches. In rat skin and possibly some human dermatological conditions, collateral endings near mast cells trigger histamine release through degranulation, augmenting the flare. (After Foreman, J. C. (1987) *Allergy*, **42**, 1–11.)

14.5 Hormonal control of the circulation

Several hormones influence the heart and circulation acutely, although they are generally less important that neural control under physiological conditions. Hormones such as adrenaline, vasopressin and angiotensin become major regulators of cardiovascular function during pathological events such as a haemorrhage, or when neural control is impaired as in transplanted hearts. The hormones **adrenaline**, **vasopressin**, **angiotensin** and **atrial natriuretic peptide** are described in Sections 14.6–14.8. The last three are also important regulators of the extracellular fluid and plasma volume through effects on renal tubular function. Other hormones with significant cardiovascular effects include **insulin**, **oestrogens**, **relaxin** and **thyroxine**.

Insulin

Insulin stimulates endothelial NO production, so it has vasodilator and antithrombotic actions. Insulin also inhibits vascular smooth muscle growth and migration. Reduction of these effects in diabetics (who either lack insulin or are resistant to it) may

contribute to their proneness to atheroma and ischaemic heart disease.

Oestrogens

The ovarian follicle hormone 17β-oestradiol causes vasodilatation in many tissues, including the female genitourinary system (uterus, vagina, kidneys), mammary glands, heart and skin. The acute vasodilatation is mediated partly by the activation of endothelial nitric oxide synthase via the protein kinase B pathway (Section 9.4) and partly through activation of vascular myocyte K_{Ca} channels. During pregnancy high levels of oestrogen cause a characteristic fall in blood pressure.

Relaxin

Relaxin is a peptide hormone secreted by the corpus luteum of the ovary during pregnancy and parturition. It has a vasodilator action on the uterus, mammary gland and heart.

Thyroxine

Thyroxine enhances myocardial contractility, in part by inducing increased β_1-adrenoceptor density on the myocytes. In addition thyroxine increases basal metabolic rate, which leads to vasodilatation, reduced peripheral resistance and tachycardia.

14.6 Adrenaline

The adrenal gland is situated at the upper pole of the kidney. Its medulla (core) secretes adrenaline (epinephrine) and noradrenaline (norepinephrine), which are known collectively as the catecholamines. Adrenaline is a methylated form of noradrenaline. Although the gland secretes both adrenaline and noradrenaline, adrenaline accounts for over three-quarters of the secreted catecholamine in man. (In diving mammals, by contrast, the secretion is mainly noradrenaline. This induces muscle vasoconstriction during dives to conserve O_2.) The plasma adrenaline and noradrenaline concentrations are 0.1–0.5 nM and 0.5–3.0 nM respectively at rest. The high level of noradrenaline is due to spillage from the tonically active sympathetic vasomotor terminals.

Adrenaline secretion is controlled by preganglionic sympathetic fibres

The adrenal medulla develops embryologically from postganglionic sympathetic neurons, and it retains an innervation by preganglionic sympathetic fibres via the splanchnic nerve (Figure 14.1). Increased firing of the preganglionic sympathetic fibres triggers the glandular secretion of catecholamines. Catecholamine secretion is increased during **exercise**, the **alerting response** (fear–flight–fight situations), **hypotension** and **hypoglycaemia**. During exercise the plasma adrenaline level can reach 5 nM and the noradrenaline level 10 nM. The latter is again due chiefly to spillover from the increasingly active sympathetic vasomotor terminals.

Adrenaline has multiple metabolic and cardiovascular effects

The cardiovascular effects of adrenaline at physiological concentrations are quite small compared with the effects of autonomic nerves and intrinsic regulatory factors. **The metabolic effects of adrenaline are at least as important as its cardiovascular effects.** Adrenaline stimulates **glycogenolysis** in the liver and **lipolysis** in adipose tissue, which releases glucose into the bloodstream. The cardiovascular effects of the catecholamines are as follows.

- Both adrenaline and noradrenaline stimulate the cardiac β_1-adrenoceptors, causing a **tachycardia and increased contractility**.

- At physiological concentrations both the catecholamines cause **arterial and venous vasoconstriction** in many tissues, e.g. skin. At high, pharmacological concentrations both cause vasoconstriction in *all* tissues due to the activation of vascular α-adrenoceptors (Figure 12.6). Many students have an ingrained belief that adrenaline necessarily causes vasodilatation, but this is untrue.

- As an exception to the rule that catecholamines cause vasoconstriction, **adrenaline at physiological concentrations causes vasodilatation in skeletal muscle, myocardium and liver**. This is due to an abundance of β_2-**adrenoceptors** in these three tissues (Table 14.1), and to the high affinity of adrenaline for β_2-receptors. The β_2-adrenoceptor is coupled to the adenylate cyclase-cAMP vasodilator cascade (Figure 12.10). After β-blockade by propranolol, adrenaline causes vasoconstriction even in skeletal muscle, because it also activates α-receptors. Noradrenaline causes vasoconstriction even in muscle, because noradrenaline has a higher affinity for α-receptors than β-receptors.

The net effects of circulating adrenaline and noradrenaline are different

As explained above, adrenaline and noradrenaline have opposite effects on skeletal muscle. Since skeletal muscle is the single most abundant tissue in the body (~40% of body weight), the overall effects of the two catecholamines on the systemic circulation differ considerably (Figure 14.10).

Intravenous noradrenaline causes a generalized vasoconstriction, which markedly **raises the peripheral resistance** and blood pressure. The raised pressure elicits a baroreceptor reflex, which reduces the sympathetic drive to the heart and increases the parasympathetic drive. Thus the baroreflex slows the heart and reduces cardiac output, offsetting the direct stimulatory effect of noradrenaline on the myocardium.

Intravenous adrenaline, by contrast, **slightly reduces the total peripheral resistance**, because the vasodilatation in muscle outweighs the vasoconstriction in other tissues. Mean blood pressure

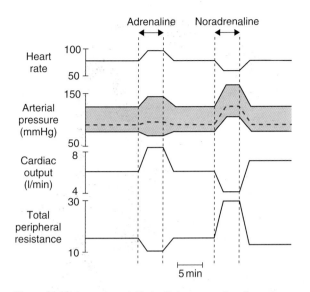

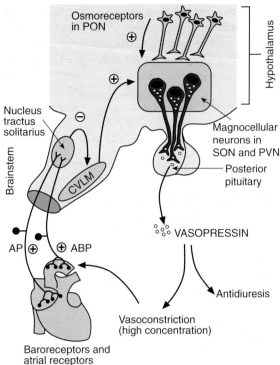

Figure 14.10 Comparison of effects of intravenous adrenaline and noradrenaline in man. For explanation, see text. An initial transient drop in blood pressure that occurs during adrenaline infusion is not shown here. (From the classic monograph of Barcroft, H. and Swan, H. J. C. (1953) *Sympathetic Control of Human Blood Vessels*, Edward Arnold, London, by permission.)

Figure 14.11 Regulation of vasopressin secretion. Relative importance of arterial baroreceptors and atrial receptors varies between species. ABP, arterial blood pressure; AP, atrial pressure; PON, pre-optic nucleus; SON, supraoptic nucleus; PVN, paraventricular nucleus; CVLM, caudal ventrolateral medulla.

therefore changes little, and the direct stimulation of the heart by circulating adrenaline proceeds without significant opposition by the baroreflex. Therefore stimulation of the adrenal medulla increases cardiac output.

A rare tumour of the adrenal medulla, the phaeochromocytoma, secretes a mixture of catecholamines and causes hypertension. The latter can be treated with α-antagonists such as phentolamine.

14.7 Vasopressin (antidiuretic hormone)

Vasopressin is a vasoconstrictor peptide produced by magnocellular neurons in the supraoptic and paraventricular nuclei of the hypothalamus (Figure 14.11). From the cell bodies the vasopressin is transported along the axons, through the pituitary stalk and into the posterior lobe of the pituitary gland, from where it is released into the bloodstream.

Osmoreceptors and cardiovascular receptors regulated vasopressin secretion

The secretion of vasopressin is regulated partly by hypothalamic cells sensitive to tissue fluid osmolarity (osmoreceptors) and partly by cardiovascular pressure receptors. Secretion is stimulated by **a rise in plasma osmolarity** (threshold 285 mOs), such as occurs

during dehydration, and by **a fall in blood pressure and volume**, such as occurs during a haemorrhage or severe dehydration. The sensitivity of vasopressin secretion to osmolarity is much greater than the sensitivity to blood volume; a 2% rise in osmolarity elicits the same vasopressin secretion as a 10% fall in blood volume.

The main role of vasopressin at normal plasma concentrations is the regulation of water excretion by the kidneys, as indicated by its common name 'anti-diuretic hormone'. The cardiovascular effects of vasopressin are seen at substantially raised concentrations, such as occur during haemorrhagic hypotension.

High levels of vasopressin support blood pressure during hypovolaemia

High concentrations of vasopressin elicit a pronounced vasoconstriction in most tissues. This helps to support arterial pressure and contributes to the characteristic pallor of hypovolaemic patients. Cerebral and coronary vessels, however, respond to vasopressin with a NO-mediated dilatation. Vasopressin thus causes a redistribution of the cardiac output in favour of the brain and heart, as is appropriate in hypovolaemia. In dogs with diabetes insipidus and in Brattleboro rats, both of which lack vasopressin, the blood pressure is abnormally depressed during dehydration or haemorrhage.

During nausea and vomiting the vasopressin levels rise to up to 50 times the antidiuresis level. This may contribute to the characteristic grey pallor of nausea.

14.8 The renin–angiotensin–aldosterone (RAA) system

Angiotensin II is a powerful vasoconstrictor hormone with important roles in hypovolaemia, hypertension and cardiac failure.

Angiotensin II formation is mediated by renin and endothelial ACE

The production of angiotensin begins with the secretion of **renin** (pronounced ree-nin,) into the blood stream of the kidney (Figure 14.12). Renin is secreted by granular cells in the walls of the afferent arterioles close to the glomeruli (juxtaglomerular cells). Renin is a proteolytic enzyme that acts on angiotensinogen, a plasma α_2-globulin, to cleave off a decapeptide called angiotensin I. Angiotensin I is then cleaved further by an enzyme situated on the surface of endothelial cells (**angiotensin converting enzyme**, ACE) to form the active octapeptide angiotensin II. The formation of angiotensin II takes place mainly in the lungs, because this is the first major area of endothelium to be encountered by venous angiotensin I.

Angiotensin II supports blood pressure

A major role of angiotensin II at normal, physiological concentration is to stimulate the adrenal cortex to secrete **aldosterone**, a steroidal hormone. Aldosterone acts on the renal tubules to promote salt and water retention. In this way the RAA system maintains the plasma volume and indirectly the blood pressure.

A second role of angiotensin II is to support blood pressure directly. The basal plasma level of angiotensin II has a **tonic vasoconstrictor action** that helps to maintain the peripheral resistance and blood pressure. Consequently, **ACE inhibitors** such as captopril and enalapril cause a fall in blood pressure, and are used to treat hypertension and cardiac failure.

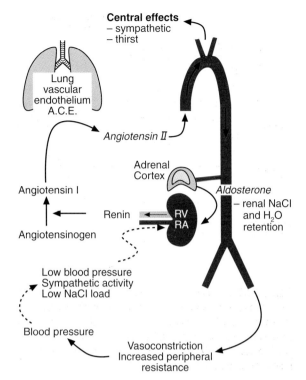

Figure 14.12 Renin–angiotensin–aldosterone system; see text. RA and RV, renal artery and vein. Central effects are stimulation of sympathetic outflow, reduction in sensitivity of baroreceptor reflex and stimulation of thirst.

In hypovolaemia and cardiac failure, angiotensin II levels are markedly elevated. The vasoconstrictor action of angiotensin contributes powerfully to supporting the blood pressure in these conditions. In addition the angiotensin II increases cardiac contractility. Its positive inotropic effect is mediated partly directly, through enhancement of the plateau Ca^{2+} current, and partly indirectly through the central stimulation of sympathetic outflow, described next.

Renin and angiotensin II levels are also raised in many but not all cases of essential hypertension.

Angiotensin II enhances sympathetic drive

The mechanisms through which angiotensin II influences the peripheral resistance are unusual, because angiotensin acts not only on the vascular myocytes but also on the sympathetic terminals and on the vasomotor region of the brainstem.

- Angiotensin II has a **direct vasoconstrictor action** on vascular smooth muscle. Angiotensin receptors evoke both electromechanical and pharmacomechanical coupling.

- Angiotensin II receptors on the varicosities of the sympathetic terminals increase the amount of noradrenaline released by sympathetic action potentials (**neuromodulation**, Figure 14.2).

- Angiotensin II also acts on the brainstem, diffusing into a region called the area postrema where the blood–brain barrier is deficient. Angiotensin receptors are abundant in the area postrema. The central effect of the angiotensin is to **increase the sympathetic vasoconstrictor outflow** and thus support the blood pressure. In addition is acts on the hypothalamus to stimulate the sensation of **thirst**.

In cardiac failure the various actions of angiotensin II contribute to high levels of sympathetic nerve activity, fluid retention (via aldosterone) and high cardiac filling pressures (Section 18.5).

Angiotensin level is controlled through negative feedback loops

The concentration of angiotensin in plasma depends on the rate of renin secretion. The factors controlling renin secretion establish negative feedback loops that help preserve blood pressure during hypovolaemia as follows:

1 **Reduced renal artery pressure** activates the RAA system. In cases of hypovolaemia this sets up a helpful negative feedback loop; the reduced arterial pressure activates the RAA system, which helps to restore the pressure. In cases of renal artery stenosis, however, inappropriate activation of the RAA system leads to clinical hypertension.

2 **Renal sympathetic nerve activity** and adrenaline stimulate β_1-adrenoceptors on the juxtaglomerular cells and thereby enhance renin secretion. Since increased sympathetic activity is part of the response to hypotension, the RAA activation reinforces the above negative feedback loop and helps to restore blood pressure.

3 **A reduced load of NaCl** flowing past the macula densa of the renal tubule promotes renin secretion. The resulting activation of the RAA system raises the aldosterone level, which stimulates the tubules to reabsorb Na^+. In this case the RAA system is part of a negative feedback loop for the homeostasis of extracellular Na^+.

14.9 Atrial natriuretic peptide

Atrial natriuretic peptide (ANP) is secreted by specialized myocytes in the atria. Secretion is stimulated by high cardiac filling pressures, and the hormone acts to reduce plasma volume and thus filling pressure. It operates as follows.

In contrast to vasopressin and the RAA system, ANP **enhances renal salt and water excretion** and causes a **moderate dilatation** of resistance vessels. The fall in plasma volume is greater than can be accounted for by the mild diuresis and is due partly to the **transfer of fluid from plasma to the interstitial compartment**. The fluid shift is brought about by a rise in capillary filtration pressure. ANP can also increase venular permeability by up to two-fold. ANP acts by raising cGMP in the vascular myocytes and endothelium.

The normal plasma level of ANP is extremely low. Even when the ANP level is raised two- to four-fold, which can be achieved by raising the central venous pressure by whole-body immersion in water, there is little consistent change in renal excretion. In heart failure, however, levels can increase as much as 20-fold, and this probably helps to mitigate the accumulation of extracellular fluid that characterizes heart failure (Chapter 18).

14.10 Special features of venous control

The venous system has been called 'the Cinderella of the circulation' because it is often neglected. The control of peripheral veins (capacitance vessels) is important because **venous tone governs the distribution of blood between the periphery and thorax, and thereby regulates cardiac filling pressure** and, indirectly, stroke volume.

Differentiation of the venous system

From a functional point of view the venous system has four distinctive compartments (Figure 14.13). The **central, thoracic compartment** is largely passive and consists of the great veins, right heart and pulmonary vessels. The central blood volume influences the cardiac filling pressure and hence stroke volume. The three peripheral compartments differ in their characteristics as follows.

Splanchnic veins

The veins of the gastrointestinal tract, liver and spleen contain ~20% of the total blood volume at rest.

They are well innervated by sympathetic constrictor nerves and possess α-adrenoreceptors. During exercise and hypotension, increased sympathetic activity and circulating adrenaline cause active contraction of the splanchnic veins (Figure 14.5). This helps to maintain the CVP at times of circulatory stress.

Skeletal muscle veins

Intramuscular veins are poorly innervated. Their volume is influenced chiefly by posture (i.e. gravity) and by the muscle pump. Although direct sympathetic control of these veins is almost non-existent, their volume is nevertheless affected indirectly by sympathetic vasomotor activity because arteriolar constriction reduces downstream pressure. The fall in venular pressure causes the venous system to recoil elastically and displace blood centrally (Figure 14.4).

Cutaneous veins

The veins of the skin are richly innervated by sympathetic noradrenergic fibres. High core temperatures lead to reduced cutaneous sympathetic activity and therefore venodilatation. Conversely, increased sympathetic activity causes cutaneous venoconstriction, for example in hypotensive patients or in cold weather. Sympathetic cutaneous venoconstriction is also triggered by emotional stress, deep inspiration and exercise (Figure 14.14).

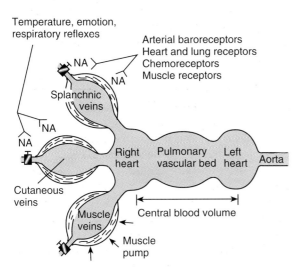

Figure 14.13 Differentiation of venous system. Changes in central blood volume and cardiac filling pressure are brought about by contraction of peripheral veins, especially splanchnic veins. NA, noradrenaline. (From Shepherd, J. T. and Vanhoutte, P. M. (1979) *The Human Cardiovascular System, Facts and Concepts*, Raven Press, New York, by permission.)

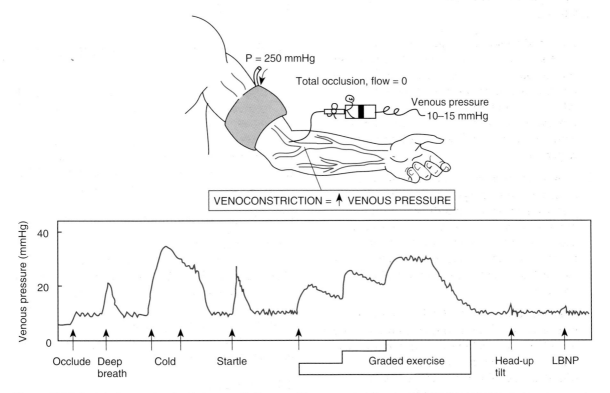

Figure 14.14 Control of venous tone in skin by sympathetic nerves. The pressure in veins when blood flow is halted by a sphygmomanometer cuff is measured as an index of changes in venous smooth muscle tension. LBNP, lower body negative pressure. (After Rowell, L. B. (1986) *Human Circulation Regulation during Physical Stress*, Oxford University Press, New York.)

Comparison of venous and arteriolar control

Veins respond in the same way as resistance vessels to many stimuli – in the skin for example both are constricted during hypotension. There are also differences in behaviour as follows.

- Most venules and veins have **little basal tone** in the absence of sympathetic activity.

- Veins generally show **little myogenic response** to stretch (with some exceptions).

- Veins can respond to hormones, autacoids and drugs differently to arterioles due to different receptor populations. **Angiotensin II**, for example, has little direct effect on veins but a powerful effect on arterioles. It does, however, act on the sympathetic terminals to potentiate the effect of sympathetic nerves on human veins (neuromodulatory action). This contributes to the intense venoconstriction of patients in cardiac failure. **Histamine** causes veins to constrict due to a predominance of H_1 receptors, whereas arterioles dilate due to their H_2 receptors (Section 13.5). **Glyceryl trinitrate** has a greater dilator effect on veins than on arterioles, and its efficacy in relieving angina is due partly to the reduction of cardiac filling pressure, and therefore cardiac work, following venodilatation.

SUMMARY

■ As summarized in Chapter 13, vascular control is achieved by a 3-tier hierarchy of interacting controls. The lowest level is the Bayliss myogenic response and autoregulation. The second level of control is exerted by local chemical factors (endothelial secretions, vasodilator metabolites in metabolic hyperaemia, and autacoids). The third level of control is the **neuroendocrine system**, which brings the vasculature under central and reflex control for the benefit of the organism as a whole.

■ **Sympathetic vasoconstrictor noradrenergic fibres** to the skin, muscle, kidney and gut are tonically active and raise vascular tone through α-adrenoceptor activation. Sympathetic regulation of resistance vessels stabilizes blood pressure, regulates local blood flow, and influences fluid partitioning between plasma and interstitium. Sympathetic fibres also regulate splanchnic and cutaneous venous tone, and thereby influence central blood volume and cardiac filling pressure. The postganglionic fibre activity is controlled by thoracic spinal preganglionic neurons, which in turn are regulated by bulbospinal fibres descending from the brainstem.

■ **Parasympathetic vasodilator nerves** occur as cranial and sacral outflow. The cranial outflow innervates the salivary glands, pancreas and gut, and evokes secretory hyperaemia. The sacral outflow innervates the genitalia (erectile tissue), bladder and colon. The main parasympathetic neurotransmitters are acetylcholine, VIP and NO.

■ A **nociceptive C-fibre axon reflex** in skin, mediated by substance P, CGRP and mast cell histamine, causes the spreading flare following trauma to the skin (the Lewis triple response). C-fibres also mediate neurogenic inflammation.

■ **Hormonal control** by adrenaline, angiotensin II and vasopressin supports blood pressure under stressful conditions such as hypovolaemia.

■ **Adrenaline** is secreted by the adrenal medulla during exercise, the alerting response and hypotension, in response to preganglionic sympathetic activity. Adrenaline promotes glucose release into the bloodstream; helps to raise cardiac output; causes β-adrenoceptor mediated vasodilatation in muscle; and causes α-adrenoceptor mediated vasoconstriction in skin.

■ **Angiotensin II** is formed in the lungs by the action of endothelial ACE on angiotensin I. The latter is generated in renal plasma by the action of the enzyme renin. Renin is secreted by the renal juxtaglomerular apparatus in response to low blood pressure, a low NaCl load and renal sympathetic activity. Angiotensin II stimulates aldosterone secretion and causes vasoconstriction by peripheral and central actions. It thus supports plasma volume and blood pressure.

■ **Vasopressin** (anti-diuretic hormone) is produced in the hypothalamus and released from the posterior pituitary in response to hypertonicity and hypotension. Its vasoconstrictor action supports blood pressure in states of hypovolaemia.

■ **Atrial natriuretic peptide** is secreted by the atria in response to distension. It reduces plasma volume by a mild diuretic action and by enhancing microvascular filtration through vasodilatation and increased permeability. Levels are high in heart failure.

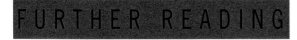

Reviews and chapters

Andersson, K-E. and Wagner, G. (1995) Physiology of penile erection. *Physiological Reviews*, **75**, 191–236.

Burnstock, G. (1986) The changing face of autonomic neurotransmission. *Acta Physiologica Scandinavica*, **126**, 67–91.

Edvinsson, L. and Uddman, R. (eds) (1993) *Vascular Innervation and Receptor Mechanisms*, Academic Press, New York.

Elser, M., Jennings, G., Lambert, G., Meredith, I., Horne, M. and Eisenhofer, G. (1990) Overflow of catecholamine neurotransmitters to the circulation: source, fate and functions. *Physiological Reviews*, **70**, 963–982.

Fitzsimons, J. T. (1998) Angiotensin, thirst and sodium appetite. *Physiological Reviews*, **78**, 583–686.

Folkow, B. and Nilsson, H. (1997) Transmitter release at adrenergic nerve endings: total exocytosis or fractional release. *News in Physiological Sciences*, **12**, 32–36.

Hainsworth, R. (1991) The importance of vascular capacitance in cardiovascular control. *News in Physiological Sciences*, **5**, 250–254.

Jänig, W. (1988) Pre- and postganglionic vasoconstrictor neurons. *Annual Reviews of Physiology*, **50**, 525–539.

Lehr, H-A. (2000) Microcirculatory dysfunction induced by cigarette smoking. *Microcirculation*, **7**, 367–384.

Lundberg, J. M., Pernow, J. and Lacroix, J. S. (1989) Neuropeptide Y: sympathetic cotransmitter and modulator? *News in Physiological Sciences*, **4**, 13–17.

Marshall, J. M. (1991) The venous vessels within skeletal muscle. *News in Physiological Sciences*, **6**, 11–15.

Mather, K., Anderson, T. J. and Verma, S. (2001) Insulin action in the vasculature: physiology and pathophysiology. *Journal of Vascular Research*, **38**, 415–422.

Monos, E., Berczi, V. and Nadasy, G. (1995) Local control of veins: biomechanical, metabolic and humoral aspects. *Physiological Reviews*, **75**, 611–666.

Reid, I. A. (1996) Angiotensin II and baroreflex control of heart rate. *News in Physiological Sciences*, **11**, 270–274.

Renkin, E. M. and Tucker, V. L. (1996) Atrial natriuretic peptide as a regulator of transvascular fluid balance. *News in Physiological Sciences*, **11**, 138–143.

Rothe, C. F. (1983) Venous system; physiology of the capacitance vessels. In *Handbook of Physiology, Cardiovascular System*, Vol. 3, *Peripheral Circulation*, Part 1 (eds Shepherd, J. T. and Abboud, F. M.), American Physiology Society, Bethesda, pp. 397–452.

Sagnella, G. A. (2000) Practical implications of current natriuretic peptide research. *Journal of Renin–Angiotensin–Aldosterone System*, **1**, 304–315.

Schmelz, M. and Petersen, L. J. (2001) Neurogenic inflammation in human and rodent skin. *News in Physiological Sciences*, **16**, 33–37.

Share, L. (1988) Role of vasopressin in cardiovascular regulation. *Physiological Reviews*, **68**, 1248–1284.

Toda, N. and Okamura, T. (1992) Regulation by nitroxidergic nerve of arterial tone. *News in Physiological Sciences*, **7**, 148–152.

Wallin, B. G. and Fagius, J. (1988) Peripheral sympathetic neural activity in conscious humans. *Annual Reviews in Physiology*, **50**, 565–576.

White, M. M., Zamudio, S., Stevens, T., Tyler, R., Lidenfeld, J., Leslie, K. and Moore, L. G. (1995) Estrogen, progesterone and vascular reactivity: potential cellular mechanisms. *Endocrine Reviews*, **16**, 739–751.

Zusman, R. M., Morales, A., Glasser, D. B. and Osterloh, I. H. (1999) Overall cardiovascular profile of sildenafil citrate ('Viagra'). *American Journal of Cardiology*, **83**(5A), 35C–44C.

Research papers

Andriantsitohaine, R. and Surprenant, A. (1992) Acetylcholine released from guinea-pig submucosal neurones dilates arterioles by releasing NO from endothelium. *Journal of Physiology*, **453**, 493–502.

Dinenno, F. A., Eisenach, J. H., Dietz, N. M. and Joyner, M. J. (2002) Post-junctional α-adrenoceptors and basal limb vascular tone in healthy men. *Journal of Physiology*, **540**, 1103–1110.

Edwards, A. V. and Garrett, J. R. (1993) Nitric oxide-related vasodilator responses to parasympathetic stimulation of the submandibular gland in the cat. *Journal of Physiology*, **464**, 379–392.

Escrig, A., Gonzalez-Mora, J. L. and Mas, M. (1999) Nitric oxide release in penile corpora cavernosa in a rat model of erection. *Journal of Physiology*, **516**, 261–269.

Hashitani, H., Windle, A. and Suzuki, H. (1998) Neuroeffector transmission in arterioles of the guinea-pig choroid. *Journal of Physiology*, **510**, 209–223.

Joyner, M. J. and Halliwill, J. R. (2000) Sympathetic vasodilatation in human limbs. *Journal of Physiology*, **526**, 471–480.

Lindqvist, M., Melcher, A. and Hjemdahl, P. (1997) Attenuation of forearm vasodilatation responses to mental stress by regional beta-blockade but not by atropine. *Acta Physiologica Scandinavica*, **161**, 135–140.

Lynn, B. and Cotsell, B. (1991) The delay in onset of vasodilator flare in human skin at increasing distances from a localized noxious stimulus. *Microvascular Research*, **41**, 197–202.

Magerl, W. and Treede, R-D. (1996) Heat-evoked vasodilatation in human hairy skin: axon reflexes due to low-level activity in nociceptive afferents. *Journal of Physiology*, **497**, 837–848.

Matsukawa, K., Shindo, T., Shirai, M. and Ninomiya, I. (1997) Direct observations of sympathetic cholinergic vasodilatation of skeletal muscle small arteries in the cat. *Journal of Physiology*, **500**, 213–225.

Modin, A., Pernow, J. and Lundberg, J. M. (1993) Sympathetic regulation of skeletal muscle blood flow in the pig: a non-adrenergic component likely to be mediated by neuropeptide Y. *Acta Physiologica Scandinavica*, **148**, 1–11.

Rosenfeld, C. R., White, R. E., Roy, T. and Cox, B. E. (2000) Calcium-activated potassium channels and nitric oxide coregulate estrogen-induced vasodilation. *American Journal of Physiology*, **279**, H319–H328.

Sugenoya, J., Iwase, S., Mano, T., Sugiyama, Y., Ogawa, T., Nishiyama, T., Nishimura, N. and Kimura, T. (1998) Vasodilator component in sympathetic nerve activity destined for the skin of the dorsal foot of mildly heated humans. *Journal of Physiology*, **507**, 603–610.

CHAPTER 15

Specialization in individual circulations

Learning objectives

In this chapter the learning objectives and summary for each circulation are combined as a Key Features Box after each section.

The relative importance of the numerous vessel-regulating factors varies from organ to organ. One aim of this chapter is to highlight the factors that predominate in a given tissue. The second aim is explain how the different circulations are specialized to contribute to the specific function of a given tissue. For example, a major function of the skin is to regulate body temperature, so the skin vessels are adapted both structurally and functionally for temperature regulation.

The five special circulations covered here, namely heart, skeletal muscle, skin, brain and lung, have been selected on the basis of pathophysiological importance and contrasting characteristics. Space prevents a full account of other major circulations such as the renal and splanchnic circulations, though the latter is described briefly under 'Feeding and digestion' (Section 17.5). To unify the topic, the same approach is adopted for each system. First, the **special tasks** imposed on the circulation by the tissue function are outlined. Next, the accomplishment of these tasks is described, under the headings '**Structural adaptation**' and '**Functional adaptation**'. Specific vascular **problems** in the given tissue are considered, and finally the **assessment** of the individual circulation in humans is outlined.

15.1 Coronary circulation

Flow at basal cardiac output	$70-80\,\mathrm{ml\,min^{-1}\,100\,g^{-1}}$
Flow at maximal output	$300-400\,\mathrm{ml\,min^{-1}\,100\,g^{-1}}$

The right and left coronary arteries arise from the aorta immediately above the cusps of the aortic valve (Figure 15.1). The left coronary artery supplies mainly the left ventricle and septum and the right artery mainly the right ventricle, although the distribution varies between individuals. Most of the coronary venous blood, 95%, drains through the coronary sinus into the right atrium (Figure 1.4). The rest drains into the cardiac chambers through the anterior coronary and Thebesian veins. Some of the Thebesian veins drain into the left side of the heart and contribute to the slight deoxygenation of arterial blood (saturation 97%). The coronary circulation is the shortest in the body and its mean transit time is only 6–8 s in a resting human.

Special tasks

- The coronary circulation must deliver O_2 at a high basal rate in order to keep pace with cardiac demand. Even in a resting subject the

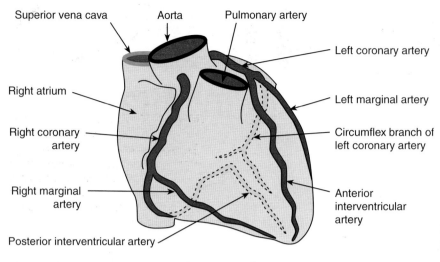

Figure 15.1 Human coronary arterial circulation, anterior view.

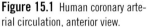

Fibre diameter $\quad$ 50 μm $\quad$ 18 μm
Capillaries per mm² $\quad$ 400 $\quad$ 3000

Figure 15.2 Density of capillaries (dots) in skeletal and cardiac muscle on same scale. Each tissue has roughly one capillary per fibre. Since the myocardial fibres are smaller, the capillary density is greater in myocardium and the diffusion distances are shorter. Open circles in skeletal muscle represent capillaries not perfused with blood at any given moment in resting muscle. (From Renkin, E. M. (1967) In *International Symposium on Coronary Circulation* (eds Marhetti, G. and Taccardi, B.), Karger, Basel, pp. 18–30, by permission.)

myocardial O_2 consumption is very high, ~8 ml O_2 per min per 100 g. This is 20 times greater than in resting skeletal muscle.

● During exercise the cardiac work rate can increase over five-fold, so the coronary circulation must increase the O_2 delivery correspondingly. This requires a tight coupling between coronary blood flow and cardiac work.

Structural adaptation

Myocardial **capillary density** is high, namely 3000–5000 capillaries per mm² cross-section. There is approximately one capillary per myocyte (Figure 15.2). The high capillary density facilitates the efficient delivery of O_2 and nutrients to the myocytes by creating a large endothelial area for exchange and by

reducing the maximum diffusion distance to 9 μm (the myocyte being 18 μm wide). Oxygen transport is also facilitated by the presence of **myoglobin** in the cardiac myocytes at 3.4 g/l (Section 10.11).

Exercise training increases the cross-sectional area of the coronary arteries and increases the number of arterioles. Ventricular myocyte mass increases, and capillary angiogenesis ensures that capillary density is maintained or even increased.

Functional adaptations

Basal flow and O_2 extraction are high

To satisfy the high metabolic rate of the heart, the blood flow per gram of myocardium is around 10 times higher than the body average. The continuous generation of **nitric oxide** by coronary endothelium helps to maintain this high basal flow. Blockage of NO production by arginine analogues reduces myocardial blood flow by 60%.

Even though the blood flow is high, the myocardium has to extract 65–75% of the arterial O_2 to meet its needs (cf. 25% for the whole body at rest). This reduces the blood O_2 content from 195 ml/l in arterial blood to 50–70 ml/l in coronary sinus blood (Figure 15.3). During heavy exercise, the oxygen extraction can reach 90%, leaving the coronary venous blood with only 20 ml O_2/l. The extraction of fatty acid from coronary blood is also high (40–70%), whereas glucose extraction is usually low (2–3%), due to the substrate preference of myocardium.

Metabolic hyperaemia is the dominant form of vascular regulation

The extra O_2 required at high work rates is supplied chiefly by increased blood flow rather than increased extraction, since extraction is already high at basal

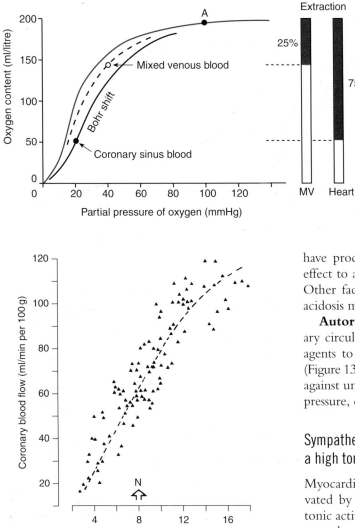

Figure 15.3 O_2 carriage curves for arterial blood (P_{CO_2}, 40 mmHg), mixed venous blood (P_{CO_2}, 46 mmHg) and coronary sinus blood (P_{CO_2}, 58 mmHg). CO_2 displaces the oxyhaemoglobin dissociation curve to the right (the Bohr shift): this markedly enhances oxygen unloading in myocardium. A, arterial point; MV, mixed venous blood (subject at rest).

Figure 15.4 Effect of cardiac work (myocardial O_2 consumption) on coronary blood flow in the dog. N, normal values at rest. Cardiac work was varied by adrenaline and by haemorrhage. (From Berne, R. M. and Rubio, R. (1979) In *Handbook of Physiology, Cardiovascular System*, Vol. 1, *The Heart* (eds Berne, R. M. and Sperekalis, N.) American Physiological Society, Bethesda, pp. 873–952, by permission.)

outputs. Coronary blood flow increases in almost linear proportion to myocardial O_2 consumption at light to moderate work rates (Figure 15.4). At high work rates the increase in flow lags a little, so O_2 extraction rises. Coronary blood flow during exercise is thus a fine example of metabolic hyperaemia (Section 13.7).

The nature of the metabolic vasodilator agent(s) 'remains a well-sought but carefully guarded secret of nature', as one investigator put it. One contender for the role is adenosine, which is generated through the breakdown of ATP. However, studies of the effects of adenosine antagonists and degrading enzymes upon myocardial metabolic hyperaemia

have produced variable results, ranging from little effect to a 50% reduction of metabolic hyperaemia. Other factors such as increased interstitial K^+ and acidosis must also contribute.

Autoregulation is well developed in the coronary circulation and is reset by metabolic vasodilator agents to operate at a higher flow during exercise (Figure 13.6). Autoregulation protects the myocardium against under-perfusion during periods of low blood pressure, down to ~50 mmHg.

Sympathetic vasomotor activity maintains a high tone at rest

Myocardial arteries and arterioles are well innervated by sympathetic vasoconstrictor fibres. Their tonic activity contributes to vascular tone and resistance through α-adrenoceptor activation. Resistance vessel tone is overcome in a graded fashion by metabolic vasodilatation during exercise. When the heart is stimulated by increased sympathetic activity, the increased cardiac work due to β_1 adrenoceptor-mediated tachycardia and increased contractility causes a metabolic vasodilatation which outweighs the α-adrenoceptor mediated vasoconstriction. Thus sympathetic activity normally raises rather than reduces myocardial blood flow; but see also 'Special Problems' later.

There is some evidence that parasympathetic cholinergic fibres too can dilate coronary arteries but this is not thought to be significant during exercise.

Adrenaline causes vasodilatation in myocardium

Adrenaline is secreted during exercise, the alerting response and hypovolaemia. Adrenaline reinforces the coronary hyperaemia by preferentially activating β_2-adrenoceptors on the coronary vascular myocytes. Activation of β_2-adrenoceptors evokes vasodilatation.

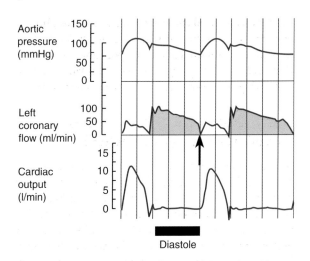

Figure 15.5 Flow in left coronary artery monitored by an electromagnetic flow meter in a conscious dog. Note the sharp curtailment of flow at the onset of systole (arrow); most coronary flow occurs during diastole (shaded area). Time lines 0.1 s. (After Khouris, E. M., Gregg, D. E. and Rayford, C. R. (1965) *Circulation Research*, **17**, 427–437.)

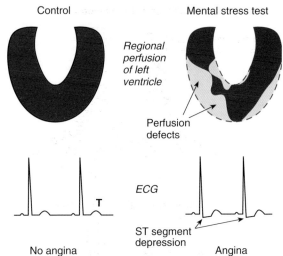

Figure 15.6 Perfusion of left ventricle wall mapped by [82]Rb uptake. *Control:* Uniform perfusion and normal ECG with patient relaxed. *Stress test (mental arithmetic):* Areas of defective myocardial perfusion, ST segment depression (ischaemia) and angina develop due to increased cardiac work and sympathetic coronary vasoconstriction. (Redrawn from Deanfield, J. E., Shea, M., Kensett, M., *et al.* (1984) *Lancet,* **2**, 1001–1005, by permission.)

Special problems

Systole interferes with coronary blood flow

The main coronary arteries run over the outer surface of the heart (Figure 15.1) but the smaller branches run within the myocardium. The intramural vessels are compressed during systole. Compression is worst during isovolumetric contraction because the coronary artery pressure is at its minimum, ~80 mmHg, and pressure inside the left ventricle wall is maximal, ~240 mmHg. The reversed vascular transmural pressure (240 mmHg outside, 80 mmHg inside) transiently closes the vessels within the ventricle wall. As a result, coronary artery flow stops briefly in early systole, or even goes into reverse (Figure 15.5). A moderate flow is restored during the ejection phase because coronary artery pressure rises and ventricle wall stress declines. Flow is only fully restored, however, in diastole. Roughly 80% of coronary flow occurs in diastole at basal heart rates.

The impairment of myocardial perfusion during systole is aggravated by aortic valve stenosis. Aortic stenosis increases the systolic stress in the left ventricle wall and can lead to collapse during exercise. See Case 5, 'The elderly man with a murmur', at the end of the book.

Stress and cold can trigger sympathetic coronary vasoconstriction and angina

Coronary sympathetic nerve activity is greatly influenced by mental stress. The effect of anger on myocardial perfusion has been studied in dogs, and the effect of mental arithmetic has been studied in man. Both stresses cause a prolonged, sympathetically mediated vasoconstriction of coronary arteries. When this is superimposed on ischaemic coronary disease due to atheroma, it causes regional ischaemia, ST-segment depression and stress-induced angina (Figure 15.6). An eminent anatomist at St George's Hospital, John Hunter, once remarked in relation to his own coronary disease 'My life is at the mercy of any rascal who chooses to annoy me'; and Hunter did indeed die after a stressful committee meeting at St George's.

Severe cold too can trigger a reflex sympathetic vasoconstriction of ischaemic coronary vessels, evoking angina.

Human coronary arteries are functional end-arteries prone to atheroma

The nature of atheroma is described in Section 9.10 and Table 17.4. Risk factors are shown in Concept Box 19. The seriousness of coronary atheroma is partly due to the fact that human coronary arteries are functional end-arteries (Figure 15.7). Although there are some arterio–arterial anastomoses between the branches of the coronary arteries, they are few in number and small in diameter (35–500 μm), so they conduct only a low flow. Consequently, when an atheromatous coronary artery is blocked by

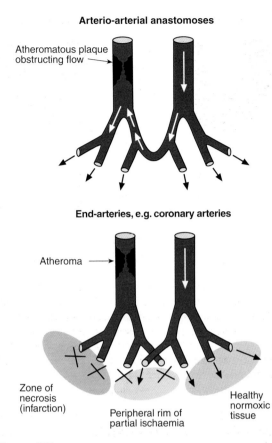

Arterio-arterial anastomoses

Atheromatous plaque
obstructing flow →

End-arteries, e.g. coronary arteries

Atheroma →

Zone of
necrosis
(infarction)

Peripheral rim of
partial ischaemia

Healthy
normoxic
tissue

Figure 15.7 Arterio-arterial connections affect susceptibility to infarction following arterial obstruction. Human and pig coronary arteries are functional end-arteries. Dog coronary circulation has better anastomoses.

thrombosis (a blood clot over an atheromatous plaque), flow to the downstream tissue falls to under 10% of normal. This is insufficient to support normal contraction and metabolism (ischaemia). Human coronary arteries are therefore called functional end-arteries.

Sudden obstruction by thrombosis causes myocardial infarction (a 'heart attack')

Sudden obstruction of an atheromatous coronary artery by thrombosis is the single commonest cause of death in the West. After a coronary thrombosis, the ischaemic myocardium becomes acidotic. The acidosis causes severe cardiac pain. Contractility is impaired and arrhythmias are common. The residual flow may be so low that myocytes begin to die after a few hours (necrosis, Figure 1.2). This sequence of events is called myocardial infarction or a 'heart attack'. Myocardial infarcts are commonest and largest in the subendocardium (inner tissue) because the wall stress during systole is greatest here, curtailing the endocardial blood flow at low perfusion pressures.

Slowly developing coronary stenosis leads to exercise-induced angina

Arteries offer negligible resistance to flow compared with arterioles, so the additional resistance caused by atheromatous narrowing (stenosis) does not affect flow until the narrowing is severe. Even then resting flow may be adequate because, when a stenosis develops gradually over months/years, the smaller, distal arterial vessels have time to enlarge and multiply. This 'arteriogenesis' is driven by growth factors. The arteriogenesis, coupled with distal dilatation due to autoregulation and the accumulation of vasodilator metabolites, maintains an adequate flow at rest; see Concept Box 20. During exercise or emotional stress, however, the fixed resistance of the stenosed artery prevents flow from increasing sufficiently to meet the increased myocardial O_2 demand. The distal vessels dilate, but the stenosis dominates the total resistance to flow. Exercise and/or mental stress therefore precipitate local myocardial ischaemia, leading to acidosis, chest pain (angina pectoris) and acute ST segment depression on the ECG. The exercise ECG test is a routine test for latent ischaemia.

Angina can also be caused by **vasospasm**, an intense, prolonged contraction of a coronary artery with atheroma. Vasospasm usually occurs downstream of the atheromatous plaque and is caused by the release of serotonin and thromboxane from platelets activated by the atheroma. The vasospasm precipitates **resting angina**. In this case the angina is due to reduced

Coronary stenosis restricts myocardial hyperaemia during exercise

■ Resistances in series summate. For example, if the normal coronary artery has a resistance of 1 unit and the rest of the coronary circulation has a resistance of 19 units, the total resistance is 20 units.

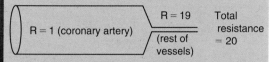

■ During exercise, metabolic vasodilatation of the myocardial resistance vessels reduces the resistance beyond the artery, e.g. to 4 units. Given a healthy artery, total resistance is now 5 units. Myocardial blood flow increases four-fold (20/5) and meets the increased O_2 demand.

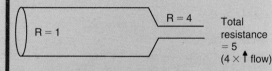

■ Consider next a severely stenosed artery of resistance 10 units. Due to distal arteriogenesis and dilatation, the distal resistance at rest falls from 19 to 10 units. Total vascular resistance is still 20 units at rest, so resting flow is normal.

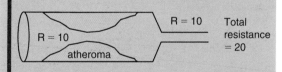

■ When the patient exercises, the reserve dilatation of resistance vessels reduces the distal resistance further, e. g. to 3 units. Total resistance, 13 units, is now dominated by the stenosis. Myocardial blood flow increases only 1½-fold (20/13). This does not meet the increased O_2 demand, so angina develops.

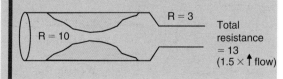

The Coronary Circulation

Special tasks

■ Maintain high basal rate of O_2 supply

■ Increase O_2 supply in proportion to cardiac work

Structural adaptations

■ High capillary density

■ Short diffusion distances (small fibres)

Functional adaptations

■ High O_2 extraction (>60%)

■ Metabolic vasodilatation dominates regulation

■ Good autoregulation

■ Vascular β_2 adrenoceptors ensure adrenaline causes vasodilatation

Special problems

■ Flow is obstruction by compression in systole; aggravated by aortic stenosis.

■ Functional end-arteries in man, so thrombosis → infarction (heart attack)

■ Gradual stenosis by atheroma → exercise-induced angina

■ Sympathetic vasoconstrictor activity and atheroma → stress-induced angina

■ Coronary artery vasospasm downstream of atheroma → resting angina

Assessment in man

■ Coronary angiography to locate stenosed segment

■ Coronary sinus thermal dilution method for absolute flows

■ Isotope imaging for distribution of perfusion

■ Exercise ECG test for latent ischaemia (ST depression on exercise)

---

myocardial O_2 *supply*, whereas exercise-induced angina is due to increased myocardial O_2 *demand*.

Angina is relieved by **nitrodilator drugs** such as glyceryl trinitrate. Glyceryl trinitrate chiefly dilates the systemic veins and systemic conduit arteries, but not the stenosed artery; it has relatively little effect on vascular resistance. Systemic venodilatation reduces the cardiac filling pressure (preload). Systemic conduit artery relaxation reduces pulse wave velocity and reflection, leading to a fall in peak systolic pressure and cardiac afterload (Section 8.4 and Figure 8.10). The venous and arterial effects together reduce cardiac work and therefore O_2 demand. **β-adrenergic blockers** such as propranolol reduce O_2 demand by reducing the heart rate and contractility.

Surgical treatments for stenosed coronary arteries include **angioplasty** (dilatation of the stenosed segment using a balloon-tipped catheter introduced through a peripheral artery) and **bypass surgery** (replacement of the stenosed region with a section of saphenous vein or internal mammary artery).

Assessment of the human coronary circulation

- **Coronary angiography** is used to locate atheromatous obstructions, often as a preliminary to vascular surgery. The artery is perfused with a radio-opaque contrast medium and monitored by X-ray.

- **Coronary sinus thermodilution** measures coronary blood flow quantitatively. The sinus is cannulated, a bolus of cold saline is injected and temperature is recorded downstream. See the thermodilution principle, Section 7.2.

- **Gamma scans** are used to assess the evenness of myocardial perfusion (Figure 15.6). A gamma-emitting isotope such as thallium or rubidium is infused into the circulation and its appearance in the myocardium is monitored by a gamma-camera. Being analogues of K^+, thallium and rubidium are pumped into the myocytes by the Na^+-K^+ pump. Regions with defective perfusion are revealed by patches of defective uptake.

15.2 Skeletal muscle circulation

Flow, resting postural (tonic) muscle	$\sim 15\ ml\ min^{-1}\ 100\ g^{-1}$
Flow, resting phasic muscle	$\sim 3-5\ ml\ min^{-1}\ 100\ g$
Max flow during phasic exercise	$>100-200\ ml\ min^{-1}\ 100\ g^{-1}$

The skeletal muscle and coronary circulations have much in common; metabolic hyperaemia is crucial to both, and both can experience atheromatous ischaemia. There are also important differences, however, such as the responsiveness of skeletal muscle vessels to cardiovascular reflexes.

Special tasks

- During exercise the muscle circulation must increase the rate of O_2 and glucose delivery and the rate of removal of metabolic waste products.

- A second important duty is to help regulate arterial blood pressure. Muscle constitutes $\sim 40\%$ of the adult body mass, so its vascular resistance has a major effect on total peripheral resistance and blood pressure.

Structural adaptation

The capillary density depends on muscle type. Postural muscles such as the soleus have a high proportion of tonically active red fibres (slow oxidative fibres). Postural muscles tend to be continuously active and have a higher **capillary density** than phasic muscles. Phasic muscles such as the forearm and gastrocnemius muscles consist chiefly of fast, glycolytic white fibres.

Endurance training causes capillary angiogenesis in muscle. The number of capillaries per muscle fibre increases in proportion to the fibre mitochondrial volume.

Functional adaptations

Resistance vessels have high tone in resting muscle

Vascular tone is a prerequisite for dilatation (loss of tone). The very high tone of resistance vessels in resting muscle is revealed by the fact that conductance and flow can increase 20 times or more in active muscle. Most of the vascular tone is evidently of a non-neural origin, since sympathetic denervation only doubles the conductance and flow.

Muscle vascular resistance helps to regulate blood pressure

The resistance vessels are richly innervated by tonically active, sympathetic vasoconstrictor fibres, whose activity is controlled reflexly through pressure receptors in the central arteries and heart (Chapter 16). Sympathetic activity is increased in orthostasis and hypovolaemia, raising muscle vascular resistance and thus helping to prevent a fall in arterial pressure. After a severe haemorrhage sympathetic activity reaches the maximum physiological rate of 6–10 impulses/sec, and the attendant vasoconstriction reduces muscle blood flow to $\sim 1/5$th normal.

Vasoconstrictor fibre activity modulates vascular tone even in the dilated resistance vessels of active muscle. This prevents excessive dilatation, which could otherwise cause arterial hypotension. The vasoconstrictor discharge to exercising muscle is regulated by the baroreceptor reflex.

Metabolic hyperaemia raises flow to active muscle

During strenuous exercise the blood flow through phasic muscle can increase more than 20 times and account for 80–90% of the cardiac output (cf. 18% at rest). The metabolic hyperaemia is so great that, if all the muscles of the body could be maximally vasodilated at the same time, the output capacity of the heart would be exceeded. The increased flow is due almost entirely to a fall in vascular resistance, not to the small rise in arterial pressure. The fall in resistance is brought about by **metabolic hyperaemia**, which is accompanied by a permissive **ascending dilatation** in feed arteries and **flow-induced dilatation** in conduit arteries (Section 13.7).

As in the myocardium blood flow increases almost linearly with local metabolic rate. Also as in myocardium the identity of the vasodilator agent is controversial. Over the first 3–5 min of exercise **K^+ ions** are released by the contracting muscle. The interstitial K^+ concentration increases in proportion to the exercise intensity and can reach 11 mM, which produces near maximal vasodilatation in some muscles. The clearance of the released K^+ into the bloodstream gradually raises the arterial plasma K^+. A rise in interstitial **osmolarity** by 20–30 mOs also contributes to the early vasodilatation, as does the release of **inorganic phosphate** by contracting muscle fibres. The vasodilator effect of these factors is potentiated by a rise in interstitial **adenosine** and tissue **acidosis**. Together these various factors probably account for much of the early hyperaemia of exercise. Nitric oxide contributes little to exercise hyperaemia.

As exercise continues the elevated K^+ level decays with a half-time of ~3 min. Osmolarity likewise decays. It is not certain what maintains the vasodilatation during prolonged exercise. Interstitial **adenosine** concentration increases in proportion to exercise intensity, and some studies using blockers indicate that adenosine accounts for up to 40% of the sustained vasodilatation in dynamic exercise. Adenosine also contributes substantially to the vasodilatation of isometric exercise.

Two other special adaptations are the vasodilator response of muscle arterioles to **adrenaline** (Section 14.6) and, in non-primates, the sympathetic cholinergic vasodilator innervation (Section 14.3).

Capillary recruitment improves solute exchange in active muscle

Due to the intermittent, asynchronous contractions of terminal arterioles (vasomotion) only a half to a third of the capillaries in resting muscle is well perfused at any one instant (Figure 15.2, left). Dilatation of the terminal arterioles during metabolic hyperaemia increases the well-perfused fraction of capillaries. This 'capillary recruitment' increases the effective **surface area** for

gas exchange and shortens the extravascular **diffusion distance (**Krogh cylinder model, Figure 10.14).

O_2 extraction increases but 'oxygen debt' and lactate accumulate

In resting muscle the intracellular P_{O_2} is ~20 mmHg and the muscle extracts 25–30% of the O_2 from the perfusing blood. In exercise the intracellular P_{O_2} falls and the O_2 extraction can reach 80–90% (Section 10.11). In severe exercise the fall in intracellular P_{O_2} leads to anaerobic glycolysis and **lactic acid formation**. Most of the lactate diffuses into the bloodstream, raising the plasma lactate from 0.5 mM at rest (plasma pH 7.4) to as much as 20 mM in extreme exercise (pH 6.9). The quantity of lactate formed is an index of the deficit in O_2 supply. This 'O_2 debt' can reach several litres. The interstitial lactic acid and K^+ stimulate nociceptive C-fibres, causing a painful burning sensation that forces the termination of violent exercise. The lactate also stimulates muscle metaboloreceptors involved in the reflex control of the circulation (Section 16.6).

After exercise has stopped, a period of **post-exercise hyperaemia** resupplies the muscle with O_2 and washes out the accumulated lactate (Figures 13.4, 13.11). The circulating lactate is taken up by the heart as a primary substrate and by the liver for re-synthesis into glycogen.

The venous muscle pump aids perfusion in rhythmic exercise

Although exercise hyperaemia is due chiefly to increased vascular conductance, the intermittent compression of deep veins in rhythmic exercise assists perfusion, particularly in the human calf. In a standing, stationary adult the arterial and venous pressures in the calf are both elevated by ~70 mmHg due to the effect of gravity (Figure 15.8). The pressures are

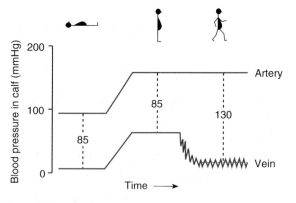

Figure 15.8 Effect of posture and muscle pump on pressure gradient driving blood through calf.

respectively ~165 mmHg and 80 mmHg. The perfusion pressure across calf muscle, i.e. the pressure drop, is thus 85 mmHg at rest. During walking, running or cycling, the muscle pump lowers the venous pressure to ~35 mmHg. This increases the pressure gradient driving flow by >50%, to 130 mmHg.

Special problems

Muscle contraction compresses the supply vessels

When a muscle contracts at over 30–70% of maximum voluntary force, compression of the intramuscular vessels impairs the blood flow. As a result the blood flow oscillates during rhythmic exercise such as running or cycling (Figure 13.4). During a strong, sustained contraction the impairment of flow is sustained. Since the O_2 store in oxymyoglobin is only sufficient for 5–10 s activity, the fibres quickly become hypoxic and lactate accumulates, leading to pain and fatigue. The rapid loss of strength during a strong sustained contraction will be familiar to anyone who has struggled along with a heavy suitcase.

Increased capillary filtration causes active muscle to swell

Fluid translocation across capillaries in exercising muscle leads to muscle swelling ('pumped' muscle) and a 10–15% fall in plasma volume, as described in Section 11.9.

Ischaemic arterial disease leads to intermittent claudication

The major leg arteries are common sites for atheroma and stenosis, and similar arguments apply to the leg as in Concept Box 20 for the heart. Ischaemic pain may occur on walking, forcing repeated rests (intermittent claudication). Severe cases progress to chronic pain at rest, ulceration, and gangrene necessitating amputation.

Measurement of human muscle blood flow

The soft tissue of a human limb consists mainly of skeletal muscle. Limb blood flow can be measured by **venous occlusion plethysmography** (Figures 8.5, 13.11) and **Doppler velocimetry** of the principal artery (Figure 13.4). Local capillary perfusion rate can be estimated by the **Kety radioisotope clearance method** (Figure 8.6).

15.3 Cutaneous circulation

Flow at thermo-neutrality (27°C)	10–20 ml min^{-1} 100 g^{-1}
Minimal flow	1 ml min^{-1} 100 g^{-1}
Maximum flow	150–200 ml min^{-1} 100 g^{-1}

Skin is the organ of temperature regulation in humans. Its surface area is ~1.8 m^2 in an adult, its weight is 2–3 kg, and the combined thickness of the epidermis and dermis is 1–2 mm. The dermis is well vascularized but the epidermis is avascular (Figure 15.9). Unlike muscle, where large fluctuations in metabolic activity govern the blood flow, skin has a relatively constant metabolic rate. Its O_2 needs are readily met by a low blood flow, aided by the direct diffusion of O_2 into the superficial 100 μm or so of epidermis. Skin blood flow is heavily influenced by sympathetic fibres whose activity is linked to core temperature.

KEY FEATURES BOX 15.2

The Skeletal Muscle Circulation

Special tasks
- To deliver O_2 and nutrients in proportion to work rate
- To help regulate blood pressure as the largest tissue mass in the body

Structural adaptations
- High capillary density, especially in postural muscles

Functional adaptations
- Metabolic vasodilatation dominates regulation during exercise
- Vasodilatation to adrenaline
- Capillary recruitment in exercise
- Skeletal muscle pump enhances local pressure gradient
- O_2 extraction increases with exercise
- Sympathetically-mediated participation in baroreflex

Special problems
- Mechanical impairment of flow, especially in isometric contractions
- Increased capillary filtration → swollen 'pumped' muscle in severe exercise
- Ischaemia due to leg artery atheroma → intermittent claudication, ulcers, gangrene

Assessment in man
- Venous occlusion plethysmography for limb blood flow
- Doppler velocity meter for clinical assessment of patency
- Kety's isotope clearance method for local capillary perfusion

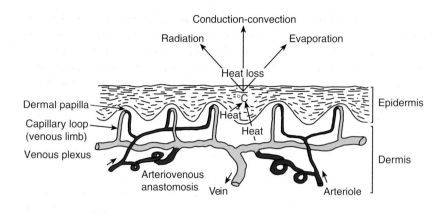

Figure 15.9 Dermal vascular architecture and heat flux in an extremity (acral skin). Skin colour is influenced by the volume and oxygenation of blood in subpapillary venous plexus.

Special tasks

The cutaneous circulation regulates core temperature

The temperature of the human core, i.e. the brain, thoracic and abdominal organs, is normally maintained at 37.0–37.5°C. This is achieved by balancing internal heat production and external heat loss. The main heat-dissipating surface is species-dependent; in humans it is the skin, in dogs the tongue and in rabbits and elephants the ears. Heat is lost by three physical processes (Figure 15.9):

- radiation
- conduction–convection
- evaporation.

With **radiation** the rate of heat loss is proportional to the difference between ambient temperature and skin temperature. Skin temperature depends on the rate at which blood delivers heat from the core, i.e. cutaneous blood flow.

With **conduction–convection**, warm skin heats up the adjacent air by conduction, and the warmed air is removed by convection (air currents). Conductive heat loss increases with skin temperature and therefore cutaneous blood flow.

In the **evaporation of sweat** 2.4 kJ of heat energy are used per gram of water evaporated (the latent heat of evaporation). Both the water and the heat are delivered to the skin by the bloodstream.

Cutaneous blood flow is thus a key regulator of heat loss by each physical process. The skin itself is poikilothermic rather than homeothermic, i.e. it has a widely varying temperature. For short periods it can tolerate temperatures as extreme as 0°C and 45°C without damage.

Cutaneous vessels participate in protection against the environment

The other major role of skin is physical protection. The cutaneous circulation participates in this role through the Lewis triple response to trauma.

Structural adaptations

Dermal arteriovenous anastomoses (AVAs) abound in the extremities

Specialized regions called 'acral skin' have numerous, direct connections between the dermal arterioles and venules, the arteriovenous anastomoses or AVAs (Figure 15.9). AVAs were discovered by R. T. Grant in the rabbit ear in 1930. Human AVAs are found in exposed regions with a high surface area/volume ratio, namely the fingers and toes, palm and sole, lips, nose and pinna of the ear. AVAs are coiled, muscular-walled vessels of diameter ~35 μm. They have little basal tone and are controlled almost exclusively by sympathetic vasoconstrictor fibres, whose activity is controlled by a temperature-regulating centre in the **hypothalamus**. AVAs also respond directly to ambient temperature, dilating to heat and constricting to cold.

In a thermoneutral environment, namely 27–28°C for a naked human, skin temperature is ~33°C and hypothalamic temperature is 37–37.5°C. Under these conditions the acral skin is subject to a high level of tonic, sympathetic vasoconstrictor tone. In the skin of the limbs and trunk, which lack AVAs, there is only slight basal sympathetic vasoconstrictor activity. This has been shown by surgical sympathectomy and local nerve block, which cause greater cutaneous hyperaemia in the limb extremity than proximally.

When core temperature is high, the hypothalamus reduces the vasomotor drive to the AVAs, allowing them to relax and dilate. This creates a low-resistance shunt into the venous plexus and therefore raises the blood flow and heat delivery. Heat readily crosses the venous wall, so skin temperature rises and heat loss increases. Conversely, the AVAs are constricted to conserve heat under cold conditions. It is worth reiterating that the dilatation of AVAs increases heat loss, since students sometimes believe the opposite. The following 'aide memoire' might well have been sung by the mud-loving hippopotamus in Flanders and Swan's famous song:

A – V – A's, let 'em flood,
There's nothing quite like them
For cooling the blood.
So dilate them widely,
Let's lose heat right blithely –
But close them up tightly
When chill is the mud.

Venous–arterial countercurrent exchangers conserve heat in limbs

The flippers of whales and the feet of wading birds possess an elaborate countercurrent heat-conserving mechanism. The cool blood from the extremity drains into deep veins, and the deep veins ramify around the limb artery. This allows heat to pass directly from the warm arterial blood into the cool venous blood. The extremity is thus fed pre-cooled arterial blood, and heat-loss to the environment is reduced. The same short-circuiting of heat occurs in human limbs but to a lesser degree.

Functional adaptations

Cutaneous blood flow is influenced by both ambient temperature and core temperature.

Ambient temperature directly affects cutaneous vascular tone

Local warming of the skin causes dilatation of the cutaneous arterioles, venules and small veins. The familiar reddening of skin in hot water is due to an increased volume of well-oxygenated blood in the dilated venular plexus. **Skin colour**, aside from that due to melanin, depends chiefly on the volume and oxygen content of blood in the dermal venous plexus. Conversely, local cooling of the skin to 10–15°C causes vasoconstriction and venoconstriction (Figure 15.10a). This reduces cutaneous heat loss and protects the core temperature.

The responsiveness to local temperature is attributed to an abundance of α_2-**adrenoceptors** in cutaneous vessels. The affinity of α_2-adrenoceptors for noradrenaline, the sympathetic transmitter,

increases as temperature falls towards 10°C. Thus the α_2-adrenoceptor blockers yohimbine and rauwolscine inhibit cold-induced vasoconstriction.

Immersion of one hand in cold water elicits a small vasoconstriction in the opposite hand. This is partly a spinal sympathetic reflex and partly due to cooled blood affecting the hypothalamic temperature sensors.

Paradoxical cold vasodilatation follows severe cold

When a hand is placed in water at 10°C or less for a long time, the initial cold-induced vasoconstriction gives way to dilatation after 5–10 min, with reddening of the skin and relief of the painful sensation (Figure 15.10c). This is called paradoxical cold vasodilatation. Paradoxical cold vasodilatation occurs in regions rich in AVAs and contributes to the cold, red noses and hands seen in frosty weather. It is attributed to the paralysis of noradrenergic neurotransmission and the release of vasodilator substances such as prostacyclin. Cold-induced vasodilatation is well developed in manual workers such as Arctic Indians and Norwegian fishermen and prevents skin damage during prolonged cold exposure.

If the exposure to cold persists, vasoconstriction recurs after a while and the skin oscillates between vasoconstriction and vasodilatation over a 15–20 min cycle. This is called the **hunting reaction**.

Core temperature influences cutaneous sympathetic vasomotor activity

Cutaneous vasomotor nerve activity is strongly influenced by core temperature. Increased core temperature, for example during exercise, is sensed by **warmth receptors** in the anterior hypothalamus. The hypothalamic neurons project to presympathetic neurons in the brainstem and these regulate the sympathetic vasomotor and sudomotor discharge to the skin. Thus a rise in core temperature elicits cutaneous vasodilatation and sweating (Figures 15.10b, 15.11).

The thermoregulatory vasodilatation is brought about by different mechanisms in acral and non-acral skin. In **acral skin** the vasodilatation is due mainly to a **reduction** of the high basal sympathetic vasoconstrictor drive to the AVAs. In the **non-acral skin** of the limbs, trunk and scalp, the dilatation is due mainly to **increased activity in sympathetic vasodilator fibres**, and is closely associated with sweating. The active nature of the limb response is demonstrated by its abolition by local nerve block (Figure 15.11). The active vasodilatation is impaired but not completely abolished by atropine, and is probably mediated by both acetylcholine and VIP.

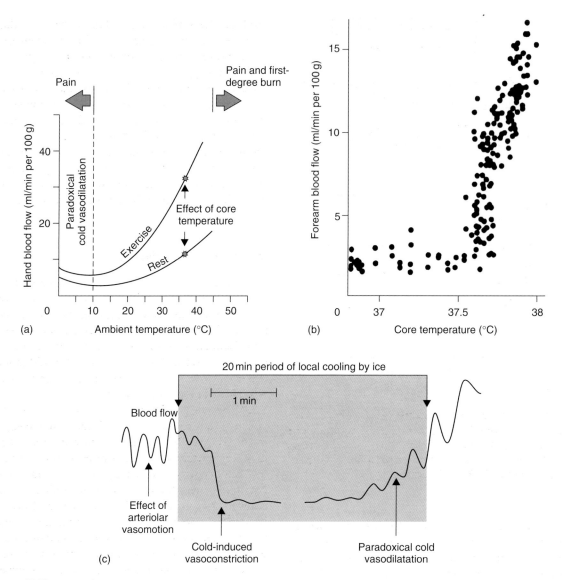

Figure 15.10 Effect of external and internal temperature on skin blood flow. (a) Response of the hand to immersion in water at various temperatures, when the internal heat load is either low (rest) or high (exercise). Note the paradoxical vasodilatation at <10°C. (b) Response of forearm blood flow, measured by plethysmography, to changes in internal temperature induced by leg exercise. The increase in blood flow arises in the skin; xenon clearance studies showed that forearm muscle flow actually decreased slightly. (c) Initial vasoconstriction of skin to cold gives way to paradoxical vasodilatation in 10–20 min. Human calf studied by laser Doppler fluxmeter; the oscillation in arteriolar tone, or vasomotion, is normal. (a) After Greenfield, A. D. M. (1963) In *Handbook of Physiology, Cardiovascular System*, Vol. III, Part II, *Peripheral Circulation* (eds Hamilton, W. F. and Dow, P.), American Physiological Society, Bethesda, pp. 1325–1352; (b) from Johnson, J. M. and Rowell, J. B. (1975) *Journal of Applied Physiology*, **39**, 920–924, by permission; (c) based on Van den Brande, P., De Coninck A. and Lievens, P. (1997) *International Journal of Microcirculation*, **17**, 55–60.)

The cutaneous response to a heat load is finely **graded** (Figure 15.10b). Maximum vasodilatation produces skin blood flows of >5 l/min in an adult, which necessitates an increase in cardiac output and compensatory vasoconstriction in the splanchnic, renal and skeletal muscle circulations to maintain arterial pressure. By contrast, in a cold environment skin blood flow can be reduced to a mere 20 ml/min. This allows the full insulating action of the subcutaneous fat to protect the core temperature.

Skin vessels help regulate arterial and central venous pressures

Hypovolaemia and acute cardiac failure cause a reflex increase in cutaneous sympathetic vasoconstrictor fibre activity and increased circulating levels of angiotensin, vasopressin and adrenaline. These changes cause a strong contraction of the cutaneous veins and arterioles, leading to the characteristic **pale, cold skin of patients in clinical shock**. The

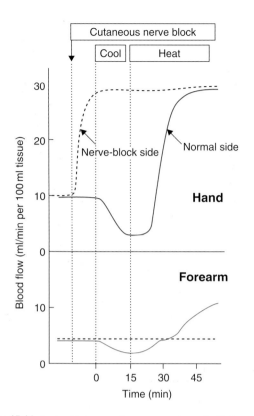

Figure 15.11 Contrast between cutaneous vascular control in human hand and arm. Dashed line shows effect of cutaneous vasomotor nerve block by local anaesthetic. Cooling or heating was indirect (legs in cold/hot water) with the upper limbs exposed to room temperature. (After Roddie, I. C. (1983); see Further Reading.)

resistance vessel contraction helps to support arterial pressure and the venoconstriction helps to support central venous pressure. The importance of these responses was revealed on the battlefields of France during World War I, when it was noticed that wounded men who were rescued quickly and warmed in blankets (producing cutaneous dilatation) survived haemorrhage less well than the men who could not be reached for some time and retained their natural cutaneous vasoconstriction.

Exercise initially evokes a sympathetically mediated cutaneous vasoconstriction, but this changes to dilatation if the core temperature subsequently rises.

Stimuli that elicit the **alerting (defence) response**, such as mental arithmetic, cause a transient cutaneous venous and arteriolar constriction (Figure 14.14). **Deep inspiration** has the same effect.

Orthostatis elicits the veni-arteriolar response

Dependency below heart level causes a strong cutaneous vasoconstriction (Figures 8.6, 11.5), which reduces skin blood flow in the foot to less than a third of the supine value. This helps to reduce dependent oedema formation, and to maintain arterial pressure during standing. The arteriolar contraction is triggered by the venous congestion, so it is called the **veni-arteriolar response**. Its mechanism is not properly understood. The myogenic response may contribute, but in addition local nerve fibres seem to be involved, because the response is abolished by local anaesthetics. The traditional view that the veni-arteriolar response is a 'sympathetic axon reflex' must be questioned, because a blocking dose of the α-antagonist phentolamine fails to block the response.

Skin is the mirror of the soul

Poets and playwrights have long emphasized the responsiveness of skin colour to emotion. Aside from pigmentation, skin colour depends on the red cell mass in the dermal venous plexus and its oxygenation. Skin colour is therefore influenced by vascular tone. We blush with embarrassment (vasodilatation) and blanch in response to stress or fear (vasoconstriction elicited by the alerting response).★

Blushing is poorly understood because it is difficult to produce on demand. Folkow and Neil, in their classic textbook 'The Circulation', recall how they were unable to make a habitual blusher blush in a laboratory setting, either by insults or rude jokes, but when they disconnected their equipment and thanked the subject, she blushed violently. Blushing is often associated with emotional sweating and may be mediated by the sympathetic cholinergic vasodilator system. Blushing affects only certain areas, namely the face, neck and upper chest. A hyperaemic response to emotional stimuli has also been observed in the gastric and colonic mucosa.

★Juliet was evidently a blusher. Her nurse, announcing Romeo's desire to marry her, remarked:

> There stays a husband to make you a wife:
> Now comes the wanton blood up in your cheeks,
> They'll be in scarlet straight at any news.
> (Romeo and Juliet, Act 2, Sc. 5)

The defence or alerting response has the opposite effect. When Salisbury tells King Richard of his army's desertion, the King pales, crying:

> But now the blood of twenty thousand men
> Did triumph in my face, and they are fled;
> And, till so much blood thither comes again,
> Have I not reason to look pale and dead?
> (Richard II, Act 3, Sc. 2)

Trauma increases skin blood flow

The response of skin to trauma is nicely illustrated by the Lewis triple response, which was covered in Section 14.4. Both flow and capillary permeability increase, thereby boosting the delivery of white cells and immunoglobulins to the injured site.

Special problems

Weight-bearing can produce pressure ulcers

Skin gets sat on, stood on and leaned on for long periods, impairing its blood flow. Ischaemic damage is normally prevented by the high tolerance of the skin to hypoxia, and by **reactive hyperaemia** when discomfort leads to a shift in position and relief of the compression. The reddening of skin following unloading is obvious in white-skinned humans. The urge to shift position is attributed to the accumulation of metabolites that stimulate skin nociceptors.

In certain groups of patients, namely the elderly, the enfeebled, the paraplegic and the comatose, there is little or no spontaneous shifting of position to relieve skin compression. If major pressure areas such as the heels and buttocks are not relieved, for example by regular turning of the patient, the skin undergoes ischaemic necrosis, resulting in deep **pressure ulcers** (**bed sores**).

Problems during hot weather

- The dilatation of cutaneous veins in a hot environment reduces the central venous pressure, which predisposes the subject to **postural fainting**. The classic example is the guardsman who faints while standing at attention in hot weather.

- Cutaneous vasodilatation increases capillary filtration pressure, leading to **tissue swelling**. Thus a ring often feels tight on the finger during hot weather.

- Heavy exercise in a hot environment can lead to hypotension and **heat exhaustion**. The combined hyperaemia of skin and muscle greatly reduces the peripheral resistance. At the same time the plasma volume falls, due to a combination of sweating and fluid filtration into the exercising muscle. The reduced cardiac filling pressure and reduced peripheral resistance lead to hypotension and collapse (heat exhaustion).

Problems during cold weather

- Paradoxical cold vasodilatation normally prevents tissue damage in cold weather. In

---

KEY FEATURES BOX 15.3

The Cutaneous Circulation

Special tasks
- Regulate body temperature
- Respond to trauma

Structural adaptations
- Arterio-venous anastomoses in acral skin (fingers, palms, toes, lips, nose, ears) dilate to increase heat dissipation

Functional adaptations
- Sympathetic nerves, rather than metabolic hyperaemia, dominate control
- Core temperature receptors in hypothalamus control sympathetic vasoconstrictor fibres to acral skin (AVAs) and sympathetic vasodilator fibres to non-acral skin
- Ambient temperature too influences vessel tone, with paradoxical cold vasodilatation at very low temperatures
- Reflex vaso- and venoconstriction follows hypotension or acute cardiac failure
- Veni-arteriolar response reduces perfusion of dependent skin
- Perfusion responds to emotional state (vasoconstriction to stress, blushing to embarrassment)
- Lewis triple response enhances perfusion and immunoglobulin escape after skin damage
- Reactive hyperaemia follows relief of compression

Special problems
- Compression during weight-bearing → pressure ulcers ('bed sores')
- Heat → tissue swelling and venodilatation. Latter aggravates postural hypotension and fainting. Heat-induced cutaneous dilatation plus strenuous exercise can lead to heat exhaustion
- In Raynaud's disease, ambient cold → sustained, damaging vasoconstriction in fingers

Assessment in man
- Laser Doppler probe for red cell flux
- Kety's isotope clearance method for local capillary perfusion

---

Raynaud's disease, however, the vessels of the fingers show an exaggerated, sustained vasoconstriction to cold, usually in women. This leads to severe blanching, numbness, tingling or pain in the finger tips, and local tissue ischaemia.

- In severe eczema or psoriasis the vasoconstrictor response to cold is prevented by inflammatory vasodilatation. Temperature regulation becomes very unstable and can occasionally necessitate hospitalization.

Measurement of human cutaneous blood flow

- The **laser–Doppler** method is widely used as a rapid, semi-quantitative measurement of the flux of red cells through the superficial dermis.

- **Thermography**, the imaging of skin surface temperature, has been used as an indirect index of flow; but epidermal temperature also depends on ambient temperature and skin thickness.

- **Venous occlusion plethysmography** of a digit measures chiefly skin blood flow.

- **Kety's isotope clearance technique** measures nutritive flow (Figure 8.6).

15.4 Cerebral circulation

Mean flow through brain	$55\,\text{ml}\,\text{min}^{-1}\,100\,\text{g}^{-1}$
Basal flow through grey matter	$100\,\text{ml}\,\text{min}^{-1}\,100\,\text{g}^{-1}$

The human brain accounts for only 2% of the body mass yet it receives 14% of the resting cardiac output. Most of the flow goes to the grey matter (chiefly neurons), which makes up 40% of the brain mass. A small proportion goes to the white matter, which is chiefly myelinated tracts.

A structural peculiarity of the cerebral circulation is that the arterioles are rather short and thin walled. As a result the large cerebral arteries account for an unusually high proportion of the vascular resistance, namely 40–50%, and have a rich autonomic innervation.

Special tasks

The cerebral circulation must provide a totally secure O$_2$ supply

Grey matter has a very high rate of oxidative metabolism, $\sim 7\,\text{ml}\,\text{O}_2\,\text{min}^{-1}\,100\,\text{g}^{-1}$. Indeed, the O_2 consumption of grey matter accounts for nearly 20% of human O_2 consumption at rest. Grey matter is exquisitely sensitive to hypoxia, and human consciousness is lost after just a few seconds of cerebral ischaemia. Irreversible neuronal damage follows within 4 minutes or so. The primary task of the cerebral circulation, therefore, is to maintain an uninterrupted O_2 delivery at all costs.

Local blood flow must respond to varying neuronal activity

Many mental functions are localized in well-defined regions of the brain. For example, visual interpretation is located in the occipital visual cortex. External monitoring of the uptake of radiolabelled glucose and O_2 shows that increased local neuronal activity raises the local metabolic rate. Illumination of the retina, for example, raises the metabolic rate of the occipital visual cortex. The cerebral vessels must therefore adjust the blood flow regionally to match the varying regional demand for O_2.

Structural adaptations

The circle of Willis helps safeguard the arterial supply

The **basilar** and **internal carotid arteries** enter the cranial cavity and immediately anatomize to form an arterial circle around the optic chiasma called the circle of Willis (Figure 15.12). (The young assistant employed by Thomas Willis to illustrate the circle later designed St Paul's Cathedral in London, being Christopher Wren.) The **anterior**, **middle** and **posterior cerebral arteries** arise from the circle of Willis. This arrangement should, in principle, maintain cerebral perfusion even if one carotid artery becomes obstructed. This is the case in young subjects, but in elderly subjects the anastomoses are less effective. The anterior, middle and posterior cerebral arteries divide into **pial arteries** that run over the surface of the brain. Pressure in the pial arteries is only ~50% of the systemic arterial pressure owing to the relatively high resistance of the large intracranial arteries. The pial arteries give rise to finer arteries that penetrate into the parenchyma and divide into the short arterioles.

A high capillary density optimizes O$_2$ transport

Grey matter contains on average 3000–4000 capillaries per mm^2 cross-section, similar to myocardium. The high capillary density provides a large surface area for O_2 exchange and reduces the extravascular diffusion distance to $\leqslant 10\,\mu\text{m}$. Tight endothelial junctions form a blood–brain barrier to lipid-insoluble solutes (see later).

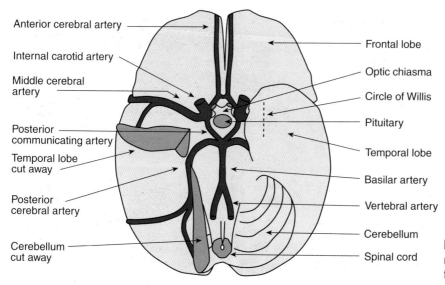

Figure 15.12 Circle of Willis and main cerebral arteries in man. View from underside of brain.

Functional adaptations

Cerebral blood flow is regulated chiefly by intrinsic mechanisms, namely autoregulation and functional hyperaemia, rather than by extrinsic factors (vasomotor nerves, hormones).

Grey matter has a very high basal blood flow

The grey matter receives a very high blood flow, about 100 ml blood min^{-1} 100 g^{-1}. This is more than 10 times the average for the whole body. The O_2 extraction of ~35% is also above average.

Cerebral perfusion pressure is safeguarded through brainstem regulation of other circulations

As in any organ cerebral blood flow depends on vascular conductance and arterial pressure. Unlike any other organ, however, the brain can safeguard its blood supply by controlling the arterial pressure, which it does through the neural regulation of cardiac output and peripheral vascular resistance. When necessary the perfusion of the peripheral organs, excepting the heart, is sacrificed through peripheral vasoconstriction to maintain arterial pressure and hence cerebral perfusion.

Cerebral autoregulation maintains perfusion during hypotension

As a further safeguard against underperfusion, autoregulation is very well developed in the brain (Figure 15.13). If blood pressure should fall, the cerebral resistance vessels dilate and thereby maintain cerebral blood flow. There is a limit, however, to this

process. Below ~50 mmHg autoregulation fails and cerebral blood flow declines steeply. Hypotension of this severity therefore leads to mental confusion and syncope. The upper limit of autoregulation is probably ~175 mmHg.

Cerebral vessels are unusually responsive to arterial CO_2

Cerebral vascular tone is very sensitive to arterial CO_2. **Hypercapnia** causes vasodilatation, which is a helpful response during asphyxia (Figure 15.13). The vasodilatation is partly mediated by endothelial NO formation, aided perhaps by a fall in vascular myocyte pH due to the carbonic acid.

Hypocapnia causes vasoconstriction. If arterial P_{CO_2} is reduced to 15 mmHg by hyperventilation (normal P_{CO_2} is 40 mmHg), vasoconstriction halves the cerebral blood flow. The vasoconstriction can be observed directly in the retina, which is embryologically an extension of the brain. The vasoconstriction is of some medical significance because **panic hyperventilation** in adults, or hyperventilation for fun by children, can lead via hypocapnia and cerebral vasoconstriction to disturbed vision, dizziness and even fainting. The traditional remedy is to hold the opening of a paper bag (not plastic) in front of the mouth to cause re-breathing of expired carbon dioxide.

Local hypoxia causes cerebral vasodilatation, due in part to adenosine formation. **Systemic hypoxia**, however, stimulates ventilation, and the resulting hypocapnia causes a counteracting cerebral vasoconstriction. As a result of the two opposing effects, systemic hypoxia has only a minor effect on human cerebral blood flow.

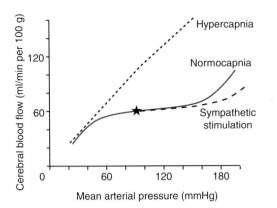

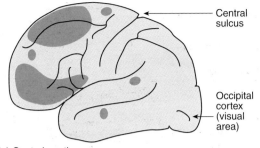

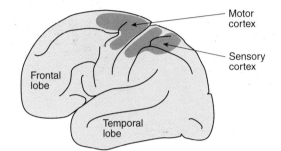

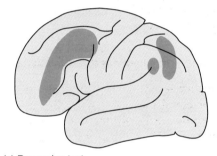

(a) Control, resting

(b) Movement of contralateral hand

(c) Reasoning test

Figure 15.13 Autoregulation of brain blood flow at normal arterial P_{CO_2} (solid line); star represents normal operating point. Flow in the autoregulated range changes by only 6% per 10 mmHg. High carbon dioxide tension causes vasodilatation (upper dashed line). Sympathetic nerve stimulation only affects flow significantly when arterial pressure is abnormally high (lower dashed line). (After Heistad, D. D. and Kontos, H. A. (1983) In *Handbook of Physiology, Cardiovascular System*, Vol. III, Part 1, *Peripheral Circulation*, (eds Shepherd, J.T. and Abboud, F.M.), American Physiological Society, Bethesda, pp. 137–181, by permission.)

Regional neuronal activity evokes regional hyperaemia

Shining a light into one eye causes a rise in temperature in the corresponding occipital cortex and an increase in local blood flow, i.e. functional (metabolic) hyperaemia. Deeper parts of the visual pathway, such as the lateral geniculate body, likewise display functional hyperaemia. Computer-assisted isotope imaging techniques have shown that increased local mental activity evokes increased local flow in many other regions of the brain in conscious humans (Figure 15.14).

The functional hyperaemia is caused partly by a rise in **interstitial K$^+$** concentration, resulting from the outward, repolarizing K$^+$ currents of the active neurons (Figure 15.15). The interstitial [K$^+$] can increase from 3 mM to 10 mM but is not well maintained. Additional factors maintaining the hyperaemia include raised interstitial adenosine and H$^+$ concentrations. **Adenosine** levels increase rapidly in response to electrical stimulation, hypoxaemia and hypotension, and are well sustained until the stimulus is withdrawn. Adenosine is a powerful vasodilator of cerebral arterioles.

Extra-cerebral arteries are innervated by both sensory and motor fibres

The intracerebral arterioles are poorly innervated, but the cerebral arteries outside the brain parenchyma

Figure 15.14 Functional hyperaemia in human cortex revealed by xenon-133 imaging. The grey areas show flows 20% above mean. (a) In the resting, pensive subject, there is frontal lobe hyperaemia. (b) On moving the contralateral hand voluntarily, there is hyperaemia of the hand area of the upper motor, premotor and sensory cortex. (c) The reasoning test evokes hyperaemia in the precentral and postcentral areas. (From Ingvar, D. H. (1976) *Brain Research*, **107**, 188–197; and Lassen, N. A., Ingvar, D. H. and Skinhoj, E. (1978) *Scientific American*, **239**(4), 50–59, by permission.)

are richly innervated by:

- nociceptive C-fibres
- parasympathetic vasodilator fibres
- sympathetic vasoconstrictor fibres.

Perivascular nociceptive C-fibres are abundant. They probably mediate the pain of **vascular headaches**, including the severe pains of meningitis, migraine and strokes. The fibres also have a motor function, for they contain the vasodilator

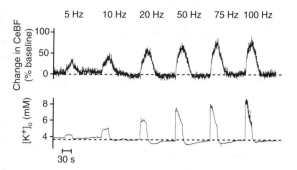

Figure 15.15 Effect of neuronal activity on rat cerebellar blood flow (CeBF), monitored by laser Doppler; and concomitant change in interstitial K^+ concentration $[K^+]_o$, monitored by an ion-sensitive electrode. Neurons were activated by remote electrical stimulation of parallel fibre system at frequency indicated in Hertz. (From Caesar, K., Akgören, N., Mathiesen, C. and Lauritzen, M. (1999) *Journal of Physiology*, **520**, 281–292, by permission.)

neurotransmitters **calcitonin gene-related peptide** (CGRP) and **substance P**, which in skin are involved in antidromic vasodilatation and neurogenic inflammation (Section 14.4). In the cranium the C-fibre vasodilators probably contribute to the hyperaemia of meningitis, seizures and the second phase of migraine.

Parasympathetic vasodilator fibres contain acetylcholine and VIP. They may contribute to the vasodilatation that causes some vascular headaches.

Sympathetic vasoconstrictor fibres release noradrenaline and neuropeptide Y. The noradrenaline evokes only a weak response because cerebral vessels have relatively few α-adrenoceptors. **Neuropeptide Y** is abundant in cerebral sympathetic varicosities and probably accounts for much of the evoked vasoconstriction. Even so, the maximal effect of sympathetic stimulation in anaesthetized humans is only a 37% rise in cerebral vascular resistance, in contrast to a 500% increase in skeletal muscle. Cerebral perfusion is favoured by the weakness of cerebral sympathetic vasoconstriction and negligible involvement in the baroreflex. The chief role of the vasoconstrictor innervation may be to protect the blood–brain barrier against disruption by sudden rises in arterial pressure.

Cerebral capillaries form a tight blood–brain barrier

Lipid-soluble molecules such as O_2, CO_2 and anaesthetics diffuse freely between the plasma and brain interstitium, but lipid-insoluble solutes such as K^+ ions, L-glucose, mannitol and catecholamines fail to penetrate from the bloodstream into most regions of the brain. The 'blood–brain barrier' to lipophobic

solutes was discovered through the simple observation that an intravenous injection of ionic dye stains all the tissues of the body except the nervous system. The functions of the blood–brain barrier are probably to protect the delicate neuronal circuits from interference by solutes such as circulating catecholamines, and to prevent the washout of neurotransmitters from the brain parenchyma. As J. Barcroft eloquently put it in his book, *Architecture of Physiological Function*, 'To look for high intellectual development in a milieu whose properties have not become stabilized is to seek music among the crashings of a rudimentary wireless, or ripple patterns on the surface of the stormy Atlantic.'

The blood–joint barrier is created by the capillary endothelium. In cerebral endothelium, multiple junctional strands form an unbroken seal between the cells. In addition the caveola–vesicle system is very scanty. These structural specialisations are probably induced by the astrocytes, the 'feet' of which envelop over 80% of the abluminal surface of a brain capillary.

Breakdown of the blood–brain barrier is common in pathological conditions such as acute hypertension, local ischaemia (strokes), haemorrhage and inflammation. Breakdown of the barrier leads to cerebral oedema.

In a few locations the blood–brain barrier is physiologically absent. These locations are regions where plasma solutes gain access to receptors. For example, in the **circumventricular region** sodium chloride gains access to the pre-optic osmoreceptors, and angiotensin II gains access to the subfornicular thirst centre. In the **area postrema** angiotensin II accesses presympathetic neurons, and circulating emetics access the vomiting centre.

Cerebral endothelium has specific carriers for metabolites and K^+

The chief energy source for neurons is D-**glucose**, the naturally occurring dextro-rotatory form of glucose (dextrose). Unlike its stereo-isomer L-glucose, D-glucose rapidly crosses the blood–brain barrier. Transport is achieved through facilitated diffusion, which involves the reversible binding of D-glucose to a specific carrier protein in the endothelial cell membrane. Although carrier-based, the transport process is one of passive diffusion down a concentration gradient set up by neuronal activity.

Carriers also exist for the **metabolic acids** lactate and pyruvate and for **adenosine**. There are three distinct carriers for **amino acids**: one for large neutral amino acids, e.g. phenylalanine: one for anionic amino acids, e.g. glutamate: and one for cationic amino acids, e.g. arginine.

There is also active $Na^+ - K^+$ **exchange** across cerebral endothelium. When brain interstitial K^+ concentration rises due to neuronal electrical activity, K^+ is pumped out across the abluminal membrane of the endothelial cell by $Na^+ - K^+$ ATPase. This helps to regulate the K^+ concentration in brain interstitium, and probably explains why cerebral endothelium has five to six times as many mitochondria as muscle endothelium.

Special problems

Orthostasis can cause transient cerebral hypoperfusion and dizziness

Gravity does not directly affect cerebral perfusion in the upright position, because the cerebral circulation is like an inverted U-tube or siphon (Figures 8.2, 8.22, bottom panel); the drag of gravity on the arterial limb is offset by the drag on the venous limb and cerebrospinal fluid. Gravity affects cerebral perfusion indirectly however, because the reduction in central venous pressure in the upright posture reduces cardiac output. The ensuing transient postural hypotension can reduce cerebral perfusion transiently, sufficiently to cause dizziness on standing, or even fainting (postural syncope, Section 17.1).

Space-occupying lesions elicit Cushing's reflex

The adult brain is enclosed in a completely rigid casing, the cranium. Consequently, a space-occupying lesion such as a cerebral tumour or haemorrhage raises the intracranial pressure and forces the brainstem (the site of vasomotor control) down into the foramen magnum, which is the opening in the base of the skull that admits the spinal cord. Compression of the vasomotor centres in the foramen magnum triggers increased sympathetic vasomotor activity, which raises arterial blood pressure (**Cushing's reflex**). The rise in blood pressure helps to maintain the cerebral blood flow in the face of raised intracranial pressure. The raised arterial pressure also evokes a bradycardia through the baroreceptor reflex, and the combination of bradycardia and acute hypertension is recognized by neurologists as the hallmark of a large, space-occupying lesion.

Arterial vasospasm can cause cerebral ischaemia

Spasm of the extracerebral arteries is triggered by a subarachnoid haemorrhage and can lead to a stroke (cerebral infarct). The causes of the cerebral vasospasm

---

KEY FEATURES BOX 15.4

The Cerebral Circulation

Special tasks

▪ Maintain high O_2 delivery to hypoxia-intolerant grey matter

▪ Increase regional O_2 supply in response to regional activity

▪ Maintain a tightly regulated neuronal environment

Structural adaptations

▪ Anastomosis of major arteries forms circle of Willis

▪ High capillary density facilitates gas exchange

▪ Tight endothelial junctions form blood–brain barrier

Functional adaptations

▪ High basal blood flow due to low arteriolar resistance

▪ Brain controls rest of circulation through baroreflex to safeguard its own perfusion pressure. The cerebral vessels themselves are 'excused' from the baroreflex and have only a weak sympathetic innervation

▪ Good autoregulation of flow if blood pressure falls

▪ Strong vasodilatation to CO_2 and asphyxia

▪ Well developed regional metabolic hyperaemia in response to neuronal activity, mediated by interstitial K^+, adenosine and H^+

▪ Blood-brain barrier creates a well-regulated neuronal environment, with specific carriers for facilitated diffusion of D-glucose etc

Special problems

▪ Postural syncope if baroreflex impaired

▪ Space-occupying lesions (tumours, bleeding) → bulbar ischaemia and Cushing reflex

▪ Vascular spasm → cerebral ischaemia

▪ Vascular dilatation → headache, migraine

Assessment in man

▪ Carotid angiography

▪ Transcranial Dopplerimetry

▪ Xenon-133 and SPECT imaging

---

are not well understood, but probably include:

- high levels of endothelin-1 (since cerebral vasospasm is ameliorated by ET_A receptor antagonists);

- release of serotonin (5-hydroxytryptamine) by platelets and perivascular nerves;

- release of neuropeptide Y by sympathetic nerves;

The vasospasm is usually treated with Ca^{2+}-channel blockers.

Cerebral vasoconstriction and vasodilatation underlie a migraine attack

A migraine attack usually begins with a **visual prodroma**, which takes the form of flickering wavy lines in the visual field. The prodroma is caused by the contraction of intracerebral vessels in the visual pathway. The prodroma is followed by a prolonged, severe **headache**, which is due to the dilatation of large extracerebral vessels such as the middle cerebral artery and inflammation around the vessel. The dilatation is thought to be caused by the release of substance P and CGRP from the perivascular sensory fibres, coupled with a local depletion of serotonin. The vasoconstrictor drug **sumatriptan** is an effective treatment for migraine headaches. Sumatriptan is a selective agonist of serotonin $5HT_1$ receptors, which are abundant on cerebral vascular myocytes.

Measurement of human cerebral blood flow

- **Carotid angiography** (arteriography) is XR imaging of the major cerebral arteries during the infusion of radio-opaque contrast medium into the internal carotid artery. The method is used to assess the patency and anatomical course of the vessels.

- **Transcranial Doppler velocimetry** assesses flow in the major cerebral arteries.

- **SPECT imaging** (single photon emission compound tomography) assesses regional perfusion by imaging the brain with a gamma-camera after the intra-arterial injection of a lipophilic, high energy gamma-emitting isotope.

15.5 Pulmonary circulation

Flow at rest, human adult	4–6 l/min
Maximum flow, non-athlete	20–25 l/min

The pulmonary circulation has very different characteristics from the various systemic circulations described above.

- Pulmonary vessels have a low basal tone.

- Autoregulation of flow is absent.

- Sympathetic vasomotor nerves, though present, have no clear physiological role.

- Metabolic factors have no regulatory role, because the entire right ventricular output flows through the alveoli, vastly exceeding their nutritional needs.

The metabolic needs of the bronchi (cf. alveoli) are met by a separate **bronchial circulation**, which is part of the systemic circulation. Some of the bronchial venous blood drains into the pulmonary veins, however. Along with the Thebesian vein input, this reduces the O_2 saturation of left ventricular blood to ~97%.

Special tasks

The primary function of the lungs is the oxygenation of blood and the removal of carbon dioxide. The pulmonary circulation has to ensure (i) that the blood equilibrates with the gas phase at both low and high cardiac outputs; and (ii) that each alveolus is perfused in proportion to its ventilation.

A secondary task is the enzymatic modification of circulating peptides such as angiotensin I.

Structural adaptations

Dense capillary packing and ultra-short diffusion distance promote efficient gas exchange

The density of capillaries in the alveolar wall is extraordinarily high (Figure 15.16). Inspection of an exposed alveolus shows an almost continuous sheet of blood flowing across it, with very little tissue separating the individual capillaries. Moreover the combined endothelium–epithelium layer is extraordinarily thin, with only ~0.3 μm separating the gas phase from the plasma (Figure 15.16). The massive capillary surface area, up to $90-126\,m^2$ in the two human lungs, and short diffusion distance together produce a very high O_2 transport capacity.

Numerous short arterioles create a low vascular resistance

Pulmonary arteries and arterioles are shorter and thinner walled than their systemic counterparts and offer less resistance to flow. This enables the pulmonary circulation to transmit the cardiac output under a low pressure gradient. The low pressures prevent stress damage to the extremely thin alveolar membrane.

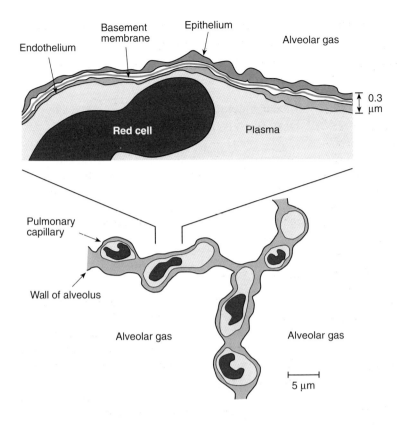

Figure 15.16 Ultrastructure of alveolar wall and pulmonary capillaries, based on electron micrographs from fixed inflated lungs.

Functional adaptations

Gas equilibration is achieved during the transit time

The volume of blood in the human pulmonary capillary bed is ~100 ml and pulmonary blood flow is ~5000 ml min^{-1} at rest. Blood therefore traverses the capillary bed with a **transit time** of 100/5000 min, or ~1 s. Because the diffusion distance across the alveolar membrane is so short, a transit time of 1 s is more than long enough for gas equilibration.

As the cardiac output increases during exercise, increased pulmonary pressure raises the pulmonary capillary volume. This helps to prevent excessively short transit times (volume/flow). Even so, the transit time falls to ~0.3 s in exercise. The blood still equilibrates with the alveolar gas in this time. Since equilibration is achieved by the end of the capillary bed, gas exchange is **flow-limited** in nature (Section 10.10). As a result, **O$_2$ uptake is directly proportional to pulmonary blood flow** (Fick's principle, Section 7.1).

In **athletes** exceptionally high cardiac outputs can be generated during extreme performance and the transit time becomes so short that full gaseous equilibration is no longer achieved. This leads to a fall in arterial O$_2$ saturation during extreme athletic effort.

Hypoxic pulmonary vasoconstriction optimizes ventilation/perfusion ratios

Local hypoxia causes contraction of pulmonary resistance vessels, in contrast to the vasodilator response of systemic resistance vessels (Section 13.4). If a small region of the lung becomes hypoxic, perhaps due to a local mucous plug, hypoxic pulmonary vasoconstriction (HPV) occurs in the under-ventilated region (Figure 15.17). This is functionally important, because it reduces local alveolar blood flow $\dot{Q}$ to match the reduced local alveolar ventilation $\dot{V}$.

The role of HPV is thus to preserve an optimum local ventilation/perfusion ratio, $\dot{V}/\dot{Q}$. For efficient oxygenation each alveolus must have roughly the same $\dot{V}/\dot{Q}$ ratio, namely 0.8 in humans (because alveolar ventilation is 4 l/min and cardiac output is 5 l/min). If the ventilation to a group of alveoli falls, for example following local bronchoconstriction or a mucous plug, the alveoli become hypoxic. The ensuing local HPV partially restores the $\dot{V}/\dot{Q}$ ratio to normal. The vasoconstriction in effect diverts blood away from hypoxic alveoli, so that relatively little under-oxygenated blood is added to arterial blood. Thus, while HPV in the lungs is the opposite of hypoxic vasodilatation in systemic vessels, each response is well suited to the needs of the organ.

In considering mechanisms it is necessary to note that isolated pulmonary arteries behave somewhat differently from the intact lung. Hypoxic vasoconstriction in an intact lung shows a lag of 1–2 min before starting, followed by a slow monophasic build-up of resistance over 20–40 min (Figure 15.17). Isolated vessels show an early, fast, but transient vasoconstriction over ~5 min (Figure 15.17, dashed line) before the more important slow, sustained vasoconstriction. Both phases involve depolarization and increased cytosolic $[Ca^{2+}]$. The initial fast vasoconstriction is due to the activation of **Ca^{2+} entry channels**. During the second phase, constriction increases progressively but cytosolic $[Ca^{2+}]$ does not, indicating a progressive **Ca^{2+} sensitization**. The slow phase is endothelium dependent. It is

thought that endothelium senses hypoxia through its mitochondrial enzyme chain and releases an agent that activates the myocyte protein kinases responsible for Ca^{2+} sensitization (Section 12.5).

The lung pressure–flow relation is passive and lacks autoregulation

Pulmonary vascular resistance is about an eighth of the systemic resistance, so pulmonary arterial pressure is low, namely 20–25 mmHg systolic and 8–12 mmHg diastolic. In isolated, perfused lungs the pressure–flow relation resembles that of a set of passive, slightly distensible tubes, unlike the highly autoregulated relations in the brain, myocardium and kidney. Autoregulation would be counterproductive in the lungs.

The lung pressure–flow curve steepens slightly with pressure because vascular distension raises the vascular conductance (Figure 15.18a). If the lungs are ventilated under positive pressure, as in humans

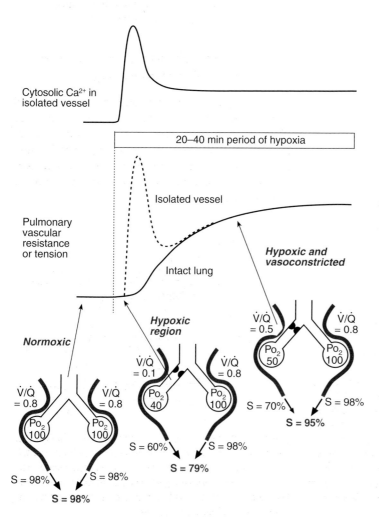

Figure 15.17 Pulmonary hypoxic vasoconstriction in whole lung (*solid curve*) or isolated rat pulmonary artery (*dashed line*). Sketches show how hypoxic vasoconstriction helps to maintain a normal ventilation/perfusion ratio ($\dot{V}/\dot{Q}$), and thus maintain the oxygen saturation (*S*) in mixed arterial blood. P_{O_2} in mmHg; size of arrows represents magnitude of flow. (Based on Robertson, T. P., Aaronson, P. I. and Ward, J. P. T. (1995) *American Journal of Physiology,* **268**, H301–H307.)

undergoing general anaesthesia, the positive airway pressure compresses some pulmonary vessels at low perfusion pressures, but the vessels open up as pulmonary blood pressure is increased. This exacerbates the curvature of the pressure–flow plot.

Total pulmonary blood volume is ~600 ml in supine humans. It can be increased transiently to ~1 l by reducing the intrathoracic pressure through forced inspiration, and can be reduced to ~300 ml by raising the intrathoracic pressure through forced expiration (the Valsalva manoeuvre, Section 17.2).

In supine exercise, pulmonary blood flow increases in proportion to pressure

During exercise the increased right ventricular output raises the pulmonary artery pressure. In **young adults** performing supine exercise the pulmonary blood flow increases almost linearly with perfusion pressure, i.e. pulmonary artery pressure minus left atrial pressure (Figure 15.18b, middle line). In **endurance-trained athletes** the pressure–flow relation is steeper because the 'trained' pulmonary vessels have a higher conductance, which enables them to transmit more flow for a given perfusion pressure (Figure 15.18b, left). Conversely, at **high altitude** the pressure–flow relation becomes flatter because chronic HPV reduces vascular conductance (Figure 15.18b, right). In **ageing** healthy men, the pulmonary venous pressure increases with exercise. This distends the vessels and raises their conductance, generating a steeper pressure–flow relation.

During upright exercise enhancement of apical perfusion boosts O_2 transfer capacity

In the upright position the lung apices are not well perfused at rest due to the effect of gravity; see Figure 15.19 and 'Special problems'. During exercise the apical perfusion is greatly improved because pulmonary artery pressure rises. The increased perfusion of apical capillaries boosts the O_2 transfer capacity of the lungs.

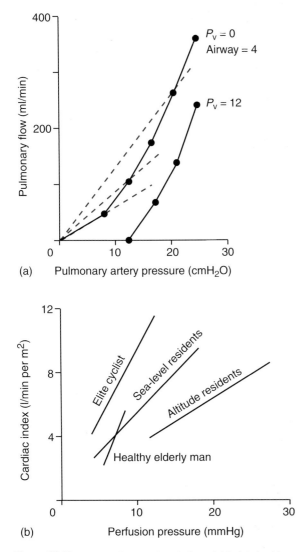

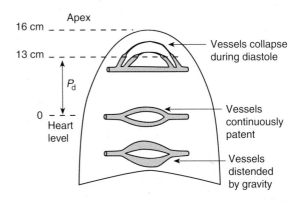

Figure 15.18 Pressure–flow relations for lung. (a) Isolated cat lung perfused with plasma. Venous pressure (P_v) was zero or 12 cmH$_2$O, and airway pressure was 4 cmH$_2$O. Dashed lines are lines of constant conductance; the lung shows increasing conductance as pressure rises. (b) Human subjects during supine exercise. Perfusion pressure is pulmonary artery pressure minus left atrial pressure. Venous pressures were greater than zero and airway pressure atmospheric. ((a) From Banister, R. J. and Torrance, R. W. (1960) *Quarterly Journal of Experimental Physiology*, **45**, 352–357; and (b) from Grover, R. F., et al. (1983); see Further Reading, by permission.)

Figure 15.19 Gradient of perfusion in human lung in upright position at rest. Scale shows vertical distance above heart. Diastolic artery pressure P_d is 13 cmH$_2$O at heart level but zero (atmospheric) 13 cm above heart. Vessels higher than this are perfused only in systole. Perfusion was measured by external gamma counting following injection of radioisotope into right heart.

Low capillary pressures reduce the pulmonary membrane stress and prevent oedema

The distribution of vascular resistance is more even in the lungs than in the systemic circulation. Pulmonary arterial vessels account for ~30% of the net resistance, the microcirculation ~50% (arterioles to venules) and veins ~20%. As a result **pulmonary capillary pressure** is roughly midway between mean arterial pressure (12–15 mmHg) and left atrial pressure (5–8 mmHg), namely 8–11 mmHg. Low capillary pressure reduces the stress in the ultra-thin alveolar-endothelial membrane to a safe level.

Although pulmonary capillary pressure is below plasma colloid osmotic pressure, the capillaries are nevertheless in a state of filtration and generate lung lymph. The filtration state is maintained by the high colloid osmotic pressure of pulmonary interstitial fluid (Sections 11.4, 11.6). Elevation of the left atrial pressure to 20–25 mmHg raises capillary pressure sufficiently to create **pulmonary oedema**, but smaller increases are within the safety margin against oedema (Section 11.10).

Pulmonary endothelium transforms some circulating vasoactive agents

As blood passes through the lungs, it is exposed to 90–126 m^2 of endothelium. This facilitates the enzymatic transformation of circulating vasoactive substances by endothelium. Endothelial angiotensin-converting enzyme (ACE) converts angiotensin I to angiotensin II in the lungs (Section 9.6). ACE also degrades circulating bradykinin. Several other vaso-active substances, including serotonin, prostaglandin E and leukotrienes, are removed by lung endothelium. Circulating hormones such as adrenaline and vasopressin are unaffected.

Special problems

Orthostasis causes a vertical gradient of perfusion in human lungs

In the upright position blood flow is distributed unevenly in the human lung (Figure 15.19). Mean pulmonary arterial pressure is ~15 mmHg at heart level, but the drag of gravity reduces it to ~3 mmHg at the apex of the lung, and raises it to ~21 mmHg at the base of the lung. The high pressure at the base distends the thin-walled vessels, increasing their conductance and hence the basal perfusion. Conversely, vessels at the apex collapse during diastole. Diastolic pressure at heart level is ~9 mmHg, or 13 cmH$_2$O. This is insufficient to distend the

apical vessels, which are ~16 cm above heart level. The apex is therefore perfused only during systole. As a result of the basal distension and apical diastolic collapse, the **mean flow through the lung apex is ~1/10th the flow through the base**, at rest.

As noted earlier, the efficiency of O$_2$ exchange depends on the **ratio of ventilation to perfusion** in each alveolus, $\dot{V}/\dot{Q}$. Ideally $\dot{V}/\dot{Q}$ should be ~0.8 throughout the lung. Although alveolar ventilation $\dot{V}$ is greater in the base than the apex, the vertical gradient of ventilation does not fully compensate for the large vertical gradient of flow $\dot{Q}$. A standing human, therefore, has a higher $\dot{V}/\dot{Q}$ at the apex than the base. This ventilation/perfusion mismatch slightly impairs the efficiency of blood oxygenation. In the supine position the apex-to-base gradients are abolished and $\dot{V}/\dot{Q}$ is more even.

Chronic hypoxic vasoconstriction can cause right ventricular failure

Although HPV is a valuable local response, minimizing local $\dot{V}/\dot{Q}$ mismatch, it can have serious consequences when the whole lung is hypoxic for a long period. This happens at high altitude and in chronic lung diseases such as emphysema. Chronic hypoxia causes a chronic increase in pulmonary vascular resistance and therefore chronic pulmonary hypertension. The high afterload on the right ventricle can lead to heart failure.

High stresses in the thin alveolar-endothelial membrane can cause leakage

The blood–gas barrier is extremely thin, so the tensile force per unit thickness of membrane (the stress) is substantial. If the membrane stress is raised by pulmonary capillary hypertension, as in patients with **mitral valve stenosis**, some membranes may break down. This causes pulmonary oedema and, in severe cases, alveolar haemorrhage. The effect of mechanical stress is seen most dramatically in the modern, thoroughbred racehorse. Racehorses are capable of very high cardiac outputs, and their pulmonary vascular pressures reach extreme values during racing, namely 120 mmHg pulmonary arterial pressure and 70 mmHg left atrial pressure. This can lead to exercise-induced pulmonary haemorrhage. In human exercise, fortunately, pulmonary capillary pressure does not rise much above 30 mmHg.

Assessment in man

The measurement of pulmonary blood flow, i.e. cardiac output, by the **Fick principle, indicator**

KEY FEATURES BOX 15.5

The Pulmonary Circulation

Special tasks

▨ Respiratory gas exchange

▨ Enzymatic modification of circulating peptides, e.g. angiotensin I

Structural adaptations

▨ Extremely high capillary density and extremely short diffusion distance

▨ Short arterioles of low resistance allow right ventricular output at low pressure

Functional adaptations

▨ Transit time of 0.3–1.0 s allows blood-alveolar gas equilibration

▨ Hypoxic pulmonary vasoconstriction matches local alveolar perfusion to local ventilation

▨ Flow increases in proportion to pressure; no autoregulation

▨ Low capillary pressure reduces membrane stress and prevents oedema

▨ Endothelial enzymes modify/degrade circulating vasoactive peptides

Special problems

▨ Apices not well perfused in orthostasis, improving on exercise

▨ At extreme flows (athletes) capillary transit time of $\leqslant 0.3$ s cause under-oxygenation

▨ Chronic hypoxia causes chronic vasoconstriction, leading to right heart failure

▨ Thin alveolar/endothelial membrane. In mitral stenosis, pulmonary capillary hypertension raises membrane stress and leads to leakage

Assessment in man

▨ Fick principle (O_2 uptake) measures pulmonary flow

▨ Indicator dilution and thermal dilution methods ditto

▨ Pulmonary wedge pressure indicates pulmonary venular pressure

dilution method and **thermal dilution method** was described in Chapter 7.

Pulmonary microvascular pressure is estimated clinically by advancing a catheter through the pulmonary artery until the tip wedges in a narrow arterial vessel, blocking the downstream flow. The pressure of the stationary distal column of blood, the **pulmonary wedge pressure**, equals that in the nearest distal perfused vessel, usually a venule.

FURTHER READING

Coronary circulation

Reviews and chapters

Feigl, E. O. (1983) Coronary physiology. *Physiological Reviews*, **63**, 1–205.

Fletcher, G. F. (1994) *Cardiovascular Response to Exercise*. Futura, New York.

Kuo, L. (1997) Coronary vasodilatation and K_{ATP} channels; independence from NO. *News in Physiological Sciences*, **12**, 246–247.

Mary, D. A. S. G. (1992) Reflex effects on the coronary circulation. *Experimental Physiology*, **77**, 243–270.

Sobel, B. E. (1988) Coronary artery and ischemic heart disease. In *Cardiovascular Pathophysiology* (ed. Ahumada, G. G.), Oxford University Press, Oxford.

Verrier, R. L. (1990) Behavioural influences on coronary blood flow and susceptibility to arrhythmias. *News in Physiological Sciences*, **5**, 108–112.

Research papers

Beckenrath, N., Cyrys, S., Dischner, A. and Daut, J. (1991). Hypoxic vasodilatation in isolated perfused guinea-pig heart: an analysis of the underlying mechanism. *Journal of Physiology*, **442**, 297–319.

Broten, T. P., Romson, J. L., Fullerton, D. A., Van Winkle, D. M. and Feigl, E. O. (1991) Synergistic action of myocardial O_2 and CO_2 in controlling coronary blood flow. *Circulation Research*, **68**, 531–542.

Schelbert, H. R. and Buxton, D. (1988) Insights into coronary artery disease gained from metabolic imaging. *Circulation Research*, **78**, 496–505.

Skeletal muscle circulation

Reviews and chapters

Gorman, M. W. and Sparks, H. V. (1991) The unanswered question. (What is the dilator substance in exercise hyperaemia?). *News in Physiological Sciences*, **6**, 191–193.

Hudlicka, O. and El-Khelly, F. (1988) The role of inorganic phosphate in functional hyperemia in skeletal muscle. In *Vasodilatation: Vascular Smooth Muscle, Peptides, Autonomic Nerves and Endothelium* (ed. Vanhoutte, P. M.), Raven Press, New York, pp. 378–381.

Intaglietta, M. and Johnson, P. C. (eds) (1995) Functional capillary density: active and passive determinants. *International Journal of Microcirculation*, **15**, 213–276.

Rowell, L. B. (1993) *Human Cardiovascular Control*, Oxford University Press, New York.

Shepherd, J. T. (1983) Circulation to skeletal muscle. In *Handbook of Physiology, Cardiovascular System*, Volume III, Part 1, *Peripheral Circulation*, (eds Shepherd, J. T. and Abboud, F. M.), American Physiological Society, Bethesda, pp. 319–370.

Wittenberg, B. A. and Wittenberg, J. B. (1989) Transport of oxygen in muscle. *Annual Review of Physiology*, **51**, 857–878.

Research papers

Goonewardene, I. P. and Karim, F. (1991) Attenuation of exercise vasodilatation by adenosine deaminase in anaesthetized dogs. *Journal of Physiology*, **442**, 65–79.

Green, S., Langberg, H., Skovgaard, D., Bülow, J. and Kjaer, M. (2000) Interstitial and arterio-venous [K^+] in human calf muscle during dynamic exercise: effect of ischaemia and relation to muscle pain. *Journal of Physiology*, **529**, 849–861.

Hargreaves, D., Egginton, S. and Hudlicka, O. (1990) Changes in capillary perfusion induced by different patterns of activity in rat skeletal muscle. *Microvascular Research*, **40**, 14–28.

Lott, M. E. J., Hogeman, C. S., Vickery, L., Kunselman, A. R., Sinoway, L. I. and MacLean, D. A. (2001) Effects of dynamic exercise on mean blood velocity and muscle interstitial metabolite responses in humans. *American Journal of Physiology*, **281**, H1734–H1741.

O'Leary, D. S., Rowell, L. B. and Scher, A. M. (1991) Baroreflex-induced vasoconstriction in active skeletal muscle of conscious dogs. *American Journal of Physiology*, **260**, H37–H41.

Poole, D. C. and Mathieu-Costello, O. (1996) Relationship between fiber capillarisation and mitochondrial volume density in control and trained rat soleus and plantaris muscles. *Microcirculation*, **3**, 175–186.

Cutaneous circulation

Reviews and chapters

Braverman, I. M. (1989) Ultrastructure and organization of the cutaneous microvasculature in normal and pathological states. *Journal of Investigative Dermatology*, **93**(Suppl.), 2S–9S.

Flanahan, N. A. (1991) The role of α_2-adrenoceptors as cutaneous thermosensors. *News in Physiological Sciences*, **6**, 251–255.

Johnson, J. M., Brengelmann, G. L., Hales, J. R. S., Vanhoutte, P. M. and Wenger, C. B. (1986) Regulation of the cutaneous circulation. *Federal Proceedings*, **45**, 2841–2850.

Roddie, L. C. (1983) Circulation to skin and adipose tissue. In *Handbook of Physiology, Cardiovascular System*, Volume III, Part 1, *Peripheral Circulation* (eds Shepherd, J. T. and Abboud, F. M.), American Physiological Society, Bethesda, pp. 285–317.

Research papers

Bergensen, T. K. (1993) A search for arteriovenous anastomoses in human skin using ultrasound Doppler. *Acta Physiologica Scandinavica*, **147**, 195–201.

Chotani, M. A., Flavahan, S., Mitra, S., Daunt, D. and Flavahan, N. A. (2000) Silent α_{2C}-adrenergic receptors enable cold-induced vasoconstriction in cutaneous arteries. *American Journal of Physiology*, **278**, H1075–1083.

Crandall, C. G., Shibasaki, M. and Yen, T. C. (2002) Evidence that the human cutaneous veno-arteriolar response is not mediated by adrenergic mechanisms. *Journal of Physiology*, **538**, 599–605.

Marshall, J. M., Stone, A. and Johns, E. J. (1991) Analysis of responses evoked in the cutaneous circulation of one hand by heating the contralateral hand. *Journal of Autonomic Nervous System*, **32**, 91–100.

Wårdell, K., Naver, H. K., Nilsson, G. E. and Wallin, B. G. (1993) The cutaneous vascular axon reflex in humans characterized by laser Doppler perfusion imaging. *Journal of Physiology*, **460**, 185–199.

Cerebral circulation

Reviews and chapters

Bevan, J. A. and Bevan, R. D. (1993) Is innervation a prime regulator of cerebral blood flow? *News in Physiological Sciences*, **8**, 149–153.

Bradbury, M. W. B. (1993) The blood–brain barrier. *Experimental Physiology*, **78**, 453–472.

Duelli, R. and Kuschinsky, W. (2001) Brain glucose transporters: relationship to local energy demand. *News in Physiological Sciences*, **16**, 71–76.

Faraci, F. M. and Heistad, D. D. (1998) Regulation of the cerebral circulation: role of endothelium and potassium channels. *Physiological Reviews*, **78**, 53–74.

Goadsby, P. J. (1993) Vasoactive peptides in migraine and cluster headaches. In *Vascular*

Innervation and Receptor Mechanisms (eds Edvinsson, L. and Uddman, R.), Academic Press, New York, pp. 415–424.

Heistad, D. D. (2001) What's new in the cerebral microcirculation? *Microcirculation*, **8**, 365–375.

Juul, R. and Edvinsson, L. (1993) Perivascular peptides in subarachnoid haemorrhage. In *Vascular Innervation and Receptor Mechanisms* (eds Edvinsson, L. and Uddman, R.), Academic Press, New York, pp. 399–414.

Research papers

Clar, C., Pedersen, M. E. F., Poulin, M. J., Tansley, J. G. and Robbins, P. A. (1997) Effects of 8 h of eucapnic and poikilocapnic hypoxia on middle cerebral artery velocity and heart rate in humans. *Experimental Physiology*, **82**, 791–802.

Coney, A. M. and Marshall, J. M. (1998) Role of adenosine and its receptors in the vasodilatation induced in the cerebral cortex of the rat by systemic hypoxia. *Journal of Physiology*, **509**, 507–518.

Delp, M. D., Armstrong, R. B., Godfrey, D. A., Laughlin, M. A., Ross, C. D. and Wilkerson, M. K. (2001) Exercise increases blood flow to locomotor, vestibular, cardiorespiratory and visual regions of the brain in miniature swine. *Journal of Physiology*, **533**, 849–859.

Guibert, C. and Beech, D. J. (1999) Positive and negative coupling of the endothelin ET_A receptor to Ca^{2+}-permeable channels in rabbit cerebral cortex arterioles. *Journal of Physiology*, **514**, 843–856.

Osol, G. and Halpern, W. (1985) Myogenic properties of cerebral blood vessels from normotensive and hypertensive rats. *American Journal of Physiology*, **249**, H914–H921.

Pulmonary circulation

Reviews and chapters

Bahkle, Y. S. (1990) Pharmacokinetic and metabolic properties of the lung. *British Journal of Anaesthesia*, **65**, 79.

Butler, J. (1991) The bronchial circulation. *News in Physiological Sciences*, **6**, 21–25.

Grover, R. F., Wagner, W. W., McMurty, I. F. and Reeves, J. T. (1983) Pulmonary circulation. In *Handbook of Physiology, Cardiovascular System*, Vol. 3, *Peripheral Circulation* (eds Shepherd, J. T. and Abboud, F. M.), American Physiological Society, Bethesda, pp. 103–136.

Hlasta, M. P. and Glenny, R. W. (1999) Vascular structure determines pulmonary blood flow distribution. *News in Physiological Sciences*, **14**, 182–186.

Leach, R. M. and Treacher, D. F. (1995) Clinical aspects of hypoxic pulmonary vasoconstriction. In *Control of the Pulmonary Circulation*. Physiological Society Symposium. *Experimental Physiology*, **80**, 865–875.

Nunn, J. F. (1993) *Nunn's Applied Respiration Physiology*. Butterworth Heinemann, Oxford.

West, J. B. and Mathieu-Costello, O. (1993) Pulmonary blood–gas barrier: a physiological dilemma. *News in Physiological Sciences*, **8**, 249–253.

Research papers

Harms, C. A., McClaran, S. R., Nickele, G. A., Pegelow, D. F., Nelson, W. B. and Dempsey, J. A. (1998) Exercise-induced arterial hypoxaemia in healthy young women. *Journal of Physiology*, **507**, 619–628.

Robertson, T. P., Hague, D., Aaronson, P. I. and Ward, J. P. T. (2000) Voltage-independent calcium entry in hypoxic pulmonary vasoconstriction of intrapulmonary arteries of the rat. *Journal of Physiology*, **525**, 669–680.

Turner, J. L. and Kozlowski, R. Z. (1997) Relationship between membrane potential, delayed rectifier K^+ currents and hypoxia in rat pulmonary arterial myocytes. *Experimental Physiology*, **82**, 629–645.

CHAPTER 16

Cardiovascular receptors, reflexes and central control

Learning objectives

After reading this chapter you should be able to:

- Sketch the locations of arterial baroreceptors and outline the receptor firing characteristics (16.1).
- State the reflex effects of baroreceptors and their importance in hypovolaemia (16.2).
- Outline the responses and roles of veno-atrial stretch receptors (16.3, 16.4).
- Give the roles of two kinds of ventricular sensory receptor and the origin of ischaemic cardiac pain (16.3).
- Outline the reflex responses to a rise in human CVP and fluid volume (16.4).
- Explain the role of the kidneys in the long term regulation of blood pressure (16.5).
- Outline the location and role of peripheral arterial chemoreceptors (16.6).
- State the cardiovascular reflex evoked by lung stretch receptors (16.6).
- Outline the nature and role of muscle work receptors (16.6).
- List the roles of the medulla in cardiovascular control (16.7).
- Define the alerting response and central command (16.8).
- Outline the central pathways that control the vagal and sympathetic outflows (16.9).

Overview. The heart and blood vessels are controlled by sympathetic and parasympathetic nerves. The nerve activity is regulated by the brain, which is guided by sensory information from peripheral receptors located within the circulation and outside it. The term 'receptor' in this context means a sensory nerve ending, not a drug-binding molecule. The three elements, namely afferent (sensory) fibres, central relays and efferent (motor) fibres, form reflex arcs (Figure 16.1). The two most important groups of **sensor** are the pressure receptors in the walls of systemic arteries (arterial baroreceptors) and the

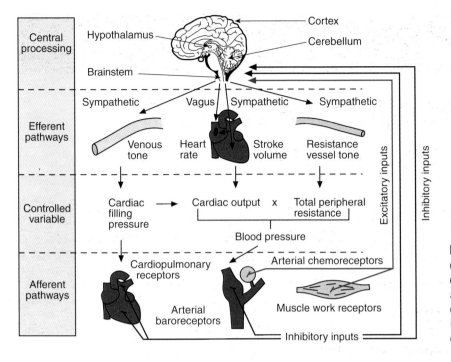

Figure 16.1 Overview of reflex control of circulation, excluding endocrine aspects. Terms 'inhibitory' and 'excitatory' refer to net effect on cardiac output and blood pressure; inhibitory reflexes are depressor, excitatory reflexes are pressor.

pressure receptors in the heart (cardiopulmonary receptors). Their afferent fibres transmit information about arterial pressure and cardiac filling to the **brainstem**, where it is integrated with information from muscle receptors, arterial chemoreceptors and other sensors. The integration of information and computation of an appropriate cardiovascular response involve up-and-down traffic between the brainstem, hypothalamus, cerebellum and cortex. **Presympathetic and parasympathetic outflows** from the brainstem are then adjusted to initiate the desired cardiovascular response.

The reflexes are often, but not invariably, directed at stabilizing blood pressure. For example, the reflex response to a rise in blood pressure is bradycardia and peripheral vasodilatation, which restores the blood pressure towards its original level (a **depressor reflex**). When a change in a variable, such as blood pressure, triggers an inhibitory response that returns the variable towards its control value or **set point**, the regulatory process is called **negative feedback**. The baroreceptor reflex is a good example of negative feedback.

Other reflexes, such as those from arterial and muscle chemoreceptors, are excitatory. They raise rather than stabilize pressure (**pressor reflexes**). Moreover, the brain can initiate non-reflex cardiovascular changes. For example, at the start of exercise a signal from the cerebral cortex, called central command, helps to increase the heart rate instantly.

This process is termed **feedforward**, in contrast to feedback.

16.1 Arterial baroreceptors

The prefix 'baro-' means pressure. A baroreceptor is a sprayed nerve ending packed with mitochondria and connected to a myelinated or non-myelinated axon. Baroreceptors are found in the adventitia of arteries at two main locations: the carotid sinus and the aortic arch (Figure 16.2).

The **carotid sinus** is a thin-walled dilatation at the start of the internal carotid artery. The afferent fibres from carotid sinus baroreceptors form the carotid sinus nerve. This joins the **glossopharyngeal nerve** (IXth cranial nerve) to reach the petrous ganglion, where the parent neurons are located. Like all afferent neurons the petrous neurons are bipolar. Their central axons pass up the glossopharyngeal nerve into the brainstem and terminate in the **nucleus tractus solitarius**.

Aortic baroreceptors are located mainly around the transverse arch of the aorta. Their fibres form the aortic or 'depressor' nerve in some species, then ascend in the **vagus** (Xth cranial nerve). Their neurons lie in the nodose ganglion. The central axons again terminate in the nucleus tractus solitarius.

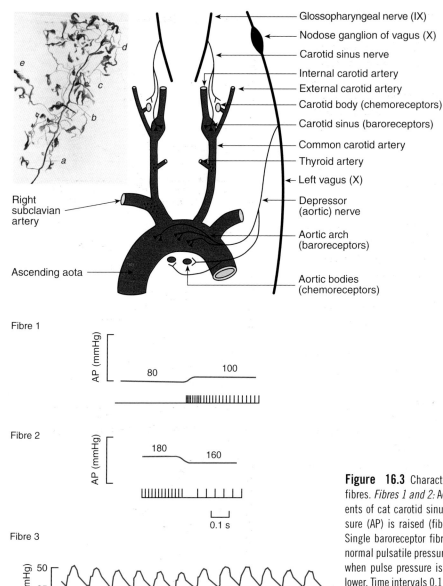

Figure 16.2 Major reflexogenic zones of arterial system. Right vagus not shown. Minor baroreceptor regions shown as dots. *Inset* shows a single baroreceptor ending in the human carotid sinus. (From Abraham, A. (1969) *Microscopic Innervation of the Heart and Blood Vessels in Vertebrates Including Man*, Pergamon Press, Oxford, by permission.)

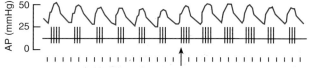

Figure 16.3 Characteristics of baroreceptor afferent fibres. *Fibres 1 and 2:* Action potentials in myelinated afferents of cat carotid sinus when non-pulsatile arterial pressure (AP) is raised (fibre 1) or reduced (fibre 2). *Fibre 3:* Single baroreceptor fibre from rabbit aorta subjected to a normal pulsatile pressure. There are four impulses per pulse when pulse pressure is high (arrow) and three when it is lower. Time intervals 0.1 s. (Fibres 1 and 2 after Landgren, S. (1952) *Acta Physiologica Scandinavica*, **26**, 1–34; fibre 3 from Downing, S. E. (1960) *Journal of Physiology*, **150**, 210–213, by permission.)

The **coronary arteries** too possess baroreceptors, at least in dogs, and the coronary baroreflex is of similar potency to the carotid sinus baroreflex.

Baroreceptors are stretch receptors

The baroreceptors are mechanoreceptors that respond to stretch. A rise in arterial pressure stretches the artery wall, and this excites the receptor. For example, the diameter of the carotid sinus, which is relatively thin and stretchy, oscillates by ~15% with each arterial pulse. If stretch is prevented by applying a plaster cast around the sinus, the baroreceptors no longer respond to changes in pressure.

Baroreceptors have both static and dynamic sensitivity

Baroreceptors are stimulated not only by the magnitude of the pressure (static sensitivity) but also by its rate of rise (dynamic sensitivity). If the carotid sinus is distended experimentally by a rapid rise in blood pressure, the baroreceptor fires an initial burst of action potentials at a high frequency, which is the dynamic response to the pressure change (Figure 16.3, fibre 1). The fibre activity then declines (**adaptation**) and settles down to a sustained, adapted discharge rate that signals the new pressure level. Adaptation may be due to mechanical creep of the receptor within its stretched environment, and/or ion channel adaptation.

Conversely, when pressure is reduced, the baroreceptor transiently falls silent, then resumes activity at a new, slower rate (Figure 16.3, fibre 2). As a result of dynamic sensitivity a baroreceptor fibre *in vivo* characteristically fires a burst of action potentials in systole and falls silent in diastole (Figure 16.3, fibre 3).

A-fibres have lower thresholds than C-fibres

The **threshold** of a baroreceptor is the lowest pressure that triggers an action potential. Based on threshold, axon myelination and conduction velocity there are two kinds of baroreceptor, the A-fibre and the C-fibre.

The **A-fibres** are large-diameter, fast-conducting myelinated fibres with low thresholds, in the range 30–90 mmHg (Figure 16.4a). A-fibres are active at normal blood pressure and fire a burst of impulses with each arterial pulse. A-fibres are less numerous, however, than C-fibres.

The more abundant **C-fibres** are narrow, slower-conducting, unmyelinated fibres with high thresholds, in the range 70–140 mmHg. Only a quarter or so are active at normal blood pressures and the rest are inactive. The active fibres fire in phase with the pulse but at a low frequency.

A-fibres have a higher sensitivity than C-fibres

The mean discharge frequency of a baroreceptor fibre increases with mean blood pressure. The steepness of this response is called the **sensitivity** of the fibre (Figure 16.4a). In the middle of their operating range the A-fibres are 2–3 times more sensitive than C-fibres. A-fibres can also achieve higher discharge frequencies than C-fibres.

C-fibres are important at high pressures owing to A-fibre saturation

At high pressures the A-fibre activity reaches a maximum (**saturation**), whereas the C-fibres remain responsive to pressure (Figure 16.4a). Therefore, C-fibres of high threshold are important for signalling graded information about high blood pressures. The A-fibres are important for signalling changes around normal blood pressure, aided by 25% or so of the C-fibres with a low enough threshold.

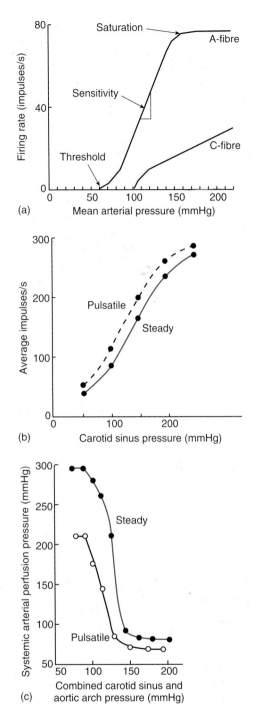

Figure 16.4 Effect of pressure on baroreceptor traffic and the resulting reflex in anaesthetized dogs. (a) Response of single A- and C-fibres to increasing pressure. (b) Average discharge rate in multi-fibre carotid sinus nerve: pulsatile pressures evoke higher activity. (c) Reflex fall in systemic pressure due to bradycardia and vasodilatation upon raising pressure in a vascularly isolated, perfused baroreceptor region. Pulsatility strengthens the depressor reflex. (From (a) Coleridge, H. M., Coleridge, J. C. G. and Schultz, H. D. (1987) *Journal of Physiology*, **394**, 291–313; (b) Korner, P. I. (1971) *Physiological Reviews*, **51**, 312–367; and (c) Angell-James, J. E. and De Burgh Daly, M. (1970) *Journal of Physiology*, **209**, 257–293, by permission.)

Fibre recruitment extends the signalling range of multi-fibre nerves

The carotid sinus and aortic nerves contain a large number of A- and C-fibres. When blood pressure rises, not only does the discharge frequency of each active fibre increase but in addition fibres of progressively higher threshold begin to fire. This is called **recruitment**. Recruitment gives the nerve a wider operating range than any one fibre, enabling it to signal a wide range of arterial pressures to the brainstem (Figure 16.4b).

Baroreceptors signal the pulse pressure as well as mean pressure

Carotid baroreceptors signal the size of the pulse, i.e. the pulse pressure, as well as mean pressure. The greater the oscillation in pressure about a given mean, the greater the aggregate activity in the nerve (Figure 16.4b). As a result, a pulsating pressure elicits a greater depressor reflex than a steady pressure (Figure 16.4c). The responsiveness of the reflex to pulsation is partly due to the dynamic sensitivity of baroreceptors, partly due to recruitment with each systole, and partly to the adaptation of brainstem neurons to a sustained signal. The signalling of pulse pressure is important during **orthostasis** and **moderate haemorrhage**, when the reduced stroke volume is often associated with a reduced pulse pressure but little or no fall in mean arterial pressure (Figure 18.2).

Carotid sinus and aortic baroreceptors have similar properties

A-fibres in the carotid sinus have slightly lower thresholds than in the aortic arch, but otherwise the receptor properties and the evoked reflexes are broadly similar for the two zones. Both regions have strong reflex effects on human heart rate, but the aortic baroreceptors have a stronger effect on vasomotor nerve activity. What, then, are the reflexes elicited by the baroreceptors?

16.2 The baroreflex

The baroreflex elicits changes in the heart and circulation that stabilize arterial pressure. Let us consider first the protection that the baroreflex provides against acute rises in pressure, and then the medically important response to hypovolaemia.

Acute elevation of blood pressure triggers a depressor reflex

The key reflexes elicited by baroreceptor activation were discovered by Ludwig and Cyon in 1886. Upon stimulating the aortic nerve they observed a reflex fall in heart rate and blood pressure – the depressor reflex. Later, Hering found that the carotid sinus nerve elicits the same reflex (Figure 16.5).

In the intact animal an acute rise in arterial pressure increases the net baroreceptor input to the brainstem through the glossopharyngeal nerves and vagi. The input activates polysynaptic central pathways that **enhance the vagal parasympathetic output** to the heart and **inhibit the sympathetic output** to the heart and the vasculature, with the following effects.

- Reduced sympathetic vasomotor activity causes **vasodilatation** and a **fall in total peripheral resistance**. Human sympathetic vasomotor activity ceases entirely if blood pressure is raised rapidly to ≥150/90 mmHg.

- Reduced cardiac sympathetic activity and increased vagal parasympathetic activity cause **bradycardia** and **reduced myocardial contractility**, which reduces cardiac output.

Since mean blood pressure equals cardiac output × peripheral resistance, the above changes return arterial pressure towards normal (Figure 16.1).

The baroreflex thus serves as a buffer against acute changes in blood pressure. The buffering process is

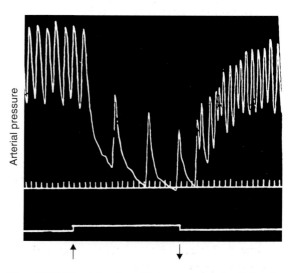

Figure 16.5 Stimulation of carotid sinus nerve in a dog elicits reflex hypotension and bradycardia. This classic smoked-drum recording is by Hering, who discovered the carotid baroreflex in 1923. Time intervals 0.2 s. (From Hering (1927) *Die Karotissinusreflexe auf Herz und Gefässe*, T. Steinkopf, Dresden.)

very rapid. The latency between baroreceptor stimulation and bradycardia is 0.5 s or less, and the latency to the onset of vascular dilatation is ~1.5 s.

Knowledge of the carotid sinus reflex can occasionally be put to practical use. In patients experiencing a supraventricular tachycardia, massage of the carotid sinus region at the angle of the jaw will sometimes stop the arrhythmia. The reflex parasympathetic activity slows pacemaker activity and slows propagation through the atrioventricular node.

Hypovolaemia triggers multiple compensatory reflexes

From both the clinical and evolutionary points of view the reflex to reduced arterial pressure is particularly important, because acute hypovolaemia is a common emergency. Hypovolaemia reduces the pulse pressure, and in severe cases the mean pressure too. The ensuing fall in baroreceptor traffic triggers the following autonomic-mediated reflex changes.

- **Tachycardia** and increased myocardial **contractility** are brought about by increased sympathetic activity and reduced vagal parasympathetic activity.

- **Resistance vessel contraction** is mediated by sympathetic vasomotor activity. This raises the total peripheral resistance. In humans the splanchnic circulation, kidneys and forearm muscles participate in the carotid sinus reflex but the skin does not. However, the skin vessels are affected reflexly by the cardiopulmonary receptors and by vasoconstrictor hormones (see below).

- **Splanchnic venoconstriction**, mediated by sympathetic fibres, displaces blood from the gut and liver into the central veins (Figures 14.5, 14.13). Blood is also expressed from skeletal muscle veins, even though they are poorly innervated, because arteriolar contraction reduces the local venous pressure (Figure 14.4), and circulating adrenaline, vasopressin and angiotensin cause venoconstriction. Venoconstriction supports the **central venous pressure** and hence stroke volume.

- **Adrenaline** is secreted by the adrenal medulla in response to increased splanchnic nerve activity. Adrenaline stimulates the heart and enhances glycogenolysis.

- **Microvascular absorption of interstitial fluid.** Contraction of the precapillary resistance vessels reduces the capillary pressure, which initiates a gradual osmotic absorption of interstitial fluid (Figures 11.4, 11.11b). This expands the plasma volume.

- **Activation of the renin–angiotensin–aldosterone system** by renal sympathetic fibres raises the circulating levels of angiotensin and aldosterone. The angiotensin II contributes to the generalized vasoconstriction. Aldosterone promotes renal salt and water retention, which helps to correct the hypovolaemia.

- **Vasopressin (ADH) secretion** from the posterior pituitary gland is stimulated by baroreceptor unloading in primates. The vasopressin causes an antidiuresis and contributes to the peripheral vasoconstriction.

The effect of the baroreflex during acute hypovolaemia is thus to stimulate the heart, raise peripheral resistance, attenuate the fall in central venous pressure, promote renal fluid retention and partially restore plasma volume. Together these responses support arterial pressure and cerebral perfusion.

The 'gain' and 'setting' of the baroreflex are not fixed

The operating characteristics of the baroreflex have been assessed in animals by observing the changes in heart rate and systemic pressure in response to the distension of vascularly isolated baroreceptor regions (Figure 16.4c). In humans the baroreflex can be studied by raising the blood pressure with the vasoconstrictor drug phenylephrine and observing the reflex changes in heart rate. Another method is to apply suction around the carotid sinus using a neck cuff, which allows reflex changes in arterial pressure as well as heart rate to be studied. Using these techniques a stimulus–response curve is obtained, from which the gain and setting of the baroreflex can be determined.

The optimal **sensitivity** or 'gain' of the reflex is the maximum slope of the response curve (Figure 16.6). In man the gain is reduced by ageing and chronic hypertension because the distensibility of the artery wall declines.

The **set point** is the pressure that the reflex strives to maintain (Figure 16.6). This can be altered by neural interactions within the central nervous system (central resetting) or by physical changes in the receptor region (peripheral resetting), as follows.

Central resetting

During exercise impulses from higher regions of the brain (central command) and from work receptors in active muscle reset the baroreflex to operate

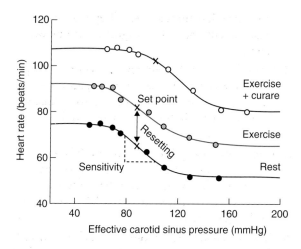

Figure 16.6 Resetting of human baroreflex during cycling exercise. Carotid sinus was distended by a suction collar around neck to chart the reflex. 'X' shows change in set point; sensitivity was unchanged. After partial neuromuscular blockade by curare, more central command was needed to achieve the same exercise level. Upward shift of reflex shows that central command contributes to exercise re-setting. (Based on Gallagher, K. M., Fadel, P. J., Strømstad, M., *et al.* (2001) *Journal of Physiology*, **533**, 861–870, by permission.)

around a higher pressure (Figure 16.6, middle curve). Consequently, arterial pressure can rise without reflexly impairing the heart rate or cardiac output, as would otherwise be the case. The baroreflex remains active during exercise and buffers the blood pressure around its new set point. If the human quadriceps are made to contract by electrical stimulation (removing central command) and the input from muscle work receptors is blocked by epidural anaesthesia, exercise no longer resets the baroreflex.

Regular central modulation of the baroreflex is responsible for sinus arrhythmia, i.e. the tachycardia associated with inspiration (Figure 5.4a). The brainstem neurons that drive inspiration inhibit the cardiac vagal motor neurons, rendering them briefly unresponsive to the baroreceptor input; see Figure 16.15 later. The resulting fall in vagal activity largely explains the tachycardia of inspiration.

Peripheral resetting

If blood pressure is raised for a substantial period, the baroreceptor threshold shifts to a new, higher pressure over the course of 15 minutes or so. The resulting right-shift of the entire stimulus−response curve reinstates the receptors on the steep part of the stimulus−response curve, where they operate most effectively. This has the advantage of **extending the range** over which the reflex can effectively operate. It has the **disadvantage**, however, that the baroreceptors do not provide the brain with reliable information about absolute blood pressure over long

periods. After peripheral resetting the new pressure may produce the same signal as the old pressure.

The ambiguity of the baroreceptor signal over the long term is exacerbated by sympathetic motor nerves that innervate the carotid sinus and can enhance the baroreceptor activity. Because the baroreceptors fail to provide unambiguous information about absolute blood pressure, they cannot by themselves control basal arterial pressure in the long term.

The baroreflex provides short-term homeostasis of blood pressure

Arterial pressure is very unstable in an animal deprived of its baroreflex, so the chief role of the baroreflex seems to be to buffer acute changes in arterial pressure over the short term (minutes). For example, walking up a 21-degree incline raises the blood pressure by only ∼10 mmHg in normal dogs, but when the dogs are deprived of the carotid sinus reflex, the same exercise protocol raises pressure by 50 mmHg (Figure 16.7). The major role of the baroreflex is thus to buffer short-term fluctuations in arterial pressure.

When the baroreceptor nerves of a dog are cut, the animal is hypertensive for a few days but the mean blood pressure then settles down to a value that

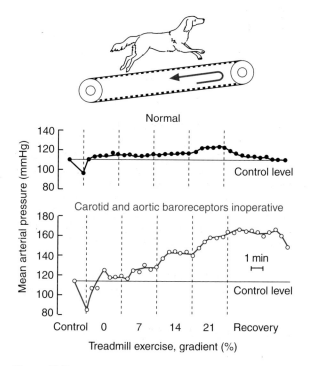

Figure 16.7 Dogs walking up an increasing steep incline normally show only a small rise in arterial pressure (mean 12 mmHg). After elimination of the carotid sinus and aortic arch reflexes, exercise caused much bigger changes in pressure (mean 51 mmHg). (Adapted from Walgenbach, S. C. and Donald, D. E. (1983) *Circulation Research*, **52**, 253–262, by permission.)

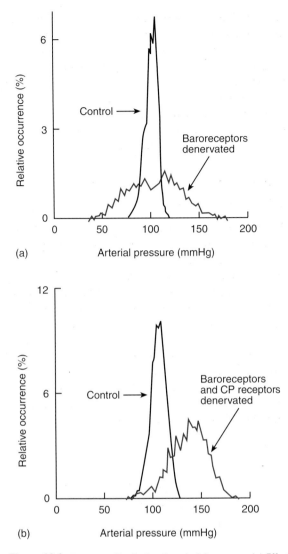

(a)

(b)

Figure 16.8 Frequency distribution for arterial pressure: (a) Effect of chronic arterial baroreceptor denervation in dogs. After some days, mean pressure has not changed much but the fluctuations about the mean increase, i.e. pressure is less stable. (b) Both the cardiopulmonary (CP) and arterial baroreceptors were denervated. There is now a marked increase in mean pressure as well as pressure instability. ((a) From Cowley, A. W., Liard, J. F. and Guyton, A. C. (1973) *Circulation Research*, **32**, 564–578; (b) Persson, P. B., Ehmke, H. and Kirchheim, H. R. (1989) *NIPS*, **4**, 56–59, by permission.)

is only ∼11 mmHg above normal, albeit with fluctuations over a wider range than normal (Figure 16.8a).

16.3 Cardiac receptors

The heart and pulmonary artery are richly innervated by afferent fibres (Figure 16.9). The cardiopulmonary afferents are of four main types:

1 **Myelinated veno-atrial mechanoreceptors.** Mechanoreceptors around the right and left veno-atrial junctions are served by myelinated vagal afferent fibres. They signal central blood volume.

2 **Non-myelinated mechanoreceptors.** Many mechanoreceptors in the ventricles, atria and pulmonary artery are served by non-myelinated fibres that travel in both the vagus and the cardiac sympathetic nerves.

3 **Coronary artery baroreceptors.** These function much like other arterial baroreceptors and travel in the vagi. Their reflex potency is several times greater than that of left ventricular mechanoreceptors.

4 **Chemosensors.** Chemosensitive afferents from the ventricles travel in both the vagus and cardiac sympathetic nerves. The vagus and cardiac sympathetic nerves are 'mixed nerves' that carry both motor and sensory fibres.

Cardiac de-afferentation studies show that the cardiopulmonary afferents have a net tonic inhibitory effect on heart rate and peripheral vascular tone, similar to that of arterial baroreceptors. Unselective stimulation of the cardiac receptors by an intra-coronary injection of veratridine causes a reflex bradycardia, vasodilatation and hypotension (the **Bezold–Jarisch response**). This kind of mass, unphysiological stimulation, however, obscures the fact that there are marked differences between the reflexes evoked by the different receptors.

Veno-atrial stretch receptors monitor atrial filling

Veno-atrial fibres are normally the most active of the non-coronary afferents, at least in animals; human data are lacking. The receptors are branched endocardial sprays resembling baroreceptor sprays. The receptors are served by large, myelinated vagal afferent fibres. An increase in **cardiac blood volume** stretches the veno-atrial receptors and increases their firing. Maximum activity can occur during atrial systole (type A pattern, Figure 16.9) or during the V wave of atrial filling (type B pattern), probably depending on the position of the receptor in the wall. The receptor thus transmits information about central venous pressure and cardiac filling.

Stimulation of the veno-atrial receptors, for example by inflating a small balloon at the veno-atrial junction, causes two reflex changes:

● tachycardia, and

● diuresis (increased urine flow).

The **tachycardia** is brought about by a selective increase in sympathetic outflow to the pacemaker

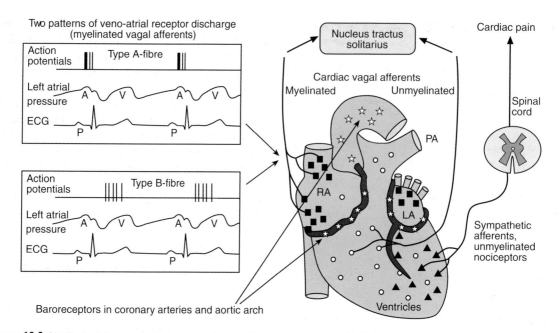

Figure 16.9 Distribution of cardiac and pulmonary artery receptors. Squares, veno-atrial stretch receptors; circles, unmyelinated mechanoreceptors; stars, arterial baroreceptors; triangles, nociceptive chemosensors; RA and LA, right and left atria, respectively; PA, pulmonary artery. Recordings of veno-atrial receptor activity in dog shown on left. (Based on Kappagoda, C. T., Linden, R. J. and Sivananthan, N. (1979) *Journal of Physiology*, **291**, 393–412, by permission.)

without a reciprocal fall in vagal parasympathetic activity – an unusual event. The reflex partly explains the '**Bainbridge effect**', discovered in 1915, namely tachycardia in response to a large, rapid infusion of saline into the venous system. (The other factor contributing to the Bainbridge effect is distension of the pacemaker.) The reflex tachycardia may serve to shift blood out of the congested venous system into the arterial system.

The **diuresis**, and with it natriuresis (increased salt excretion), is due in part to reduced renal sympathetic nerve activity, which causes renal vasodilatation; and partly to changes in the circulating levels of vasopressin (anti-diuretic hormone), angiotensin, aldosterone and atrial natriuretic peptide. The reflex diuresis establishes a negative feedback loop that helps to regulate plasma volume.

Unmyelinated mechanoreceptors signal overdistension

Around 80% of cardiac afferents are small-diameter, unmyelinated fibres, and some of these subserve mechanoreception. They form a network of fine fibres in the left ventricle and atria. The activity of the unmyelinated left ventricular mechanoreceptors is weak unless the heart is distended. Similarly the unmyelinated atrial mechanoreceptors fire only when atrial filling is at its highest, namely during inspiration coincident with the V wave.

The reflex effect of the unmyelinated mechanoreceptors is depressor, i.e. bradycardia and peripheral vasodilatation. In laboratory animals, where the reflex can be studied rigorously, the reflex is weak and probably of little regulatory importance. The reflex may be stronger in humans (see below).

Chemosensitive fibres mediate ischaemic cardiac pain

Most unmyelinated left ventricular fibre endings are chemosensitive rather than mechanosensitive. They fire in response to adenosine, bradykinin, prostaglandins, lactic acid and K^+ ions, which are released in ischaemic myocardium. The afferent fibres travel in the cardiac sympathetic nerves and vagi.

The sympathetic chemosensitive afferents are known to mediate the pain of **angina** (and presumably myocardial infarction), because surgical interruption of the cardiac sympathetic pathway relieves chronic ischaemic cardiac pain in over 80% of cases. The sympathetic afferents ascend the spinal cord in the cervical spinothalamic tract, in which there is considerable convergence with somatic afferent fibres. The convergence may explain why cardiac pain is usually experienced as emanating from the chest wall and arms (**referred pain**). The reflex effect of the sympathetic afferents is mainly excitatory, producing a rise in blood pressure.

16.4 Cardiac receptor reflexes in man

Most of our knowledge of cardiac receptors and reflexes comes from animal studies (preceding section). It is difficult, for obvious reasons, to establish the roles of the various cardiac receptors in humans. Indirect evidence indicates that the human heart possesses sensors of cardiac blood volume ('**central volume receptors**'), and that their activity has a substantial reflex effect on peripheral vessels. Studies of patients with transplanted, denervated ventricles indicate that **left ventricular mechanoreceptors** may have a significant reflex effect on vascular tone in humans, unlike laboratory animals.

Central blood volume reflexly influences peripheral vascular tone

Increases in human intrathoracic venous pressure and blood volume, accompanied by only small changes in arterial pressure, evoke a graded reflex **vasodilatation** in skin and skeletal muscle (Figure 16.10). To perform the converse experiment, intrathoracic blood volume can be reduced by applying suction around the lower body, distending the peripheral veins. This causes central hypovolaemia. Even

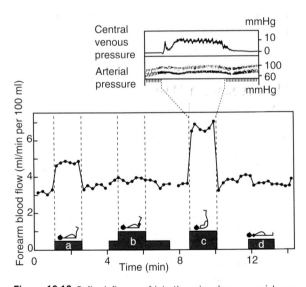

Figure 16.10 Reflex influence of intrathoracic volume on resistance vessels of human forearm muscle. (a) Legs alone raised, raising intrathoracic blood volume; vasodilatation follows. (b) Legs raised but pneumatic cuff around thigh at 180 mmHg prevents blood translocation; no change in forearm flow. (c) Legs and lower trunk raised: *inset* shows how central venous pressure rises; large reflex vasodilatation. (d) Pneumatic cuff around neck inflated to 30 mmHg to reduce carotid sinus distension; very little reflex change in forearm blood flow. (From Roddie, I. C., Shepherd, J. T. and Whelan, R. F. (1957) *Journal of Physiology*, **139**, 369, by permission.)

when the lower body negative pressure is so mild as not to change arterial pressure detectably, there is reflex vasoconstriction in the muscle, splanchnic and coronary circulations, increased circulating noradrenaline, and stimulation of the renin–angiotensin–aldosterone system. In cardiac transplant patients with intact posterior atrial innervation but denervated ventricles, the reflex to mild lower body negative pressure is greatly attenuated. For this reason it is thought that **human left ventricular mechanoreceptors** may contribute importantly to the regulation of vascular tone, unlike their minor role in laboratory animals.

Human extracellular fluid volume is controlled partly through cardiovascular reflexes

A role for cardiovascular receptors in controlling human extracellular fluid volume has been demonstrated by immersing subjects in water in the feet-down position. The water pressure displaces ~700 ml blood into the thorax, simulating an acute expansion of body fluid volume (Figure 8.21). The total diastolic volume of the heart rises by ~180 ml, stroke volume increases by ~30% due to the Frank–Starling mechanism, and arterial pressure rises by ~10 mmHg. Therefore both the cardiopulmonary mechanoreceptors and arterial baroreceptors are stimulated. A substantial diuresis ensues, caused by **renal vasodilatation**, reduced circulating **vasopressin**, reduced **renin–angiotensin–aldosterone** activation and increased **atrial natriuretic peptide**.

In astronauts subjected to **zero gravity**, the redistribution of venous blood from legs to thorax leads to a diuresis and fall in extracellular fluid volume. The reduced plasma volume, coupled with a weakened baroreflex, causes severe orthostatic intolerance on returning to earth, i.e. postural hypotension.

16.5 Long-term regulation of arterial blood pressure

As indicated earlier, the baroreflex is primarily a short-term buffer of blood pressure. In the longer term the maintenance of a normal basal blood pressure depends on the maintenance of a normal blood volume. Since plasma is part of the extracellular fluid compartment, this entails maintaining a **normal extracellular fluid volume** and **sodium mass**, which is the job of the kidneys. The renal excretion of salt and water is linked to blood pressure through two kinds of mechanism:

(i) **pressure natriuresis**; and (ii) **diuretic hormones** whose secretion is influenced by cardiovascular reflexes.

Raised renal artery pressure directly increases salt and water excretion

Pressure natriuresis is the increase in renal salt and water excretion that follows a rise in renal arterial pressure. The proposed mechanism is as follows. A rise in renal arterial pressure raises the pressure in the renal medullary capillaries, because the autoregulation of medullary capillary pressure is reported to be poor, unlike the excellent autoregulation of glomerular pressure. Increased medullary capillary pressure leads to a rise in renal interstitial fluid pressure, which in turn impairs the reabsorption of glomerular filtrate by renal tubules.

Arterial blood pressure reflexly regulates diuretic hormone levels

The chief hormones that regulate the renal excretion of salt and water are as follows.

- The **renin–angiotensin–aldosterone** system strongly promotes salt and water retention. The system is activated by reduced renal afferent arteriole pressure and by increased renal sympathetic activity following baroreceptor unloading (Figure 14.12).

- **Antidiuretic hormone** (vasopressin) strongly promotes water retention. Vasopressin secretion in primates is increased reflexly by arterial baroreceptor unloading (Figure 14.11).

- **Atrial natriuretic peptide** promotes salt excretion and diuresis. It is released in response to atrial distension but its effect is weak at physiological concentrations (Section 14.9).

Cardiac and arterial receptors together underpin long-term pressure homeostasis

Vasopressin, angiotensin and aldosterone levels are influenced reflexly by the combined inputs from the cardiac mechanoreceptors and arterial baroreceptors, which therefore contribute to the long-term regulation of mean blood pressure. If the input from either group of receptors is interrupted, the basal blood pressure rises only a little in the long term (Figure 16.8a). This is fortunate for patients with transplanted hearts, who have little problem regulating their blood pressure. Evidently one group of receptors can largely compensate for lack of the other group. (This illustrates Comroe's principle; if a job is worth doing, the body

The regulation of blood pressure

☐ Mean arterial pressure equals cardiac output × total peripheral resistance. Depressor reflexes (e.g. baroreflex) adjust cardiac output and peripheral resistance to stabilise pressure from minute to minute.

☐ Baroreceptor stimulation by increased arterial pressure evokes increased vagal parasympathetic outflow and decreased sympathetic outflow. The ensuing bradycardia, reduced contractility and resistance vessel relaxation return pressure towards its set point.

☐ The set point can be raised by central neuronal interactions, e.g. in exercise.

☐ The baroreflex is supplemented by a depressor reflex from unmyelinated cardiac mechanoreceptors.

☐ In the long term, cardiac output and blood pressure depend also on extracellular fluid volume regulation by the kidneys through (a) pressure natriuresis (increased renal artery pressure increases salt and water excretion) and (b) changes in vasopressin, aldosterone and atrial natriuretic peptide levels as a reflex response to altered cardiovascular receptor signalling.

CONCEPT BOX 21

has more than one way of doing it!) If, however, both groups of receptors are denervated, there is a sustained elevation of renin–angiotensin–aldosterone levels and sustained hypertension develops (Figure 16.8b).

16.6 Excitatory inputs: arterial chemoreceptors, lung stretch receptors and muscle work receptors

As well as the depressor reflexes that stabilize blood pressure, there are excitatory reflexes that help the cardiovascular system to respond positively to challenges such as hypoxia or exercise. The following receptor groups elicit excitatory or 'pressor' reflexes:

- arterial chemoreceptors
- lung stretch receptors
- muscle work receptors
- the external senses.

Arterial chemoreceptors support blood pressure in asphyxia and clinical shock

Arterial chemoreceptors are stimulated by arterial blood hypoxaemia, hypercapnia, acidosis and hyperkalaemia. The arterial chemoreceptors are located mainly in the **carotid bodies** (not to be confused with the carotid sinus) and the **aortic bodies**. The carotid and aortic bodies are small, highly vascularized nodules adjacent to the carotid sinus and aorta (Figure 16.2). Their afferent fibres accompany the baroreceptor afferents in the IXth (glossopharyngeal) and Xth (vagus) cranial nerves.

The chief role of the arterial chemoreceptors is to regulate breathing. Their influence on the circulation is slight at normal gas tensions but becomes important in **asphyxia** and **clinical shock**. When excited by hypoxia and hypercapnia, the chemoreflex elicits the following cardiovascular changes:

- **Resistance vessels constriction** is mediated by reflexly increased sympathetic vasomotor activity.

- **Venoconstriction of the splanchnic circulation** is likewise sympathetically mediated.

- **Blood pressure increases** due to the above two effects.

- **Tachycardia** is induced indirectly. If breathing is controlled by artificial ventilation, the chemoreflex elicits a moderate **bradycardia**. During spontaneous breathing, however, the chemoreflex stimulates breathing, which in turn stimulates lung stretch receptors. The **lung inflation reflex** (see below) evokes a marked tachycardia and overrides the moderate chemoreflex bradycardia.

The cardiovascular effects of the chemoreflex are important in the following situations.

Asphyxia is the combination of hypoxia and hypercapnia. Asphyxia strongly stimulates the chemoreceptors, leading to a reflex rise in blood pressure and enhanced cerebral perfusion and O_2 delivery.

Clinical shock. In clinical shock due to severe haemorrhage or other causes, there is reduced perfusion of the carotid and aortic bodies. The resulting 'stagnant hypoxia', in combination with metabolic acidosis (which is a feature of hypotension, Chapter 18), excites the arterial chemoreceptors. The resulting reflex vasoconstriction supports the blood pressure. The support of the chemoreflex is particularly important at pressures below the operating range of the baroreflex. Most baroreceptor fibres fall silent below ~70 mmHg. The chemoreceptors, by contrast, become progressively more excited the lower the perfusion pressure. The importance of the chemoreflex following a severe haemorrhage has been demonstrated in dogs by cutting the chemoreceptor nerves. This causes a sharp plunge in blood pressure and increased mortality. The chemoreflex

also initiates the **rapid breathing** that characterizes patients in hypotensive shock.

Diving reflex. The chemoreceptors contribute to the bradycardia of diving (Chapter 17).

Lung stretch receptors cause reflex tachycardia

Lung mechanoreceptors are activated by each inspiration. Their input to the brainstem inhibits the cardiac vagal parasympathetic neurons and thus elicits tachycardia. The inhibition is powerfully reinforced by inspiratory neurons in the brainstem. The combined inhibitory inputs causes **sinus arrhythmia**, which is an increase in heart rate during each inspiration (Figure 5.4a).

The **tachycardia of asphyxia** is caused by the lung inflation reflex. This overpowers the bradycardia of the arterial chemoreflex.

Deep inspiration also elicits reflex vaso- and venoconstriction in human skin (Figure 14.14). This **inspiratory gasp reflex** can be used to test human sympathetic function.

Muscle work receptors elicit tachycardia and the exercise pressor reflex

The cardiovascular responses to exercise include tachycardia and increased blood pressure (the exercise pressor response). These changes are driven partly by reflexes from muscle 'work receptors'. If sensory information from human muscle afferents is blocked by anaesthesia of the major limb nerves, the tachycardia and pressor response to exercise are reduced, though not abolished (Figure 16.11). There are two kinds of muscle work receptor, the mechanoreceptor and the chemoreceptor (metaboreceptor).

Muscle mechanoreceptors are served mainly by small myelinated fibres (group III). They are stimulated by local pressure and muscle contraction. Muscle mechanoreceptors reflexly inhibit cardiac **vagal tone**, and thereby contribute to the rapid increase in heart rate in the first few seconds of exercise. Muscle spindle afferents (group I) do not contribute to cardiovascular control.

Muscle metaboreceptors are served mainly by unmyelinated, group IV fibres. Metaboreceptors are activated by chemicals released during exercise, notably K^+ ions, $H_2PO_4^-$ ions, and to a lesser extent H^+ ions due to lactic acid formation. Since the accumulation of these stimulants is more pronounced during **isometric exercise**, the exercise pressor response is bigger in isometric exercise than dynamic exercise (Figure 17.6).

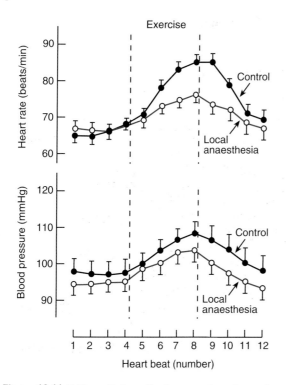

Figure 16.11 Evidence that a reflex from muscle work receptors contributes to exercise tachycardia and the exercise pressor response in humans. The response to 4 s of maximal voluntary handgrip was attenuated by local anaesthesia of axillary and radial nerves. (From Lassen, A., Mitchell, J. H., Reeves, D. R., Rogers, H. B. and Secher, J. (1989) *Journal of Physiology*, **409**, 333–341, by permission.)

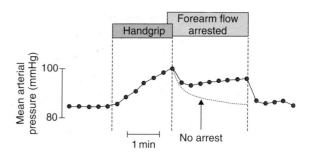

Figure 16.12 Evidence for human muscle metaboreceptors. Isometric handgrip raises blood pressure. If blood is then trapped in the exercised arm by inflating a brachial cuff to suprasystolic pressure, the exercise pressor response is partly maintained until cuff release. (Adapted from Rusch, N. J., Shepherd, J. T., Webb, R. C. and Vanhoutte, P. M. (1981) *Circulation Research*, **48**(Suppl 1), 118–125, by permission.)

External receptors can influence heart rate and blood pressure

Cardiovascular responses can be evoked by receptors not concerned primarily with cardiovascular control. **Somatic pain**, for example, causes tachycardia and hypertension. Severe **visceral pain** causes bradycardia, hypotension and even fainting. **Ambient cold** causes a rise in blood pressure, which increases left ventricular work and can trigger angina in susceptible patients.

The **special senses** too influence the cardiovascular system. The alerting response, for example to a sudden loud noise or the sight of a bus bearing down on one, produces a brisk tachycardia. Sexual stimulation evokes tachycardia and hypertension (Figure 8.13). Stimulation of facial receptors by cold water elicits bradycardia (the diving reflex, Chapter 17).

16.7 Central pathways; role of medulla

In 1854 the celebrated French physiologist Claude Bernard showed that transection of the cervical spinal cord causes peripheral vasodilatation and an abrupt fall in blood pressure to ~40 mmHg. This established that normal sympathetic vasomotor activity depends on a tonic, net excitatory drive from the brain to the spinal sympathetic neurons. The tonic excitatory drive arises within the medulla oblongata, the most caudal (tail-end) part of the brainstem (Figure 16.13). However, the medulla is by no means the only region involved in cardiovascular regulation. In addition the hypothalamus,

The reflex from chemical stimuli in muscle was discovered by Alam and Smirk in 1937. They inflated a pneumatic cuff around the human arm before stopping forearm exercise, in order to trap blood and chemical stimulants within the limb (Figure 16.12). The exercise pressor response is then partly maintained after the cessation of exercise, and only subsides when the cuff is released.

The metaboreceptors detect the under-perfusion of an active muscle and initiate an appropriate reflex, namely increased sympathetic outflow. The ensuing tachycardia, increased myocardial contractility and general peripheral vasoconstriction raise the arterial blood pressure. Raised pressure is advantageous during isometric exercise, because isometric contraction compresses the intramuscular vasculature, and vascular compression is opposed by a rise in arterial pressure. The pressor reflex can thereby maintain muscle perfusion at isometric contractions up to 50% of maximum voluntary contraction. More forceful contractions, however, impede the local perfusion.

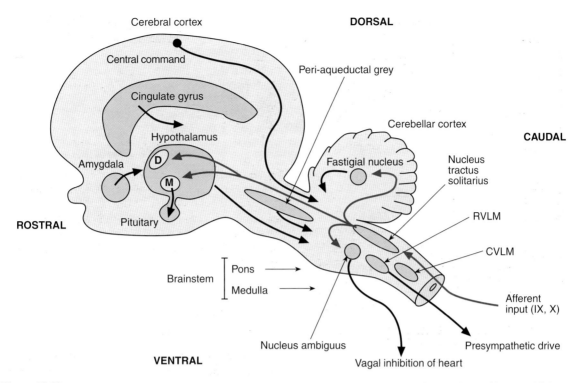

Figure 16.13 Longitudinal pathways for cardiovascular regulation in cat brain. D, depressor region of hypothalamus; M, magnocellular neurons of supraoptic and paraventricular hypothalamic nuclei that synthesize vasopressin; RVLM and CVLM, rostral and caudal ventrolateral medulla, respectively.

limbic system, cerebellum and cerebral cortex all play a role. The complex central pathways are only partly understood at present.

The traditional idea that the medulla has a dorsal 'vasomotor centre' is no longer tenable. The modern view emphasizes transverse traffic between a number of different regions of the medulla, and also up and down traffic between the medulla and higher regions. The roles of the medulla in circulatory control are as follows.

The nucleus tractus solitarius receives and integrates the cardiovascular receptor traffic

The dorso-medial medulla contains an elongated nucleus of cells, the **nucleus tractus solitarius** (Figures 16.13, 16.14). Nearly all the cardiovascular afferents – baroreceptor and cardiopulmonary afferents, arterial chemoreceptors, pulmonary stretch receptors and muscle work receptors – terminate in the nucleus tractus solitarius. Consequently, destruction of the nucleus tractus solitarius causes sustained hypertension. Muscle afferents also project to the lateral reticular nucleus (Figures 16.14, 16.16),

so destruction of the lateral reticular nucleus impairs the exercise pressor response.

The nucleus tractus solitarius is more than just a relay station; the processing of the sensory information begins here. An individual neuron receives many inputs, so its output is influenced by many different signals. This is called **sensory integration**.

The nucleus tractus solitarius relays integrated afferent information to other regions

The output of the nucleus tractus solitarius is relayed to other parts of the medulla, hypothalamus and cerebellum (Figure 16.13). Within the medulla a polysynaptic path projects to the **nucleus ambiguus**, which contains the vagal cardiac motor neurons, and to the **caudal ventrolateral medulla** (CVLM), which influences presympathetic output (Figure 16.13). The nucleus tractus solitarius also projects to the **hypothalamus**, sending cardiovascular information to a depressor area and to the vasopressin-producing, magnocellular neurons of the supraoptic and paraventricular nuclei (Figures 14.11, 16.13).

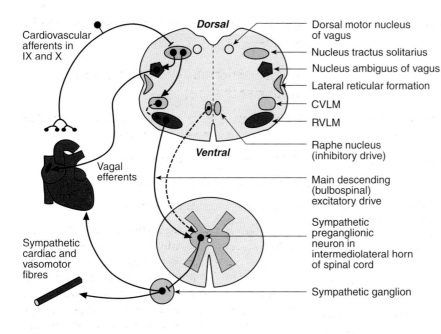

Figure 16.14 Schematic transverse section through the medulla to show lateral traffic and relative positions of cardiovascular nuclei in the dorsoventral plane. RVLM, rostral ventrolateral medulla group; CVLM, caudal ventrolateral medulla group. Dashed lines indicate inhibitory pathways. The structures occur at various rostrocaudal levels and would not in reality all be present in a single anatomical section.

The nucleus ambiguus generates the tonic vagal parasympathetic outflow to the heart

The cell bodies of the vagal parasympathetic fibres to the heart are located chiefly in the **nucleus ambiguus** and to a lesser extent the dorsal motor nucleus (Figures 16.13, 16.14). The vagal nuclei used to be known collectively as the 'cardioinhibitory centre'. Their activity is regulated by inputs from the nucleus tractus solitarius, from inspiratory neurons, and from the hypothalamus.

Rostral ventrolateral medulla generates the tonic presympathetic outflow to the spinal cord

When the anaesthetic pentobarbitone is applied to the surface of the **rostral ventrolateral medulla** (RVLM), there is a sharp fall in blood pressure, similar to that produced by cervical cord transection. This led to the discovery of the RVLM vasomotor neurons. The RVLM neurons give rise to **bulbospinal fibres** that run down the dorsolateral funiculus of the spinal cord and exert a tonic excitatory (glutaminergic) effect on the sympathetic preganglionic neurons of the **thoracic spinal cord** (Figure 16.14). The medullary vasomotor neurons are topographically organized; the most rostral neurons control renal sympathetic activity and a separate region controls the output to limb vessels.

The tonic output of the RVLM is continuously restrained by an inhibitory input from the **caudal ventrolateral medulla** (CVLM), mediated by the

inhibitory neurotransmitter γ-aminobutyric acid (GABA). The CVLM itself receives a regulatory input from the nucleus tractus solitarius (Figure 16.14). There is also a direct, descending inhibitory influence from the **raphe nuclei** of the brainstem to the spinal sympathetic neurons.

The **area postrema** is a small patch on the dorsal surface of the medulla where the blood–brain barrier is deficient. Angiotensin II gains access to area postrema neurons here, increasing their activity. Projections to the RVLM lead to an increased vasomotor presympathetic outflow.

16.8 Central pathways; role of higher regions

The central defence area co-ordinates the alerting response

'Alerting' is a pattern of responses to an unusual environmental stimulus, such as danger or a sudden noise, and is vital to survival in the wild. The alerting response has a behavioural component (head raised, ears pricked in dog and cats) and a cardiovascular component that prepares the animal for action. The alerting response was first described by Cannon in 1929, and is also known as the **defence** or **fear–fight–flight response**. 'Alerting response' seems the best description because in humans its cardiovascular manifestations can be elicited by quite mild arousal such as performing mental arithmetic to the beat of a metronome.

The cardiovascular response is highly stereotyped and comprises:

- **tachycardia** and increased cardiac output;

- **vasodilatation in skeletal muscle**;

- sympathetic-mediated **vasoconstriction** in the skin, splanchnic and renal circulations;

- **increased blood pressure** accompanied by inhibition of the baroreflex.

The muscle vasodilatation is mediated partly by circulating adrenaline, partly by reduced sympathetic vasoconstrictor activity to muscle, and in many non-primates by sympathetic cholinergic nerves (Chapter 14).

Brain stimulation experiments show that the alerting response is generated by an extensive system of neurons distributed along the **central long axis** of the brain. The neurons are located in three zones, namely the amygdala, a part of the **limbic system** that generates emotional behaviour patterns; the perifornical region of the **hypothalamus;** and the **periaqueductal grey matter** of the pons and medulla (Figure 16.13). These regions are influenced by inputs from the frontal cortex, and their output modulates the nucleus tractus solitarius (Figure 16.15), cardiac vagal motor neurons and RVLM vasomotor neurons to produce the characteristic cardiac and vasomotor changes of alerting. Electrical stimulation of the periaqueductal grey matter evokes the cardiovascular pattern listed above and also, in conscious animals, the behavioural manifestations of fear and rage, such as spitting, snarling and piloerection.

Hypertensive humans show a greater renal vasoconstriction to a mental stress test than normal subjects, and also less habituation to repeated stress. This led to the suggestion that an overdeveloped alerting response may contribute to the development of clinical hypertension.

The limbic system co-ordinates the 'playing dead' response

The 'playing dead' response is a behaviour pattern exhibited by the opossum and many young creatures faced with danger. Its cardiovascular components are profound **bradycardia** and **hypotension**, i.e. the opposite of the alerting response. The response originates in the cingulate gyrus of the **limbic system** (Figure 16.13). It is thought that **human fainting** in response to an intolerable psychological stimulus ('swooning') is a manifestation of the same response, namely the avoidance of a threatening situation by collapse.

The hypothalamus integrates several cardiovascular responses

Several regions of the hypothalamus are involved in cardiovascular regulation, including:

- the temperature-regulating area

- the vasopressin-secreting nuclei

- the hypothalamic depressor area.

The **temperature regulating area** in the anterior hypothalamus co-ordinates the sympathetic vasomotor and sudomotor outflow to skin (Section 15.3).

The supraoptic and paraventricular nuclei contain magnocellular neurons that produce **vasopressin**. These neurons receive inputs from local osmoreceptors, and from baroreceptors via a polysynaptic nucleus tractus solitarius–CVLM pathway (Figure 14.11).

The **hypothalamic depressor area** is in the dorsal anterior hypothalamus (Figure 16.13). It receives an input from the nucleus tractus solitarius. When stimulated electrically, the depressor area mimics the baroreflex, i.e. it activates the cardiac vagal fibres and inhibits sympathetic outflow. Lesions of the depressor area impair but do not abolish the baroreflex.

The cerebellum helps to co-ordinate cardiovascular changes during exercise

The main function of the cerebellum is to co-ordinate muscular movement. During exercise the cerebellum also co-ordinates the cardiovascular changes. The cerebellar fastigial nucleus and the associated vermal cortex receive projections from the medulla (Figure 16.13). Destruction of the fastigial nucleus reduces the tachycardia and pressor response of dogs to exercise. Stimulation of the vermal cortex in laboratory animals elicits renal vasoconstriction and muscle vasodilatation, a pattern characteristic of exercise.

The cerebral cortex initiates 'central command' in exercise

In 1913 Krogh and Lindhard postulated the 'central command' hypothesis to explain the rapid cardiovascular response to exercise. The central command hypothesis proposes that the cerebral cortex not only initiates muscular exercise, but also initiates many of the cardiovascular responses through projections to the brainstem (Figure 16.13). When stimulated electrically the frontal sensorimotor and temporal areas of the cortex elicit multiple cardio-vascular changes.

Support for the central command hypothesis in humans comes from experiments in which the arm muscles are completely paralysed by anaesthetizing the motor nerves. Voluntary attempts to carry out a maximum hand grip generate no force, but there is an immediate rise in heart rate and blood pressure.

16.9 Overview of central control

Figures 16.15 and 16.16 provide a highly simplified overview of the central cardiovascular pathways.

Control of vagal outflow to the heart

Two main routes link the baroreceptor input and the vagal motor neurons that control heart rate. One route, of short latency, remains within the medulla and passes from the nucleus tractus solitarius to the vagal motor nuclei, possibly via interneurons (Figure 16.15). The other route, of longer latency, passes from the nucleus tractus solitarius up to the hypo-thalamic depressor centre and from there to the vagal motor neurons.

During inspiration a projection of the brainstem respiratory neurons to the vagal nuclei hyperpolar-izes the cardiac motor neurons. The hyperpolariza-tion causes a loss of vagal neuronal responsiveness to the baroreflex during each inspiration (**gating** of the baroreflex). The inhibition of vagal activity causes a tachycardia in synchrony with inspiration (**sinus arrhythmia**). The inspiratory tachycardia helps to compensate for the fall in left ventricular stroke vol-ume during inspiration, which is due to expansion of the pulmonary blood capacity during inspiration.

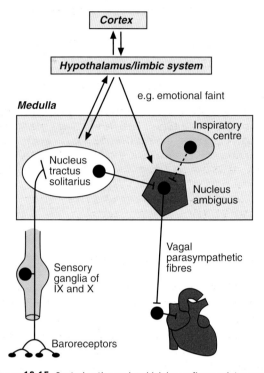

Figure 16.15 Central pathways by which baroreflex regulates vagal parasympathetic drive to heart. Inspiratory inhibition (dashed line) generates sinus arrhythmia. Inputs from muscle work receptors (exer-cise pressor reflex) and face (diving reflex) not shown. (Based on Spyer, K. M. (1994); see Further Reading.)

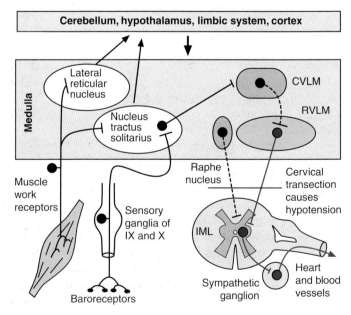

Figure 16.16 Simplified central pathways governing sympathetic drive (red neurons) to heart and vessels. Dashed lines denote inhibitory pathways. Excitatory cen-tral pathways from chemoreceptors are not shown. CVLM, RVLM, caudal and rostral ventrolateral medulla, respec-tively; IML, intermediolateral horns of thoracic spinal cord with sympathetic preganglionic neurons.

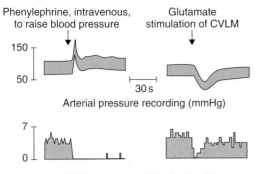

Phenylephrine, intravenous, to raise blood pressure

Glutamate stimulation of CVLM

Arterial pressure recording (mmHg)

RVLM neurone activity (spikes/s)

Figure 16.17 Reflex control of presympathetic neurons in rostral ventrolateral medulla (RVLM). (*Left*) Raising blood pressure by i.v. phenylephrine evokes a baroreflex inhibition of RVLM. (*Right*) Stimulation of the caudal ventrolateral medulla (CVLM) by a glutamate injection (excitatory neurotransmitter) inhibits the RVLM. This reduces spinal sympathetic activity, leading to a fall in blood pressure. The sequence of events mimics the baroreflex. (After Blessing, W. W. (1991); see Further Reading.)

Control of sympathetic outflow

The inhibitory pathway from the nucleus tractus solitarius to the spinal sympathetic neurons is more complex and less well understood than the vagal pathway (Figure 16.16). Several intermediate pathways, some involving higher regions of the brain, mediate inhibition of RVLM neurons. One pathway passes from the nucleus tractus solitarius to the caudal ventrolateral medulla, which then inhibits the RVLM (Figure 16.17).

The net effect of the nucleus tractus solitarius projection is that many RVLM neurons fall silent during the pulse. The baroreflex thus inhibits the descending excitatory drive from the RVLM to the spinal preganglionic sympathetic neurons. The spinal sympathetic neurons also receive an inhibitory input via bulbospinal fibres from the brainstem raphe nuclei.

Blood pressure is maintained but labile in spinal patients

The activity of the spinal sympathetic preganglionic neurons depends chiefly on the activity of the descending excitatory and inhibitory bulbospinal fibres, and to a lesser degree on local inputs within the spinal cord. As Claude Bernard showed, sectioning the cervical spinal cord cuts off the net excitatory influence of the brainstem and causes an abrupt hypotension. Sherrington and others soon pointed out, however, that over several weeks the **blood pressure gradually recovers in patients with spinal transection**. This is due to the ability of the sympathetic preganglionic neurons to generate an output by local mechanisms when brainstem control is removed.

Some reflex modulation of sympathetic activity still occurs in cervical transection patients, due to local pathways in the spinal cord. A full bladder or somatic pain, for example, may both cause a reflex rise in blood pressure. Moreover, spinal patients retain baroreflex control of the **heart rate** via the vagus. However, they **lack the vasomotor component of the baroreflex**, and therefore suffer from a labile blood pressure and proneness to postural hypotension. Compensation during orthostasis is provided by the **myogenic constrictor response to dependency** (Figures 8.6, 11.5) and by **angiotensin formation** in response to a fall in renal artery pressure (Section 14.8).

SUMMARY

■ Heart rate, contractility, vascular tone and blood pressure are regulated through cardiovascular reflexes. The reflex can be **depressor** (pressure-lowering, e.g. baroreflex) or **pressor** (pressure-raising e.g. chemoreflexes). The afferent inputs from cardiovascular receptors relay in the brainstem and modify the autonomic outflow to the heart and vessels.

■ **Arterial baroreceptors** in the carotid sinus and aortic arch are dynamically sensitive stretch receptors. They signal pulse pressure and mean pressure. The myelinated, low-threshold A-fibres and non-myelinated, higher threshold C-fibres travel in the glossopharyngeal and vagal nerves to the medulla. Baroreceptor excitation elicits a depressor reflex comprising bradycardia, reduced contractility and dilatation of resistance and capacitance vessels.

■ The baroreflex is a negative feedback loop that **stabilizes blood pressure**. 'Resetting' enables the baroreflex to buffer pressure around different levels during exercise (central resetting) or clinical hypertension (peripheral resetting).

■ During **hypovolaemia**, baroreceptor unloading elicits tachycardia, increased contractility, vaso- and venoconstriction, interstitial fluid absorption and renal fluid retention (via renin–angiotensin–aldosterone stimulation and ADH suppression). These responses help to maintain the arterial blood pressure.

■ **Cardiac receptors** fall into several classes. **Chemosensitive ventricular afferents** mediate ischaemic heart pain. **Myelinated veno-atrial stretch receptors** monitor atrial distension and evoke reflex tachycardia and diuresis, which reduce cardiac distension and extracellular fluid volume. **Non-myelinated mechanoreceptors** in the left ventricle, atria and pulmonary artery elicit a depressor reflex (vasodilatation), which is weak in dogs but may be more important in humans.

■ In humans **increased CVP and extracellular fluid volume** triggers a reflex via the cardiopulmonary and arterial receptors. The reflex comprises skin, muscle and renal vasodilatation, reduced vasopressin secretion and reduced renin–angiotensin–aldosterone. Atrial distension also stimulates atrial natriuretic peptide secretion.

■ **Long-term regulation of arterial pressure** depends on the regulation of extracellular salt and water mass by the kidneys. Renal excretion is controlled partly by pressure natriuresis and partly by vasopressin and aldosterone, the levels of which are regulated reflexly by the combined baroreceptor and cardiopulmonary receptor inputs.

■ **Peripheral arterial chemoreceptors** in the carotid and aortic bodies are excited by hypoxia, acidosis, asphyxia and hyperkalaemia. Besides stimulating ventilation, they elicit a pressor reflex through peripheral vasoconstriction. This supports the blood pressure during severe haemorrhage and asphyxiation. A reflex from **lung stretch receptors** elicits a concomitant tachycardia.

■ **Muscle metaboreceptors** are excited by K^+, phosphate and acidity during exercise and evoke the exercise pressor reflex (tachycardia, increased myocardial contractility, vasoconstriction). Along with muscle mechanoreceptors they help to drive the cardiovascular response to exercise, especially isometric exercise.

■ All the above afferents relay in the **nucleus tractus solitarius** of the brainstem (medulla). Projections from the nucleus tractus solitarius pass via the medulla, hypothalamus and cerebellum to modulate (i) cardiac vagal motor neuron activity in the **nucleus ambiguus**; and (ii) the presympathetic excitatory outflow from the **rostral ventrolateral medulla**.

■ Higher centres elicit co-ordinated responses. The **central defence axis** elicits the alerting response (tachycardia, muscle vasodilatation and splanchnic, renal and cutaneous vasoconstriction) in preparation for fight or flight. The **hypothalamic temperature-regulating area** controls cutaneous sympathetic outflow. The **cerebral cortex** issues a 'central command' in exercise that raises heart rate and blood pressure.

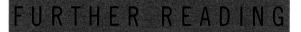

FURTHER READING

Reviews and chapters

Andresen, M. C. (1994) Nucleus tractus solitarius – gateway to neural circulatory control. *Annual Reviews of Physiology*, **56**, 93–116.

Bisset, G. W. and Chowdrey, H. S. (1988) Control of release of vasopressin by neuroendocrine reflexes. *Quarterly Journal of Experimental Physiology*, **73**, 811–872.

Blessing, W. W. (1991) Inhibitory vasomotor neurons in the caudal ventrolateral medulla oblongata. *News in Physiological Sciences*, **6**, 139–141.

Calaresu, F. R. and Yardley, C. P. (1988) Medullary basal sympathetic tone. *Annual Review of Physiology*, **50**, 511–524.

Cowley, A. W. (1992) Long-term control of arterial blood pressure. *Physiological Reviews*, **72**, 231–278.

Dampney, R. A. L. (1994) Functional organization of central pathways regulating the cardiovascular system. *Physiology Reviews*, **74**, 323–364.

De Burgh Daly, M. (1997) *Peripheral Arterial Chemoreceptors and Respiratory–Cardiovascular Integration*. Oxford Medical Publications, OUP, Oxford (Monographs of The Physiological Society No. 46).

Dorward, P. K. and Korner, P. I. (1987) Does the brain 'remember' the absolute blood pressure? *News in Physiological Sciences*, **2**, 10–13.

Eckberg, D. L. and Fritsch, J. M. (1993) How should human baroreflexes be tested? *News in Physiological Sciences*, **8**, 7–12.

Eckberg, D. L. and Sleight, P. (1992) *Human Baroreflexes in Health and Disease*, Oxford University Press, Oxford.

Foreman, R. D. (1999) Mechanisms of cardiac pain. *Annual Review of Physiology*, **61**, 143–167.

Hainsworth, R. (1991) Reflexes from the heart. *Physiological Reviews*, **71**, 617–658.

Jordan, D. (1995) CNS integration of cardiovascular regulation. In *Cardiovascular Regulation* (eds. Jordan, D. and Marshall, J.), Portland Press, London, pp. 1–14.

Kumada, M., Terui, N. and Kuwaki, T. (1990) Arterial baroreceptor reflex: its central and peripheral neural mechanisms. *Progress in Neurobiology*, **35**, 331–361.

Marshall, J. M. (1994) Peripheral chemoreceptors and cardiovascular regulation. *Physiological Reviews*, **74**, 543–594.

Marshall, J. M. (1995) Cardiovascular changes associated with behavioural alerting. In *Cardiovascular Regulation* (eds Jordan, D. and Marshall, J.), Portland Press, London, pp. 37–60.

Mitchell, J. H. and Schmidt, R. F. (1983) Cardiovascular reflex control by afferent fibres from skeletal muscle receptors. In *Handbook of Physiology, Cardiovascular System*, vol. 3 (eds Shepherd, J. T. and Abboud, F. M.), American Physiological Society, Bethesda, pp. 623–658.

Rowell, L. B. (1986) *Human Circulation. Regulation during Physical Stress*, Oxford University Press, New York.

Seller, H. (1991) Central baroreceptor reflex pathways. In *Baroreceptor Reflexes, Integrative Functions and Clinical Aspects* (eds Persson, P. B. and Kirchheim, H. R.), Springer, Berlin, pp. 5–74.

Spyer, K. M. (1994) Central nervous system mechanisms contributing to cardiovascular control. *Journal of Physiology*, **474**, 1–19.

Stone, H. L., Dormer, K. J., Foreman, R. D., Thies, R. and Blair, R. W. (1985) Neural regulation of the cardiovascular system during exercise. *Federal Proceedings*, **44**, 2271–2278.

Sved, A. F. and Gordon, F. J. (1994) Amino acids as central neurotransmitters in the baroreceptor reflex pathway. *News in Physiological Sciences*, **9**, 243–246.

Wallin, B. G. and Elam, M. (1994) Insights from intraneural recordings of sympathetic nerve traffic in humans. *News in Physiological Sciences*, **9**, 203–207.

Williams, J. L., Barnes, K. L., Brosnihan, K. B. and Ferrario, C. M. (1992) Area postrema: a unique regulator of cardiovascular function. *News in Physiological Sciences*, **7**, 30–34.

Research papers

Boushel, R., Madsen, P., Nielsen, H. B., Quistorff, B. and Secher, N. H. (1998) Contribution of pH, diprotonated phosphate and potassium for the reflex increase in blood pressure during handgrip. *Acta Physiologica Scandinavica*, **164**, 269–275.

Coleridge, H. M., Coleridge, J. C. G. and Schultze, H. D. (1987) Characteristics of C fibre baroreceptors in the carotid sinus of dogs. *Journal of Physiology*, **394**, 291–313.

Edfeldt, H. and Lundvall, J. (1993) Sympathetic baroreflex control of vascular resistance in comfortably warm man. Analyses of neurogenic constrictor responses in resting forearm and in its separate skeletal muscle and skin tissue compartments. *Acta Physiologica Scandinavica*, **147**, 437–447.

Jacobsen, T. N., Morgan, B. J., Scherrer, U., *et al.* (1993) Relative contributions of cardiopulmonary and sinoaortic baroreflexes in causing sympathetic activation in human skeletal muscle circulation during orthostatic stress. *Circulation Research*, **73**, 367–378.

McIlveen, S. A., Hayes, S. G. and Kaufman, M. P. (2001) Both central command and exercise pressure reflex reset carotid sinus baroreflex. *American Journal of Physiology*, **280**, H1454–1463.

Sanders, J. S., Mark, A. L. and Ferguson, D. W. (1989) Importance of aortic baroreflex in regulation of sympathetic responses during hypotension: evidence from direct sympathetic nerve recordings in humans. *Circulation*, **79**, 83–92.

Thoren, P., Munch, P. A. and Brown, A. M. (1999) Mechanisms for activation of aortic baroreceptor C-fibres in rabbits and rats. *Acta Physiologica Scandinavica*, **166**, 167–174.

Tjen-A-Looi, S. C., Pan, H.-L. and Longhurst, J. C. (1998) Endogenous bradykinin activates ischaemically sensitive cardiac visceral afferents through kinin B_2 receptors in cats. *Journal of Physiology*, **510**, 633–641.

Vissing, S. F., Scherrer, U. and Victor, R. G. (1994) Increase of sympathetic discharge to skeletal muscle but not to skin during mild lower body negative pressure in humans. *Journal of Physiology*, **481**, 233–241.

Wright, C. I., Drinkhill, M. J. and Hainsworth, R. (2000) Reflex effects of independent stimulation of coronary and left ventricular mechanoreceptors in anaesthetised dogs. *Journal of Physiology*, **528**, 349–358.

Zhang, J. and Miflin, S. W. (2000) Responses of aortic depressor nerve-evoked neurones in rat nucleus of the solitary tract to changes in blood pressure. *Journal of Physiology*, **529**, 431–443.

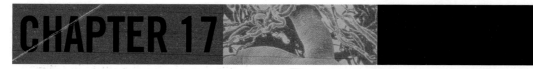

CHAPTER 17

Co-ordinated cardiovascular responses

Learning objectives.

After reading this chapter you should be able to:

Regarding posture:

• Explain how orthostasis reduces cardiac output.

• Describe the compensatory reflexes that prevent postural dizziness.

Regarding the Valsalva manoeuvre:

• Explain how forced expiration affects cardiac output and blood pressure.

Regarding exercise:

• Explain how pulmonary O_2 uptake is increased.

• Describe the changes in stroke volume and heart rate and how they are induced.

• Outline how solute exchange is raised between blood and active muscle.

• Contrast the effects of static and dynamic exercise on blood pressure.

• State the roles of central command and peripheral reflex during exercise.

Regarding training:

• List the cardiovascular changes induced by training.

Regarding feeding:

• State the changes in cardiac output, splanchnic and limb blood flow after a meal.

Regarding diving:

• Name the three key features of the diving response and the receptors responsible.

Regarding ageing:

• Define arteriosclerosis and state how arterial pressure changes with ageing.

• Outline the changes in cardiac performance with ageing.

Regarding sleep and alerting:

• Contrast the cardiovascular responses to sleep and alerting (stress).

All the individual elements of the circulation have been covered in the preceding chapters, but as with a jigsaw puzzle it is not enough to view the separate pieces; what matters is how they fit together to produce a functional whole. The purpose of this chapter is to show how the components of the cardiovascular system respond in a co-ordinated pattern to the demands of everyday life.

A general principle will emerge, namely that **each major adaptation is achieved by the integration of several smaller responses**. For example, a 13-fold increase in the rate of O_2 absorption by the pulmonary circulation during strenuous exercise is achieved, typically, by the combination of a 1½-fold rise in stroke volume, a 3-fold rise in heart rate, and a 3-fold increase in the arteriovenous concentration difference for O_2. Other examples of 'adaptation by integration' will be found below.

17.1 Posture

Orthostasis triggers an initial postural hypotension

Orthostasis, the adoption of an upright position, is a severe challenge to the human circulation due to the effect of gravity on venous blood distribution. Gravity causes a 10-fold rise in transmural pressure in the most dependent veins (Figures 8.2, 11.5), which increases the volume of blood in the dependent veins by ~500 ml (Figure 8.21). The redistribution of blood reduces the intrathoracic blood volume by 20% over ~15 seconds. Central venous pressure falls from 5–6 mmHg supine to around zero, which reduces the energy of contraction of the heart through the Frank–Starling mechanism (Figure 6.10b). The stroke volume declines initially by 30–40%, from ~70 ml to 45 ml, reducing the pulse pressure. Mean pressure falls transiently.

Although mean pressure is quickly restored through the operation of the baroreflex (see below), the transient hypotension can be severe enough to impair cerebral perfusion transiently. The reduced cerebral perfusion causes dizziness and visual fading for a few seconds. Most healthy individuals occasionally experience this postural giddiness. Postural giddiness is exacerbated by **warmth**, which causes cutaneous venodilatation and hence a low central filling pressure; **prolonged bedrest**; and exposure to **zero gravity** (returning astronauts). Postural hypotension does not progress to postural syncope (fainting) unless the baroreflex is blocked by an autonomic neuropathy or by pharmacological agents such as α-adrenoceptor blockers.

Neuroendocrine responses quickly restore mean arterial pressure

In healthy subjects the reflexes elicited by the unloading of arterial baroreceptors and cardiopulmonary mechanoreceptors restore the mean arterial pressure sufficiently rapidly to prevent postural dizziness. The reflexes are outlined in Figure 17.1. **Carotid baroreceptor traffic** is reduced by the fall in pulse pressure, and also by the fall in sinus pressure. Being located close to the base of the skull, the carotid sinus is raised 25 cm or so above heart level during orthostasis, so gravity directly reduces the sinus pressure (Figure 8.2). **Cardiopulmonary receptor traffic** is reduced by the fall in cardiac blood volume. The reduced inputs to the nucleus tractus solitarius inform the brain of the gravity of the situation (!) and elicit a reduction in cardiac vagal outflow and an increase in sympathetic outflow, with the following effects.

- **Heart rate increases** by 15–20 beats/min (Figure 17.2).

- **Stroke volume** remains below the supine value despite increased myocardial contractility and splanchnic venoconstriction. Pulse pressure is therefore reduced (Figure 17.2).

- **Cardiac output falls**, but the reflex tachycardia limits the fall to ~20%.

- **Peripheral resistance increases** by 30–40% due to sympathetic-mediated vasoconstriction in the skeletal muscle, splanchnic and renal vascular beds.

- **Mean arterial pressure** is not only restored by the increased peripheral resistance but is actually **raised 10–14 mmHg above the supine** value (Figure 17.2).

The above responses normally take less than a minute to complete. Over the next half-hour or so the orthostatic increase in capillary filtration pressure in the dependent tissues causes a **12–13% (375 ml) fall in plasma volume** (Section 11.9). This reduces systolic pressure and elicits an additional tachycardia. To compensate, the **excretion of salt and water is reduced** through renal vasoconstriction, sympathetic activation of the renin–angiotensin–aldosterone system and reflexly increased vasopressin secretion.

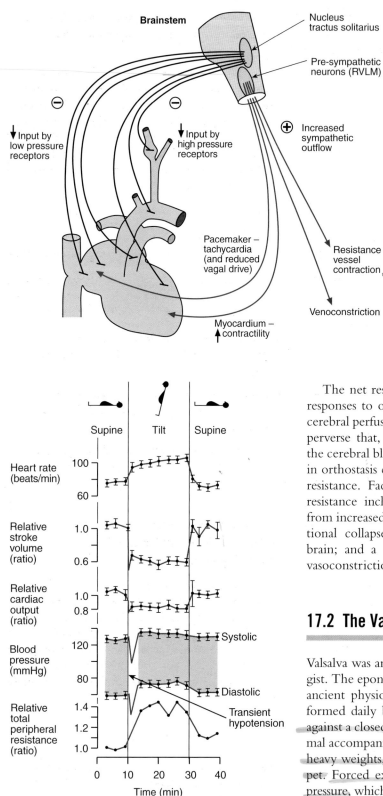

Figure 17.1 Reflex sympathetic response to orthostasis in humans.

Figure 17.2 Response of young adults to a 20-min head-up tilt. Points represent means, bars are standard errors. (From Smith, J. J., Bush, J. E., Weideier, V. T. and Tristani, F. E. (1970) *Journal of Applied Physiology*, **29**, 133, by permission.)

The net result of the combined neuroendocrine responses to orthostasis is that arterial pressure and cerebral perfusion pressure are safe-guarded. It seems perverse that, despite all this physiological 'effort', the cerebral blood flow actually declines by 10–20% in orthostasis due to an increase in cerebral vascular resistance. Factors that raise the cerebral vascular resistance include a fall in arterial P_{CO_2} resulting from increased ventilation in orthostasis; the gravitational collapse of extracranial veins draining the brain; and a slight sympathetic-mediated cerebral vasoconstriction.

17.2 The Valsalva manoeuvre

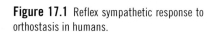

Valsalva was an eighteenth-century Italian physiologist. The eponymous manoeuvre is not, however, an ancient physiological rite but a natural event performed daily by all of us. It is a forced expiration against a closed or narrowed glottis, and this is a normal accompaniment to defaecation, coughing, lifting heavy weights, singing a top A or playing the trumpet. Forced expiration creates a high intrathoracic pressure, which evokes a complex circulatory response with four phases (Figure 17.3).

1 Arterial pressure immediately rises (**phase 1**), because the aorta is compressed by the high intrathoracic pressure.

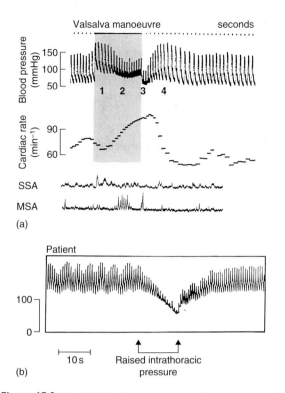

(a)

(b)

Figure 17.3 Effect of Valsalva manoeuvre on blood pressure and heart rate. (a) Normal subject. (b) Patient suffering from idiopathic orthostatic hypotension, caused by an autonomic defect. The patient's pressure failed to stabilize during phase 2, and there was no reflex bradycardia in phase 4. SSA and MSA, sympathetic nerve activity to skin and muscle, respectively. ((a) From Bannister, Sir R. (1980) In *Arterial Blood Pressure and Hypertension* (ed. Sleight, P.), Oxford University Press, Oxford, pp. 117–121 and Wallin, B. G. and Elam, M. (1994); see Further Reading, Chapter 16; (b) from Johnson, R. H. and Spalding, J. M. K. (1974) *Disorders of the Autonomic Nervous System*, Blackwell, London, by permission.)

2 In **phase 2** the mean pressure and especially pulse pressure fall, because the raised intrathoracic pressure impedes venous return and therefore stroke volume. A reflex increase in sympathetic outflow causes **tachycardia** and **peripheral vasoconstriction**, which arrest the fall in blood pressure (Figure 17.3a).

3 **Phase 3** marks the termination of the Valsalva manoeuvre. Arterial pressure drops abruptly as intrathoracic pressure falls to normal, decompressing the aorta.

4 In **phase 4** the pulse pressure and mean pressure increase rapidly, because the normalized intrathoracic pressure allows venous blood to surge into the thorax, distending the heart and increasing the stroke volume.

The increase in arterial pressure stimulates the baroreflex, causing a characteristic **reflex bradycardia**.

The sudden bradycardia in phase 4 of the Valsalva response is used as a **clinical test of baroreflex competence** in humans. If the reflex is interrupted by a neurological disorder, the Valsalva test shows a continuing pressure fall in phase 2 and neither pressure overshoot nor bradycardia in phase 4 (Figure 17.3b). Individuals with such a response are prone to postural hypotension.

17.3 Exercise

For the survival of the fittest in the wild the most important circulatory response is that to exercise. Exercise imposes three tasks on the circulation.

- **Pulmonary blood flow** must increase in order to raise O_2 uptake and CO_2 removal (Figure 17.4).

- **Blood flow through active muscle** must increase to raise O_2 and glucose delivery (Figure 17.4).

- **Arterial pressure** must be stabilized despite huge changes in cardiac output and vascular resistance.

Pulmonary O_2 uptake is raised by increased flow and reduced venous O_2 content

Increased O_2 consumption by active muscle must be matched by increased O_2 uptake in the lungs. The increased O_2 uptake, $\dot{V}_{O_2}$, is achieved partly through increased pulmonary blood flow i.e. increased cardiac output CO, and partly through an increase in the amount of O_2 that is added to each litre of blood, in accordance with the **Fick principle** (Section 7.1):

$$\dot{V}_{O_2} = CO(C_A - C_V)$$

where C_A and C_V are the arterial and mixed venous O_2 contents of the blood.

The cardiac output of an untrained human can increase maximally about four-fold, from 5 l/min at rest to 20 l/min in heavy exercise. The O_2 uptake per litre of blood, $(C_A - C_V)$, can increase approximately three-fold, because the mixed venous blood entering

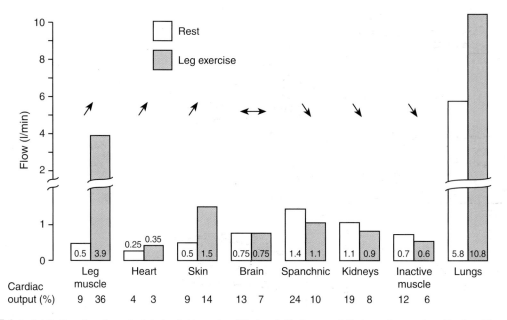

Figure 17.4 Redistribution of cardiac output during light exercise of the legs in the human adult at room temperature. Number at base of each column is blood flow in l/min. (After Wade, O. L. and Bishop, J. M. (1962) *Cardiac Output and Regional Blood Flow*, Blackwell, Oxford; and Blair, D. A., Glover, W. E. and Roddie, I. C. (1961) *Circulation Research*, **9**, 264.)

the lungs has less O_2 remaining in it during exercise (Figure 17.5). Typical values are as follows:

- Mixed venous blood at rest (C_V) = 145 ml O_2/l

- Mixed venous blood in heavy exercise (C_V) = 40 ml O_2/l

- Arterial blood at rest and in exercise (C_A) = 195 ml O_2/l.

It follows from the Fick principle that the O_2 uptake of an untrained human can increase about 13-fold, from a basal level of 0.25 l O_2/min to a maximum of just over 3 l O_2/min in severe exercise ($\dot{V}_{O_2max}$, Table 17.1).

O_2 consumption is widely used as an objective measure of work rate. Basal O_2 consumption by a resting adult is ~0.25 l/min. Subjectively light work, such as walking on the level at 3 km/h, raises consumption to 0.4–0.8 l O_2/min. Subjectively moderate work corresponds to 0.8–1.6 l O_2/min, and hard work to 1.6–2.4 l O_2/min. Subjectively severe work such as running at 12 km/h corresponds to 2.4–3.0 l O_2/min.

Cardiac output is raised through tachycardia and increased stroke volume

Cardiac output increases in proportion to whole-body O_2 consumption (Figure 17.5). The tight coupling between cardiac output and $\dot{V}_{O_2}$ indicates that the brainstem regulatory regions are kept well-informed about muscle O_2 consumption, but how this is achieved is not well understood. The increased output is achieved mainly through tachycardia, and to a lesser extent through increased stroke volume.

Heart rate is a linear function of work rate in the steady state (Figure 17.5). The rapid onset of tachycardia at the start of exercise (Figure 16.11) is due to the withdrawal of vagal inhibition of the pacemaker, under the direction of central command and the muscle mechanoreceptor reflex. Later, sympathetic stimulation contributes to the tachycardia. Maximum rate is 180–200 beats/min in a young adult human.

Stroke volume is raised partly through increased filling pressure, which increases the ventricular end-diastolic volume (EDV), and partly through increased ejection fraction, which reduces the end-systolic volume (ESV) (Figure 6.24, Table 17.2).

Filling pressure rises by ~1 mmHg during moderate, sustained, upright exercise. The rise is brought about by the skeletal muscle pump and sympathetically mediated splanchnic venoconstriction. During an explosive burst of cycling, however, the muscle pump can transiently raise the right atrial pressure by 12 mmHg. Consequently, increased EDV makes a greater contribution during a sudden,

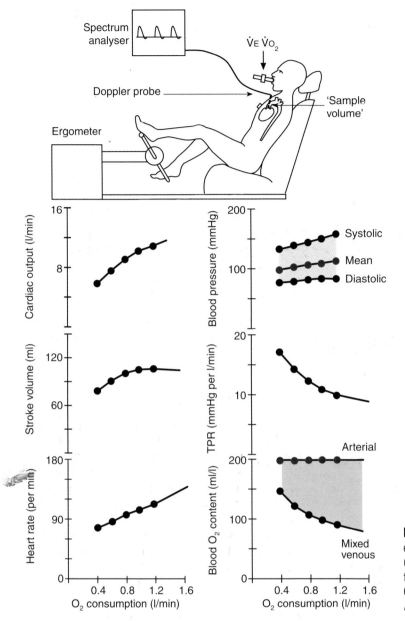

Figure 17.5 Human cardiovascular response to exercise, measured by pulsed Doppler method (Section 6.3) and expired gas analysis. (Adapted from Innes, J. A., Simon, T. D., Murphy, K. and Guz, A. (1988) *Quarterly Journal of Experimental Physiology*, **73**, 323–341, by permission.)

Table 17.1 Cardiovascular and pulmonary function capacities during maximal exercise in college students and Olympic athletes. *

	Exercising students			Olympic athletes
	Control	After bedrest	After training	
Maximal oxygen uptake (l/min)	3.30	2.43	3.91	5.38 [†]
Maximal voluntary ventilation (l/min)	191.0	201.0	197.0	219.0
Transfer coefficient for O_2 (ml min^{-1}mmHg^{-1})	96.0	83.0	86.0	95.0
Arterial O_2 capacity (vol %)	21.9	20.5	20.8	22.4
Maximal cardiac output (l/min)	20.0	14.8	22.8	30.4 [†]
Maximal stroke volume (ml)	104.0	74.0	120.0	167.0 [†]
Maximal heart rate (beats/min)	192.0	197.0	190.0	182.0
Systemic arteriovenous O_2 difference (vol %)	16.2	16.5	17.1	18.0

* Mean values, $n = 5$ and 6, respectively. Age, height and weight similar.
[†] Significantly different from college students after training, $P < 0.05$.
(After Blomqvist, C. G. and Saltin, B. (1983) *Annual Review of Physiology*, **45**, 169–189.)

Table 17.2 Ventricular volume during upright submaximal exercise in 30 normal subjects and 20 patients with multiple coronary artery disease.

	Normal		Coronary disease	
	Rest	Exercise	Rest	Exercise
Cardiac output (l/min)	6.0	17.5	5.7	11.3
Heart rate (beats/min)	81	170	75	119
Stroke volume (ml)	76	102	76	96
End-diastolic volume (ml)	116	128	138	216
End-systolic volume (ml)	40	26	62	120
Ejection fraction	0.66	0.8	0.6	0.46

Upright submaximal bicycle exercise. Left ventricle dimensions determined by radionuclide angiocardiography. (After Rerych, S. K., Scholz, P. M., Newman, G. E. *et al.* (1978) *Annals of Surgery*, **187**, 449–458.)

Table 17.3 Supine exercise *versus* upright exercise in 8 healthy subjects.

	Stroke volume (ml)	Heart rate (beats/min)	Cardiac output (l/min)
Supine			
Rest	111	60	6.4
Exercise	112	91	9.7
Upright			
Rest	76	76	5.6
Exercise	92	95	8.4

Response to pedalling at 30% of maximum oxygen consumption. Stroke volume measured by the aortic Doppler flow technique. (After Loeppky, J. A., Green, E. R., Hoekenga, D. E. *et al.* (1981) *Journal of Applied Physiology*, **50**, 1173–1182.)

maximal effort than during sustained, moderate exercise. Increases in EDV are also important in elderly subjects; see 'Ageing'.

Ejection fraction is raised and ESV thereby reduced through sympathetic enhancement of contractility. Ejection fraction can exceed 80% in heavy exercise. Patients with severe coronary disease cannot achieve this increase in ejection fraction and have a poor cardiac output during exercise (Table 17.2).

The relative contributions of increased heart rate and stroke volume to cardiac output depend on **posture** (Table 17.3). In supine exercise the increased output is due almost entirely to tachycardia. Filling pressure and EDV are already high at rest, and the stroke volume increases at most by 10–20%, due to a reduction in ESV. In the upright position by contrast the stroke volume starts from a lower value and can increase by 50–100% through a combination of increased EDV and reduced ESV. Most of the

increase in stroke volume occurs at low work rates (Figure 17.5).

Muscle blood flow and capillary exchange are raised by metabolic vasodilatation

In a fit man the total blood flow to muscle can increase from 1 l/min at rest (20% of the cardiac output) to ~19 l/min during hard dynamic exercise (>80% of cardiac output). Even during hard exercise many muscle groups are used only lightly (e.g. arm muscles during strenuous running), so it is estimated that the blood flow to the maximally active groups may increase 40-fold. Besides enhancing the transport of O_2 and glucose to the active muscle, the fall in vascular resistance has a vital permissive effect on the cardiac output. Without a fall in peripheral resistance, increased left ventricular output would raise arterial pressure to high levels, which in turn would limit the stroke volume (Section 6.9).

The muscle hyperaemia is due chiefly to **metabolic vasodilatation**, aided by the muscle pump during upright exercise (Figure 15.8). Metabolic dilatation of terminal arterioles not only increases **flow** but also causes **capillary recruitment**, which increases the area available for gas exchange and shortens the diffusion distances (Figures 10.14, 15.2 left). These changes greatly increase the rate of transport between blood and muscle fibre. The changes in glucose and O_2 transport were covered in Sections 10.10–10.11.

Arteriolar dilatation also raises capillary pressure. This, along with interstitial fluid hyperosmolarity, raises capillary filtration rate. As a result the **plasma volume** can fall by as much as 600 ml during prolonged heavy exercise (Section 11.9). The ensuing haemoconcentration raises the O_2-carrying capacity of the blood modestly. Arterial saturation falls slightly, however, due to the Bohr shift (effect of increased temperature and acidity). Also, in endurance athletes the pulmonary transit time becomes excessively short. Due to the opposing effects of haemoconcentration and reduced saturation, the arterial O_2 content during maximal exercise is unchanged in non-athletes and reduced in athletes.

As emphasized above, vasodilatation in active muscle is induced by intrinsic metabolic control, not by extrinsic autonomic control. If stress is involved, however, as at the start of a race, then the alerting response is evoked. **Feedforward** by the alerting response causes an autonomic-mediated muscle vasodilatation and anticipatory tachycardia.

Blood flow to many other tissues is adjusted during exercise

Blood flow to most of the tissues of the body is altered during exercise (Figure 17.4).

- **Coronary blood flow** increases in proportion to cardiac work due to metabolic vasodilatation.

- **Respiratory muscle perfusion** increases due to the increased work of breathing, and can account for up to 16% of the cardiac output in heavy exercise.

- **Skin** is a battleground of conflicting demands. Initially the cutaneous vessels are constricted to support the blood pressure, but as exercise raises the core temperature the thermoregulatory role of skin supervenes and dilatation develops. This requires a further rise in cardiac output. Since cutaneous venodilatation reduces the cardiac filling pressure, the stroke volume tends to decline during prolonged hard exercise, and the heart rate increases further to compensate.

- The **splanchnic vascular bed and non-exercising muscle groups** undergo sympathetic-mediated vasoconstriction to maintain blood pressure.

The fall in peripheral resistance occasioned by vasodilatation in the active muscle, respiratory muscles, myocardium and skin is so great during hard exercise that blood pressure would fall by 12–40 mmHg, despite the raised cardiac output, were it not for the compensatory vasoconstriction of inactive vascular beds. During leg exercise, for example, vascular resistance rises in the forearm muscle. Textbooks commonly state that vasoconstriction in the resting tissues 'diverts' blood to working muscle, but a simple tally of the changes in Figure 17.4 shows that the diverted flow, 0.6 l, makes a trivial contribution to the active hyperaemia. The real importance of the vasoconstrictor response lies in maintaining the arterial pressure.

Static exercise raises arterial pressure more than dynamic exercise

Systemic blood pressure depends on the severity of the exercise (Figure 17.5), its duration, the muscle mass involved, and especially the type of exercise (Figure 17.6).

In **dynamic exercise**, where muscles alternately contract and relax, mean blood pressure increases only

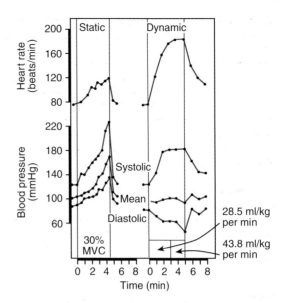

Figure 17.6 Effects of static compared with dynamic exercise. Static exercise caused a bigger rise in mean pressure. Dynamic exercise caused a bigger rise in pulse pressure and heart rate. MVC, maximal voluntary static contraction; arrowed numbers refer to oxygen consumption. (From Lind, R. A. and McNicol, G. W. (1967) *Canadian Medical Association Journal*, **96**, 706, by permission.)

moderately, because the raised cardiac output is counterbalanced by the reduced total peripheral resistance. Typically the mean pressure rises by 20 mmHg or less, and rarely exceeds 120 mmHg. Systolic pressure and pulse pressure increase much more than the mean due to the rise in stroke volume and ejection velocity. Systolic pressure can reach 200 mmHg. Diastolic pressure increases relatively little (Figure 17.5) or even falls (Figure 17.6, right panel).

Static exercise such as a sustained handgrip causes much bigger increases in diastolic pressure and mean pressure (Figure 17.6, left panel). The increases are caused by a rise in total peripheral resistance. Resistance rises because isometric contraction compresses the muscle vessels, which activates the muscle metaboreflex (exercise pressor reflex, Section 16.6) and directly attenuates the fall in muscle resistance. Supporting a 20 kg suitcase for 2–3 min can raise diastolic pressure by 30 mmHg. Since the **work of the left ventricle** is dominated by pressure, isometric exercise is best avoided by patients with ischaemic heart disease.

The last comment applies also to **resistive exercise**, which is a combination of static and heavily loaded dynamic exercise, e.g. weight lifting. Blood pressures as high as 350/250 mmHg (! – yes, really) have been recorded in young adults using a large mass of muscle at maximum effort. The high pressures are due to a combination of the Valsalva phase 1 effect (i.e. aortic compression by a raised intrathoracic pressure), the exercise pressor reflex, and compression of muscle vessels. A rise in cerebrospinal fluid pressure helps to protect the brain vessels during these extreme pressure rises.

The rise in **pulmonary blood pressure** during exercise was described in Section 15.5.

Circulating catecholamines drive the response of denervated hearts to exercise

Under normal circumstances the cardiac output during exercise is driven chiefly by the cardiac autonomic nerves. Animals and humans with denervated, transplanted hearts can, however, still increase the cardiac output during exercise. This is due to a **redundancy of control mechanisms**. The chief back-up mechanisms are the circulating catecholamines and the muscle pump.

The supportive role of **circulating catecholamines** has been studied in racing greyhounds subjected to chronic cardiac denervation. Exercise still causes a tachycardia in these animals, albeit a smaller one of slower onset (Figure 17.7). The tachycardia is due to a rise in plasma adrenaline and noradrenaline. As a result of this back-up the track speed of the cardiac-denervated greyhound is only 5% less than normal. If the back-up effect of the catecholamines is blocked by a β-adrenoceptor antagonist, exercise tachycardia is abolished in the denervated greyhounds (Figure 17.7, lower panel). Track speed now falls markedly and the greyhound finishes in a state of extreme exhaustion.

In hard human exercise **plasma noradrenaline** rises from ~1 nM to 10–20 nM, due chiefly to spillage from sympathetic vasomotor junction gaps. **Plasma adrenaline** shows little change during light to moderate exercise in humans (concentration 0.2 nM) but rises to 2–5 nM during maximal dynamic exercise owing to secretion by the adrenal medulla. These inotropic influences more than offset the negative inotropic effects of exercise-induced hyperkalaemia (up to 8 mM K^+) and lactic acidosis (plasma pH as low as 6.9).

Cardiac transplant patients also benefit from back-up by the **skeletal muscle pump**. This raises the cardiac filling pressure, and hence the stroke volume by the Frank–Starling mechanism. The above examples of redundancy of mechanisms illustrate a general principle enunciated by the respiratory physiologist, Julius H. Comroe: if a job is worth doing, the body generally has more than one way of doing it.

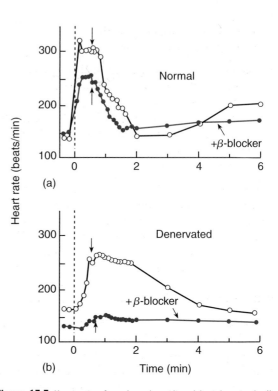

Figure 17.7 Heart rate of greyhound monitored by telemetry (radio transmitter) during a race: (a) normal; (b) after cardiac denervation. Red lines show effect of β-adrenoceptor blockade using propanolol. Response of denervated heart depended on circulating catecholamines. Arrows show time to 5/16th mile mark. (From Donald D. E., Ferguson, D. A. and Milburn, S. E. (1968) *Circulation Research*, **22**, 127–133, by permission.)

What initiates the circulatory adjustments in exercise?

With the important exception of metabolic vasodilatation the cardiovascular responses to exercise are brought about by the autonomic nervous system. What causes the brainstem to alter the autonomic outflow? Two main hypotheses have been put forward: the central command hypothesis and the peripheral reflex hypothesis. Both processes seem to contribute.

Central command

Central command was proposed by Krogh and Lindhard in 1913 (Section 16.8). It is thought that regions of the cerebral cortex, and/or related motor regions of the thalamus and basal ganglia, not only initiate voluntary movement but also 'command' the cardiovascular and respiratory centres of the medulla. A role for central command is supported by the following observations:

- The heart rate increases at the first beat after the onset of exercise (Figure 16.11). This response is so brisk that it implies 'feedforward' by the central nervous system.

- After partial neuromuscular blockade by curare, voluntary attempts to contract the partially paralysed muscle presumably require an exaggerated central command signal. The result is an enhanced tachycardia, an enhanced pressor response and enhanced resetting of the baroreflex (Figure 16.6).

Central command does not, however, readily explain a quintessential feature of the cardiac response, namely the almost linear relation between cardiac output and skeletal muscle O_2 consumption (Figure 17.5). This coupling seems to demand information from the active muscle.

Peripheral reflexes from muscle work receptors

The muscle work receptors could provide the missing link that couples cardiac output to muscle work rate. Muscle mechanoreceptors and metaboreceptors reflexly increase the heart rate and blood pressure during exercise (Figures 16.11, 16.12). Muscle mechanoreceptors contribute to the initial vagal inhibition and instant tachycardia. The progressive interstitial accumulation of chemicals such as K^+ may drive the gradual increase in tachycardia and blood pressure that is seen in the 1–2 min after the start of the exercise (Figure 17.6).

It seems likely therefore that central command and muscle work receptors, acting by **feedforward** and **feedback** respectively, drive the cardiac response to exercise. Central command and muscle mechanoreceptors produce the initial, rapid-onset tachycardia by suppressing the cardiac vagal motor neurons; and the muscle chemoreflex contributes to the subsequent slower, sympathetically mediated rise in cardiac output and peripheral vasoconstriction. Signals from joint mechanoreceptors contribute only slightly, perhaps 10%, to the increased drive to the heart.

17.4 Physical training

Endurance training leads to performance-enhancing circulatory adaptations, including increased maximum cardiac output. In an endurance event such as a medium-distance race the maximal rate of O_2 transport from the lungs to muscle mitochondria has an important influence on performance. The maximum transport rate is limited by (i) the maximum rate of O_2 uptake from the lungs, $\dot{V}_{O_2max}$; and (ii) the resistance of the diffusion pathway from capillary to muscle. For brief, power events such as sprints and shot-putting, cardiovascular adaptations are less important.

Endurance training raises maximum cardiac output and $\dot{V}_{O_2max}$

The $\dot{V}_{O_2max}$ is determined by the maximum cardiac output and haematocrit. $\dot{V}_{O_2max}$ is ~3 l O_2/min in untrained students and over 5 l O_2/min in Olympic athletes (Table 17.1). The increased $\dot{V}_{O_2max}$ of athletes is due their raised maximal cardiac output. The **cardiac output** can reach ~30 l/min in athletes, cf. 20 l/min in untrained students. The maximum output of an athlete is so high that the reduced alveolar transit time curtails gas equilibration and arterial O_2 saturation falls to ~90%.

It is interesting to compare human maximal exercise with that of an athletic animal such as a racehorse or dog. Unlike humans, many species have a contractile spleen that pumps red cells into the circulation during exercise, raising the **haematocrit**. In a galloping racehorse the haematocrit can increase by 50%, to 0.65. The arterial O_2 saturation falls to ~77%, however, at maximum effort due to the short pulmonary transit time. Moreover the high pulmonary blood flow in a galloping racehorse generates a very high pulmonary artery pressure, ~120 mmHg, and this causes a tendency to pulmonary haemorrhage.

Training-enhanced cardiac output is achieved through increased stroke volume

Dynamic training leads to:

- enlargement of the ventricular cavities
- increased myocardial vascularity
- increased blood volume by 5–10%, raising central venous pressure
- increased stroke volume
- resting bradycardia.

Left ventricle mass can increase by ~20% due to hypertrophy of the myocytes under the influence of local growth factors such as IGF (insulin-like growth factor). The cavities enlarge because new sarcomeres are added in series inside the myocyte, elongating the cells and the end-diastolic dimensions. By contrast, pressure overload in **hypertensive patients** or **isometric trained** athletes causes replication of the sarcomeres in parallel. This thickens the left ventricle wall and normalizes the wall stress, but does not increase end-diastolic dimensions.

The enlarged cavities of dynamically-trained athletes, coupled with the increased blood volume and central venous pressure, raises the ventricular EDV from ~120 ml in untrained adults to as much as 220 ml in the athlete at rest. **Stroke volume** at rest increases from the normal 70–80 ml to 100–125 ml, but the resting cardiac output is unchanged. The high stroke volume is offset at rest by a low heart rate, 40–50 beats/min. The **resting bradycardia** is produced by tonic vagal inhibition of the pacemaker. Mean blood pressure is little changed.

During maximal exercise athletes achieve up to 70% bigger stroke volumes (167 ml) than untrained subjects (Table 17.1). The maximum heart rate is unaltered (180–190 beats/min), but since athletes start with a slower heart rate, they can achieve a proportionately greater increase in rate. An increase from 40 beats/min to 180 beats/min provides a 4.5-fold increase in output, whereas an increase from 70 beats/min to 180 beats/min in an untrained human provides only a 2.6-fold increase in output.

As a result of the enhanced stroke volume and resting bradycardia, athletes can increase the right and left ventricular outputs up to seven-fold, greatly enhancing $\dot{V}_{O_2max}$. Maximal outputs of 35 l/min have been recorded in some individuals.

Exchange in muscle is enhanced by capillary angiogenesis

Endurance training improves O_2 transport in skeletal muscle by stimulating capillary growth. Capillary angiogenesis increases the exchange area and reduces diffusion distance or, if the muscle fibres hypertrophy, prevents an increase in diffusion distance. Muscle mitochondria become more abundant, especially at subsarcolemmal sites close to capillaries, and myoglobin concentration increases.

The conduit arteries too respond to endurance training. The femoral artery of a trained human has a 7–9% wider lumen and thinner wall than that of a sedentary subject.

17.5 Feeding, digestion and the splanchnic circulation

The splanchnic circulation comprises the gastrointestinal tract, spleen and pancreas, which are fed by the coeliac artery, superior and inferior mesenteric arteries (Figure 1.6). The arrival of food in the gastrointestinal tract triggers **mucosal hyperaemia**, which lasts 1–3 h. Mucosal hyperaemia is initiated partly by local hormones such as gastrin and cholecystokinin, partly by the glucose and fatty acids produced by digestion, and partly by vagal parasympathetic activity. Pancreatic secretion is accompanied by parasympathetic-mediated **pancreatic hyperaemia** (Section 14.2). As a result of these changes human splanchnic blood flow increases from a basal 1.5 l/min to 2.5 l/min after a carbohydrate meal. Conversely, splanchnic flow can be reduced to 0.3 l/min by sympathetic-mediated vasoconstriction, for example in response to hypovolaemia.

The postprandial hyperaemia evokes a **tachycardia** and **increased cardiac output** of ~1 l/min by 30–60 min after a meal. The increased cardiac work can sometimes trigger **postprandial angina** in patients with severe ischaemic heart disease. Carbohydrate meals cause the greatest hyperaemia and cardiac change.

Reflex vasoconstriction in vascular beds such as the forearm and calf prevents significant postprandial changes in blood pressure. However some elderly subjects and patients with autonomic dysfunction (e.g. diabetics) can experience **postprandial hypotension** after carbohydrate meals or oral glucose. This is due to a failure of the reflex tachycardia and limb vasoconstriction.

17.6 Diving response

Diving animals such as the duck, seal and whale show remarkable cardiovascular changes during a dive. Humans show the same responses to a lesser degree. The diving response comprises three reflexes:

- apnoea
- intense bradycardia
- peripheral vasoconstriction.

The cardiovascular changes conserve O_2 for the benefit of the heart and brain, allowing prolonged dives. The Weddell seal can survive 70 min immersion and the whale 2 h, though feeding dives are usually shorter than this. By contrast human pearl divers remain underwater for only 40–50 s. The vastly superior performance of diving animals is achieved by a combination of larger O_2 stores in blood and muscle myoglobin (Figure 17.8, bottom), more extreme cardiovascular responses and greater toleration of asphyxia. The arterial gas values in a harbour seal after a prolonged dive are 10 mmHg O_2 and

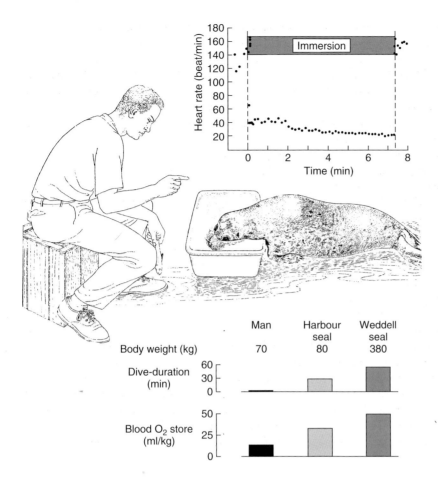

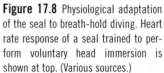

Figure 17.8 Physiological adaptation of the seal to breath-hold diving. Heart rate response of a seal trained to perform voluntary head immersion is shown at top. (Various sources.)

100 mmHg CO_2. These gas levels vastly exceed the human breath-hold breaking point and would probably be fatal to humans.

The diving response is initiated by cold water touching the **facial receptors** of the trigeminal nerve, especially around the eyes, nose and nasal mucosa. Immersion of the body but not the face, or immersion of the face wearing a breathing tube, fails to elicit the reflex. As the dive progresses, asphyxia develops and **arterial chemoreceptors** reinforce the cardiovascular responses.

Facial immersion causes human bradycardia

The heart rate of a seal can fall to 20 beats/min during a dive due to vagal inhibition of the pacemaker (Figure 17.8). Many humans too display a pronounced reflex bradycardia to facial immersion in cold water (Figure 17.9). Indeed, facial immersion has been used as a homely remedy to correct supraventricular tachycardia in patients. The reflex may also contribute to sudden deaths associated with water or foreign bodies in the airways.

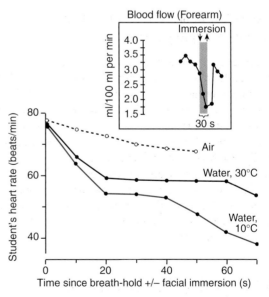

Figure 17.9 Human diving response; bradycardia in a medical student following breath-hold and facial immersion in cold water. The experiment was stopped in alarm when heart rate fell to <40/min. Boxed inset illustrates concomitant vasoconstriction in forearm. (Courtesy of J. R. Henderson (unpublished). Inset from Heistad, D. D., Abboud, F. M. and Eckstein, J. W. (1968) *Journal of Applied Physiology*, **25**, 542–549, by permission.)

Peripheral vasoconstriction diverts flow to the heart and brain

Humans respond to facial immersion with vasoconstriction in the skin and skeletal muscles (Figure 17.9 inset). Diving animals show a profound, sympathetically mediated vasoconstriction in the splanchnic, renal and skeletal muscle circulations. This overrides metabolic vasodilatation in the active muscles. Peripheral vasoconstriction maintains the blood pressure despite the extreme bradycardia, and diverts the low cardiac output to the heart and brain. Large arteries, which are safely upstream of metabolic vasodilator agents, contract strongly. A large quantity of lactic acid accumulates in the swimming muscles, leading to a sharp vasodilatation when the animal resurfaces.

17.7 Ageing

Ageing is associated with changes in vessel wall structure, raised arterial pressure (especially systolic), reduced baroreflex sensitivity and impaired cardiac performance during exercise. The changes seem to be an inevitable accompaniment of ageing and are not due to atheroma.

Elastic arteries show diffuse sclerosis of the tunica media (arteriosclerosis)

Ageing is accompanied by diffuse changes in the media of elastic arteries, leading to reduced elasticity. The elastic lamellae of the tunica media, shown in Figure 1.10, become thin, broken and disordered, possibly due to repetitive strain injury. The diffuse fracturing of the elastic lamellae weakens the elastic arteries and causes them to **dilate**. The aorta dilates by ~50% between the ages of 40 and 70 years. As the wall stretches, the wall stress is transferred to the **collagen fibres** (Figure 8.15). With advancing age more collagen is laid down, and since collagen is much stiffer than elastin, the dilated vessel becomes increasingly **stiff**. Calcium salts may also be deposited in the media, and there is intimal hyperplasia. These changes occur irrespective of whether atheroma develops.

The above degenerative changes are called arteriosclerosis. 'Sclerosis' meaning fibrous hardening, and the popular term for the condition is 'hardening of the arteries'. The condition is one of elastic vessels, not muscular arteries. Arteriosclerosis is important because it raises the pulse pressure and cardiac work, as described below.

Table 17.4 Characteristics of arteriosclerosis compared with those of atheroma.

	Arteriosclerosis of ageing	Atheroma
Epidemiology	All societies, West and East	Western lifestyle and diet
Distribution along vessel	Diffuse	Focal
Layer primarily affected	Media	Intima
Key biochemical change	Elastin fragmentation and loss	Cholesterol plaque
Effect on lumen	Dilatation	Stenosis
Effect on blood flow	None	Impaired
Resulting pathophysiology	↑ systolic pressure ↑ ventricular O_2 consumption	Tissue ischaemia

Arteriosclerosis is not atheroma

Arteriosclerosis is quite distinct from atheroma (Section 9.9), both biochemically and pathologically. Confusingly, however, atheroma is often called 'atherosclerosis' – a self-contradictory term meaning 'porridge-like hardening'! Even worse, and generating maximum confusion, atheroma is sometimes called arteriosclerosis – in which case one has to look at the context to see which condition is really meant. The differences, summarized in Table 17.4, include **distribution** (arteriosclerosis is diffuse, atheroma forms plaques), **location** (media vs intima), **biochemistry** (elastin fragmentation vs subintimal cholesterol deposition), effect on **vessel diameter** (arteriosclerotic dilatation vs atheromatous narrowing), **pathological consequence** (raised pulse pressure in arteriosclerosis, distal ischaemia in atheroma), and **epidemiology** (loss of elasticity with ageing in all cultures cf. atheroma associated with Western lifestyle).

Arterial blood pressure increases with age

The pattern of pressure change with ageing has not altered from early in the last century to the present day, and is the same in Eastern and Western populations.

Mean blood pressure increases moderately with age due to a rise in total peripheral resistance (Figure 17.10). The increased resistance may be due at least in part to a rise in peripheral sympathetic activity, as indicated by neural recordings and by an enhanced dilator response to the α-adrenoceptor blocker phentolamine.

Systolic pressure increases much more than mean pressure owing to the reduced compliance of

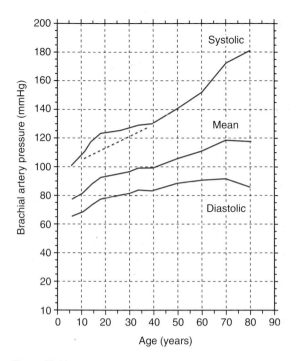

Figure 17.10 Effect of ageing on brachial artery pressure in a British population. Systolic pressure (mmHg) is roughly 100 + age here. Recent Australian and American surveys show the same pattern but a less steep climb after 40 years, reaching ~145/85 mmHg at 70 years. Dashed line shows inferred aortic systolic pressure (see text). (Data from Miall and Oldham (1936) *British Medical Journal*, I, 75.)

the elastic vessels, i.e. arteriosclerosis. In the brachial artery, where pressure is normally measured, **systolic pressure** increases steeply from childhood until age 20, levels off until age 30–40, then climbs thereafter, rising by 30–40 mmHg at age 80. The levelling off of brachial systolic pressure at 20–40 years is attributed to the gradual loss of distal pressure amplification, a phenomenon illustrated in Figure 8.11. **Aortic systolic pressure** probably pursues a more even climb. Aortic systolic pressure is more important than brachial systolic pressure because it represents the afterload against which the ventricle must eject the stroke volume.

Systolic pressure is raised through reduced compliance and fast wave reflection

Systolic pressure and pulse pressure increase disproportionately with ageing due to two effects of arteriosclerosis:

1 Pulse pressure is approximately equal to stroke volume divided by arterial compliance (Section 7.4). Therefore a fall in compliance

due to arteriosclerosis raises the pulse pressure. Clinical hypertension accelerates the ageing process and exaggerates this effect (Figure 18.8).

2 The velocity of propagation of the pulse is related to wall stiffness. In the aorta, where the increase in wall stiffness is greatest, the pulse wave velocity more than doubles from ~4 m/s at 25 years to ~10 m/s at 70 years. The reflected wave now travels so fast that it returns to the aorta during systole, adding to aortic systolic pressure (Figure 8.10). Reflection is estimated to add ~25 mmHg to systolic pressure between age 30 and age 60.

High systolic pressures impair left ventricular performance

Systolic pressure in the aorta represents the afterload against which the left ventricle has to eject the stroke volume. A high systolic pressure reduces the ability of the ventricle to eject the stroke volume, particularly in exercise. Also, by raising cardiac work it raises the O_2 demand of the ageing heart. Arteriosclerosis can therefore contribute to heart failure in the elderly. The severity of cardiovascular disease is more closely related to systolic than diastolic pressure, and cardiovascular disease is reduced by the therapeutic reduction of systolic hypertension.

Cardiac performance during exercise is impaired

Ageing has little effect on stroke volume and heart rate at rest, though myocardial O_2 demand increases as explained above. Also ventricular relaxation and early diastolic filling slow down. The chief effect of ageing on the heart is to reduce its ability to respond to stresses such as exercise.

Maximum heart rate in exercise

The maximum attainable heart rate decreases with advancing age. As a rule-of-thumb the maximum beats/min is approximately 220 minus age in years. The decline in maximum rate is probably due to a reduced pacemaker response to β_1-adrenoceptor activation (see below). The responsiveness of the heart to the baroreflex is also reduced.

Maximum stroke volume in exercise

The ability to raise the ventricular ejection fraction, i.e. reduce the ESV, is progressively impaired despite ample adrenoceptor stimulation. Stroke volume can still be raised during exercise, but this is achieved through a rise in EDV and the Frank–Starling mechanism.

The decline in maximum heart rate and ejection fraction is due to impaired responsiveness to β-adrenoceptor stimulation. There is ample catecholamine release but the β_1-adrenoceptors do not trigger as big a rise in intracellular cAMP in the ageing heart as in a young heart. The decline in contractile power with ageing is also partly of anatomical origin. Counts of nuclei in the myocardium indicate that many millions of myocytes are lost each year, though there is some compensatory hypertrophy of the remaining myocytes (>1000 million cells).

17.8 Sleep and the alerting response

Sleep involves a fall in metabolic rate and reduced O_2 consumption. This is accompanied by a characteristic pattern of cardiovascular and respiratory changes, namely:

- bradycardia and a low cardiac output
- reduced blood pressure (e.g. 80/50 mmHg, Figure 8.13)
- splanchnic vasodilatation
- reduced ventilation.

During the non-rapid-eye-movement phase on first falling asleep (non-REM) bradycardia accounts for the hypotension. Later, in REM sleep, dilatation of the splanchnic circulation also contributes. Cerebral blood flow is increased to many regions despite the low blood pressure.

The **alerting response** to unusual or threatening environmental stimuli was described in Section 16.8. It originates from the central long axis of the brain and is in many respects the opposite of the sleep response, being characterized by:

- tachycardia
- increased blood pressure
- splanchnic, renal and cutaneous vasoconstriction
- muscle vasodilatation
- increased ventilation.

The alerting response is clearly an appropriate preparation for imminent physical action.

SUMMARY

Posture

■ On standing, distension of dependent veins by gravity redistributes ~500 ml blood from the thorax into the lower limbs. The reduced cardiac filling pressure leads via the Frank–Starling mechanism to a 30–40% fall in stroke volume and arterial pulse pressure. A transient fall in mean pressure can cause postural hypotension and dizziness in warm, venodilated subjects.

■ The fall in pulse pressure and carotid sinus pressure reduce arterial baroreceptor activity. This evokes a reflex peripheral vasoconstriction, splanchnic venoconstriction and increase in heart rate by 15–20 beats/min, which together restore the mean arterial pressure.

■ Over long periods increased capillary filtration into the dependent limbs reduces plasma volume by ~12%. Reflex increases in plasma vasopressin and renin–angiotensin–aldosterone reduce the excretion of salt and water.

Valsalva manoeuvre

■ Forced expiration against a closed glottis raises intrathoracic and arterial pressure by mechanical compression (phase 1).

■ The impeded venous return results in a progressive fall in stroke volume and arterial pressure. The latter elicits a reflex tachycardia and peripheral vasoconstriction, leading to pressure stabilization (phase 2).

■ On resumption of normal breathing, intrathoracic and arterial pressure immediately fall (phase 3).

■ The inrush of accumulated venous blood raises stroke volume (Frank–Starling mechanism). The resulting rise in pulse pressure triggers reflex bradycardia (phase 4), which is used as a clinical test of autonomic function.

Exercise

■ **Muscle metabolic hyperaemia** (increased blood flow), along with **capillary recruitment** and **steepened concentration gradients**, speed up O_2 and glucose delivery to active fibres. The increased blood flow is due chiefly to metabolic vasodilatation, aided by the muscle pump in upright exercise and a relatively small rise in arterial pressure.

■ **Increased cardiac output** provides the increased muscle perfusion and increases gas exchange in the lungs (Fick's principle). Output rises in proportion to muscle O_2 consumption. Output can increase four times to ~ 20 l/min in untrained students. Pulmonary O_2 uptake can increase more (12–13 times) because the mixed venous O_2 content falls (Fick's principle).

■ The **tachycardia** (max 180–190 beats/min) is driven by withdrawal of vagal tone and increased sympathetic activity. **Stroke volume** increases mainly in upright, dynamic exercise. Increases of 50–100% result from sympathetic-mediated increased contractility (reducing end-systolic volume) and increased end-diastolic volume (effect of muscle pump and reflex venoconstriction).

■ The autonomic outflow driving the raised cardiac output is elicited by **central command** from the forebrain (feedforward) and by a **pressor reflex from work receptors** in active muscle (feedback).

■ **Reflex adjustment of other vascular beds** regulate blood pressure and core temperature. Sympathetic-mediated vasoconstriction in the splanchnic circulation, renal circulation and inactive muscles counters the hypotensive effect of vasodilatation in active muscle, respiratory muscles, myocardium and, later, skin (for heat dissipation). Mean arterial pressure, controlled by a reset baroreflex, can rise by $\sim 20\%$ in hard dynamic exercise but more in static (isometric) exercise due to a stronger muscle metaboreflex. Severe isometric or resistive exercise is best avoided by patients with ischaemic heart disease.

Maintain bp

Training

■ Improved cardiovascular performance is of value chiefly in dynamic, endurance events.

■ Endurance training enlarges the ventricular cavities through sarcomere addition. End-diastolic volume and stroke volume are increased at rest and in exercise.

■ Resting cardiac output is unaltered because a vagally-mediated bradycardia of 40–50 beats/min offsets the rise in stroke volume. Maximum heart rate remains 180–190/min. Thus the heart rate can increase 4-fold on exercise, in contrast to the normal 2½-fold. Cardiac outputs of 35 l/min are possible in athletes.

■ Capillary angiogenesis in endurance-trained muscle and myocardium promotes diffusional exchange.

Response to feeding

■ Mucosal hyperaemia is most pronounced after a carbohydrate meal but more prolonged after a fatty meal. The hyperaemia is mediated by local hormones (gastrin, vasoactive intestinal polypeptide) and vagal parasympathetic activity.

■ The hyperaemia of up to 1 l/min necessitates increased cardiac output. Blood pressure is also supported by vasoconstriction in the limbs. If the latter fails, as in some elderly subjects and those with autonomic neuropathy, postprandial hypotension can develop.

Diving response

■ Stimulation of facial and nasal mucosal receptors by cold water evokes a reflex bradycardia, peripheral vasoconstriction and apnoea.

■ As asphyxia develops, arterial chemoreceptors reinforce the cardiovascular changes.

■ The cardiovascular changes conserve the O_2 store for the benefit of the brain and heart. In man, active dives of up to 40–50 seconds are possible; in whales, up to 2 h.

Ageing

■ Arteriosclerosis is elastin fragmentation and fibrosis of the media in ageing elastic arteries. The reduced compliance (increased stiffness) and early return of the reflected wave raise systolic pressure and hence cardiac work.

■ Mean pressure rises too, probably due to a sympathetic-mediated increase in peripheral resistance.

■ The cardiac response to exercise is impaired. Maximum heart rate and the ability to raise the ejection fraction decline due to impaired responsiveness to β_1-adrenoceptor stimulation (reduced coupling of receptors to second messenger production). Stroke volume is raised instead by increasing the end-diastolic volume.

The alerting response and sleep

■ The alerting response to stress involves tachycardia, increased blood pressure, splanchnic, renal and cutaneous vasoconstriction, muscle vasodilatation and increased ventilation.

■ Sleep evokes bradycardia, reduced low cardiac output, reduced blood pressure, splanchnic vasodilatation and reduced ventilation.

FURTHER READING

Posture (orthostasis)

Huisman, H. W., Pretorius, P. J., Van Rooyen, J. M., Malan, N. T., Eloff, F. C., Laubscher, P. J. and Steyn, H. S. (1999) Haemodynamic changes in the cardiovascular system during the early phases of orthostasis. *Acta Physiological Scandinavica*, **166**, 145–149.

Jacob, G., Ertl, A. C., Shannon, J. R., Furlan, R., Robertson, R. M. and Robertson, D. (1998) Effect of standing on neurohumoral responses and plasma volume in healthy subjects. *Journal of Applied Physiology*, **84**, 914–921.

Smit, A. A. J., Halliwill, J. R., Low, P. A. and Wieling, W. (1999) Pathophysiological basis of orthostatic hypotension in autonomic failure. *Journal of Physiology*, **519**, 1–10.

Wieling, W., Halliwill, J. R. and Karemaker, J. M. (2002) Orthostatic intolerance after space flight (Perspective). *Journal of Physiology*, **538**, 1.

Valsalva

Smith, M. L., Beightol, L. A., Fritsch-Yelle, J. M., Ellenbogen, K. A., Porter T. R. and Eckberg, D. L. (1996) Valsalva's maneuver revisited: a quantitative method yielding insight into human autonomic control. *American Journal of Physiology*, **271**, H1240–1249.

Exercise, training and stress

Reviews and chapters

Blomqvist, C. G. and Saltin, B. (1983) Cardiovascular adaptations to physical training. *Annual Review of Physiology*, **45**, 169–189.

Bove, A. A. (1989) Hormonal responses to acute and chronic exercise. *News in Physiological Sciences*, **4**, 143–146.

Christensen, N. J. and Galbo, H. (1983) Sympathetic nervous activity during exercise. *Annual Review of Physiology*, **45**, 139–153.

Coote, J. H. and Bothams, V. F. (2001) Cardiac vagal control before, during and after exercise. *Experimental Physiology*, **86**, 811–815.

Fletcher, G. F. (ed.) (1994) *Cardiovascular Response to Exercise*, American Heart Association Monograph, New York, Futura.

Jones, J. H. and Linstedt, S. L. (1993) Limits to maximal performance. *Annual Reviews of Physiology*, **55**, 547–569.

Rowell, L. B. and Shepherd, J. T. (eds) (1996) *Exercise: Regulation and Integration of Multiple Systems*. Handbook of Physiology Section 12, Oxford University Press, New York.

Research papers

Dinenno, F. A., Tanaka, H., Monahan, K. D., Clevenger, C. M., Eskurza, I., DeSouza, C. A. and Seals, D. R. (2001) Regular endurance exercise induces expansive arterial remodelling in the trained limbs of healthy men. *Journal of Physiology*, **534**, 287–295.

Friedman, D. B., Jensen, F. B., Mitchell, J. H. and Secher, N. H. (1990) Heart rate and arterial blood pressure at the onset of static exercise in man with complete neural blockade. *Journal of Physiology*, **423**, 543–550.

Gandevia, S. C. and Hobbs, S. F. (1990) Cardiovascular responses to static exercise in man: central and reflex contributions. *Journal of Physiology*, **430**, 105–117.

Harms, C. A., McClaran, S. R., Nickele, G. A., Pegelow, D. F., Nelson, W. B. and Dempsey, J. A. (1998) Exercise-induced arterial hypoxaemia in healthy young women. *Journal of Physiology*, **507**, 619–628.

Jensen-Urstad, M., Bouvier, F., Nejat, M., Saltin, B. and Brodin, L-A. (1998) Left ventricular function in endurance runners during exercise. *Acta Physiologica Scandinavica*, **164**, 167–172.

Kjaer, M., Perko, G., Secher, N. H., *et al.* (1994) Cardiopulmonary and ventilatory responses to electrically induced cycling with complete epidural anaesthesia in humans. *Acta Physiologica Scandinavica*, **151**, 199–207.

Perko, M. J., Nielsen, H. B., Skak, C., Clemmesen, J. O., Schroeder, T. V. and Secher, N. H. (1998) Mesenteric, coeliac and splanchnic blood flow in humans during exercise. *Journal of Physiology*, **513**, 907–913.

Wieling, W., Harms, M. P. M., ten Harkel, A. D. J., van Lieshout, J. J. and Sprangers, R. L. H. (1996) Circulatory responses evoked by a 3 s bout of dynamic leg exercise in humans. *Journal of Physiology*, **494**, 601–611.

Feeding

Kearney, M. T., Cowley, A. J. and MacDonald, I. A. (1995) The cardiovascular responses to feeding in man. *Experimental Physiology*, **80**, 683–700.

O'Donovan, D., Feinle, C., Tonkin, A., Horowitz, M. and Jones, K. L. (2002) Postprandial hypotension in response to duodenal glucose delivery in healthy older subjects. *Journal of Physiology*, **540**, 673–679.

Waaler, B. A. and Eriksen, M. (1992) Post-prandial cardiovascular responses in man after ingestion of carbohydrate, protein or fat. *Acta Physiologica Scandinavica*, **146**, 321–327.

Diving response

Butler, P. J. and Jones, D. R. (1997) Physiology of diving of birds and mammals. *Physiological Reviews*, **77**, 837–899.

de Burgh Daly, M. (1997) *Peripheral Arterial Chemoreceptors and Respiration–Cardiovascular Integration*, Oxford, Clarendon Press.

Ageing

Fleg, J. L. (1994) Effects of aging on the cardiovascular response to exercise. In Fletcher, G. F. (ed.) *Cardiovascular Response to Exercise*, New York, Futura. pp. 387–404.

Folkow, B. and Svanborg, A. (1993) Physiology of cardiovascular aging. *Physiological Reviews*, **73**, 725–745.

Nichols, W. W. and O'Rourke, M. F. (1998) *McDonald's Blood Flow in Arteries*, 4th Edition, Arnold, London.

Olivetti, G., Melissari, M., Capasso, J. M. and Anvers, P. (1991) Cardiomyopathy of the aging human heart. *Circulation Research*, **68**, 1560–1568.

Seals, D. R. and Esler, M. D. (2000) Human ageing and the sympathoadrenal system. *Journal of Physiology*, **528**, 407–417.

Sleep

Franzini, C., Zoccoli, G., Cianci, T. and Lenzi, P. (1996) Sleep-dependent changes in regional circulations. *News in Physiological Sciences*, **11**, 274–280.

Marshall, J. M. (1995) Cardiovascular changes associated with sleep. In *Cardiovascular Regulation* (eds Jordan, D. and Marshall, J.), Portland Press, London, pp. 61–76.

CHAPTER 18

Cardiovascular responses in pathological situations

Learning objectives

After reading this chapter you should be able to:

- Outline the cardiovascular responses to systemic hypoxaemia (18.1).
- List the principal causes of acute circulatory failure (clinical shock) (18.2).
- Describe the reflexes supporting blood pressure and plasma volume during hypovolaemia (18.2).
- State the cardiovascular events that precipitate fainting (18.3).
- Define 'hypertension' and list its clinical consequences (18.4).
- Draw the hypertensive pressure pulse and state the vascular changes that underlie (i) the increased mean pressure; and (ii) the disproportionate increase in systolic pressure (18.4).
- Outline the chief aetiological theories for hypertension (18.4).
- Define chronic cardiac failure and sketch the altered ventricular function curve (18.5).
- Outline the changes in excitation–contraction coupling and electrophysiology of failing myocytes (18.5).
- List the changes in cardiac performance at rest and in exercise in heart failure (18.5).
- Describe the peripheral circulatory response to heart failure (18.5).
- Explain how and where oedema arises in heart failure (18.5).

The previous chapter described co-ordinated cardiovascular response to physiological challenges. This final chapter considers how the circulation reacts to pathological situations, taking examples from the field of human disease. The first example, systemic hypoxaemia, is encountered both in chronic lung disease and in healthy individuals at high altitudes.

18.1 Systemic hypoxaemia

Systemic hypoxaemia is a subnormal partial pressure of O_2 in arterial blood. It can be due to high altitude, asphyxiation, lung diseases such as chronic emphysema or pulmonary oedema, and right-to-left shunts through congenital heart defects. The following account focuses on high altitude hypoxaemia, which can be simulated in the laboratory by reducing the O_2 content of the inspired air (Figure 18.1).

Arterial P_{O_2} falls with increasing altitude

Oxygen makes up 21% of the atmosphere. Since atmospheric pressure at sea level is $\sim$760 mmHg or 100 kPa, the partial pressure of inspired oxygen, P_{O_2}, is 160 mmHg or 21 kPa. Alveolar P_{O_2} is lower, namely 100 mmHg or 13 kPa, due to oxygen extraction by blood. Arterial P_{O_2} is virtually the same as alveolar P_{O_2}, and the resulting haemoglobin saturation is 97% at sea level.

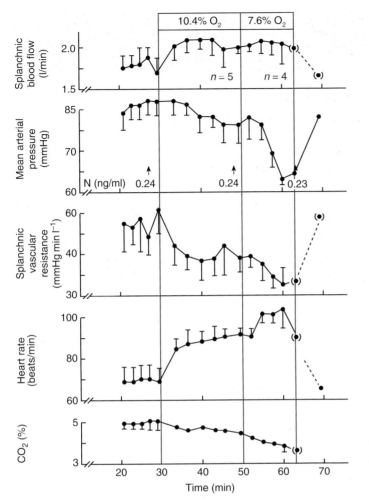

Figure 18.1 Human responses to moderate and severe hypoxaemia. Inspired O_2 (normally 21%, with an arterial P_{O_2} of 100 mmHg) was reduced to 10.4% (equivalent altitude 5500 m), then to 7.6% (equivalent to a major Himalayan summit; arterial P_{O_2} 27 mmHg). Alveolar CO_2 falls due to hyperventilation. N, noradrenaline. (After Rowell, L. B. (1986); see Further Reading.)

Atmospheric pressure and P_{O_2} fall with increasing altitude. Oxygen saturation shows little change up to 2000 m owing to the plateau on the haemoglobin dissociation curve (Figure 15.3). Saturation begins to fall significantly when arterial P_{O_2} drops below 60 mmHg (8 kPa), at 3000 m and above. Such altitudes are commonly experienced by cable-car-borne skiers, tourists and Alpinists and raise the ventilation and cardiac output at rest. On major Alpine summits ~4000 m above sea level the arterial P_{O_2} drops to 45 mmHg (6 kPa), about half normal. Even so, there is permanent human habitation up to 5000 m in the Andes, and acclimatized individuals have survived several days without supplementary O_2 on Himalayan peaks above 8000 m.

Humans respond to arterial hypoxaemia with increased cardiac output, peripheral vasodilatation and hyperventilation, as follows.

Resting hyperventilation improves arterial P_{O_2}

The hypoxic stimulation of arterial chemoreceptors (Section 16.6) causes a reflex increase in ventilation at rest. The hyperventilation **increases alveolar P_{O_2}** towards the inspired level, and **reduces alveolar P_{CO_2}** (hypocapnia, Figure 18.1). The hypocapnia shifts the haemoglobin dissociation curve to the left (**reverse Bohr shift**), which enables arterial blood to take up more O_2 at the prevailing alveolar P_{O_2} but reduces O_2 unloading in the tissues. Hypocapnia also attenuates the central and peripheral chemoreceptor activity and therefore **attenuates the ventilatory response**. This is an important difference between altitude hypoxaemia and asphyxia; in **asphyxia** the arterial P_{CO_2} rises, adding to the ventilatory stimulus.

Resting cardiac output is raised

A fall in arterial P_{O_2} reduces the blood-to-tissue gradient for O_2. As a result, less O_2 is extracted from each millilitre of blood and the **arteriovenous O_2 difference falls**. For example, at 7.5% inspired O_2 (a Himalayan degree of hypoxia) the arterial O_2 content is 120 ml/l (normal 195 ml/l) and the mixed venous O_2 is 90 ml/l (normal 145 ml/l). The $(A-V)_{O_2}$ is 30 ml/l as opposed to 50 ml/l at sea level. The increase in cardiac output at rest compensates for the fall in $(A-V)_{O_2}$. The increased cardiac output (8 l/min in the above case) multiplied by the reduced $(A-V)_{O_2}$ allows a normal resting O_2 uptake and consumption, ~ 250 ml/min (**Fick's principle**, Section 7.1).

The cardiac output is raised by a **resting tachycardia**, up to 100 beats/min (Figure 18.1). The tachycardia is due to the withdrawal of vagal inhibition of the pacemaker. This cannot be attributed to the arterial chemoreflex (Section 16.6), nor to pacemaker hypoxia, both of which cause bradycardia. Reduced vagal activity might be due to central suppression of cardiac vagal motor neurons by the hyperactive inspiratory neurons (Figure 16.15).

Reduced peripheral resistance raises tissue perfusion

In humans, arterial hypoxaemia dilates the systemic resistance vessels, particularly in the coronary and splanchnic circulations (Figure 18.1). The dilatation is due to adenosine and adrenaline. Increased sympathetic activity due to the arterial chemoreflex restrains the degree of dilatation, as shown by enhanced hypoxic vasodilatation after α-adrenoceptor blockade.

Cerebral vessels show little vasodilatation, because hypocapnia increases cerebrovascular tone.

Pulmonary arterial pressure rises, systemic arterial pressure falls

Hypoxia reduces systemic arterial pressure through peripheral vasodilatation (Figure 18.1). In the lungs, by contrast, hypoxic pulmonary vasoconstriction leads to pulmonary hypertension (Section 15.5). Resting mean pressure in the pulmonary artery can double to ~ 30 mmHg, which improves apical perfusion and the ventilation–perfusion ratio (Figure 15.19). If pulmonary hypertension is prolonged, however, as in chronic emphysema, the increased right ventricular workload eventually leads to **right heart failure**. Failure is exacerbated by the negative inotropic effect of hypoxaemia (Section 6.12).

Hypoxaemic exercise requires exaggerated cardiac outputs

During submaximal hypoxaemic exercise the cardiac output is higher than normal for a given work rate and O_2 consumption. Blood flow to the active muscle is likewise higher than normal. Maximal heart rate and output are reduced, however, by hypoxic pacemaker depression. Consequently the maximum O_2 transport rate $V_{O_2 max}$ is reduced, severely limiting exercise performance at Himalayan altitudes.

Altitude can cause mountain sickness and pulmonary oedema

Unacclimatized subjects who ascend too rapidly to >3000 m (10 000 ft) often experience **acute mountain sickness** after 8–24 h. Acute mountain sickness comprises headache, dizziness, sweating, nausea, vomiting, sleeplessness and irritability. The cerebral symptoms are attributed to the effects of hypoxaemia and acute respiratory alkalosis (low P_{CO_2}) on neuronal function. Treatment includes descent to a lower altitude, supplementary O_2, acetazolamide (to stimulate renal excretion of bicarbonate and so counterbalance the respiratory alkalosis) and in severe cases the steroid dexamethasone to reduce cerebral oedema.

Acute pulmonary oedema is distinct from acute mountain sickness. It can occur in subjects with predisposing factors, such as ischaemic heart disease, on rapid ascent to high altitude. Pulmonary oedema is also common in climbers exposed for too long to extreme altitude.

Acclimatization develops during chronic exposure to hypoxaemia

Slow, progressive exposure to altitude over several days allows time for acclimatization and prevents acute mountain sickness. Acclimatization involves the following adaptations.

- There is a further **increase in resting ventilation** above the acute hypoxaemic level. The extra drive to breathing is traditionally attributed to the renal correction of respiratory alkalosis.

- Production of 2,3-diphosphoglycerate in the red cells shifts the haemoglobin dissociation curve to the right (**Bohr shift**). This improves O_2 unloading in the tissues.

- The **blood O_2-carrying capacity** is increased by a rise in haematocrit, which can reach 0.6. The erythropoiesis is stimulated by renal erythropoietin. The attendant high viscosity increases the risk of a thrombotic event such as a **high-altitude stroke**.

18.2 Shock and haemorrhage

Clinical shock is an acute failure of the circulation

The term 'shock' is used by the medical profession and general public in different senses. In general conversation the term refers to an emotional reaction to a traumatic experience, perhaps with physical manifestations such as muscle tremor, but without organic pathology. Clinical shock, by contrast, is a potentially fatal, **pathophysiological disorder characterized by acute failure of the cardiovascular system to perfuse the tissues of the body adequately.** This acute circulatory failure results in the following characteristic signs:

- The skin is pale, cold, sweaty and venoconstricted.

- The pulse is rapid and weak, due to a tachycardia and small stroke volume.

- Mean arterial pressure may be reduced or normal but pulse pressure is always reduced.

- Breathing is rapid and shallow.

- Urine output is reduced.

- There may be reduced mental awareness or confusion, muscular weakness and collapse.

The causes of clinical shock

Clinical shock can be divided into four categories:

1 **Hypovolaemic shock** is caused by a fall in blood or plasma volume, which may be due to external fluid loss (haemorrhage, diarrhoea, vomiting, dehydration) or internal fluid loss (extensive burns, crushing injuries, pancreatitis).

2 **Septic shock** is caused by cardiovascular toxins such as endotoxin released by infecting bacteria.

3 **Cardiogenic shock** is caused by the acute impairment of cardiac function by myocardial infarction, myocarditis or an arrhythmia.

4 **Anaphylactic shock** is caused by an intense allergic reaction to antigens to which the patient has become sensitized, e.g. foodstuffs, antibiotics, insect bites.

Although the pathophysiological responses vary to some extent with the cause, there is a common pattern which is illustrated below by considering a very common medical emergency, acute haemorrhage.

Haemorrhagic shock triggers compensatory reflexes

A 10% blood loss represents a standard blood donation and does not threaten the cardiovascular system significantly. A rapid 20–30% blood loss may or may not reduce the mean arterial pressure, depending on the compensatory responses, but it causes clinical shock. With prompt treatment a 20–30% loss is not usually life-threatening. A 30–40% blood loss reduces arterial pressure to 50–70 mmHg and causes severe, sometimes irreversible shock, with anuria and impaired cerebral and coronary perfusion.

The immediate effect of acute hypovolaemia is to reduce the central blood volume and hence ventricular end-diastolic volume. This reduces the contractile energy through the **Frank–Starling mechanism**, so the stroke volume and pulse pressure decline. A large, rapid blood loss will also reduce the mean arterial pressure. Arterial hypotension, it will be noted, is mediated by the Frank–Starling mechanism and is in no way analogous to the loss of pressure in a punctured tyre!

A set of reflex responses helps to support the arterial pressure in shock and thus safeguard cerebral and myocardial perfusion. The activity of **cardiopulmonary stretch receptors** and **arterial baroreceptors** declines or ceases (Figure 18.2). **Arterial chemoreceptor** activity is raised by a metabolic acidosis (Figure 18.3, bottom) and by reduced

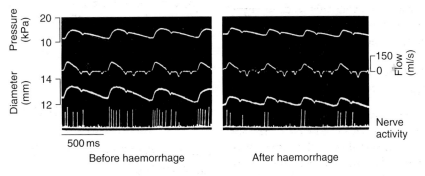

Before haemorrhage   After haemorrhage

Figure 18.2 Aortic baroreceptor discharge (single fibre), aortic diameter and aortic pressure before (left) and after (right) a slow haemorrhage of 20% blood volume in dog. Note that pulse pressure is reduced, due to fall in stroke volume, but *mean* pressure is unchanged (compensated phase). The reduced baroreceptor activity is attributed to the fall in pulse pressure and aortic diameter (presumably the result of active constriction). (After Hartikainen, J., *et al.* (1990) *Acta Physiologia Scandinavica*, **140**, 181–190.)

chemoreceptor perfusion (stagnant hypoxia). The arterial chemoreflex input drives the characteristic rapid ventilation of shock. The abnormal pattern of inputs into the **nucleus tractus solitarius** evokes a reflex increase in **sympathetic outflow** and raised levels of **circulating vasoactive hormones**, namely angiotensin II, adrenaline, noradrenaline and vasopressin.

With blood losses of 20% or less the increased neuroendocrine outflow maintains the mean blood pressure near normal. This is called a **compensated haemorrhage**. With blood losses over 30% a second phase may develop in which blood pressure falls rapidly – the **decompensated phase**.

The body defences during compensated, non-hypotensive hypovolaemia occur over three time scales: rapid reflexes that act within seconds; intermediate responses that act over 5–60 min; and slow responses that act over days–weeks, as follows.

Rapid reflexes immediately support arterial pressure

A reflex increase in sympathetic vasomotor activity constricts the resistance vessels in the cutaneous, skeletal muscle, splanchnic and renal vascular beds.

The resulting **increased total peripheral resistance** provides immediate support to the arterial pressure. However the **reduced tissue perfusion** causes muscular weakness, lactic acidosis, oligura (low urine flow) and skin pallor. Increased sympathetic cholinergic discharge to skin causes sweating and the characteristic cold, clammy skin. White cell adhesion in microvessels contributes to the poor tissue perfusion in severe shock.

Reflex **venoconstriction** in the splanchnic and cutaneous circulations partially restores the thoracic blood volume and cardiac filling pressure. The attending physician becomes acutely aware of the cutaneous venoconstriction when he or she attempts to cannulate a vein for intravenous fluid replacement!

Filling pressure remains subnormal despite the venoconstriction, so the stroke volume remains low. The reduction of cardiac output is partly counteracted by increased cardiac sympathetic activity, which causes **tachycardia** and enhances **myocardial contractility**.

The above sympathetic-mediated responses are reinforced by increased levels of **circulating vasoconstrictor hormones**, namely angiotensin II, adrenaline, noradrenaline and vasopressin. Angiotensin II and catecholamine levels increase substantially during

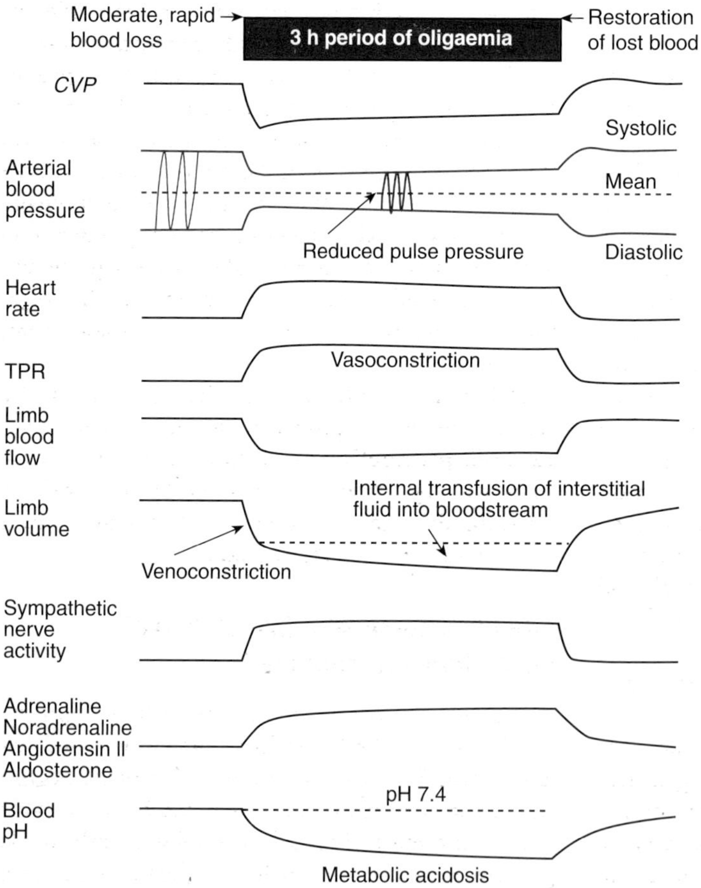

Figure 18.3 Compensated haemorrhage, showing responses to a blood loss of ≤20%. Mean blood pressure is maintained, although pulse pressure falls. Slow fall in limb volume, below dashed line, is due to capillary absorption of interstitial fluid into circulation. With a more severe oligaemia, mean arterial pressure falls, and retransfusion may fail to halt a progressive fall in pressure (decompensated phase), leading to death. (Adapted from Chien, S. (1967) *Physiological Reviews*, **47**, 214–288; and Jacobsen, J, *et al.* (1990); see Further Reading; and Länne, T. and Lundvall, J. (1992); see Further Reading.)

compensated, normotensive haemorrhage, whereas vasopressin only reaches high enough levels to cause vasoconstriction during hypotensive haemorrhage.

Studies using ACE inhibitors indicate that **angiotensin II** accounts for ~30% of the initial recovery of arterial pressure in venesected dogs. The renin−angiotensin system is activated by the increased renal sympathetic activity, reduced renal artery pressure and reduced sodium load at the macula densa. Angiotensin II contributes to the peripheral vasoconstriction by both local and central actions (Section 14.8).

Vasopressin contributes significantly to vasomotor tone only in severe, hypotensive haemorrhage. Vasopressin is secreted by the hypothalamic magnocellular neurons as a reflex response to the fall in baroreceptor input.

Because of the compensation provided by the increased peripheral resistance, reduced venous capacitance and increased cardiac performance, mean arterial pressure may be well maintained following a moderate haemorrhage. This means that **arterial pressure is not a reliable index of blood loss**.

Capillary absorption causes a slow internal transfusion of fluid

The fall in venous pressure and the sympathetic-mediated increase in pre- to postcapillary resistance ratio R_A/R_V reduce capillary blood pressure (Figure 11.4). This allows the plasma colloid osmotic pressure (COP) to predominate and results in a **transient absorption of interstitial fluid** called the 'internal transfusion' (Figure 11.11b). Up to 500 ml of fluid can be absorbed into the human vascular compartment within an hour, partially restoring the depleted plasma volume but reducing the haematocrit and plasma protein concentration. Much of the internal transfusion comes from skeletal muscle, because muscle accounts for 40% of the body weight. Fluid return is also helped by increased lymphatic pumping. The internal transfusion explains why most haemorrhagic patients have a reduced haematocrit by the time they reach hospital. The internal transfusion is halted within an hour by a fall in interstitial fluid pressure, rise in interstitial COP and fall in plasma COP (haemodilution).

The substantial size of the internal transfusion is partly due to a second mechanism that brings the much bigger **intracellular fluid compartment** into play. Increased levels of adrenaline and glucagon trigger glycogenolysis in the liver. The hepatic output of glucose rises sharply, raising the osmolarity of the plasma and interstitial compartments by up to 20 mOsm. The increased interstitial osmolarity draws fluid osmotically from the big intracellular compartment into the smaller interstitial compartment. The replenishment of the interstitial compartment allows capillary absorption to continue for 30−60 min, much longer than would otherwise be possible. It is estimated that about half of the internal transfusion comes indirectly from the intracellular compartment.

The internal transfusion helps to raise the low cardiac filling pressure. The attendant haemodilution reduces the blood viscosity and improves tissue perfusion, but also reduces the O_2-carrying capacity of blood.

Long-term renal and biosynthetic responses restore blood volume

In compensated shock the above responses preserve the perfusion of the heart and brain. The patient is left, however, with a reduced perfusion of other organs due to a subnormal mass of body water, electrolytes, plasma protein and red cells. These deficiencies are corrected gradually over days and weeks.

The water and salt deficits are corrected first, through reduced renal excretion and increased fluid intake. **Glomerular filtration rate** is reduced by a sympathetic-mediated contraction of the afferent arterioles. **Salt and water reabsorption** are stimulated by increased plasma aldosterone and vasopressin levels. The high plasma angiotensin II not only stimulates aldosterone secretion but also stimulates the subfornical organ of the brain to cause intense **thirst**. The combination of increased water intake and oliguria quickly replenishes the body water content. The normal dietary intake of 2−10 g salt per day, combined with salt retention by the renal tubules, replenishes the extracellular salt mass within a few days.

Albumin synthesis by the liver gradually restores the plasma protein mass over a week or so. **Red cell production** by the bone marrow is stimulated by erythropoietin secreted by the kidney. Erythropoiesis restores a normal haematocrit in a few weeks if iron intake is adequate.

The decompensated (hypotensive) phase leads to organ failure

The above events are typical of reversible, compensated shock. If the blood loss exceeds 30% and has lasted over 3−4 h before fluid replacement begins, shock enters a second phase that can be irreversible even if the entire blood loss is subsequently made good by transfusion. In such cases the blood pressure may be partially maintained for a while by the high sympathetic outflow, but pressure then begins to fall (decompensated phase), leading to myocardial hypoperfusion and possibly death.

The collapse of blood pressure in the decompensated phase is caused chiefly by a profound **peripheral vasodilatation**, except in skin. The switch from vasoconstriction to vasodilatation is due chiefly to a reduction in sympathetic vasoconstrictor outflow. This outweighs the effects of the raised plasma angiotensin II, adrenaline and vasopressin. The cause of the reduced sympathetic drive is uncertain, but central pathways involving **δ-opiate receptors** may be involved. The release of endogenous opioids such as enkephalins and β-endorphins may depress the medullary vasomotor regions. In support of this hypothesis, the administration of the opioid antagonist **naloxone** into the fourth ventricle of the brain helps to restore the sympathetic outflow and prevent decompensation.

A second factor contributing to the irreversible decline in blood pressure is **acute cardiac failure**. Reduced coronary blood flow and acidosis impair myocardial contractility. This reduces cardiac output, which further reduces blood pressure and coronary perfusion. Thus a **positive feedback loop** is set up.

The following complications can result from severe, prolonged hypotension.

- **Acute tubular necrosis** is a common complication in which damage to the renal tubules causes acute renal failure. Acute tubular necrosis is suspected if urine output fails to improve after a day or so. Urine output is therefore monitored closely.

- **Myocardial infarction** can develop in patients with pre-existing ischaemic heart disease. Infarction is triggered by the fall in perfusion pressure and increase in blood coagulability. **Blood coagulability** is increased in the early stages of haemorrhage. This can lead to

microthrombi in small vessels, further reducing local tissue perfusion.

- **Acute cardiac failure** may develop even in the absence of coronary disease, due to the low perfusion pressure, microthrombi and white cell adhesion in microvessels. In severe cases **multi-organ failure** can occur.

18.3 Fainting (syncope)

Syncope is a sudden, transient loss of consciousness due to a reduction in cerebral blood flow to less than half normal following an abrupt fall in arterial pressure. The critical cerebral artery pressure is ~40 mmHg, which corresponds to ~70 mmHg mean arterial pressure at heart level in orthostasis. The initiating factor may be a pathophysiological stress such as severe hypovolaemia or orthostasis (Figure 18.4); or it may be a psychological stress such as fear, pain or horror (Figure 18.5). The sight of blood, especially one's own, often induces emotional fainting in young adults.

In psychogenic fainting (the 'swoon' of Victorian novels) the circulation initially evinces an alerting response, namely tachycardia, muscle vasodilatation, cutaneous vasoconstriction and sweating. During this pre-faint period the subject looks pale and sweaty, hyperventilates and, very characteristically, yawns. Then a sudden increase in vagal outflow causes **a profound bradycardia**. In the medical student of Figure 18.4, for example, there was no heartbeat for 8 s. At the same time there is a sudden **peripheral vasodilatation**, probably due to a fall in sympathetic vasoconstrictor drive. As a result, the blood pressure falls precipitously (Figure 18.5). The reduced cerebral perfusion is followed within seconds by loss of consciousness. This sequence is sometimes called a '**vasovagal attack**'.

The mechanism that triggers the sudden changes in vagal and vasomotor activity is not clear. In

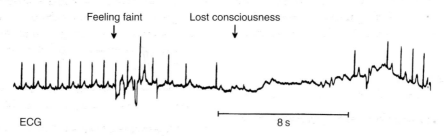

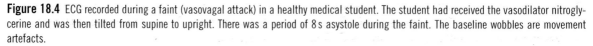

Figure 18.4 ECG recorded during a faint (vasovagal attack) in a healthy medical student. The student had received the vasodilator nitroglycerine and was then tilted from supine to upright. There was a period of 8 s asystole during the faint. The baseline wobbles are movement artefacts.

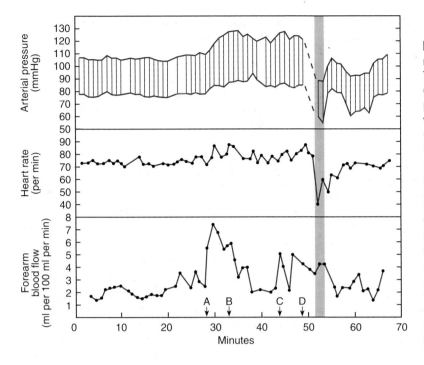

Figure 18.5 Circulatory changes in a male student during an emotional faint. The student showed forearm vasodilatation (alarm response) while watching the preparation for venepuncture (A) and venepuncture of a colleague (B), but did not faint as the experimenter intended. Insertion of a needle into his arm (C) again produced vasodilatation, but no faint. The subject was, therefore, asked to drink some blood taken from his colleague (D). He became pale, yawned, said 'I'm going' and fainted (tinted area). No heart beat was detected by ECG for 11 s and heart rate then averaged 37/min. Forearm blood flow remained above resting level despite the slump in blood pressure, showing that vasodilatation had occurred. Consciousness was regained after 2 min. (From Greenfield, A. D. M. (1951) *The Lancet*, p. 1303, by permission.)

psychogenic fainting the response could be related to the 'playing dead' response of small animals, which emanates from the cingulate gyrus (Section 16.8). In the case of orthostatic or post-haemorrhagic syncope, the response used to be attributed to a reflex from ventricular mechanoreceptors in near-empty hearts. This now seems unlikely, because echocardiography shows no pre-syncopal fall in cardiac volume, and fainting can occur in cardiac transplant patients with denervated ventricles. Activation of the depressor opioid pathway in the brainstem has been proposed as a possible mechanism.

Recovery. The supine position during a faint raises the intrathoracic blood volume and filling pressure. Along with the baroreflex this soon restores the cardiac output and arterial pressure. Consciousness is recovered in about 2 min. It is a mistake to prop the patient up during a faint, because it deprives him/her of the benefit of the Frank–Starling mechanism. Fainting occurs almost exclusively when in the upright position, i.e. fainting requires a low CVP; so sound advice for a person feeling faint is to lie down.

18.4 Hypertension

Definition and classification of hypertension

Clinical hypertension is a chronic, usually progressive, raised arterial pressure. The choice of the dividing line between normal and raised pressure is difficult because the distribution of arterial pressure in the population is unimodal. Most physicians diagnose hypertension if repeated measurements of resting pressure exceed 140/90 mmHg in a patient under 50 years old, or 160/95 mmHg in an older patient. These criteria are based on evidence of increased morbidity at pressures above these levels.

Hypertension can be divided into the following groups. **Essential** or **primary hypertension** is hypertension without any obvious predisposing organic cause, and can take two courses.

- **Benign essential hypertension**, the commonest form, is slowly progressive, almost symptomless, and generally comes to light though a routine check-up. Otherwise it may present much later through its serious consequences, namely heart failure, renal failure and cerebral pathology.

- The rarer **malignant hypertension** is rapidly progressive and quickly induces cardiac failure and oedema, renal damage and proteinuria, and cerebral damage with papilloedema and retinopathy.

Secondary hypertension has an identifiable pathological cause. Examples are as follows:

- In **hyperaldosteronism** (Conn's syndrome) the hypertension is caused by excessive salt and water retention due to excessive aldosterone secretion.

- **Renal artery stenosis** causes hypertension by activating the renin−angiotensin−aldosterone system.

- A **phaeochromocytoma** is a catecholamine-secreting tumour that raises pressure by α-adrenoceptor activation. The above three causes are all uncommon however.

- **Pre-eclamptic toxaemia** is much the commonest form of secondary hypertension. It develops during 7−10% of pregnancies and remits on delivery. Invasion of the spiral arteries of the placenta by the cytotrophoblast causes placental ischaemia. This causes the placenta to release unknown agents that cause endothelial dysfunction, vasoconstriction and reduced pressure natriuresis, leading to hypertension. Rapidly progressive, severe hypertension can lead to cerebral pathology and fits (eclampsia) if untreated.

Except for pre-eclamptic toxaemia, secondary hypertension is uncommon. In >90% of cases no organic cause is found and the disease is classed as primary or essential hypertension. The increased blood pressure in essential hypertension is due to changes in both the **small arterial resistance vessels** and the **large elastic vessels** as follows.

Small artery pathology raises peripheral resistance and mean pressure

Mean blood pressure equals cardiac output × peripheral resistance (Section 8.5). A raised mean pressure must therefore be the result of an imbalance between cardiac output and peripheral resistance. In the early stages, when hypertension is marginal and labile, the cardiac output is raised and the peripheral resistance is only slightly above normal. In well established disease, however, the cardiac output is normal or slightly reduced. Established hypertension is therefore due to an increase in peripheral resistance (Figure 18.6). The increase in vascular resistance affects virtually every organ, including the kidney, and is caused partly by narrowing of the small arteries and partly by rarefaction.

Rarefaction is a reduction in the number of vessels per unit volume of tissue. Rarefaction has been demonstrated in the retina, skin and intestine.

Narrowing of the small arteries is caused by increased vascular tone in the early stages, and is fully reversible by vasodilator drugs at this stage. As time passes, however, the smooth muscle of the tunica media responds to the chronically raised pressure load by hypertrophy. Medial hypertrophy narrows the

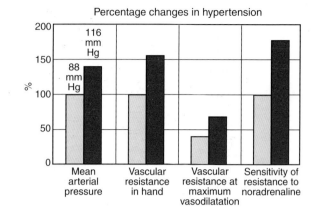

Percentage changes in hypertension

Figure 18.6 Changes in resistance vessels of hand in hypertensive subjects (red) relative to normal (grey). Resistance is above normal at rest and after maximum vasodilatation. Vasoconstrictor response to noradrenaline is raised. (Results of Sivertsson, R. and Olander, B. (1968) *Life Science*, **7**, 1291–1297.)

lumen, even during maximal vasodilatation, so the elevated resistance can no longer be fully abolished by vasodilators (Figure 18.6). Medial hypertrophy takes only a few weeks to develop when hypertension is induced in rats by clipping a renal artery (to stimulate the renin−angiotensin−aldosterone system).

The **baroreflex** remains functional in hypertensive patients, but operates around a higher set point due to peripheral resetting (Section 16.2) and shows reduced sensitivity due to stiffening of the artery wall. It is generally accepted, however, that the changes in the baroreflex are a consequence of hypertension, not its cause.

The stiffening of big elastic arteries contributes to the systolic hypertension

Although increased peripheral resistance is the primary pathology, secondary changes in the large elastic arteries raise the systolic pressure and pulse pressure further (Figure 18.7). This is important because epidemiological studies show that cardiovascular disease correlates more closely with systolic pressure than diastolic pressure.

The elastic arteries in hypertension show elastin fragmentation, dilatation and increased wall stiffness like that which normally occurs in much older vessels. The picture is, in effect, one of **accelerated ageing**. Muscular arteries such as the brachial and radial arteries are not affected; their stiffness is normal if the pressure is normalized. The stiffening of the central elastic vessels has two effects.

- **Arterial compliance** is reduced. Since pulse pressure is approximately equal to stroke

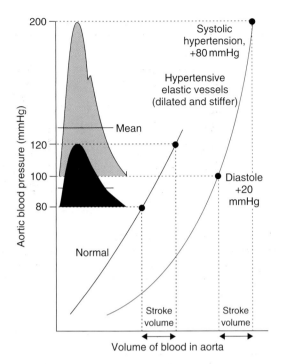

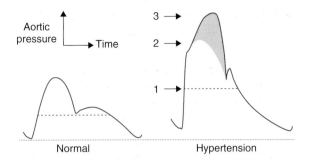

Figure 18.8 Change in aortic pressure in hypertension. *Arrow 1* and dashed lines show increase in mean pressure due to increased resistance of small arterial vessels. *Arrow 2:* reduced compliance of elastic vessels increases size of incident wave (clear area). *Arrow 3:* early return of large reflected wave augments late systolic pressure peak (pink area). Augmentation can account for over half the systolic hypertension. (Based on Nichols W. W. and O'Rourke M. F. (1998); see Further Reading.)

Figure 18.7 Reduced compliance of elastic vessels contributes to systolic hypertension. The central elastic arteries are dilated but stiffer. Dilatation due to elastin fragmentation shifts the curve to the right with ageing or hypertension. The steepened slope is due to collagen deposition and distension by the raised mean pressure. The same stroke volume causes a bigger pulse pressure; diastolic pressure was raised 20 mmHg by increased peripheral resistance but systolic pressure increased by 80 mmHg, even neglecting augmentation by reflection. (Based on Nichols, W. W. and O'Rourke, M. F. (1998); see Further Reading.)

volume divided by arterial compliance, a fall in compliance raises the pulse pressure (Figure 18.7). As a result, the incident systolic pressure increases much more than the diastolic pressure.

- **Pulse wave velocity** increases in stiffening vessels, so the reflected wave returns to the ascending aorta at an earlier point in the cycle (Figure 8.10). Moreover the degree of reflection is enhanced by the raised peripheral resistance. The early return of a bigger reflected pressure wave greatly augments the original or incident systolic pressure wave (Figure 18.8). The reflected wave in hypertensive patients can add as much as 50 mmHg to the systolic pressure, a process known as **augmentation**.

Aortic systolic hypertension is thus the product of three biophysical mechanisms, namely an increase in peripheral resistance, a fall in central artery compliance, and the rapid return of a large, reflected pressure wave. The first two mechanisms increase the incident wave, and the third mechanism increases the augmentation by wave reflection (Figure 18.8).

The left ventricle wall hypertrophies and may fail

The high systolic pressures increase the work of the left ventricle myocytes. This stimulates the release of growth factors that elicit a compensatory hypertrophy of the myocytes and an increase in wall thickness. Although this helps to normalize the stress on a given myocyte, cardiac failure may eventually supervene. This is one of several reasons for initiating treatment to reduce the systolic pressure. Left ventricle hypertrophy is reversed particularly effectively by ACE inhibitors and calcium channel blockers.

What initiates the small vessel changes?

The answer to this question remains uncertain despite huge research efforts. There are **familial and racial tendencies** to hypertension, indicating a genetic component. There are also epidemiological associations between hypertension and **salt intake, alcohol intake** and **obesity**, indicating an environmental component. These observations, coupled with direct experimental work, have led to a number of causative theories.

Neurogenic or stress hypothesis

The neurogenic hypothesis proposes that an excessive sympathetic outflow in response to stress, i.e. an exaggerated alerting response, initiates bouts of reversible hypertension. Repeated periods of hypertension induce hypertrophy of the small vessel media, which perpetuates the condition. In support, repeated exposure of laboratory animals to psychogenic stress can cause chronic hypertension. Also, experimental lesions of the nucleus tractus solitarius raise the sympathetic outflow and lead to chronic hypertension.

Salt imbalance/renal hypothesis

The salt hypothesis proposes that a small but sustained discrepancy between renal salt excretion and dietary salt intake raises the extracellular salt mass and, owing to the osmotic effect of the salt, the extracellular water. This raises the plasma volume, cardiac filling pressure, stroke volume and blood pressure, which evokes medial hypertrophy and a non-reversible rise in peripheral resistance. The association of hypertension with a high-salt diet, both epidemiologically and by intervention, supports this hypothesis. Salt-sensitivity may have a genetic component; Dahl salt-sensitive rats develop hypertension on a salt intake that is harmless to ordinary rats.

How could an imbalance between salt intake and renal excretion arise? Normally a high salt intake and fluid retention reduce the circulating levels of angiotensin II and aldosterone, which reduces renal salt and water retention and restores a balance. However, angiotensinogen, angiotensin II and aldosterone levels are raised rather than depressed in a subgroup of hypertensive patients. Extracellular fluid volume is increased or normal, but plasma volume is reduced in established hypertension.

Depression of Na^+–K^+–ATPase in cell membranes

The activity of the cell membrane Na^+–K^+–ATPase pump is reduced in red and white cells from hypertensive subjects. Whether this is due to a circulating digoxin-like factor or an intrinsic pump abnormality is unclear, and its relevance to vascular tone and blood pressure remains unproven.

Endothelin in hypertension

Endothelin levels are high in pre-eclamptic toxaemia but generally only slightly raised in essential hypertension. In a subgroup of severe hypertensives, however, there is overexpression of the endothelin-1 gene in subcutaneous small arteries, so endothelin may contribute to hypertension in this group.

Multifactorial hypothesis

The long-term control of blood pressure involves neural, endocrine and renal mechanisms and many workers suspect that hypertension develops only if more than one regulatory process is abnormal, usually in a genetically susceptible individual. Whatever the initial cause, the process is thought to involve a self-perpetuating positive feedback once media hypertrophy develops, because a rise in pressure evokes media hypertrophy, which raises pressure, and so on.

Course of hypertension and therapeutic strategies

Hypertension itself is virtually symptomless and contrary to popular belief rarely presents with nose bleeds or headaches. If not treated, hypertension (and especially systolic hypertension) damages the heart, brain and kidneys, leading to:

- hypertensive heart failure
- atheromatous coronary artery disease
- cerebrovascular accidents (strokes)
- hypertensive retinopathy
- chronic renal failure.

It is important, therefore, to treat hypertension at the symptomless stage. There are four main therapeutic avenues.

- Peripheral vasodilators such as calcium-channel blockers (nifedipine) and α_1-adrenoreceptor blockers (prazosin) reduce the peripheral resistance.
- Diuretic drugs reduce the extracellular fluid volume and hence blood pressure.
- Captopril blocks the angiotensin-converting enzyme and therefore reduces both angiotensin II and aldosterone levels. This reduces vascular tone and extracellular fluid volume.
- β-adrenoceptor blockers such as propranolol and atenolol reduce the cardiac output and hence blood pressure.

The aim is to reduce systolic pressure to 135–145 mmHg and diastolic to 85 mmHg. This greatly reduces the mortality and morbidity. Untreated the outlook is grave, with about 50% of patients eventually developing heart failure, 25% renal failure and 25% cerebral complications (retinopathy, encephalopathy, strokes).

18.5 Chronic cardiac failure

Chronic or congestive cardiac failure (CCF) is a chronic inability of the heart to maintain an adequate

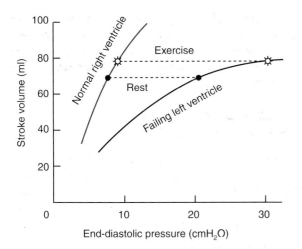

Figure 18.9 The operation of the Frank–Starling mechanism in a patient with a failing left ventricle, but relatively healthy right ventricle. The left ventricle function curve is depressed. Under resting conditions (closed circles) the left ventricle requires an elevated filling pressure to match the right ventricle stroke volume. In exercise (open symbols) the disparity in filling pressure becomes extreme owing to the near-plateau on the function curve of the failing left ventricle.

perfusion of the tissues at a normal filling pressure. Starling, working with the isolated heart–lung preparation, observed that when the heart begins to fail, it requires a higher filling pressure and higher end-diastolic volume to maintain its stroke volume (Figure 18.9). At a normal filling pressure the stroke volume declines. Thus the immediate cause of cardiac failure is a fall in the energy of contraction at any given end-diastolic volume. In other words, **cardiac failure is an abnormal reduction of myocardial contractility**.

In many patients a recognisable pathology initiates cardiac failure. Examples include diffuse coronary artery disease, reduced myocardial mass following an infarct, chronically increased afterload due to hypertension, aortic valve disease and cardiomyopathy. A diagnosis of 'heart failure' is associated with a 50% mortality over 5 years, and the deaths arise from (i) **pump failure** and (ii) an increased proneness to **ventricular arrhythmia**.

Failing myocytes have reduced Ca^{2+} transients and electrophysiological abnormalities

Energy supply is normal in failing hearts, as indicated by normal ATP and creatine phosphate levels at resting outputs. The low contractility is caused by a **reduced systolic Ca^{2+} transient**, secondary to a reduction in the size of the sarcoplasmic reticulum

Ca^{2+} store. The fall in store size is due in part to a **reduced expression of the sarcoplasmic reticulum Ca^{2+} pump**. Reduced pumping also leads to a slow relaxation of the failing heart. A second factor contributing to Ca^{2+} store reduction is **upregulation of the sarcolemmal Na^+–Ca^{2+} exchanger**, which increases the Ca^{2+} expulsion from the myocyte through the current i_{Na-Ca}.

As noted above, ventricular arrhythmia is a major cause of death in failing hearts. The arrhythmia is often triggered by a **delayed afterdepolarization (DAD)**, which is generated by the Na^+–Ca^{2+} **exchanger current** i_{Na-Ca} that follows a spontaneous Ca^{2+} store discharge (Section 3.9). Store discharge may follow temporary overloading by a burst of sympathetic activity; there appears to be an association between sympathetic activity and arrhythmia, and arrhythmias become less common as the responsiveness to β_1-adrenoceptors deteriorates in late-stage failure. Due to the upregulation of the Na^+–Ca^{2+} exchanger, only half as much Ca^{2+} discharge is needed to generate a given amplitude of DAD in failing myocytes. The size of the DAD is also increased by **downregulation of the inward rectifier K^+ channel**. The reduction of outward K^+ current i_{K1} means that a given inward current i_{Na-Ca} generates a bigger DAD. This increases the likelihood of triggering an arrhythmogenic action potential (Figure 3.15).

The **action potential** is prolonged in severe cardiac failure, probably due to a downregulation of the K^+ channel genes. Electrical repolarization depends on an outward K^+ current, so a reduced outward K^+ current and increased inward current i_{Na-Ca} cause a long plateau, long refractory period and delayed repolarization (Section 3.5). Variations in the refractory period between myocytes would increase the possibility for **re-entry circuits** to arise (Figure 5.10).

It is presently thought, therefore, that the upregulation of the Na^+–Ca^{2+} exchanger and downregulation of K^+ channels contribute to the high incidence of arrhythmia in failing hearts, by facilitating the development of DADs that trigger arrhythmias and re-entry circuits that sustain them.

Cardiac output may/may not be reduced at rest

The reduced contractility of the failing heart depresses the ventricular function curve (Figure 18.9). The pump function curve, i.e. the plot of stroke volume as a function of arterial pressure, is likewise depressed as illustrated in Figure 6.15. These changes may or may not reduce the resting stroke volume depending on compensatory responses, as described next.

The **ejection fraction** falls from 66% to as little as 10–20%, so the end-systolic volume (ESV) and end-diastolic volume (EDV) increase, i.e. the heart swells. In mild failure the increase in filling pressure and EDV shift the heart up the depressed ventricle function curve and thereby maintain an almost normal **stroke volume** (Figures 6.13, 18.9, 18.10). In severe failure, however, the fall in ejection fraction and depression of the ventricular function curve are so great that stroke volume falls despite the increased EDV. The resting **cardiac output** may thus be within the normal range (compensated failure, Figure 18.10) or subnormal (decompensated failure). In both cases the EDV and ESV are raised, so the heart is dilated.

Output fails to increase normally on exercise; exercise intolerance

An **exercise test** reveals cardiac failure even when the output is compensated at rest, because the failing heart cannot raise its output to a normal degree. In Figure 18.10 the output of healthy hearts increased to 17.5 l/min in response to a standard exercise test on a bicycle ergometer, whereas the output of failing hearts increased to only 11.3 l/min. The patient's exercise tolerance is poor and he/she complains of **excessive fatigue**. Exercise intolerance, **breathlessness** due to pulmonary congestion and **ankle swelling** due to oedema are the usual presenting symptoms of chronic cardiac failure.

The poor cardiac response to exercise is due to the impairment of not only the stroke volume response but also, more surprisingly, the heart rate response (Figure 18.10).

Stroke volume fails to increase adequately for several reasons. (i) The Frank–Starling mechanism is impaired, so stroke volume becomes less responsive to filling pressure, as shown by the reduced slope of the ventricular function curve (Figure 18.9). (ii) The ventricle ejects less well against the raised arterial pressure of exercise, as shown by the depression of the pump function curve in Figure 6.15. (iii) The β_1-mediated contractility response to catecholamines is impaired (see below), so the ejection fraction fails to increase in exercise (Figure 18.10).

The impaired **heart rate** response is due partly to a depletion of noradrenaline from the cardiac sympathetic nerve terminals, associated with a fall in tyrosine hydroxylase activity, and partly to a downregulation of β_1-adrenoceptors in the pacemaker. Downregulation is due to phosphorylation of the β_1-adrenoceptor by receptor kinases. The phosphorylated receptors become uncoupled from adenylyl cyclase and then internalized.

Exercise intolerance is due in part to the impaired cardiac response described above, and to the exertional dyspnoea caused by pulmonary congestion (see later). However, the patients experience increased fatigue even when using small hand muscles that do not put much demand on the heart and lungs. It is becoming increasingly evident that Ca^{2+} handling by **skeletal muscle fibres** as well as cardiac fibres is abnormal, and that this contributes to the exercise intolerance. Slow fibres have the same SR Ca^{2+}–ATPase isoform as the heart and show slowed Ca^{2+} reuptake, slowed relaxation and impaired fatigue resistance in animal models of heart failure.

The **responses of the body** to chronic cardiac failure include compensatory influences on the heart, a redistribution of the cardiac output, the retention of salt and water by the kidneys, and oedema formation, as described next.

Compensatory mechanisms help to support the failing output

The output of the failing heart is supported to a limited degree by an increase in **circulating catecholamines**, as well as by the increase in **filling pressure** noted above. The compensation may be quite effective in mild failure at rest, but not in severe failure or during exercise.

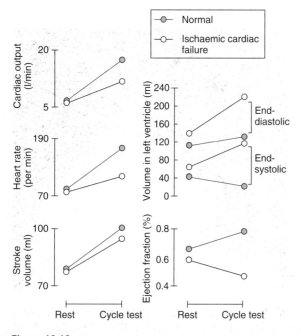

Figure 18.10 Effect of chronic cardiac failure on cardiac performance at rest and during a standard exercise test (submaximal bicycle ergometry). Data from Table 17.2.

Circulating catecholamines versus β_1-adrenoceptor downregulation

The cardiac nerves become depleted of catecholamine but the plasma levels of adrenaline and noradrenaline increase markedly in heart failure. Their inotropic action helps to support the stroke volume in mild failure. However, the uncoupling and downregulation of myocardial β_1-adrenoreceptors vitiates their inotropic effect as the disease progresses.

Raised filling pressure: friend or foe?

Cardiac filling pressure rises to >12 cmH$_2$O in chronic cardiac failure due to plasma volume expansion and peripheral venoconstriction (see later). Cardiac distension is readily detected by measuring the **cardiothoracic ratio** in a chest radiogram (Figure 18.11). The width of the cardiac shadow is normally <50% of the width of the thoracic cavity from inside rib to inside rib, whereas in cardiac failure the ratio exceeds 50%. In mild failure the end-diastolic distension improves the contractile energy by the Frank–Starling mechanism and stroke volume is almost normal (Figure 18.9); see also Guyton's analysis of cardiac failure (Figure 6.13).

Although end-diastolic distension shifts the ventricle along the ventricular function curve, this brings no benefit once on the plateau of the flattened curve that characterizes severe failure. On the contrary, cardiac dilatation and increased filling pressure then have the following deleterious effects.

1 The **mechanical efficiency** of contraction is impaired. As dictated by **Laplace's law**, the active tension required to generate a given systolic pressure increases with ventricular radius (Figure 6.14). Cardiac dilatation thus raises the energy cost of systole.

2 **Atrioventricular valve leakage** can result from widening of the atrioventricular orifices in a grossly dilated heart. This reduces the effective ejection fraction.

3 **Peripheral oedema** develops, due to the high central venous pressures associated with right ventricular failure.

4 **Pulmonary vascular congestion** (Figure 18.11) and extra-alveolar oedema develop as a result of the high filling pressures associated with left ventricular failure. The stiffened lungs require more effort to inflate, which generates a sensation of difficulty in breathing called **dyspnoea**.

There are thus many reasons for therapeutically lowering the filling pressure and cardiac distension.

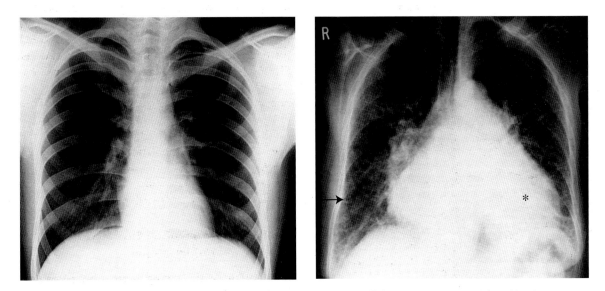

Figure 18.11 Anteroposterior radiograph of the chest. (*Left*) Normal subject; cardiothoracic ratio 0.45. (*Right*) Patient with left ventricular failure; cardiothoracic ratio 0.72. Asterisk marks grossly dilated left ventricle. Arrow: septal line caused by interstitial oedema (Kerley B lines). Radiating opacities due to pulmonary interstitial oedema are present in the lung field (Kerley A lines). Also note 'air bronchogram', the outlining of the major bronchi by surrounding oedema, and blunting of the costophrenic angle images by oedema. (Courtesy of Dr A. Wilson, St George's Hospital, London.)

Peripheral vasoconstriction redistributes the output and supports blood pressure

The limited cardiac output is preferentially distributed to the coronary, cerebral and skeletal muscle circulations through intense vasoconstriction in other tissues (Figure 18.12). The cutaneous, renal and splanchnic vascular beds are strongly vasoconstricted and venoconstricted by increased **sympathetic vasomotor activity**, which is probably elicited by the baroreflex. Plasma **angiotensin II** and **endothelin-1** levels are also raised. The peripheral vasoconstriction maintains the arterial pressure, which would otherwise be threatened by a low cardiac output. The venoconstriction contributes to the rise in cardiac filling pressure.

Although venoconstriction and vasoconstriction may be beneficial in mild failure, they cause problems in severe failure because excessive cardiac dilatation is harmful as described above, and because the stroke volume of a failing ventricle is substantially impaired by ejection against a normal arterial pressure (Figure 6.15).

Renal salt and water retention expands the extracellular fluid compartment

The kidneys retain salt and water in cardiac failure. This expands the extracellular fluid compartment by up to 30%, and the increased extracellular fluid volume contributes to the cardiac dilatation and oedema formation. The salt and water retention is due to the pronounced **renal vasoconstriction** (Figure 18.12) and the activation of the **renin–angiotensin–aldosterone** system through increased sympathetic activity. The plasma aldosterone level is further elevated by reduced degradation of aldosterone by the congested, underperfused liver. The liver may be palpably swollen following right ventricular failure.

Plasma levels of **atrial natriuretic factor** (ANF) are high in cardiac failure due to the atrial distension. The ANF may have a beneficial role in attenuating the renal over-retention of salt and water. Despite this the extracellular fluid volume is increased in cardiac failure.

Cardiac failure causes peripheral and/or pulmonary oedema

Oedema of the lungs and/or periphery is a prominent feature of cardiac failure. The oedema is due primarily to **increased capillary pressure**. Since capillaries drain into veins, increased venous pressure inevitably raises capillary pressure. In right ventricular failure the pressure in the venous limb of human skin capillaries reaches 20–40 mmHg (normal 12–15 mmHg).

Oedema formation is exacerbated by a fall in **plasma colloid osmotic pressure**. Plasma colloid osmotic pressure falls by ~7 mmHg due to the expansion of plasma volume following renal salt and water retention. The imbalance of Starling forces across the venous capillary wall is thus shifted in the direction of increased filtration, leading to oedema formation. The oedema may be worse in the periphery or lungs depending on whether the right side or left side filling pressure is more severely affected.

Pulmonary congestion and oedema cause dyspnoea

Ischaemic heart disease primarily affects the left ventricle. The Frank–Starling mechanism ensures that the output of a failing left ventricle remains equal to that of the right ventricle, but at the expense of increased pulmonary venous pressure. Pulmonary venous pressure increases because, if the left side transiently pumps out less blood than the right, some blood accumulates in the lungs. The pulmonary congestion continues to increase until, through the Frank–Starling mechanism, the output of the left ventricle equals that of the right (Figure 18.9). The pulmonary congestion is obvious in radiographs (Figure 18.11).

The rise in pulmonary microvascular pressure causes **pulmonary oedema**. In moderate pulmonary oedema the excess fluid collects in the pulmonary

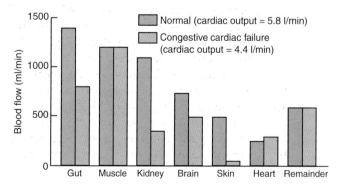

Figure 18.12 Redistribution of cardiac output in a resting patient with chronic cardiac failure and an output of 4.4 l/min (grey columns). Note the poor perfusion of kidney, gut and skin. (From Wade, O. L. and Bishop, J. M. (1962) *Cardiac Output and Regional Bloodflow*, Blackwell, Oxford, by permission.)

interstitium and inside the bronchi. Fluid in the bronchi gives rise to crackles (**crepitations**) during breathing, audible through a stethoscope. In severe pulmonary oedema, fluid accumulates in the alveoli too, impairing O_2 transport with potentially fatal results.

The net effect of pulmonary vascular congestion and oedema is to make the lungs stiffer and therefore more difficult to inflate. This causes one of the characteristic symptoms of left ventricular failure, **dyspnoea** (difficulty in breathing). Dyspnoea of cardiac origin becomes worse in bed, and a severe attack of dyspnoea may wake the patient up during the night (**paroxysmal nocturnal dyspnoea**). The paroxysm is the result of the supine position, which increases pulmonary congestion and leads to increasing pulmonary oedema as the night wears on. The patient therefore finds it more comfortable to sleep propped up by several pillows.

Peripheral oedema arises from right ventricle failure

If the right ventricle fails – for example, following pulmonary hypertension due to chronic lung disease – central venous pressure and venous pressure throughout the systemic circulation increase, due to the operation of the Frank–Starling mechanism and the renal retention of salt and water. Raised pressure in venous capillaries results in peripheral oedema, usually in dependent regions such as the ankles or, in bed-ridden patients, over the sacrum. Such patients show a characteristic combination of **distended jugular veins** and **pitting peripheral oedema**.

Failure occurs not infrequently in both the right and left ventricles, and such patients may have both peripheral and pulmonary oedema.

The treatment of heart failure is based on physiological principles

The treatment of cardiac failure is an interesting exercise in applied physiology. The physiological objectives are to:

- reduce cardiac O_2 demand by reducing cardiac work;
- improve stroke volume by reducing arterial pressure (afterload);
- improve mechanical efficiency by reducing cardiac dilatation (Laplace's law);
- reduce peripheral oedema and pulmonary congestion by reducing plasma volume and filling pressure;
- improve myocardial contractility.

Cardiac work can be reduced by bed-rest, by lowering the arterial pressure and hence afterload, and by lowering the cardiac filling pressure and hence preload. **Arterial pressure** can be reduced by peripheral vasodilators such as prazosin, an α_1-adrenoceptor blocker. **Filling pressure** can be reduced by venodilators such as nitroglycerine and nitroprusside, and by angiotensin-converting enzyme (ACE) inhibitors such as captopril and enalapril, which are widely used to relax both resistance and capacitance vessels. Endothelin levels are raised in cardiac failure, and the endothelin antagonist bosentan is reported to improve peripheral blood flow and reduce peripheral venoconstriction, arterial pressure and pulmonary pressures in cardiac failure.

Stroke volume and ejection fraction can be markedly improved by reducing the pressure opposing ejection using peripheral vasodilators. Due to the steepness of the pump function curve quite a small reduction in arterial pressure can produce a substantial improvement in stroke volume, as shown by point 4 in Figure 6.15.

Cardiac distension, plasma volume expansion and **oedema** are reduced by diuretic drugs such as frusemide and the thiazides. ACE inhibitors help to reduce the plasma volume by lowering the angiotensin II level and hence aldosterone level. The advantage of reducing cardiac dilatation is that the heart wall then operates at a better mechanical advantage (Laplace's law).

Treatment with vasodilator and diuretic drugs is in effect reversing physiological compensations that are overdone in cardiac failure.

Myocardial contractility can be partially restored using the inotropic drug digoxin. The discovery of digoxin by William Withering in 1785 is a nice example of the roles of chance and a prepared mind in scientific discovery. Dr Withering was journeying through Shropshire when he was asked to see a woman suffering from severe 'dropsy' (cardiac failure). He could do little for her and on his return journey was astonished to find her not only alive but much improved. On enquiring he discovered that she had been taking a local folklore remedy, an infusion of the leaves of the foxglove, *Digitalis purpurea*. The efficacy of a digitalis infusion is illustrated in Figure 3.14, and the mechanism by which it enhances the intracellular Ca^{2+} store is explained there. The increased Ca^{2+} store can trigger afterdepolarization and arrhythmia unless the digoxin level is carefully controlled, so digoxin is prescribed with restraint. In many cases good responses are obtained simply by a combination of rest, an ACE inhibitor and a diuretic.

Other drugs that enhance contractility, such as the phosphodiesterase inhibitor milrinone or the β_1-agonists dobutamine and dopamine, are used in emergency situations. Temporary mechanical support of the cardiac output can also be provided in an acutely ill patient by intra-aortic balloon counterpulsation. A sausage-shaped balloon in the ascending aorta is inflated during diastole (to raise diastolic pressure and enhance coronary perfusion) and deflated in systole (to reduce systolic pressure and cardiac work).

SUMMARY

Systemic hypoxaemia

■ Systemic hypoxaemia occurs at high altitude, in asphyxiation, chronic emphysema, severe pulmonary oedema and right-to-left shunts through congenital heart defects.

■ Increased arterial chemoreceptor activity causes reflex resting hyperventilation, which improves arterial P_{O_2} but causes hypocapnia and a reversed (left) Bohr shift.

■ Resting tachycardia raises cardiac output, which maintains resting O_2 delivery despite reduced arterial O_2 saturation and extraction. Tissue perfusion is enhanced by systemic vasodilatation to hypoxaemia. In the brain this is offset by the vasoconstrictor response to hypocapnia.

■ In the lungs hypoxic vasoconstriction promotes apical perfusion but causes pulmonary hypertension, which can lead to right ventricular failure in the long term.

■ Maximum cardiac output is reduced, and since arterial O_2 saturation is reduced, V_{O_2max} and exercise ability are impaired.

■ Acclimatization involves correction of the respiratory alkalosis, a further increase in resting ventilation, increased haematocrit and a right Bohr shift that facilitates O_2 unloading in the tissues.

Shock and haemorrhage

■ Acute circulatory failure or clinical 'shock' is caused by hypovolaemia (e.g. haemorrhage), septicaemia, acute cardiac failure or anaphylaxis.

■ Hypovolaemia reduces CVP, stroke volume and pulse pressure through the Frank–Starling mechanism. Reduced cardiopulmonary and baroreceptor

activity plus increased arterial chemoreceptor activity evoke a reflex increase in sympathetic outflow, circulating catecholamines, angiotensin II and in severe cases vasopressin.

■ After ⩽20% hypovolaemia the reflex tachycardia, increased contractility, increased peripheral resistance and venoconstriction maintain the mean blood pressure near normal (compensated, non-hypotensive phase), but the skin is pale, cold and sweaty and lactic acidosis drives an arterial chemoreflex-mediated hyperventilation.

■ Over 30–60 min the reduced capillary pressure allows plasma oncotic pressure to draw ~500 ml interstitial fluid into the circulation. This internal transfusion is aided by a shift of intracellular fluid into the interstitial compartment following increased extracellular fluid osmolarity due to adrenaline-induced hepatic glycogenolysis.

■ Renal conservation of salt and water results from increased renal sympathetic nerve activity, aldosterone and vasopressin (ADH). Coupled with increased fluid intake due to angiotensin II-stimulated thirst, renal conservation restores the extracellular fluid volume over a few days. Plasma proteins and red cells are resynthesized more slowly.

■ In severe or late-treated hypotensive haemorrhage, an irreversible, decompensated phase sets in. Peripheral vessels relax, causing a sharp collapse of blood pressure. Poor coronary perfusion sets up a positive feedback leading to acute cardiac failure. Poor renal perfusion leads to acute renal failure, signalled by anuria.

Fainting

■ Emotional stress, hypovolaemia or prolonged orthostasis trigger an abrupt, profound, vagally mediated bradycardia and a peripheral vasodilatation (vasovagal attack).

■ As the mean arterial pressure falls below ~70 mmHg, reduced cerebral perfusion causes loss of consciousness. Spontaneous restoration of the normal heartbeat is followed by recovery in 2 minutes or so.

Essential hypertension

■ Resting blood pressures in excess of 140–160 mmHg/90–95 mmHg, depending on age, lead to cardiac, cerebral, retinal and renal disease. Systolic hypertension is particularly harmful.

■ Mean pressure is raised by an increase in peripheral resistance, caused by rarefaction and narrowing of small resistance arteries. Narrowing is initially due to reversible vasoconstriction and later to medial hypertrophy.

■ Systolic pressure increases more than diastolic pressure due to a stiffening of the elastic arteries. The reduced compliance raises pulse pressure, and the increased wave conduction velocity causes systolic augmentation by an early reflected wave.

■ The aetiology of essential (primary) hypertension may be multifactorial, involving genetic predisposition, stress, high salt intake and inappropriate renin–angiotensin–aldosterone or endothelin secretion in some subgroups.

■ Hypertension is controlled using ACE inhibitors, peripheral vasodilators, diuretics, and β-adrenoceptor blockers to reduce cardiac output.

Chronic cardiac failure

■ Chronic cardiac failure is a reduced ventricular contractility secondary to ischaemic heart disease, pulmonary or systemic hypertension, valve defects or cardiomyopathy. Failure results in **exercise intolerance**, **dyspnoea** and **oedema**. Death is due to pump failure or arrhythmia.

■ Contractility is low due to a **reduced systolic Ca^{2+} transient** and Ca^{2+} store following downregulation of the sarcoplasmic reticulum Ca^{2+} pumps and upregulation of the sarcolemmal Na^+–Ca^{2+} exchangers.

■ **Action potentials** and refractory periods are prolonged by K^+ channel downregulation. The Na^+–Ca^{2+} exchanger upregulation and K^+ channel downregulation contribute to the high incidence of arrhythmia by increasing the size of **delayed after-depolarizations**.

■ The ventricular function curve, pump function curve and ejection fraction are depressed. The heart is swollen (cardiothoracic ratio >50%) due to increased filling pressure. **Resting stroke volume** and output may be almost normal in mild, compensated failure due to the Frank–Starling mechanism and stimulation by raised plasma catecholamines. In severe failure resting output is reduced by deterioration of the Frank–Starling effect, mechanical inefficiency due to an excessive radius (Laplace's law) and β_1-adrenoceptor downregulation.

■ In **exercise** both the heart rate and stroke volume fail to increase adequately, due to noradrenaline depletion from cardiac sympathetic fibres, β_1-adrenoceptor downregulation and the plateau of the ventricular function curve. **Exercise intolerance** results from the inadequate cardiac response, dyspnoea and skeletal muscle Ca^{2+} handling abnormality.

■ **Vasoconstriction** of the cutaneous, splanchnic and renal circulations supports blood pressure and **venoconstriction** contributes to the elevated CVP. Vascular constriction is due to sympathetic-activity, raised angiotensin II and raised endothelin.

■ High aldosterone levels and renal vasoconstriction cause **salt and water retention**, despite raised atrial natriuretic peptide levels. The plasma volume expansion and venoconstriction raise cardiac filling pressures. Increased central venous pressure in right ventricular failure raises systemic capillary pressure, leading to **peripheral oedema** of the legs and sacrum. Increased pulmonary vein pressure in left ventricular failure causes **pulmonary congestion**, oedema and dyspnoea.

■ **Treatment** is based on reduction of the oedema, plasma volume and excessive cardiac dilatation using diuretics and ACE inhibitors; reduction of cardiac O_2 demand by rest and peripheral vasodilators; improvement of stroke volume by afterload reduction via peripheral vasodilators; and improvement of contractility using inotropic drugs such as digoxin.

FURTHER READING

Hypoxaemia

Johnson, R. L., Grover, R. F. and DeGraff, A. C. (1994) Effects of high altitude and training on O_2 transport and exercise performance. In *Cardiovascular Response to Exercise* (ed. Fletcher G. F.), New York, Futura, pp. 223–252.

Marshall, J. M. (1999) The integrated response to hypoxia: from circulation to cells. *Experimental Physiology*, **84**, 449–470.

Rowell, L. B. (1986) *Human Circulation Regulation during Physical Stress*, Oxford University Press, New York.

Savard, G. K., Areskog, N.-H. and Saltin, B. (1995) Cardiovascular responses to exercise in humans following acclimatization to extreme altitude. *Acta Physiologica Scandinavica*, **154**, 499–509.

Weissbrod, C. J., Minson, C. T., Joyner, M. J. and Halliwill, J. R. (2001) Effects of regional phentolamine on hypoxic vasodilatation in healthy humans. *Journal of Physiology*, **537**, 613–621.

Shock and haemorrhage

Courneya, C. A. and Korner, P. I. (1991) Neuro-humoral mechanisms and the role of arterial baroreceptors in the reno-vascular response to haemorrhage in rabbits. *Journal of Physiology*, **437**, 393–407.

Hartikainen, J., Ahonen, E., Nevalaines, T., Sikanen, A. and Hakumaki, M. (1990) Haemodynamic information encoded in the aortic baroreceptor discharge during haemorrhage. *Acta Physiologica Scandinavica*, **140**, 181–189.

Jacobsen, J., Søfelt, S., Sheikh, S., Warberg, J. and Secher, N. H. (1990) Cardiovascular and endocrine responses to haemorrhage in the pig. *Acta Physiologica Scandinavica*, **138**, 167–173.

Länne, T. and Lundvall, J. (1992) Mechanisms in man for rapid refill of the circulatory system in hypovolaemia. *Acta Physiologica Scandinavica*, **146**, 299–306.

Schadt, J. C. and Ludbrook, J. (1991) Hemodynamic and neurohumoral responses to acute hypovolaemia in conscious mammals. *American Journal of Physiology*, **260**, H305–318.

Fainting

Hainsworth, R. (1989) Fainting. In *Autonomic Failure* (ed. Bannister, R.), Oxford University Press, Oxford, pp. 142–158.

Ludbrook, J. and Evans, R. (1989) Posthemorrhagic syncope. *News in Physiological Science*, **4**, 120–133.

Novak, V., Honos, G. and Schondorf, R. (1996) Is the heart empty at syncope? *Journal of Autonomic Nervous System*, **60**, 83–92.

Hypertension

Alexander, B. T., Bennett, W. A., Khalid, R. A. and Granger, J. P. (2001) Preeclampsia: linking placental ischaemia with cardiovascular renal dysfunction. *News in Physiological Science*, **16**, 282–286.

Blaustein, M. P. (1993) Physiological effects of endogenous ouabain: control of intracellular Ca^{2+} stores and cell responsiveness. *American Journal of Physiology*, **264**, C1367–1387.

Bohr, D. F. (1989) Cell membrane in hypertension. *News in Physiological Science*, **4**, 85–88.

Cowley, A. W., Barber, W. J., Lombard, J. H., Osbom, J. and Liard, J. F. (1986) Relationship between body fluid volume and arterial pressure. *Federal Proceedings*, **45**, 2864–2870.

Dickhout, J. G. and Lee, R. M. K. W. (2000) Increased medial smooth muscle cell length is responsible for vascular hypertrophy in young hypertensive rats. *American Journal of Physiology*, **279**, H2085–2094.

Haddy, F. J. (1989) Humoral factors in hypertension. *News in Physiological Sciences*, **4**, 202–205.

Heagerty, A. M., Aalkjaer, C., Bund, S. J., Korsgaard, N. and Mulvany, M. J. (1993) Small artery structure in hypertension. Dual processes of remodelling and growth. *Hypertension*, **21**, 391–397.

Nichols, W. W. and O'Rourke, M. F. (1998) *McDonald's Blood Flow in Arteries*, London, Arnold.

Prewitt, R. L., Stacy, D. L. and Ono, Z. (1987) The microcirculation in hypertension: which are the resistance vessels? *News in Physiological Sciences*, **2**, 139–141.

Chronic cardiac failure

Reviews and chapters

Bers, D. M. (2002) Calcium and cardiac rhythms. Physiological and pathophysiological. *Circulation Research*, **90**, 14–17.

Francis, G. S. and Cohn, J. N. (1990) Heart failure: mechanisms of cardiac and vascular dysfunction and the rationale for pharmacologic intervention. *FASEB Journal*, **4**, 3068–3075.

Homy, C. J., Vatner, S. F. and Vatner, D. E. (1991) β-adrenergic receptor regulation in the heart in pathophysiological states: abnormal adrenergic responsiveness in cardiac disease. *Annual Review of Physiology*, **53**, 137–159.

Niggli, E. (1999) Ca^{2+} sparks in cardiac muscle: is there life without them? *News in Physiological Science*, **14**, 129–134.

Sutch, G., Wenzel, R., Kiowski, W. and Luscher, T. F. (1997) Endothelin and its role in vascular physiology/biology. In *Vascular Endothelium* (eds Born, G. V. R. and Schwartz, C. J.), Schattauer, Stuttgart, pp. 221–242.

Winaver, J., Hoffman, A., Abassi, Z. and Haramati, A. (1995) Does the heart's hormone ANP help in congestive heart failure? *News in Physiological Sciences*, **10**, 247–253.

Research papers

Gwathmey, J. K., Copelas, L., MacKinnon, R., Schoen, F. J., Feldman M. D., Grossman, W. and Morgan, J. R. (1987) Abnormal intracellular calcium handling in myocardium from patients with end-stage heart failure. *Circulation Research*, **61**, 70–76.

Li, Q., Biagi, B., Hohl, C., Starling, R., Stokes, B. and Altschuld, R. (1990) Effects of isoprotenerol and caffeine on calcium transients and action potentials in human ventricular cardiomyocytes. *Progress in Clinical Biology Research*, **327**, 743–750.

Lunde, P. K., Verburg, E., Eriksen, M. and Sejersted, O. M. (2002) Contractile properties of *in situ* perfused skeletal muscles from rats with congestive heart failure. *Journal of Physiology*, **540**, 571–580.

Pogwizd, S. M., Schlotthauer, K., Li, L., Yuan, W. and Bers, D. M. (2001) Arrhythmogenesis and contractile dysfunction in heart failure: roles of sodium–calcium exchange, inward rectifier potassium current, and residual beta-adrenergic responsiveness. *Circulation Research*, **88**, 1159–1167.

Schwinger, R. H. G., Bohm, M., Koch, A., Schmidt, U., Morano, I., Eissner, H. J., Uberfuhr, P., Reichart, B. and Erdmann, E. (1994) The failing heart is unable to use the Frank–Starling mechanism. *Circulation Research*, **74**, 959–969.

Zelis, R. and Flaim, S. F. (1982) Alterations in vasomotor tone in congestive heart failure. *Progress in Cardiovascular Diseases*, **24**, 437–459.

The end but not the end

'Begin at the beginning', said the King, very gravely, to the White Rabbit, 'and go on till you come to the end: then stop'. Heart failure seems to offer a natural ending to this text, but the scientific investigation of the circulation is far from at an end – too many mysteries remain unsolved. The discerning reader will have recognized the superabundance of unresolved problems from the frequent use of 'may be', 'probably', 'is thought to' and so on. Our subject began essentially with the work of William Harvey over three centuries ago, yet a comment by Harvey still makes an apt conclusion to today's textbook: 'I see a field of such vast extent – that my whole life perchance would not suffice for its completion.'

(A. Mallock (1929) *William Harvey*, Hoeber, New York.)

CLINICICAL CASES

for problem-based learning

CASE 1 The Breathless Woman

A 70-year-old woman complains of tiredness on exercise and shortness of breath. She can no longer do her housework without frequent rests and gets very breathless. At night she wakes up struggling to breathe, and finds that sleeping propped up by several pillows helps. Her ankles swell as the day progresses but improve after a night's rest.

On examination the doctor notes that her breathing is rapid. Chest auscultation reveals fine crackling sounds (crepitations). The pulse is regular and arterial blood pressure is within the normal range, but the neck veins are distended even in the upright position. The doctor estimates the central venous pressure to be ~18 cmH$_2$O. The apex beat is felt faintly in the anterior axillary line of the 5th intercostal space. Examining the puffy ankles, he presses on the skin over the tibia for a minute and observes that a deep pit forms.

A chest X-ray shows a cardiothoracic ratio of 0.69, congested pulmonary vessels and the thin horizontal lines of interseptal oedema. ECG is normal. A diagnosis of biventricular cardiac failure is made. She is treated with digoxin and a diuretic, which relieve her symptoms.

Questions

1 How can inspection of the neck veins estimate central venous pressure (CVP)?
2 What is the relation between CVP and stroke volume?
3 What are the chief effects of Starling's law in humans?
4 Which factors govern the size of the CVP?
5 Why is distension disadvantageous in a failing heart?
6 How would lowering the arterial pressure help a failing heart?
7 What is the molecular basis of cardiac contraction and the effect of stretch?
8 Draw a pair of ventricular function curves to illustrate the meaning of 'impaired contractility'.
9 What process can raise contractile energy besides Starling's law?
10 How can cardiac contractility be assessed in humans?
11 What is the link between pulmonary vessel distension and dyspnoea?
12 What causes crepitations (crackles) in the lungs?
13 Why was the dyspnoea worse at night (paroxysmal nocturnal dyspnoea), and why did sleeping propped up help?

14 Why do normal tissues not pit?

15 What principle governs the distribution of fluid between the vascular and interstitial compartment? Which terms in the principle account for oedema of cardiac origin?

16 What other system is vital for tissue fluid balance besides the capillary network?

17 Why did the ankle swelling worsen during the day?

18 What might account for the patient's poor exercise tolerance?

19 How does digoxin act?

Answers

1 The jugular vein serves as a manometer connected to the right atrium without intervening valves (Section 8.10). Veins collapse when their luminal pressure is just below atmospheric pressure. If the point of venous collapse is, say, 18 cm vertically above the right atrium, atrial pressure equals atmospheric pressure plus 18 cm of H_2O, due to the effect of gravity on the fluid column.

2 CVP governs right ventricle distension in diastole, which governs the energy of contraction (Section 6.4). Figures 6.10 and 6.19 show that stroke volume increases with filling pressure (Starling's law of the heart) but plateaus at high distending pressures.

3 (i) Starling's law equalizes the outputs of the right and left ventricles. (ii) It contributes to the rise in stroke volume at the onset of exercise. (iii) It can cause postural hypotension on standing (Section 17.1). (iv) It mediates the arterial hypotension of hypovolaemia (Section 18.2).

4 CVP is governed by the blood volume and how the volume is distributed between the thoracic and peripheral veins. Distribution depends on posture (effect of gravity), movement (effect of muscle pump), and peripheral venous tone (regulated by sympathetic nerves, circulating catecholamines and angiotensin II).

5 On the plateau of the failing ventricular function curve there is no gain in contractile energy with distension, but due to the operation of Laplace's law the contractile energy is less effectively converted into stroke work (Figure 6.14). Excessive distension can also cause functional incompetence of the atrioventricular valves.

6 The greater the arterial pressure, the greater the energy used in raising intraventricular pressure, leaving less energy for ejection; see the 'pump function curve' (Figure 6.15). Reducing arterial pressure improves output.

7 Contraction is brought about by the sliding filament mechanism, triggered by a systolic Ca^{2+} transient. The transient is due to Ca^{2+}-induced Ca^{2+} release from the sarcoplasmic reticulum store plus some Ca^{2+} current from the action potential plateau (Sections 3.2, 3.5). Stretching the sarcomere reduces actin-actin interference (Figure 6.3) and raises Ca^{2+} sensitivity (Figure 6.6). Also, after an interval, the systolic Ca^{2+} transient increases (Figure 6.4).

8 The patient's ventricular function curve is depressed (Figure 18.9). Impaired contractility is a reduced force of contraction for a given filling pressure or cardiac distension.

9 Increased contractility due to increased sympathetic activity raises contractile energy (Section 6.10). Noradrenaline activates β_1-adrenoceptors which, via the adenylate cyclase-cAMP-protein kinase A pathway, increase the plateau Ca^{2+} current, Ca^{2+} store and systolic Ca^{2+} transient. In cardiac failure β_1-adrenoceptor downregulation weakens this mechanism (Section 18.5).

10 Human ventricular contractility is assessed by (i) the ejection fraction measured by radionuclide angiography (<66%, normally) and (ii) ventricular dP/dt_{max} measured through an intracardiac catheter (Figure 2.5).

11 The pulmonary vessels are distended because left atrial pressure is raised by left ventricle failure, renal salt and water retention and peripheral venoconstriction. Congestion and oedema stiffen the lungs, increasing the work of breathing.

12 Crepitations indicate oedema of the conducting airways. The pulmonary oedema is due to increased capillary pressure caused by the raised pulmonary venous and left atrial pressure.

13 The supine position redistributes peripheral venous blood into the thorax (Figure 8.21), which exacerbates pulmonary congestion and oedema. Drainage of oedema from the legs overnight further exacerbates the problem. Sleeping propped up helps prevent these gravity-based problems.

14 Although interstitial fluid makes up ~16% of normal tissue, it does not pit because the glycosaminoglycan matrix offers a high resistance to flow (Fig. 11.9). In oedema the glycosaminoglycans are diluted, so fluid is easily displaced.

15 Fluid exchange is governed by the Starling principle of fluid exchange (Section 11.1).

Capillary pressure is increased because it depends on venous pressure (Figure 11.5), which is raised in cardiac failure. Also, plasma dilution due to renal salt and water retention causes a moderate fall in plasma colloid osmotic pressure.

16 The lymphatic system maintains tissue fluid balance (Section 11.8). Lungs produce lymph despite their low capillary pressure (Section 11.6).

17 In orthostasis gravity raises capillary pressure in the legs (Figure 11.5), so the ankle swelling worsens during the day. It improves overnight because capillary pressure falls in the supine position, allowing lymphatic drainage to outpace fluid filtration.

18 The exercise intolerance is due to the inability of stroke volume and heart rate to increase normally in response to exercise (Figure 18.10), and to dyspnoea, and to increased skeletal muscle fatigability.

19 Digoxin partly restores contractility by increasing the Ca^{2+} store and systolic Ca^{2+} transient. Digoxin inhibits the sarcolemmal Na^+-K^+ pump. This reduces the Na^+ gradient that drives the Na^+–Ca^{2+} exchanger and Ca^{2+} expulsion.

CASE 2 The Man with Chest Pain

A collapsed 60-year-old bus driver was brought into Casualty complaining of a severe, sustained crushing pain in a band across the chest, spreading into the arms. Previously he had been well, though he smoked 10 cigarettes a day.

On examination he was pale, with cold, sweaty skin. His pulse was weak, with occasional extrasystoles (ventricular ectopic beats). His arterial blood pressure was 95/70 mmHg. Heart sounds were normal. An ECG revealed large Q waves and ST segment elevation. He was admitted with a provisional diagnosis of myocardial infarction due to coronary artery thrombosis. Plasma analysis showed raised cardiac enzymes (lactic dehydrogenase, creatine phosphokinase, aspartate aminotransferase).

He was given O_2 and morphine. A streptokinase infusion was set up to lyse the coronary thrombus, and he was also started on a regular, low dose of aspirin.

Questions

1 Name the major coronary arteries, state the regions supplied and define 'functional end-artery'.

2 What is the probable underlying coronary pathology here and the role of endothelium?

3 Which sensory fibres mediate ischaemic cardiac pain?

4 How can the myocardium be ischaemic when the left ventricle contains fully oxygenated blood?

5 If the arterial oxygenation was 190 ml O_2 per litre, the mixed venous content 90 ml O_2 per litre, and the O_2 consumption 300 ml/min, what was the patient's cardiac output? Name the principle involved.

6 How do you account for the low cardiac output and blood pressure?

7 What makes the skin pale, cold and sweaty (clammy)? What general response is this a characteristic of?

8 Draw a normal ECG (Lead II) and show how it aligns with atrial and ventricular action potentials. What causes the delay between the P wave and QRS complex?

9 What causes ST-segment displacement in myocardial ischaemia?

10 Sketch the relation between the ECG, heart sounds and left ventricular pressure over one cardiac cycle.

11 How does low-dose aspirin improve the prognosis?

12 What are the roles of lactic dehydrogenase and creatine phosphokinase in cardiac energy metabolism?

13 What are the dangers of abruptly restoring blood flow to a tissue after prolonged ischaemia?

14 What is a ventricular ectopic beat, how does it affect stroke volume, and what might cause it?

Answers

1 The left coronary artery supplies mainly the left ventricle and septum. The right coronary artery supplies mainly the right ventricle. A functional end-artery is one with insufficient arterial anastomoses to maintain tissue viability if the main vessel is obstructed (Section 15.1).

2 Myocardial infarction is usually due to a thrombus (organized blood clot) forming on an atheromatous plaque in the artery wall. Atheroma originates with the trans-endothelial passage of lipoproteins, fibrinogen and monocytes (Section 9.9). Endothelial NO, an inhibitor of platelet aggregation, is low in atheromatous regions. Platelet aggregation initiates the thrombosis.

3 Chemosensitive sympathetic afferents in the myocardium mediate cardiac ischaemic pain (Section 16.3). Convergence of the cardiac nociceptive pathway with pathways from the arm in the spinal column may explain why cardiac pain radiates into the arms.

4 The time needed for O_2 diffusion from the ventricle lumen increases as distance squared (Section 1.1). At more than $\sim100\ \mu m$, diffusion is too slow to support myocyte metabolism (Table 1.1). The left ventricle wall is $\sim1\,cm$ thick.

5 For an $(A-V)_{O_2}$ of $100\,ml/litre$ (i.e. $190-90$) and an O_2 uptake of $300\,ml/min$, the cardiac output must be $3\,litre/min$ (i.e. $300/100$). This is the Fick principle (Section 6.1). The output is subnormal.

6 Impaired contractility reduces the stroke volume and blood pressure (Section 6.12). The reduced contractility is due in part to intracellular acidosis (Figures 6.22, 6.23).

7 The patient's skin is pale and cold due sympathetic-mediated veno- and vaso-constriction respectively (Section 15.3). The 'clamminess' (cold sweat) is due to sympathetic sudomotor activity. The patient is in cardiogenic shock (Section 18.2) and is showing the effects of a reflex increased in sympathetic outflow.

8 See Figure 5.3. The 'P' wave corresponds to atrial depolarization, 'QRS' to ventricular depolarization and 'T' to ventricular repolarization. The PR interval is due chiefly to slow transmission through the atrioventricular node.

9 The ST segment is displaced by injury currents (Section 5.2). Injury currents develop because the resting potential of the ischaemic myocytes is less negative than that of surrounding normal myocytes, and the action potential less positive than normal (Figure 6.22).

10 See Figure 2.5.

11 Platelet aggregation, the initial event in thrombosis, is promoted by platelet thromboxane, formed via cyclo-oxygenase (Section 13.5). Low doses of aspirin inhibit platelet cyclo-oxygenase and thus protect against renewed thrombosis.

12 Lactic dehydrogenase is used to oxidize circulating lactate, an important myocardial energy source normally (Section 7.14). Creatine phosphokinase transfers high-energy phosphate from creatine phosphate to ADP to form ATP (the Lohmann reaction). ATP 'cocks' the myosin head prior to crossbridge formation (Section 3.2).

13 Paradoxically, abrupt reperfusion causes reperfusion injury (Sections 6.12, 13.9). Reperfusion injury is caused by contracture following cytosolic Ca^{2+} overload, white cell activation and free oxygen radical generation.

14 A ventricular ectopic beat is a premature systole triggered from within the ventricle (Figure 5.4b). The trigger is often a delayed afterdepolarization (Section 3.9). Excitation does not follow the normal pathway, so the contraction is ill co-ordinated and generates little output. The pulse appears to miss a beat. Due to the prolonged filling time before the next beat (compensatory pause), the ensuing beat is unusually strong.

CASE 3 The Haemorrhagic Alcoholic

A 60-year-old civil servant collapsed at work after vomiting copious fresh blood (haematemesis). When seen in the Emergency department he was confused, with a pale, clammy skin. Enquiries revealed that he was a chronic, heavy drinker and that his colleagues were concerned at his progressively deteriorating work performance.

On examination his pulse was weak and rapid (120 beats/minute) but regular. The recumbent blood pressure was 100/75 mmHg. On being sat up (he could not stand), blood pressure fell to 80/65 mmHg and he felt faint. His history of alcoholism, coupled with a firm, palpably enlarged liver and characteristic skin changes, indicated hepatic cirrhosis. Rectal examination revealed black 'tarry' stools characteristic of melaena (old blood from a bleed high in the gastrointestinal tract). The diagnosis, confirmed by endoscopy, was bleeding from oesophageal varices (distended veins in the lower oesophagus), resulting from portal vein hypertension induced by alcoholic cirrhosis (fibrosis) of the liver.

A transfusion cannula was inserted into the dorsal vein of the hand with difficulty, the vein being small and collapsed. While waiting for cross-matched blood he received an intravenous infusion of a colloidal plasma volume substitute (Gelatin 40 g/l; molecular mass 30000, osmotic pressure 36 mmHg). A central venous line inserted through the internal jugular indicated a central venous pressure (CVP) of −4 cmH₂O (subatmospheric). The line was used to infuse vasopressin. His haematocrit on admission was 0.36 and his haemoglobin 11.8 g/dl. Urine output was low, 20 ml/hour, and the patient complained of thirst.

Subsequent treatment involved rehydration and blood transfusion followed by injection of a sclerosant solution into the varices near the gastro-oesophageal junction (to induce local thrombosis). On discharge the patient was placed on daily propranolol medication.

Questions

1 What is a 'portal circulation'? Illustrate it by sketching the blood supply to the liver.
2 Why does portal vein hypertension cause oesophageal bleeding?
3 Was the CVP normal, and how did it affect stroke volume? (Hint: consider the pulse pressure.)
4 What was the patient's mean blood pressure when supine? Was he severely hypotensive when supine?
5 Why did the doctor check the arterial pressure in orthostasis, and why did the pressure fall?
6 Which class of blood vessel regulates mean blood pressure? Did the skin provide any evidence of vascular regulation?
7 Why was venipuncture difficult? Is the peripheral venous response beneficial?
8 What cardiac responses helped maintain mean arterial pressure, and what induced them?
9 Name three reflexes that drive the cardiovascular responses to hypovolaemia.
10 What accounts for the low haematocrit and haemoglobin concentration on admission, assuming that they were normal previously?
11 Would you expect an artificial colloid solution to be of greater benefit than 0.15 molar saline?
12 Why was the urine output monitored?
13 What mechanism might account for the patient's thirst?
14 How might the infusion of vasopressin help?
15 What is propranolol and how might it help?

Answers

1 The liver has a dual blood supply (Figure 1.5) – a small arterial supply from the hepatic artery and a much larger supply of intestine-derived venous blood through the portal vein. The liver drains into the hepatic vein. A portal circulation is one in series, i.e. one that receives venous blood drained from another organ (Section 1.8).
2 Portal vein pressure is normally 5−6 mmHg, but cirrhosis distorts the liver structure and raises the vascular resistance. This forces portal vein pressure up to >12 mmHg. Venous collaterals link the lower oesophageal veins to the portal vein, so swollen oesophageal veins (varices) develop. Being very superficial, they readily bleed.
3 The patient's CVP was low (−4 cmH₂O) due to hypovolaemia. CVP is typically around +4 cmH₂O. The low CVP reduced stroke volume (Starling's law of the heart), as shown by the low pulse pressure, 25 mmHg. Pulse pressure depends on stroke volume and arterial compliance (Section 7.4).
4 Mean blood pressure is diastolic pressure plus one-third of the pulse pressure (eqn 8.4), so the

mean was 83 mmHg, which is within the normotensive range. The patient is in compensated haemorrhagic shock (Figure 18.3).

5 The doctor was assessing the severity of the hypovolaemia, which is not apparent from the well-preserved supine mean pressure. Orthostasis causes blood to accumulate in the gravity- distended veins of the lower limbs. The extra fall in CVP reduced stroke volume further, as shown by the fall in pulse pressure to 15 mmHg.

6 Resistance vessels regulate mean blood pressure (Section 1.6). The resistance vessels are identified as arterioles and terminal arteries because the biggest pressure drop occurs across them (Figure 1.9). The low skin temperature and pallor indicated cutaneous vaso- and venoconstriction. This is due to increased sympathetic activity (Section 14.1), circulating catecholamines (Section 14.6), angiotensin II (Section 14.8) and vasopressin in severe cases (Sections 14.7 and 18.2).

7 Venipuncture was difficult due to venoconstriction. Peripheral venoconstriction displaces blood into the thorax and thus limits the fall in CVP following hypovolaemia.

8 Tachycardia (120 beats/min) and increased contractility helped to maintain cardiac output and therefore arterial pressure. The tachycardia is induced by increased cardiac sympathetic activity and decreased vagal parasympathetic activity, which increase the slope of the pacemaker potential (Sections 4.4–4.6). Increased ventricular contractility is due to increased sympathetic activity.

9 Baroreceptor input is reduced by the fall in pulse pressure (Figure 18.2). Cardiopulmonary receptor input is reduced by the reduced cardiac filling (Sections 16.3–16.4). Peripheral arterial chemoreceptor activity is increased by hypoperfusion and metabolic acidosis (Section 16.6, Figure 18.3). The altered input into the nucleus tractus solitarius from the three classes of receptor triggers the reflex increase in sympathetic activity (Figure 16.16).

10 Haemodilution is due to the absorption of interstitial fluid by capillaries and venules – the 'internal transfusion' (Figure 18.3). Capillary pressure is reduced by the venous hypotension and precapillary resistance vessel contraction (Figure 11.4), allowing plasma colloid osmotic pressure to predominate and draw water into the circulation (Starling's principle of fluid exchange, Sections 11.1, 11.6). The interstitium is topped-up with water drawn osmotically from the intracellular compartment by extracellular fluid hyperglycaemia (Section 18.2).

11 Saline expands the plasma volume temporarily but is not well retained because it reduces plasma colloid osmotic pressure, which enhances fluid filtration (Section 11.3). This is avoided by the use of a colloid solution.

12 Urine output is monitored to check renal function. A potentially fatal complication of hypotensive haemorrhage is acute renal failure due to acute tubular necrosis.

13 Thirst is partly due to the action of angiotensin II on the subfornicular organ near the hypothalamus (Section 18.2). Angiotensin levels are high due to the renal secretion of renin in response to sympathetic nerve activity, low perfusion pressure and low salt load (Figure 14.12).

14 Vasopressin contracts the splanchnic resistance vessels, which feed the portal vein. This reduces portal vein pressure.

15 Propranolol is a non-selective β-adrenoceptor blocker. It reduces heart rate and cardiac output by blocking cardiac β_1-receptors, and it raises splanchnic vascular resistance by blocking vascular β_2-receptors. Together these effects reduce portal vein pressure.

CASE 4 The Hypertensive Fainter

A 45-year-old travelling salesman had a minor accident while away from home. While attending the local Casualty his blood pressure was noted to be 180/110 mmHg.

Back home, his general practitioner recorded supine brachial artery pressures of 185/110 and 165/105 mmHg on two visits. On the latter visit the pressure in the standing position was 155/110 mmHg, and heart rate increased from 75 to 85 beats/minute on standing. The patient was obese and admitted to a regular, moderately heavy alcohol intake. Cardiac signs were normal. After checking the retina and excluding secondary causes the doctor diagnosed essential hypertension. He started the patient on prazosin, and advised the patient to lose weight, reduce his alcohol intake and avoid adding salt at the table.

The patient returned after a few days on prazosin because he became faint and dizzy on standing up, and on one occasion had collapsed for a few minutes. Exercise too made him feel faint and dizzy. The doctor found the supine pressure was now 145/95 mmHg. On standing, the pressure fell to 90/65 mmHg and a feeling of faintness and fading vision caused the patient to lie down again. The doctor stopped the prazosin and started the patient on nifedipine. This resolved the problem.

Questions

1 How is human brachial artery pressure measured?
2 What were the mean pressure and pulse pressure on the first visit to the GP? Why did the GP insist on a second visit?
3 At what systolic and diastolic pressures is morbidity significantly increased?
4 What two parameters determine mean blood pressure, and which is responsible for established hypertension?
5 Does the baroreflex fail in hypertension?
6 Why was the patient advised to avoid salt?
7 What changes occur in the resistance vessels in hypertension?
8 List the principal factors that regulate vascular tone.
9 What changes occur in elastic arteries in hypertension and what aspect of blood pressure does this affect?
10 How might stress contribute to essential hypertension?
11 What are the long-term effects of systemic hypertension on the heart?
12 Under what circumstances does pulmonary rather than systemic hypertension develop?
13 All drugs have side-effects, so why treat symptomless hypertension?
14 Prazosin is an α_1-adrenoceptor antagonist. What is the role of α_1-adrenoceptors in vascular control?
15 Explain how prazosin caused dizziness (i) on standing and (ii) on exercise.
16 How does nifedipine act?
17 Name three other classes of drug used to reduce moderate, essential hypertension, and their modes of action.

Answers

1 By sphygmomanometry and auscultation (Figure 8.12). As sphygmomanometer cuff pressure is lowered, the onset of Korotkoff sounds marks systolic pressure and the sudden reduction in Korotkoff sounds marks diastolic pressure. The sounds are caused by turbulent spurts of blood through the partially compressed artery.
2 For a pressure recording of 185/110 mmHg the pulse pressure is 75 mmHg and the mean is 135 mmHg (110 + (75/3), Section 8.5). The alerting response (Section 16.8) can raise pressure on an initial visit to the doctor ('white-coat hypertension'), hence the repeat visit.
3 Brachial artery pressure in normal 45-year-old white subjects averages ~130/85 mmHg (Figure 17.10), or a little higher in Afro-Caribbean subjects. Systolic pressures above 160 mmHg and diastolic pressures above 90–95 mmHg in young to middle-aged subjects increase the risk of heart failure, ischaemic heart disease, cerebrovascular accidents (haemorrhages and thrombosis), retinopathy and renal failure.
4 Mean blood pressure = cardiac output × total peripheral resistance (Section 8.5). In established hypertension, cardiac output is normal. The hypertension is due to increased vascular resistance.
5 The baroreflex remains operative but is reset to a higher pressure (peripheral resetting, Section 16.2). Evidence that the baroreflex is intact comes from the patient's tachycardia in orthostasis.
6 Long-term pressure regulation involves the renal regulation of the extracellular salt and water masses via pressure natriuresis, the renin-angiotensin-aldosterone system, vasopressin and atrial natriuretic peptide (Section 16.5). Hypertension is related epidemiologically to salt

intake, and one theory ascribes hypertension to an imbalance between salt intake and renal salt excretion (Section 18.4). The patient was therefore advised to reduce his salt intake.

7 The myocytes of small arteries undergo hypertrophy, which thickens the media and narrows the lumen (Section 18.4). Resistance is inversely proportional to the fourth power of the lumen radius (Poiseuille's law, Section 8.7). A mere 10% narrowing causes a 46% increase in resistance.

8 Vascular tone is regulated by intrinsic and extrinsic factors (Section 13.1). Intrinsic influences include endothelin and the myogenic constrictor response to blood pressure (Section 13.2), the vasodilator effects of shear stress mediated by endothelial NO (Section 13.3), tissue-derived metabolic vasodilator agents (Section 13.4), and autacoids. Extrinsic influences include the ubiquitous sympathetic noradrenergic vasoconstrictor nerves (Section 14.1) and the circulating vasoactive hormones adrenaline, angiotensin II and vasopressin (Sections 14.6–14.8).

9 Hypertension accelerates the ageing of elastic vessels, causing elastin fragmentation, dilatation and increased stiffness. The reduced compliance and rapid return of an increased reflected wave contribute substantially to the systolic hypertension (Figure 18.8).

10 Stress evokes the alerting response, which comprises tachycardia, vasodilatation in muscle, vasoconstriction in the renal, splanchnic and cutaneous circulations, and increased blood pressure (Section 16.8). The stress hypothesis proposes that an exaggerated alerting response leads to repeated episodes of transient hypertension which evoke medial hypertrophy.

11 Systemic hypertension increases left ventricular work (Section 7.5), tension–time index (Section 7.14) and O_2 demand. Growth factors trigger hypertrophy of the left ventricle myocytes, thickening the wall. Eventually, by mechanisms not yet understood, hypertrophy is followed by left ventricular failure.

12 Pulmonary hypertension occurs when pulmonary vascular resistance is raised by the hypoxic pulmonary vasoconstriction (Section 15.5), e.g. at high altitude. Pulmonary vascular resistance can also be increased by tissue destruction, e.g. in chronic emphysema. Pulmonary hypertension leads eventually to right ventricular failure.

13 Treatment is justified by the increased mortality and morbidity from heart failure, ischaemic atheromatous disease of coronary, cerebral and peripheral arteries, cerebral haemorrhage, retinopathy and renal failure.

14 The α_1-adrenoceptors mediate vasoconstriction due to sympathetic fibre activity (noradrenaline) and circulating adrenaline. α_1-adrenoceptor activation leads, via multiple pathways, to increased cytosolic Ca^{2+} and increased sensitivity of the contractile machinery to Ca^{2+} (Sections 12.5 and 12.6). Since sympathetic fibres are tonically active, α_1-adrenoceptors contribute to basal tone and resistance (Section 14.1). Consequently, α_1 blockers reduce blood pressure.

15i Prazosin is not normally the drug of first choice because it blocks a major component of the reflex responses to orthostasis, namely sympathetic-mediated reflex vasoconstriction of resistance vessel to support blood pressure (Section 17.1). Blood pressure falls because venous pooling in the legs reduces filling pressure (Section 8.11) and therefore stroke volume (Starling's law of the heart). The postural hypotension reduced cerebral blood flow, leading to dizziness and visual fade.

15ii The reduced resistance in active muscle due to metabolic vasodilatation tends to lower blood pressure. This is normally counterbalanced by sympathetic-mediated vasoconstriction in inactive tissues (Section 17.3). Also, increased sympathetic output to resistance vessels in the active muscle prevents overdilation. When these effects are blocked by prazosin, exercise can cause hypotension, leading to cerebral hypoperfusion and giddiness.

16 Nifedipine blocks voltage-sensitive L-type Ca^{2+} channels (VSCCs) in vascular myocytes (Section 12.4). This reduces Ca^{2+} entry and causes relaxation of the resistance vessels, which reduces arterial pressure. Sympathetic neurotransmission is not impaired and postural hypotension is not a problem.

17 (1) β-adrenoceptor blockers such as propranolol reduce cardiac output, and hence blood pressure, by blocking the tonic stimulatory effect of sympathetic nerves on heart rate and contractility. β-blockers also reduce the sympathetic-mediated stimulation of the renin–angiotensin–aldosterone system. They also act centrally to reduce sympathetic outflow. (2) ACE inhibitors such as captopril reduce angiotensin II formation (Section 14.8). (3) Thiazide diuretics such as bendrofluazide cause salt and water excretion, which helps to reduce blood pressure. They also dilate resistance vessels (mechanism uncertain).

CASE 5 The Elderly Man with a Murmur

A 70-year-old man visited his doctor because he experienced the sensation of a tight, constricting band across his chest when he exercised, relieved by rest. He also complained of excessive breathlessness and dizziness on exercise, and had recently fainted while exercising.

On examination his pulse was regular but slow-rising and of small amplitude. A blood pressure measurement, 115/80 mmHg, confirmed a low pulse amplitude for his age. Palpation of the chest showed that the apex beat was in the 5th interspace midclavicular line, but a palpable 'thrill' (vibration) could be felt with each systole. Auscultation revealed a systolic crescendo—decrescendo murmur (diamond shaped murmur, Figure 2.8) which was loudest over the aortic area. The second heart sound was soft, with reversed splitting, i.e. splitting on expiration.

A chest X-ray showed no increase in cardiothoracic ratio but the ascending aorta was dilated. An ECG showed left axis deviation, ST-segment depression and T wave inversion. An echocardiogram showed concentric hypertrophy of the left ventricle and poorly mobile, calcified aortic valve cusps. Cardiac catheterization with a pressure transducer showed a peak systolic pressure of 170 mmHg in the left ventricle but only 115 mmHg in the aorta. A diagnosis of aortic valve stenosis was made and the patient referred to a cardiac surgeon for aortic valve replacement. In the meantime he was advised against over-exertion and given a β-blocker, atenolol, to prevent angina.

Questions

1 Which valves create the second heart sound and why was it soft here?
2 What is the structure of the aortic valve and what lies just behind the cusps?
3 Why did splitting of the 2nd sound increase on expiration, rather than on inspiration as normal?
4 Does respiration affect stroke volume and/or heart rate?
5 How big is the pressure gradient across the normal aortic valve during (i) ejection and (ii) diastole, and why was the systolic gradient so big in this patient?
6 What arterial pressure values might be typical of a normal 70-year-old?
7 How does the coronary circulation respond to exercise?
8 How is systolic coronary blood flow affected by increased ventricular systolic pressure?
9 How can exercise-induced angina arise in a patient with aortic stenosis but no coronary artery disease?
10 What is the effect of left ventricular hypertrophy on pulmonary venous pressure? Could this contribute to the patient's dyspnoea?

11 How does the heart normally respond during exercise, and what drives the response?
12 How might aortic valve stenosis lead to dizziness and fainting on exercise?
13 How does aortic stenosis give rise to a murmur or thrill?
14 Do systolic murmurs inevitably indicate valvular lesions?
15 Which ECG feature immediately precedes the first heart sound, and what sarcolemmal ionic current generates it?
16 What is the meaning of electrical axis, and how does left ventricular hypertrophy affect it?
17 Which ECG feature immediately precedes the second heart sound, and what sarcolemmal ionic current generates it?
18 How does ischaemia lead to displacement of the ST segment?
19 How will a non-specific β-blocker help to relieve exercise-induced angina?

Answers

1 The second heart sound is caused by vibration of the aortic and pulmonary valve cusps on closing.

If cusp mobility is impaired, as in the calcified valves of the patient, there is less vibration and a softer sound.

2 All heart valves except the mitral have three cusps normally, but aortic stenosis often develops in a congenitally bicuspid valve. Each cusp is a thin, flexible sheet of fibrous connective tissue covered by endothelium. The openings of the right and left coronary arteries lie immediately behind the valve cusps, in the sinuses of Valsalva.

3 The aortic component of the second sound normally precedes the pulmonary component slightly (Figure 2.5), because left ventricular ejection stops slightly earlier than right ventricular ejection. The splitting is normally increased by inspiration due to prolongation of right ventricular ejection by a transiently increased venous return (Figure 8.24) and shortening of left ventricular ejection by expansion of the pulmonary vascular bed, which transiently reduces return to the left side (Section 2.5). In aortic stenosis the slow ejection of the left ventricle reverses the splitting; the aortic component comes second. The split is amplified by expiration because expiration reduces venous return and thus shortens right ventricular ejection.

4 Heart rate increases during inspiration due to vagal inhibition of the pacemaker (sinus arrhythmia, Figure 5.4a). Stroke volume increases on the right and decreases on the left with inspiration – see (3) above.

5 The pressure gradient across the open aortic valve during ejection is normally only a few mmHg due to its low resistance (Figure 2.5). The gradient across the closed valve is diastolic aortic pressure (80 mmHg) minus diastolic left ventricular pressure (5–10 mmHg). The large systolic pressure gradient in aortic valve stenosis (55 mmHg here) is due to the high resistance of the narrowed valve (Figure 2.8).

6 Ageing raises mean blood pressure moderately and systolic pressure substantially. The average for a 70-year-old white male is ~165/90 mmHg (Figure 17.10). As a very rough rule the systolic pressure (mmHg) is 90 + age in years. The exaggerated systolic rise with ageing is due to arteriosclerosis. Arteriosclerosis raises the pulse pressure through reduced arterial compliance (Figure 18.7) and systolic augmentation by wave reflection (Figure 18.8).

7 Myocardial metabolic hyperaemia normally increases the coronary blood flow in proportion to the increased myocardial O_2 consumption during exercise (Figures 13.6, 15.4).

8 Coronary blood flow is normally reduced during systole because the tensed myocardium compresses the intramural coronary vessels (Figure 15.5). An exaggerated increase in ventricular systolic pressure, to 170 mmHg here, further curtails the systolic perfusion.

9 Angina is ischaemic myocardial pain. Ischaemia arises when the myocardial O_2 demand exceeds supply. The patient's exercise angina is due to an excessively increased myocardial O_2 demand as the ventricle attempts to raise its output through the narrowed outlet, while at the same time the increased ventricular wall tension impedes systolic coronary flow and O_2 delivery (see 8 above).

10 Left ventricle hypertrophy stiffens the wall. To achieve passive diastolic filling, the left ventricular diastolic and atrial pressures must rise. This raises pulmonary venous pressure, congesting the lungs and increasing their stiffness. Lung stiffness causes dyspnoea, as in Case 1.

11 Stroke volume increases during upright exercise due to increased diastolic filling (Starling's law) and sympathetic-mediated increased ejection fraction (Figure 6.24). Heart rate increases due to increased sympathetic and reduced vagal outflow to the pacemaker. The altered autonomic outflow is the result of central command and a reflex from muscle mechano- and metaboreceptors (Sections 16.6, 17.3).

12 Normally the increased cardiac output maintains arterial pressure despite a fall in peripheral resistance caused by muscle metabolic vasodilatation (Figure 17.5). Mean arterial pressure = cardiac output × peripheral resistance. Severe aortic stenosis prevents an adequate increase in cardiac output, so pressure falls on exercise. If pressure falls below the limit of cerebral autoregulation (Figure 15.13), cerebral hypoperfusion leads to dizziness or even fainting on exercise.

13 Aortic blood flow is normally laminar and silent. Aortic stenosis causes turbulent flow, which sets up vibrations heard as a crescendo-decrescendo murmur (Figure 2.8) or felt as a thrill. Turbulence is favoured by the abrupt change in diameter at the stenosed valve exit, and by a high Reynolds number (fluid velocity × diameter × density/ viscosity, Section 8.2), due to high velocity of blood in the narrowed valve aperture.

14 No. Benign systolic murmurs are not uncommon, for example, in pregnancy due to the increased cardiac output and moderate anaemia (low viscosity). If the Reynolds number exceeds

~2000 during peak systolic flow, turbulence develops and creates a benign (i.e. non-valvular) systolic murmur.

15 The QRS complex precedes the first heart sound (Figure 2.5). It is caused by the upstroke (depolarization) of the ventricular action potentials (Figure 5.3), which is due to an inward Na^+ current (Figure 3.7).

16 The electrical axis is the direction of the largest dipole during ventricular depolarization (Figure 5.7). The axis depends on the orientation of the heart in the chest and on the relative bulk of the left ventricular muscle mass versus right ventricular mass. Left ventricular hypertrophy increases the magnitude of left-side current relative to the right side, shifting the electrical axis to the left.

17 The T wave precedes the second heart sound (closure of the aortic and pulmonary valves, Figure 2.5). The T wave is caused by ventricular repolarization (Figure 5.8). Repolarization is due to an outward K^+ current (Figure 3.7).

18 Hypertrophy can cause endocardial ischaemia, which reduces the resting potential and action potential. Local differences in potential between ischaemic and non-ischaemic regions now cause injury currents to flow. The injury current shifts the level of the ST segment.

19 Blockage of the β_1-adrenoceptors on the pacemaker and ventricular myocytes interrupts the tonic stimulatory effect of the cardiac sympathetic nerves on rate and contractility. The fall in cardiac output reduces myocardial work and O_2 demand, which helps to prevent angina.

FURTHER READING

Colbert, D. (1993) *Fundamentals of Clinical Physiology*, Prentice Hall, London.

Kumar, P. and Clark, M. (1994) *Clinical Medicine*, Ballière Tindall, London.

Lille, L. S. (ed.) (1998) *Pathophysiology of Heart Disease*, Williams and Wilkins, Baltimore.

Cardiovascular parameters

Values refer to young, resting human adult at heart level unless otherwise specified

Aortic parameters

Area at root	$4-5\,cm^2$
Reynolds number at peak flow	~4600
Stroke distance	$15-20\,cm$
Stroke volume, rest	$70-80\,cm^3$
Stroke volume, exercise	$110-120\,cm^3$
Velocity, mean during ejection	$50\,cm/s$
Velocity, mean over 1 cycle	$20\,cm/s$
Velocity, peak during cycle	$70\,cm/s$
Velocity, mean during ejection, heavy exercise	$250\,cm/s$

Areas

Body surface, 70 kg adult	$1.8\,m^2$
Capillary bed of skeletal muscle	$280\,m^2$
Capillary bed of two lungs	$90\,m^2$

Arterial parameters

Brachial artery pressure	$120/80\,mmHg$
Compliance, elastic artery system	2 ml per mmHg
Foot artery, standing, mean	$183\,mmHg$
Pulmonary artery pressure	$25/10\,mmHg$
Pulse velocity, young	$4-5\,m/s$
Pulse velocity, elderly	$10-15\,m/s$
Systolic pressure, ageing effect	$90-100\,mmHg$ + age in years

Blood parameters

Haematocrit, female	0.40
Haematocrit, male	0.45
Blood volume, total	5 l
Blood volume, venous	$\sim3\,l$
Blood volume, pulmonary	0.6 l
Density ρ	$1.06\,g/cm^3$
Oxygen – see 'Oxygen'	
Viscosity, water at 37°C	$0.69\,mPa\,s$
Viscosity, blood/water	~4
Viscosity, plasma/water	1.7

Cardiac parameters

Cardiac index	$3\,l/min$ per m^2
Cardiac output, rest	$4-7\,l/min$
Cardiac output, maximum	$20-35\,l/min$
Electrical axis	$-30°$ to $+110°$
Weight of heart	$300-350\,g$

Timings

Cardiac cycle, typical, rest	$0.9\,s$
ECG, P wave	$0.08\,s$
ECG, PR interval	$<0.2\,s$
ECG, QRS wave	$<0.1\,s$
ECG, ST segment	$0.2-0.4\,s$
Heart rate, rest	$50-100\,min^{-1}$
Heart rate, maximum	$180-200\,min^{-1}$
Intrinsic pacemaker rate	$105\,min^{-1}$
Isovolumetric contraction	$0.05\,s$
Isovolumetric relaxation	$0.08\,s$
Ventricular filling	$0.5\,s$
Ventricular systole	$0.35\,s$
Ventricular ejection	$0.30\,s$

Pressures

Central venous pressure	$0-10\,mmHg$
L. ventricle, end-diastole, supine	$9\,mmHg$
L. ventricle, end-diastole, orthostasis	$4-5\,mmHg$
L. ventricle, peak systolic	$120\,mmHg$
R. ventricle, end-diastole, supine	$4\,mmHg$
R. ventricle, end-diastole, orthostasis	$0\,mmHg$
R. ventricle, peak systolic	$25\,mmHg$

Volumes (resting subject)

End-diastolic volume, ventricle	120 ml
End-systolic volume	$40-50\,ml$
Ejection fraction	67%
Stroke volume	$70-80\,ml$
Stroke work	1 joule

Cellular/subcellular dimensions

Actin (thin) filament	6 nm diam $\times$ 1.05 μm
Cardiac myocyte	10–20 μm diam $\times$ 50–100 μm
Desmosome gap (cadherin)	25 nm
Gap junction (nexus, connexon)	2–4 nm
Myosin (thick) filament	11 nm diam $\times$ 1.6 μm
Purkinje fibre diameter	40–80 μm
Red cell diameter	8 μm
Sarcomere, normal diastole	1.8–2.0 μm
Sarcomere, maximum stretch	2.2–2.3 μm

Density at 20°C

Blood	1.06 g/ml
Mercury	13.55 g/ml
Water	1.00 g/ml

Diameters

Aortic root	2.5 cm
Arteriole	10–100 μm
Arteriovenous anastomosis	20–130 μm
Capillary	4–8 μm
Large named artery	1–2 cm
Medium to small named artery (e.g. radial, cerebral, coronary)	0.2–0.5 cm
Postcapillary (pericytic) venule	15–40 μm
Resistance artery	100–500 μm
Venule	50–200 μm

Distances and thickness

Aortic valve to iliac bifurcation	0.5 m
Capillary to cell	10–20 μm
Sympathetic neuromuscular gap	0.1 μm
Wall of L. ventricle	1.0 cm
Wall of R. ventricle	0.5 cm
Wall of capillary	0.3 μm

Flows per 100 g tissue

Cerebral, grey matter	100 ml/min
Coronary, resting subject	70–80 ml/min
Coronary, maximum	300–400 ml/min
Skeletal muscle, rest (phasic)	3–5 ml/min
Skeletal muscle, rest (postural)	15 ml/min
Skeletal muscle, maximum	100–200 ml/min
Skin, thermoneutral	10–20 ml/min
Skin, maximum	150–200 ml/min
Transit time, systemic capillary bed	0.5–2.0 s

Velocity, aortic peak	70 cm/s
Velocity, capillary	0.05–0.1 cm/s

Ionic and other concentrations

ATP	~5 mM
Ca^{2+}, free, extracellular	1.2 mM
Ca^{2+}, cytosolic, cardiac diastole	0.1 μM
Ca^{2+}, cardiac systole	2 μM
Cl^-, extracellular	120–134 mM
Cl^-, intracellular (vascular)	54 mM
K^+, extracellular	3.5–5.5 mM
K^+, intracellular	140 mM
Myoglobin, cardiac	3.4 g/l
Na^+, extracellular	135–145 mM
Na^+, intracellular	10 mM
pH, extracellular	7.4
pH, intracellular	7.0–7.1

Oxygen (rest)

Blood content, arterial	195 ml O_2/l
Blood content, mixed venous	150 ml O_2/l
Extraction, whole body	25%
Extraction from coronary blood	65–75%
Consumption, basal, 70 kg adult	250 ml/min
Consumption, maximum (V_{O_2max})	~3000 ml/min
Partial pressure, inspired	160 mmHg (21 kPa)
Partial pressure, arterial	100 mmHg (13 kPa)
Partial pressure, mixed venous	40 mmHg
Partial pressure, cardiac myocyte	5–20 mmHg
Saturation, arterial	97%
Saturation, mixed venous	72%

Electrophysiology

Cardiac resting potential	−80 mV to −90 mV
Cardiac action potential	+20 mV to +30 mV
Cardiac pacemaker potential	−50 to −70 mV
Cardiac plateau potential	0 to −20 mV
Cardiac action potential duration	200–400 ms
Conduction velocity, atrial	1 m/s
Conduction velocity, AV node	0.05 m/s
Conduction velocity, Purkinje	3–5 m/s
Conduction velocity, ventricle wall	0.5–1.0 m/s
Equilibrium potential, Ca^{2+}	+124 mV
Equilibrium potential, Cl^- (vascular)	−23 mV
Equilibrium potential, K^+	−94 mV
Equilibrium potential, Na^+	+70 mV
Vascular myocyte, basal state	−50 mV to −60 mV

Pressures

See Arterial parameters, Venous pressure, Cardiac parameters

Capillary, arterial limb, heart level	32–36 mmHg
Capillary, venous limb, heart level	12–25 mmHg
Capillary, foot in orthostasis	95 mmHg
Mean circulatory pressure (arrested)	7 mmHg
Pressure drop across capillary bed	20–30 mmHg
Pressure drop across resistance vessels	40–50 mmHg

Resistances

Pulmonary circulation	0.003 mmHg min/ml
Systemic circulation, rest	0.02 mmHg min/ml

Venous pressures

Foot vein, standing	90 mmHg
Named vein (femoral, antecubital), heart level	8–10 mmHg
Venule, heart level	12–20 mmHg
Veno-atrial junction	0–10 mmHg

Weight of soft tissues in 70 kg human

Blood	5 kg
Brain	1.5 kg
Gastrointestinal tract and liver	4 kg
Heart	0.35 kg
Kidneys	0.3 kg
Skeletal muscle	40 kg
Skin	2–3 kg

APPENDIX 2

Biophysical parameters and physiological mechanisms

The following units are based mainly on the standard international (SI) system of metres, kilograms and seconds. Some of the literature is based on centimetres, grams and seconds, the c.g.s. system.

Acidosis and vasodilatation Acidosis causes vasodilatation by multiple mechanisms (Wray, S., 1997, *Journal of Physiology*, **503**, 235). (i) Intracellular acidosis hyperpolarizes the vascular myocytes, probably due to the pH sensitivity of K_{ATP} channels. Hyperpolarization causes relaxation through closure of voltage-sensitive Ca^{2+} channels. (ii) Even when the myocyte is depolarized by K^+, acidosis reduces cytosolic Ca^{2+} (Figure 13.8), perhaps because acidosis affects Ca^{2+} channels. (iii) CO_2 causes endothelium to release NO in mesentery, but less certainly in the brain (Carr *et al.* 1993, *Pfluger's Archiv*, **423**, 343–345; You *et al.* 1994, *Acta Physiologica Scandinavica*, **152**, 391–398). Lactate has a non-endothelium dependent action (McKinnon *et al.* 1996, *Journal of Physiology*, **490**, 783–792).

Adenosine and vasodilatation Adenosine is formed in hypoxic myocardium, skeletal muscle and cerebral tissue, and elicits vasodilatation through multiple pathways. (i) A_{2A} receptors on vascular myocytes activate the adenylate cyclase–cAMP–protein kinase cascade (Chen, Chang and Hsiue, 2000, *American Journal of Physiology*, **279**, H2210–17). (ii) A_1 receptors are coupled to K_{ATP} channels, leading to hyperpolarization-mediated relaxation (Dart and Standen, 1993, *Journal of Physiology*, **471**, 767–786). (iii) Adenosine reduces noradrenaline release from sympathetic varicosities (Figure 14.2).

Arterial input impedance Resistance is the ratio of mean pressure drop to mean flow. Since arterial pressure and flow oscillate out of phase, the pressure/flow ratio alters from instant to instant. To take account of this, the concept of 'impedance' has been adapted from the theory of alternating electrical currents. Arterial input impedance is a measure of the opposition of the circulation to an oscillating input, i.e. stroke volume. Input impedance depends on peripheral vascular resistance, arterial viscoelastic compliance and oscillation frequency (heart rate).

Avogadro's number, N, N_A This is the number of molecules in 1 mole (1 gram-molecule), namely 6.0×10^{23} molecules per mole.

Brownian motion The random movements of particles in water was first observed in a pollen suspension by the Scottish botanist Robert Brown in 1828. The movement is due to the kinetic, diffusional motion of water molecules.

Capillary concentration profile and extraction Under idealized conditions of uniform permeability and uniform or zero interstitial solute concentration, solute concentration in a capillary falls exponentially with axial distance. The mean plasma concentration is *not* the arithmetic average but equals $[(C_a - C_v)/\ln((C_a - C_i)/(C_v - C_i))] + C_i$ (notation as in Fig. 10.8). Substitution into the permeability eqn 10.3 and Fick principle (eqn 10.4) gives the Renkin–Crone extraction equation: extraction $E = 1 - \exp(-PS/\dot{Q})$ at $C_i = 0$ (eqn 10.6). This tells us that extraction $(C_a - C_v)/C_a$ varies non-linearly with permeability and capillary blood flow.

Density ρ (rho) Density is mass per unit volume. Water 1.00 g/ml (20°C), blood 1.06 g/ml, mercury 13.55 g/ml.

Diffusion **Fick's first law of diffusion** (1855) states that diffusion rate dm/dt across a body of liquid of area A and thickness Δx equals $-DA(\Delta C/\Delta x)$, where $\Delta C/\Delta x$ is the concentration gradient and D is diffusion coefficient. The **diffusion coefficient** (Table 10.1) indicates the solute velocity through solvent. Due to frictional effects D varies inversely with solvent viscosity and is inversely proportional to the cube root of solute molecular weight. D is often used to assess the effective radius a of a molecule idealized as a sphere; see **Stokes–Einstein radius**.

D is reduced in narrow pores (radius r) due to increased **hydrodynamic drag** (Figure 10.6b). The reduced coefficient is called the restricted diffusion coefficient D_{res} and it equals $D \times [1 - 2.1a/r + 2.09(a/r)^3 - 0.95(a/r)^5]$.

Diffusion through pores is reduced further by **steric exclusion** (Figure 10.6a). Exclusion reduces the space available for solute diffusion in a cylindrical pore by the factor $(r - a)^2/r^2$. This is also the **partition coefficient** ϕ (phi) for an uncharged solute. In a membrane of surface area S and pore area A_p, the fractional area available for diffusion is $A_p\phi/S$.

The effective diffusion coefficient D_m, relative to free diffusion coefficient D is the product of steric exclusion and hydrodynamic restriction, as stated by the **Renkin equation** (solid line, Figure 10.6) $D_m/D = [(r - a)^2/r^2] \times [1 - 2.1a/r + 2.09(a/r)^3 - 0.95 (a/r)^5]$.

Taking into account the increase in pathlength along an oblique pore of length $\Delta x'$ through a membrane of thickness Δx, Fick's law (eqn 10.1) for diffusion through a porous membrane becomes

$$J_s = \frac{D_{res} A_p\ \phi \Delta C}{\Delta x'}$$

Comparison with the permeability equation $J_s = P S \Delta C$ (eqn 10.3) shows that **membrane permeability** P equals $(D_{res}/\Delta x')(A_p/S)\phi$. In other words membrane permeability is governed by the restricted intra-pore diffusion coefficient, the pore length, the fractional pore area A_p/S, and partition coefficient ϕ.

Electrical conductance G in a membrane permeable to ions

The electrical conductance G depends on the ionic permeability P thus:

$$G = \frac{P(V_m CF)}{(RT/F)^2 \cdot (1 - \exp(-V_m F/RT))}$$

where V_m is the membrane potential, R the gas constant, F the Faraday constant, T the absolute temperature and C is ion concentration.

Equilibrium

A system is in equilibrium when its components have the same free energy level. For example, two solutions containing solute at the same concentration or, more accurately, at the same chemical potential, are in equilibrium. Equilibrium should not be confused with steady state (see below).

Extraction, E

Fractional extraction E is defined as the fraction of solute that is removed as plasma passes through the capillary bed. Solute delivery to the capillary bed per unit time equals plasma flow $\dot{Q} \times$ arterial concentration C_a. Solute transmission into the veins is $\dot{Q} \times$ venous concentration C_v. Solute loss from the plasma is therefore $\dot{Q}(C_a - C_v)$ (Fick's principle). From its definition, E equals $\dot{Q}(C_a - C_v)/\dot{Q}C_a$, i.e. arterio-venous concentration difference $C_a - C_v$ as a fraction of the arterial concentration C_a. Solute flux J_s equals $\dot{Q} \times C_a \times E$.

Faraday's constant, F

F is the charge carried by one mole of monovalent ion, 96 484 coulombs/mole. The term RT/F in the **Nernst equation** equals 26.7 mV at 37°C (310°K). 1 volt is 1 joule per coulomb.

Flux

Flux is strictly the rate of movement of a material (e.g. a diffusing solute) across unit area of surface. In physiology the word is often used loosely, omitting the 'per unit area of surface' aspect.

Force, work, energy and power

A **force** of 1 newton (N) accelerates 1 kg mass at 1 m/s^2. The c.g.s. unit of force, the dyne (1 g cm/s^2) is 10^{-5} N. **Work** is force $\times$ distance moved. **Energy** is the capacity to do work and has the same units as work. One joule of work or energy (J) equals a force of 1 newton displaced over 1 metre (1 N-m). It equals 10^7 ergs, the c.g.s unit of energy (1 dyne-cm). **Power** is rate of work or rate of change of energy. Its unit the watt, W, is 1 J/s.

Free radicals

Normal chemical bonds consist of a pair of electrons. A free radical is a molecule with an odd number of electrons – effectively a half-bond. The **superoxide radical** O_2^- is an O_2 molecule that has gained an extra electron, making it highly reactive. For example, O_2^- reacts with NO to form peroxynitrite, ONOO$^-$, thus destroying NO. Superoxide is formed during oxidative metabolism. Superoxide is also formed by the reaction of O_2 with haemoglobin; ferrous Fe^{2+} donates an electron to O_2 and becomes ferric Fe^{3+}, turning haemoglobin into useless **methaemoglobin.** A scavenger enzyme, **superoxide dismutase**, protects against superoxide by catalysing its conversion to hydrogen peroxide, which in turn is degraded by catalase and glutathione peroxidase.

Gas constant, R

This is the energy of one mole of gas per unit absolute temperature; 8.316 joules K^{-1} mole^{-1}.

Goldman constant field equation The potential V_m across a membrane permeable to multiple monovalent ions depends on the ionic concentrations inside (subscript i) and outside (subscript o) and the permeability to each ion.

$$V_m = (RT/F)\ln\left[\frac{P_K[K]_o + P_{Na}[Na]_o + P_{Cl}[Cl]_i}{P_K[K]_i + P_{Na}[Na]_i + P_{Cl}[Cl]_o}\right]$$

An analogous but more complex expression applies to mixtures of monovalent and divalent ions.

Gravity, g The force of gravity varies with latitude and altitude. Gravitational acceleration is $9.81\,m/s^2$ at latitude 50° North (e.g. Land's End in Cornwall, England).

Hypoxia and vascular tone In **systemic resistance vessels**, local hypoxia causes vasodilatation. In *isolated* vascular myocytes the relaxation is due to hyperpolarization (Figure 12.1) through activation of K_{ATP} channels by reduced ATP and increases ADP and H^+ levels (Dart, C. and Standen, N. B., 1995, *Journal of Physiology*, **483**, 29–39). Hyperpolarization closes L-type Ca^{2+} channels. In *intact tissues* additional parenchymal factors contribute. (i) The vasodilator adenosine is formed in hypoxic myocardium, skeletal muscle and brain (Skinner, M. R. and Marshall, J. M., 1996, *Journal of Physiology*, **495**, 553–560), and the formation of the vasoconstrictor 20-HETE by cytochrome P450ω hydroxylase (Section 13.2) in the parenchymal and vascular cells is reduced (Frisbee, J. C. and Lombard, J. H., 2002, *Microvascular Research*, **63**, 340–343). (ii) The sensitivity of the contractile process to Ca^{2+} is reduced (Soloviev, M. J. and Basilyuk, S., 1993, *Experimental Physiology*, **78**, 395–402), so hypoxic vasodilatation can occur with little fall in cytosolic Ca^{2+} (Taggart, M. J. and Wray, S., 1998, *Journal of Physiology*, **509**, 315–325).

In **large systemic arteries** severe hypoxia can cause vasoconstriction (Siegel *et al.*, 1991, *Journal of Vascular Medicine and Biology*, **3**, 140–149) due to noradrenaline released from hypoxic sympathetic fibres, and the local release of autacoid vasoconstrictors such as platelet activating factor.

In **pulmonary resistance vessels** hypoxia causes vasoconstriction (Section 15.5).

Love's equation for tension in a thick-walled tube Love's equation for mechanical equilibrium in a thick-walled tube of internal radius r_i and external radius r_o is derived by analogous reasoning to that for eqn 8.8, and states $T = P_i r_i - P_o r_o$, where T is the absolute circumferential tension (force) in the wall. In physiology we are more interested in the increase in tension as P_i (blood pressure) rises above atmospheric pressure P_o. For this purpose, Laplace's law (eqn 8.8) is a more convenient approximation.

Osmole An osmole is the mass of solute that, when distributed in 22.4 l of solvent at 0°C, exerts an osmotic pressure of 1 atmosphere (760 mmHg, 1030 cmH$_2$O). This definition stems from **van't Hoff's law**; osmotic pressure $\pi = RTC$, where C is molal concentration (moles/kg solvent), T is absolute temperature and R is the gas constant. A one **osmolal** solution contains 1 osmole per kilogram of solvent. A one **osmolar** solution contains 1 osmole of solute per litre of solution. Mammalian body fluids contain ~0.3 osmole/kg water and have a potential osmotic pressure of 5800 mmHg at body temperature, since $22.4 \times 0.3 \times 310/273 = 7.6$ atmospheres = 5800 mmHg. Human plasma proteins (60 − 80 g/l) by contrast exert an osmotic pressure of only ~25 mmHg.

Potassium and vasodilatation Increases in extracellular $[K^+]$ up to ~10 mM (normal 4 mM) cause vasodilatation. Higher, **pharmacological** concentrations, >20 mM, cause contraction. A plot of vascular tone versus extracellular K^+ is thus U-shaped. Pharmacological K^+ levels depolarize the myocyte (Nernst equation, Section 3.1), activating voltage-sensitive Ca^{2+} channels and causing Ca^{2+}-induced contraction (Figure 13.8).

Physiological increases in extracellular K^+ paradoxically hyperpolarizes the cell, leading to Ca^{2+} channel closure and relaxation. The hyperpolarization is due to (i) stimulation of the electrogenic $3Na^+-2K^+$ pump by extracellular K^+. The pump inhibitor ouabain attenuates the vasodilator response to K^+. (ii) Increased extracellular K^+ increases the open-state probability of inward rectifying K^+ channels (K_{IR}), which shifts the membrane potential closer to the Nernst E_K, i.e. hyperpolarizes the cell (eqn 3.4).

Pressure Pressure is the force exerted by a gas or liquid upon unit area of surface. Pressure acts equally in all directions, unlike stress. The SI unit of pressure, the Pascal (Pa), equals 1 newton per square metre (N/m^2). One atmosphere pressure is 100 100 Pa (100.1 kPa, kilopascals). This supports a column of mercury 760 mm high, i.e. 1 atmosphere = 760 mmHg pressure. Body fluid pressures are expressed relative to atmospheric pressure; a venous pressure of '0 mmHg' is an absolute pressure of 760 mmHg; an interstitial pressure of '−5 mmHg' is an absolute pressure of 755 mmHg. 1 mmHg = 133 Pa = 1.36 cmH$_2$O at

20°C = fluid height × density × gravity. A 1 cm column of water ($1\,cmH_2O$) exerts a pressure of 98.1 Pa ($981\,dynes/cm^2$) at 20°C.

Quantity of ions exchanged during an action potential

A cylindrical myocyte $10^{-2}\,cm$ long × $10^{-3}\,cm$ radius has a volume of $3.14 \times 10^{-8}\,cm^3$ and a surface area of $6.28 \times 10^{-5}\,cm^2$. Each cm^2 of cell membrane requires 1 microcoulomb of charge to alter its potential by 1 volt; this is its **capacitance**. An action potential of 0.1 V (from $-80\,mV$ to $+20\,mV$) requires a net transfer of 6.28×10^{-6} microcoulombs per cell. One mole of monovalent ion carries 96 500 coulombs (Faraday's constant) so the quantity of ions transferred is 6.51×10^{-17} moles or, applying Avogadro's number, 3.9×10^7 ions. From the cell volume and intracellular concentrations in Table 3.1, the cell actually contains $1.9 \times 10^{11}\,Na^+$ ions and $2.6 \times 10^{12}\,K^+$ ions. The fractional change in ion concentration after a single action potential is thus tiny.

Reflection coefficient, σ (sigma)

The reflection coefficient σ is a measure of the difficulty that a solute experiences in entering a pore (Figure 10.7). It depends on steric exclusion (Figure 10.6a). For a spherical neutral solute of radius a entering a cylindrical pore of radius r, the available space in the pore is $(r - a)^2/r^2$. It can be shown that σ equals the square of the excluded space; $\sigma = [1 - (r - a)^2/r^2]^2$. For albumin ($a = 3.6\,nm$) and an endothelial pore of radius 4 nm, σ is 0.975. Measurements of σ have been used to estimate pore size.

Solute transport by convection (wash along or 'solvent drag') depends on σ, filtration rate J_v and bulk solute concentration C. The convective transport through a pore equals $J_v(1 - \sigma)C$.

Sodium–calcium exchanger

The exchanger swaps three Na^+ ions for one Ca^{2+} ion and can operate in either direction. In general Ca^{2+} is removed from the sarcoplasm and Na^+ added to it, with an attendant net inward positive current. Being electrogenic, the exchanger is influenced by membrane potential as well as concentration gradient. For ion species X, the driving force is $(V_m - E_x)$, where V_m is intracellular potential and E_x is the Nernst equilibrium potential, which depends on the ion concentrations (Section 3.3). Due to the 3:2 charge exchange, the net exchanger current i_{Na-Ca} is proportional to $3(V_m - E_{Na}) - 2(V_m - E_{Ca})$. In **diastole** $V_m = -80\,mV$, $E_{Na} = 69\,mV$ and $E_{Ca} = 130\,mV$ (Table 3.1), so the force on the exchanger is equivalent to an internal potential of $-27\,mV$. This draws a net positive charge into the cell, i.e. three Na^+ ions in exchange for each Ca^{2+} ion expelled.

Immediately after **depolarization** the exchanger switches briefly into reverse, i.e. Ca^{2+} entry, because an action potential $+20\,mV$ results in a net force of $+73\,mV$ on the exchanger (calculated as $3(20 - 69) - 2(20 - 130)$). The brief exchanger-mediated Ca^{2+} entry may contribute a little to the early systolic Ca^{2+} transient and calcium-induced calcium release.

During the **plateau**, cytosolic Ca^{2+} is high, reducing E_{Ca}, and membrane potential is almost zero. The balance of forces now switches the exchanger back to Na^+-in, Ca^{2+}-out mode.

If intracellular Na^+ is raised, e.g. by inhibiting the Na–K pump with digoxin, E_{Na} declines. The net force driving the exchanger therefore falls; Ca^{2+} expulsion falls, the SR Ca^{2+} store increases, and contractility improves.

Steady state

When two components at different energy levels are brought into contact, material or energy flows from the higher level to the lower. When the transfer occurs at a steady rate and without change in the energy level at either end, the system is said to be in a steady state. This should not be confused with an equilibrium state (see earlier). A flowing river may be in a steady state but it is not at equilibrium. If there is a very slow, almost negligible change in energy levels, the system is said to be in a quasi steady state (Latin *quasi*, 'as if').

Stokes–Einstein radius, *a*, r_{se}

The hydrodynamic resistance experienced by a solute particle as it diffuses through a solvent depends on its size and shape. The solute can be represented by an equivalent sphere that would generate the same hydrodynamic resistance and hence diffusion rate. The radius of this equivalent sphere is called the diffusion radius, hydrodynamic radius or Stokes–Einstein radius. Stokes and Einstein showed that the solute free diffusion coefficient D is inversely proportional to the equivalent sphere radius:

$$a = \frac{RT}{DN_A 6\pi\eta}$$

where η (eta) is solvent viscosity and T is absolute temperature. Thus solute radius can be determined by measuring diffusion coefficient.

Strain and stress

When a solid body is subjected to a force, the force per unit cross-sectional area of material is called the **stress** (N/m^2). The resulting change in size, as a fraction of the original size, is called the **strain** (dimensionless). The ratio stress/strain is **Young's modulus of elasticity**.

Work See Force

van't Hoff's law for crystalloid osmotic pressure

Osmotic pressure is a 'colligative' property like freezing point depression – it depends primarily on the solute concentration, not chemical identity. The osmotic pressure π of an 'ideal' solution is described by van't Hoff's law, namely $\pi = R \times T \times C$, where R is the gas constant, T is absolute temperature and C is molal concentration of solute. RT is 25.4 atmospheres for a 1 molal solution at 37°C. Since plasma solute concentration is ~0.3 molal, mostly as sodium, chloride and bicarbonate ions (crystalloids), the van't Hoff osmotic pressure is 7.6 atmospheres (5800 mmHg). This **crystalloid osmotic pressure** is not generally effective across the capillary wall because (i) the wall is highly permeable to electrolytes (except in the brain), so plasma and interstitial concentrations are almost identical; and (ii) the mean reflection coefficient of endothelium to electrolytes is ~0.1. Only the plasma proteins ('colloids') at a mere 0.001 molar concentration exert a sustained osmotic pressure across the capillary wall (25 mmHg).

Plasma protein osmotic pressure is non-ideal, because it greatly exceeds the van't Hoff law value (Figure 11.7). The excess COP is partly due to the large self-volume of protein molecules (0.7 ml/g), which increases the effective concentration per ml of solution, and partly due to the charge. The albumin molecule carries a net negative charge of -17 units at pH 7.4. The charge attracts a slight excess of Na^+ ions into the plasma (the **Gibbs–Donnan distribution**). These ions are retained electrostatically in the plasma, so they are osmotically effective and account for ~1/3rd of the albumin osmotic pressure.

Viscoelasticity

When a perfectly elastic body is subjected to a stress (e.g. a spring with a suspended weight) the strain is linearly proportional to stress and does not change with time. On removing the stress the original conformation is at once restored. Biological materials such as the artery wall behave differently. Stress causes an initial rapid elastic deformation, which is followed by a slower, ever-decreasing deformation as time passes (**creep**). On removal of the stress, the recovery of shape follows a non-symmetrical pathway (**hysteresis**) due to a dissipation of energy. Viscoelasticity is due to elastic elements (springs) in series and parallel with viscous, flowing elements (dashpots).

Viscosity

Viscosity is the internal friction between two moving planes of fluid. Formally viscosity is the shear stress needed to generate one unit of shear rate. **Shear stress** is the sliding force applied to unit area of contact between two laminae (Newtons/m^2). Shear stress is proportional to the pressure gradient along a blood vessel. **Shear rate** is the change in velocity per unit distance radially; its units are (m/s)/m, that is to say s^{-1}. The viscosity of water is 0.001 Newton-s/m^2, or 1 mPa-second (1 centiPoise) at 20°C and 0.69 mPa.s at 37°C. The viscosity of a fluid relative to water is easily measured in a capillary viscometer; the time taken for the fluid to drain between two marks in a capillary tube is divided by the time for water under the same pressure head. Albumin and globulin in plasma raise the viscosity of water by 70% to 1.2 mPa.s at 37°C.

Index